Medicinal Plants of the World

Medicinal Plants

of the
World

Volume 1

Chemical Constituents, Traditional and Modern Medicinal Uses

SECOND EDITION

By

Ivan A. Ross

Humana Press ✳ Totowa, New Jersey

Production Editor: Kim Hoather-Potter.
Cover design by Patricia F. Cleary.

For additional copies, pricing for bulk purchases, and/or information about other Humana titles, contact Humana at the above address or at any of the following numbers: Tel.: 973-256-1699; Fax: 973-256-8341; E-mail: humana@humanapr.com; or visit us at www.humanapress.com

Library of Congress Cataloging in Publication Data

Ross, Ivan A.
    Medicinal plants of the world: chemical constituents, traditional and modern medicinal
    uses / by Ivan A. Ross.--2nd ed.
        p.cm.
    Includes bibliographical references and index.
    ISBN 1-58829-281-9 (alk. paper)   eISBN 1-59259-365-8
        1. Medicinal plants--Encyclopedias. I. Title.

RS164.R676 2003
615'.32--dc21

2002032933

Preface

Since the publication of the first edition of *Medicinal Plants of the World: Chemical Constituents, Traditional and Modern Medicinal Uses* in 1999, there has been a significant growth in the amount of new data on the herbs covered in this volume. The references used to compile this new edition have more than doubled.

As a biologist with the US Food and Drug Administration I have been involved in toxicological research. On one occasion, while investigating herbal products sold in the United States as foods or food supplements, I realized that there was an abundance of information on plants that are commonly used as food and medicine. However, the material available was not compiled to optimally serve my interest. Most such books addressed the subject as folklore, and their information was not prepared as an educational resource on plant materials that are used as foods and food supplements by the general public. As a result, to obtain a fair knowledge of any specific plant, information from several books and journal articles had to be put together. It is this experience that guided me to compile Medicinal Plants of the World. The feedback I have received from readers of the first edition has inspired me to update the information on this important collection of plants.

No current text describes the traditional medicinal uses, the chemical constituents, the pharmacological activities, and the clinical trials of those plants that are commonly used around the world as medicine. The objectives that guided the writing of this book were to create a reference for research scientists, phytochemists, toxicologists, physicians, pharmacists, and other health care providers; to integrate traditional and modern pharmacopoeias in order to develop a more efficient medicine; to build confidence and self-reliance in the use of medicinal plants; to revive an awareness of the importance of plants as sources of medicine; and to encourage their utilization and conservation.

Around the world, and even within countries, different names are used for the same plant, and different plants may be referred to by the same name. In an effort to familiarize readers with the International Code of Botanical Nomenclature system, the code's Latin binomial is used for each plant. The common names, together with the countries with which they are associated, are also listed. Color illustrations of the plants are provided to assist in their identification by those who are not familiar with the botanical name or any of the common names. For the non-botanist, the chapter on nomenclature and descriptive terminology, the botanical description, and the origin and distribution of each plant will be useful in the practical identification of the plants.

Since medical doctors are often reluctant to prescribe medicinal plants without supporting scientific data, the sections on pharmacological activities and clinical trials, as well as those on chemical constituents, constitute most useful references. These sections will also be of value to scientists with an interest in drug development. The section on traditional medicinal uses, listed by countries, will provide support and build confidence and self-reliance in the traditional uses of medicinal plants. Throughout, the book presents vital information that will find much use by students, practitioners, or researchers interested or engaged in the development, evaluation, or use of herbal medicines. The text presumes that the reader has had little to no experience or knowledge of medicinal plants. A bibliography of approximately 3000 references is presented for readers interested in more detailed information. It represents a diversity of disciplines that reflect the complexity of the field and the variety of interests in medicinal plants.

It is my hope that readers will find in *Medicinal Plants of the World* a wealth of practical ideas and theoretical information that will expose new information and little-known facts, as well as the significant applications of plants in medicine, thereby helping us become healthier people, better students, teachers, farmers, clinicians, researchers, and entrepreneurs.

Ivan A. Ross, PhD

Contents

Preface v

Contents of Companion Volume xiii

List of Color Plates xv

1 Nomenclature and Descriptive Terminology 1

    Compound Leaves 3

    Leaf Shapes 4

    Leaf Margins 4

    Leaf Tips 5

    Leaf Bases 7

    Attachment to Stem 7

    Leaf Surfaces 7

    Types of Inflorescence 8

    Dry Fruits 12

    Fleshy Fruits 13

    Abbreviations and Chemical Constituents 14

2 *Abrus precatorius* 15

    Common Names 15

    Botanical Description 16

    Origin and Distribution 16

    Traditional Medicinal Uses 16

    Chemical Constituents 17

    Pharmacological Activities and Clinical Trials 19

    References 25

3 *Allium sativum* 33

    Common Names 33

    Botanical Description 34

    Origin and Distribution 34

    Traditional Medicinal Uses 34

    Chemical Constituents 36

    Pharmacological Activities and Clinical Trials 38

    References 77

4 *Aloe vera* 103

    Common Names 103
    Botanical Description 104
    Origin and Distribution 104
    Traditional Medicinal Uses 104
    Chemical Constituents 106
    Pharmacological Activities and Clinical Trials 108
    References 122

5 *Annona muricata* 133

    Common Names 133
    Botanical Description 133
    Origin and Distribution 133
    Traditional Medicinal Uses 134
    Chemical Constituents 134
    Pharmacological Activities and Clinical Trials 136
    References 138

6 *Carica papaya* 143

    Common Names 143
    Botanical Description 144
    Origin and Distribution 145
    Traditional Medicinal Uses 145
    Chemical Constituents 148
    Pharmacological Activities and Clinical Trials 150
    References 156

7 *Cassia alata* 165

    Common Names 165
    Botanical Description 165
    Origin and Distribution 166
    Traditional Medicinal Uses 166
    Chemical Constituents 167
    Pharmacological Activities and Clinical Trials 167
    References 171

8 *Catharanthus roseus* 175

    Common Names 175
    Botanical Description 175
    Origin and Distribution 176
    Traditional Medicinal Uses 176
    Chemical Constituents 177
    Pharmacological Activities and Clinical Trials 179
    References 185

9   *Cymbopogon citratus* 197
  Common Names 197
  Botanical Description 197
  Origin and Distribution 198
  Traditional Medicinal Uses 198
  Chemical Constituents 198
  Pharmacological Activities and Clinical Trials 199
  References 204

10 *Cyperus rotundus* 209
  Common Names 209
  Botanical Description 210
  Origin and Distribution 210
  Traditional Medicinal Uses 210
  Chemical Constituents 212
  Pharmacological Activities and Clinical Trials 213
  References 219

11 *Curcuma longa* 227
  Common Names 227
  Botanical Description 228
  Origin and Distribution 228
  Traditional Medicinal Uses 228
  Chemical Constituents 230
  Pharmacological Activities and Clinical Trials 231
  References 242

12 *Hibiscus rosa-sinensis* 253
  Common Names 253
  Botanical Description 254
  Origin and Distribution 254
  Traditional Medicinal Uses 254
  Chemical Constituents 256
  Pharmacological Activities and Clinical Trials 257
  References 262

13 *Hibiscus sabdariffa* 267
  Common Names 267
  Botanical Description 267
  Origin and Distribution 268
  Traditional Medicinal Uses 268
  Chemical Constituents 268
  Pharmacological Activities and Clinical Trials 269
  References 272

14 Jatropha curcas.. 277
    Common Names 277
    Botanical Description 278
    Origin and Distribution 278
    Traditional Medicinal Uses...................................278
    Chemical Constituents 280
    Pharmacological Activities and Clinical Trials 280
    References 284

15 Lantana camara 289
    Common Names 289
    Botanical Description 290
    Origin and Distribution 290
    Traditional Medicinal Uses...................................290
    Chemical Constituents 291
    Pharmacological Activities and Clinical Trials 292
    References 298

16 Mucuna pruriens 305
    Common Names 305
    Botanical Description 305
    Origin and Distribution 306
    Traditional Medicinal Uses...................................306
    Chemical Constituents 307
    Pharmacological Activities and Clinical Trials 307
    References 311

17 Mangifera indica.. 315
    Common Names 315
    Botanical Description 316
    Origin and Distribution 316
    Traditional Medicinal Uses...................................316
    Chemical Constituents 317
    Pharmacological Activities and Clinical Trials 319
    References 324

18 Manihot esculenta 329
    Common Names 329
    Botanical Description 329
    Origin and Distribution 329
    Traditional Medicinal Uses...................................329
    Chemical Constituents 330
    Pharmacological Activities and Clinical Trials 330
    References 334

19 *Momordica charantia* 337

Common Names 337

Botanical Description 338

Origin and Distribution 338

Traditional Medicinal Uses 338

Chemical Constituents 341

Pharmacological Activities and Clinical Trials 343

References 354

20 *Moringa pterygosperma* 367

Common Names 367

Botanical Description 368

Origin and Distribution 368

Traditional Medicinal Uses 368

Chemical Constituents 370

Pharmacological Activities and Clinical Trials 371

References 376

21 *Persea americana* 383

Common Names 383

Botanical Description 384

Origin and Distribution 384

Traditional Medicinal Uses 384

Chemical Constituents 385

Pharmacological Activities and Clinical Trials 386

References 389

22 *Phyllanthus niruri* 393

Common Names 393

Botanical Description 393

Origin and Distribution 393

Traditional Medicinal Uses 394

Chemical Constituents 395

Pharmacological Activities and Clinical Trials 395

References 399

23 *Portulaca oleracea* 405

Common Names 405

Botanical Description 406

Origin and Distribution 406

Traditional Medicinal Uses 406

Chemical Constituents 407

Pharmacological Activities and Clinical Trials 407

References 410

24 *Psidium guajava* 415

     Common Names 415
     Botanical Description 416
     Origin and Distribution 416
     Traditional Medicinal Uses 416
     Chemical Constituents 417
     Pharmacological Activities and Clinical Trials 419
     References 424

25 *Punica granatum* 431

     Common Names 431
     Botanical Description 431
     Origin and Distribution 432
     Traditional Medicinal Uses 432
     Chemical Constituents 433
     Pharmacological Activities and Clinical Trials 434
     References 439

26 *Syzygium cumini* 445

     Common Names 445
     Botanical Description 445
     Origin and Distribution 445
     Traditional Medicinal Uses 446
     Chemical Constituents 446
     Pharmacological Activities and Clinical Trials 447
     References 451

27 *Tamarindus indica* 455

     Common Names 455
     Botanical Description 455
     Origin and Distribution 456
     Traditional Medicinal Uses 456
     Chemical Constituents 457
     Pharmacological Activities and Clinical Trials 458
     References 460

Glossary 465
Index 477
About the Author 491

Contents of Companion Volume (Vol. 2)

1 *Allium cepa*
2 *Althaea officinalis*
3 *Anacardium occientale*
4 *Ananas comosus*
5 *Angelica sinensis*
6 *Azadirachta indica*
7 *Echinacea angustifolia*
8 *Ephedra sinica*
9 *Eucalyptus globulus*
10 *Ginkgo biloba*
11 *Glycyrrhiza glabra*
12 *Hypericum perforatum*
13 *Laurus nobilis*
14 *Lycopersicon esculentum*
15 *Matricaria chamomilla*
16 *Morinda citrifolia*
17 *Musa sapientum*
18 *Myristica fragrans*
19 *Nelumbo nucifera*
20 *Pimpinella anisum*
21 *Ricinus communis*
22 *Tanacetum parthenium*
23 *Tribulus terrestris*
24 *Vitex agnus-castus*

List of Color Plates

Color plates appear as an insert following page 240.

Plate 1. *Abrus precatorius* (*see* full discussion in Chapter 2).
Plate 2. *Allium sativum* (*see* full discussion in Chapter 3).
Plate 3. *Aloe vera* (*see* full discussion in Chapter 4).
Plate 4. *Annona muricata* (*see* full discussion in Chapter 5).
Plate 5. *Carica papaya* (*see* full discussion in Chapter 6).
Plate 6. *Cassia alata* (*see* full discussion in Chapter 7).
Plate 7. *Catharanthus roseus* (*see* full discussion in Chapter 8).
Plate 8. *Cymbopogon citratus* (*see* full discussion in Chapter 9).
Plate 9. *Cyperus rotundus* (*see* full discussion in Chapter 10).
Plate 10. *Hibiscus rosa-sinensis* (*see* full discussion in Chapter 12).
Plate 11. *Hibiscus sabdariffa* (*see* full discussion in Chapter 13).
Plate 12. *Jatropha curcas* (*see* full discussion in Chapter 14).
Plate 13. *Lantana camara* (*see* full discussion in Chapter 15).
Plate 14. *Mucuna pruriens* (*see* full discussion in Chapter 16).
Plate 15. *Mangifera indica* (*see* full discussion in Chapter 17).
Plate 16. *Momordica charantia* (*see* full discussion in Chapter 19).
Plate 17. *Moringa pterygosperma* (*see* full discussion in Chapter 20).
Plate 18. *Persea americana* (*see* full discussion in Chapter 21).
Plate 19. *Phyllanthus niruri* (*see* full discussion in Chapter 22).
Plate 20. *Portulaca oleracea* (*see* full discussion in Chapter 23).
Plate 21. *Psidium guajava* (*see* full discussion in Chapter 24).
Plate 22. *Punica granatum* (*see* full discussion in Chapter 25).
Plate 23. *Syzygium cumini* (*see* full discussion in Chapter 26).
Plate 24. *Tamarindus indica* (*see* full discussion in Chapter 27).

1 | Nomenclature and Descriptive Terminology

For centuries, the only names of plants known by most lay people have been the common names. These common names are often simple, descriptive, and easy to pronounce and remember. These names may be words, phrases, and even sentences. Some favorites are *"ram goat dash around"* in Jamaica, and *"piss a bed"* in Guyana. However, there are disadvantages in using the common names, especially with intention of sharing information. Common names can be different from country to country, and even within a country. The same plant may be referred to by different names, and different plants may be referred to by the same name.

Common names are not decided upon by any logical system. Their origin can seldom be determined. During the First International Botanical Congress in Paris in 1867, the International Code of Botanical Nomenclature (ICBN) evolved. This system created a single valid universally recognized scientific name for each plant. Scientific names have thus facilitated the free transfer of ideas and information by botanists all over the world. The principle of this new system is that each plant be given a two-element name or binomial. The two elements of the binomial that make up the scientific name are derived from the taxonomic hierarchy. The first element is called the genus and the second element is called the specific epithet; together, the genus and the specific epithet form the species name. The binomial, for accuracy, is followed by the abbreviation of the name of the person or persons who first applied that name to the plant. Most of the words that make up scientific names are derived from Latin or Greek, although there is no requirement that they must be. However, for technical purposes, the elements of the binomial are treated as Latin, no matter what their source. Most specific epithets indicate something characteristic about a species, such as growth pattern, habitat, season, shape of leaves, discoverer of the species, place of discovery, or type or color of flowers and fruit.

Our knowledge of the plants in our environment is far from complete. There are regions around the world, especially the tropical rain forest, where the plants have not been cataloged. This is a serious deficiency, considering the potential importance of the unknown species in terms of conservation, to establish natural preserves, and to locate and protect species that may provide germplasm resources or that may possess medically useful chemical compounds. Without knowledge of the present botanical names of plants, it will be very difficult, if not impossible, to identify, classify, and assign new names to newly discovered species.

From: *Medicinal Plants of the World, vol. 1: Chemical Constituents, Traditional and Modern Medicinal Uses, 2nd ed.*
By: Ivan A. Ross © Humana Press Inc., Totowa, NJ

Because the identification and classification of plants is based somewhat on the details of their external features, a knowledge of the terminology of plant morphology is essential. Some commonly encountered terminology for descriptive plant taxonomy is illustrated in this chapter. Understanding these terms will help one to fully understand the botanical description of the plants.

Leaves are the most important plant organs in the identification and classification of a species. They are generally broad, flattened, and are borne at the nodes of a stem. Leaves are either simple-the blade is a single part-or compound-the blade is divided into smaller, blade-like parts (*see* Fig. 1). Just above the point of attachment of the leaf base or petiole, there is an axillary bud. A complete leaf is composed of the **blade**, the expanded flattened part; **petiole**, the supporting stalk, and **stipules**, appendages that, if present, may be leaf-like, scale-like, or tendrils. Any one of these parts of the leaf may be lacking or highly modified. The arrangement of the veins of the leaf blade is referred to as *venation*. The venation may be parallel or net. Net venation may be *palmate*, the main veins radiating from the point where they join the petiole, or *pinnate*, with one central vein or midrib that has lateral veins arising along its length and at angles from it. Leaves are generally arranged in one of three ways: *alternate*, having one leaf at each node, usually arranged in spirals around the stem; *opposite*, having leaves paired at each node on opposite sides of the stem; and ventricillate, or *whorled*, having three or more leaves at each node. The edge of a leaf is also referred to as the *margin*.

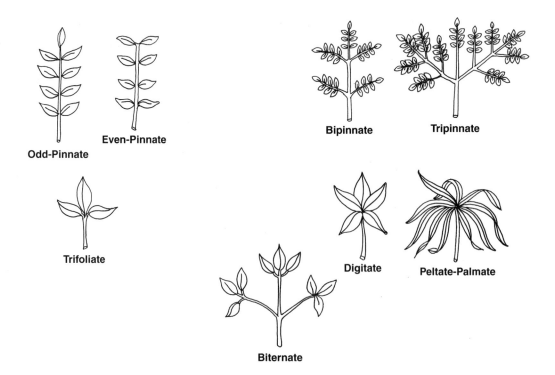

Fig. 1. Compound leaves.

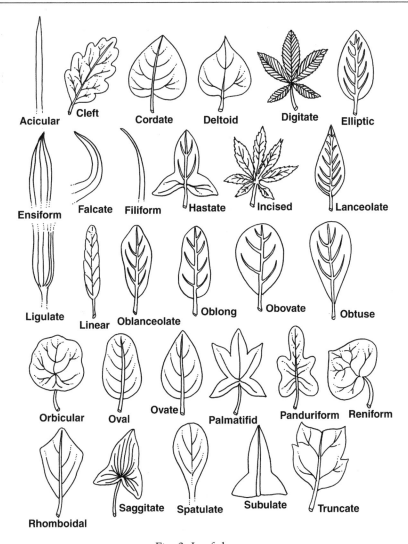

Acicular — Cleft — Cordate — Deltoid — Digitate — Elliptic

Ensiform — Falcate — Filiform — Hastate — Incised — Lanceolate

Ligulate — Linear — Oblanceolate — Oblong — Obovate — Obtuse

Orbicular — Oval — Ovate — Palmatifid — Panduriform — Reniform

Rhomboidal — Saggitate — Spatulate — Subulate — Truncate

Fig. 2. Leaf shapes.

Some common types of leaves, stems, flowers and fruits, and their shapes, characteristics and arrangements are listed below:

COMPOUND LEAVES *(Figure 1)*

Odd-pinnate. A pinnate leaf with a terminal leaflet, the number of leaflets being odd.

Even-pinnate. The condition in a compound leaf when an even number of leaflets is present, a terminal leaflet lacking.

Bipinnate A leaf that is twice pinnately compound.

Tripinnate. Three times pinnately compound.

Trifoliate. Having three leaves.

Biternate. A ternate leaf in which the first order leaflets are themselves ternately compound.

Digitate. A compound leaf in which the leaflets arise from a single point at the end of the petiole; also referred to as *palmately compound.*

Peltate-Palmate. Attached to a supporting stalk at a point inside the margin, as in the petiole of a leaf of the stalk of certain cone scales.

LEAF SHAPES *(Figure 2)*

Acicular. Needle-like, round, or grooved in a cross-section.

Cordate. Heart-shaped.

Cuneate. Wedge-shaped, tapering toward the point of attachment.

Deltoid. Triangular.

Digitate. A compound leaf in which the leaflets arise from a single point at the end of the petiole; also referred to as *palmately compound.*

Elliptical. Having the shape of flattened circle, usually twice as long as broad.

Ensiform. Sword-shaped.

Falcate. Sickle-shaped.

Filiform. Thread-like.

Hastate. Arrowhead-shaped.

Incised. Cut deeply, sharply, and often irregularly into a leaf or petal margin.

Lanceolate. Lance-shaped, tapering from a broad base to the apex; much longer than wide.

Ligulate. Shaped like a strap or narrow band, as in a petal or the corolla.

Linear. Long and narrow with almost parallel sides.

Oblanceolate. Lanceolate, but with the broadest part near the apex.

Oblong. Much longer than broad, the sides being parallel.

Obovate. Ovate, but with the broadest part near the apex.

Obtuse. An apex formed by two lines which meet at more than a right angle.

Orbicular. Having a flat body with a circular outline.

Oval. Rounded at both ends, about twice as long as broad.

Ovate. Egg-shaped, with the broadest part toward the base.

Palmatifid. Lobed, cleft, parted, divided or compounded so that the sinuses or leaflets point to the apex of the petiole.

Panduriform. Fiddle-shaped.

Reniform. Kidney-shaped.

Rhomboidal. Parallelogram-shaped with opposing acute and obtuse angles.

Sagittate. Term describing basal lobes drawn into points on either side of the petiole.

Spatulate. Shaped like a spatula.

Subulate. Tapering from a broad base to a sharp point, awl shaped.

Truncate. A straight base or apex which appears to have been cut off.

LEAF MARGINS *(Figure 3)*

Ciliate. Having hairs on the margins.

Cleft. The condition in which the leaves are palmately or pinnately cut to about the midpoint.

Crenate. With low rounded or blunt teeth.

Crenulate. Having margins with very small rounded teeth; diminutive of crenate.

Dentate. Having sharp marginal teeth pointing outward.

Denticulate. Minutely toothed.

Entire. Smooth; devoid of any indentations, lobes, or teeth.

Incised. Cut deeply, sharply, and often irregularly into the leaf margin.

Lacerate. Torn or irregularly cleft.

Lobed. Divided into parts separated by rounded sinuses extending one-third to one-half the distance between the margin and the midrib.

Palmately Lobed. Like an open hand.

Parted. Cut or dissected almost to the midrib.

Pectinate. Parts are arranged like the teeth of a comb.

Pinnatisect. Cleft almost down to the midrib in a pinnate manner.

Serrate. Having marginal teeth pointing toward the apex.

Double-serrate. With small serration on larger serration.

Serrate. Minutely serrate.

Sinuate. Having a deeply wavy margin.

Spinose. With a spine at the top.

Undulate. Having a slightly wavy margin.

Bi-serrate. The condition in which serration are themselves serrate; also referred to as *doubly serrate.*

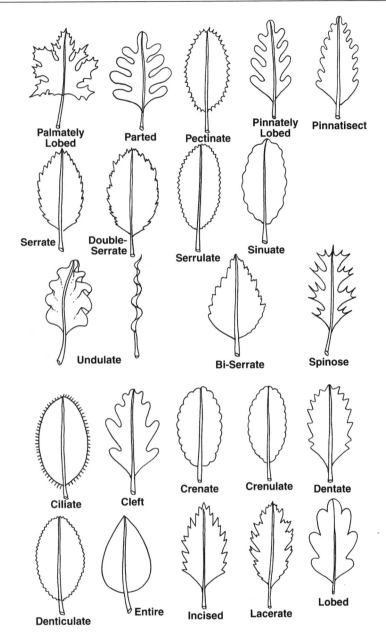

Fig. 3. Leaf Margins

LEAF TIPS *(Figure 4)*

Acuminate. Tapering gradually to a prolonged point.

Acute. Ending in a point that is less than a right angle, but one that is not acuminate; distinct and sharp, but not drawn out.

Apiculate. A leaf apex which bears a short flexible point .

Aristate. With a bristle at the tip.

Caudate. Tailed.

Cirrhose. Tendril-like.

Cleft. The condition in which the leaves are palmately or pinnately cut to about the midpoint.

Cuspidate. Tipped with a sharp and rigid point.

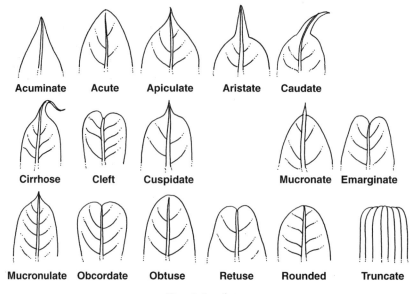

Fig. 4. Leaf tips.

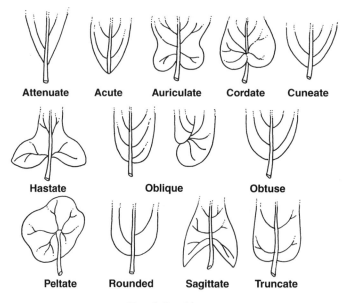

Fig. 5. Leaf bases.

Emarginate. Callously notched and indented at the apex.

Mucronate. Abruptly tipped with a small point, projecting from the midrib.

Mucronulate. Having a sharp terminal point or spiny tip.

Obcordate. The shape of an inverted heart.

Obtuse. An apex formed by two lines that meet at more than a right angle.

Retuse. With a shallow notch at a rounded apex.

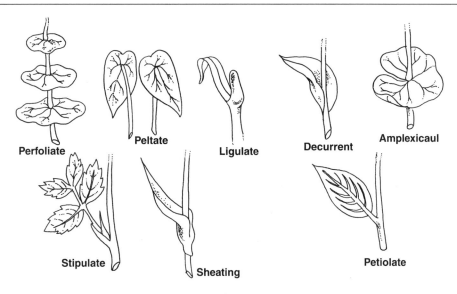

Fig. 6. Attachment to stem.

Rounded. An apex that is gently curved.

Truncate. Cut squarely across at the apex.

LEAF BASES *(Figure 5)*

Attenuate. Characterized by a long gradual taper.

Acute. Ending in a point that is less than a right angle but one that is not acuminate; distinct and sharp, but not drawn out.

Auriculate. With ear-like appendages at the base.

Cordate. Heart-shaped, with a notch at the base.

Cuneate. Wedge-shaped, gradually narrowed toward point of attachment.

Hastate. Having the general shape of an arrowhead, but with the basal lobes turned outward at right angles.

Oblique. Slanting or unequal-sided.

Obtuse. With a blunt or rounded tip.

Peltate. Attached to a supporting stalk at a point inside the margin.

Rounded. With a broad arch.

Sagittate. Basal lobes drawn into points on either side of the petiole.

Truncate. Cut squarely across at the base.

ATTACHMENT TO STEM *(Figure 6)*

Amplexicaul. Sessile with the base clasped around the stem.

Decurrent. Leaf bases that extend downward and are adnate to a stem.

Ligulate. Shaped like a strap or narrow band.

Peltate. Attached to a supporting stalk at a point inside the margin.

Perfoliate. The base surrounds the stem so that it appears that the stem penetrates the leaf.

Petiolate. Having a petiole or leaf stalk.

Sessile. Without a stalk; seated directly on the supporting structure.

Sheathing. The enclosure of the stem by a sheath-like leaf.

Stipulate. Having stipules.

LEAF SURFACES

Papillate. Having small pimple or nipple-like protuberances.

Pitted. Having small cavities or depressions; also referred to as *punctate*.

Scurfy. Covered with scales.

Uncinate. Hooked.

Barbellate. Hairs of barbs down the sides.

Glochidiate. Having apical barbed hair or bristle.

Velutinous. Velvety.

Tomentose. With densely matted soft hairs; woolly in appearance.

Lanate. Woolly, with long, intertwined, coiled hairs.

Floccose. Covered with tufts of soft woolly hairs that are easily removed by rubbing.

Scabrous. Rough to the touch.

Strigose. Stiff hairs often appressed (i.e., pressed next to the stem) and pointing in one direction.

Glandular. Having glands or small secretory structures.

Farinose. Covered with mealiness.

Hirsute. With long shaggy hairs, often stiff or bristly to the touch.

Hirtellous. Minutely hirsute.

Hispid. With stiff, rough hairs.

Echinate. With straight, often comparatively large, prick-like hairs.

Puberulent. Somewhat or minutely pubescent.

Pubescent. Covered with short, soft hairs.

Pilose. With scattered long slender soft hairs.

Villous. Covered with long fine soft hairs.

Sericeous. With soft silky hairs, usually all pointing in one direction.

Dolabriform. With forked hairs attached at the middle.

Stellate. With star-shaped hairs.

Flowers are highly modified shoots with specialized appendages. Flowers may arise in the axil of a leaf or, more often, in the axil of a reduced leaf, which is called a bract. The major components of the unmodified flower are the **perianth**, **androecium**, and the **gynoecium**. The perianth is subdivided into the **calyx** and the **corolla**. A group of **stamens**, wherein the pollen is produced, is called the androecium. The gynoecium consists of the **carpel**, the innermost ovule-bearing part of the flower. The arrangement of the flowers on the plant is referred to as the inflorescence. Some inflorescences are simple and readily distinguishable, but others are complicated and difficult to characterize. Some common types of inflorescence are listed below.

TYPES OF INFLORESCENCE *(Figure 7)*

Solitary. With a single flower.

Axillary. Growing out of the angle between the stem and the leaf stalk.

Terminal. Situated at the apex of a flowering stalk.

Axillary & Terminal. Growing out at the axil, as in axillary and also at the apex of the plant or the tip of the growing point.

Spike. An inflorescence with a single axis and flowers without pedicels.

Spikelet. A small spike; the flowers inconspicuous and more or less hidden by bracts, as in grasses and sedges.

Spadix. A thick or fleshy spike-like inflorescence with very small flowers that are massed together and usually enclosed in a spathe.

Catkin. A soft spike or raceme of small unisexual flowers, the inflorescence usually falling as a unit.

Helicoid cyme. Formed like a spring or snail shell.

Verticel. Flowers arranged in whorls at the nodes.

Head. A dense cluster of stalkless flowers.

Raceme. An inflorescence with a single axis and the flowers arranged along the main axis on pedicels.

Umbel. An inflorescence of few to many flowers on pedicels of approximately equal length arising from the top of a peduncle.

Corymb. A broad inflorescence in which the lower pedicels are successively elongate, giving the inflorescence a flat-topped appearance; indeterminate.

Dichasium. A terminal flower carried between two roughly equally branches.

Panicle. A compound inflorescence in which the main axis is branched one or more times and may support spikes, racemes, or corymbs.

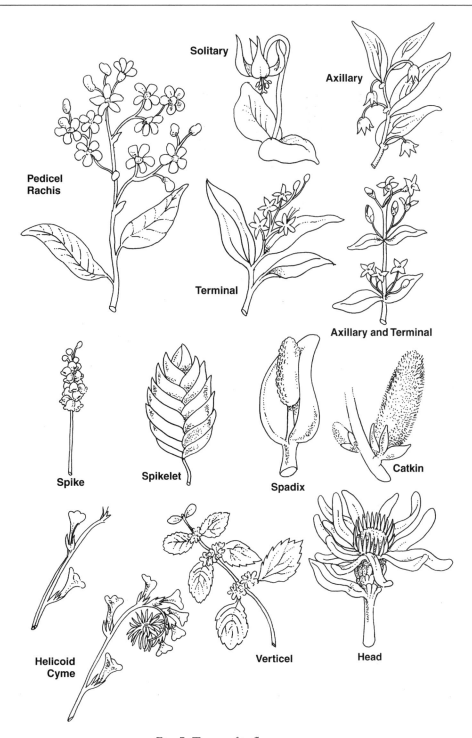

Fig. 7. Types of inflorescence.

Thyrse. A compound, compact panicle with an indeterminate main axis and laterally determinate axes.

Compound umbel. A flower head in which the flower stems spring from a common point.

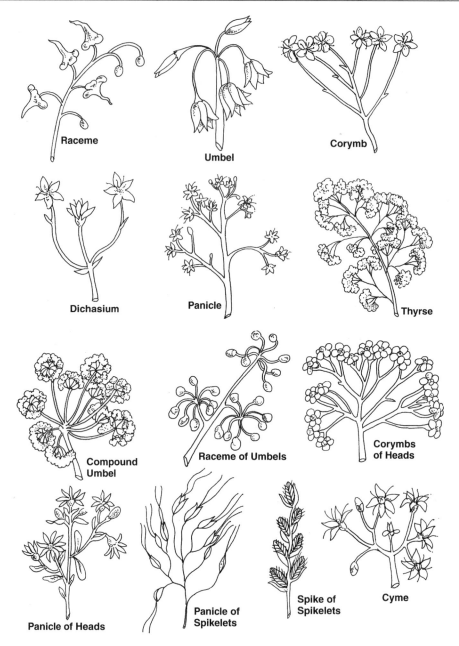

Fig. 7. Types of inflorescence (*Continued*).

Raceme of umbels. An elongated inflorescence in which the umbels are inserted along a rachis.

Corymbs of heads. A flat-topped flower cluster in which the flower stalks emanate from different parts of the main stem as different from **umbel** where they radiate from a single point.

Panicle of heads. A flower head with several branches, either opposite or alternate.

Panicle of spikelets. Panicle in which the branchlets terminate in spikelets

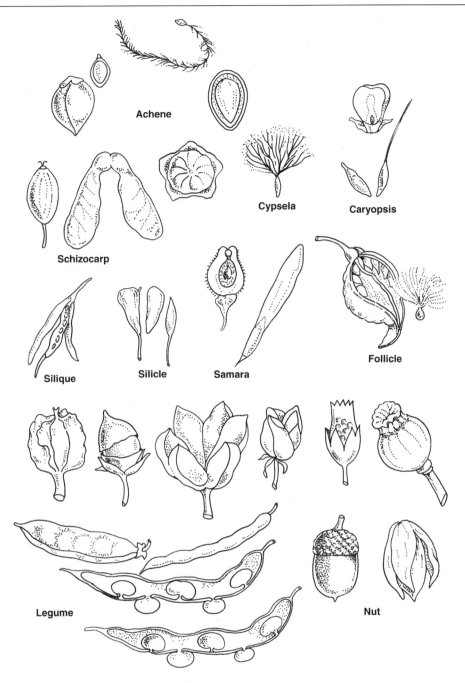

Fig. 8. Dry fruits.

rather than individual flowers, as in many grasses.

Spike of spikelets. Spikelets are sessile along an unbranched rachis.

Cyme. A broad, more or less flat-topped inflorescence with the main axis terminating in a single flower that opens before the lateral flowers, determinate.

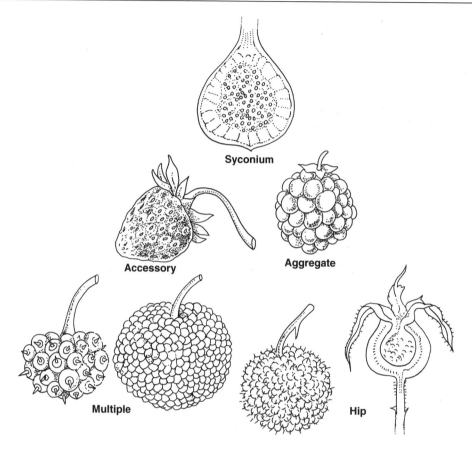

Fig. 9. Fleshy fruits.

Fruits develop from ripened ovaries in the flower. Fruits may have other floral structures associated with them and normally contain seeds, which are ripened ovules. The seed germinates and produces a new plant. Many taxonomists restrict the use of the term "fruit" to the flowering plants and do not refer to the matured female reproductive structures in gymnosperms as fruits. The botanical definition is not very clear in common usage. Corn "seeds" are actually the fruit of this plant. Fruits such as squash, eggplant, and tomatoes are called vegetables. There are many kinds of fruits, some easy to classify, and others more difficult. Two of the major groups

of fruits are dry and fleshy. Some types of dry and fleshy fruits are listed below.

DRY FRUITS *(Figure 8)*

Achene. Seed and pericarp attached only at the funiculus, the seed usually tightly enclosed by the fruit wall, as in the sunflower.
Cypsela. An achene with an adnate calyx.
Casryopsis. Seed and pericarp completely fused, as in the grass family.
Schizocarp. The carpels separating from one another into one-seeded indehiscent segments.
Silique. The walls peeling away from a papery central partition.
Silicle. A silique that is not longer than it is wide.

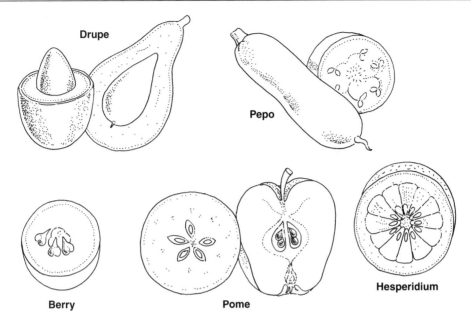

Fig. 9. Fleshy fruits (*Continued*).

Samara. A winged achene.

Follicle. A unicarpellate dehiscent dry fruit that opens along one suture.

Utricle. A small bladdery achene-like fruit with the seed loosely surrounded by the fruit wall, as in the pigweed.

Pyxis. Opening by a lid, as in the purslane.

Septicidal. A capsule that dehisces by means of openings along or within the septations.

Loculicidal. A capsule that dehisces by means of openings into locules, about midway between the partitions.

Denticidal. A capsule dehiscing by a series of teeth.

Poricidal. A capsule or anthler that opens by means of a pore or series of pores.

Legume. Unicarpellate, dehiscing along both sutures; the fruit type of the pea family.

Nut .A dry hard indehiscent one-seeded fruit derived from a syncarpous gynoecium.

FLESHY FRUITS *(Figure 9)*

Drupe. A fleshy indehiscent fruit, having its single seed enclosed in a stony endocarp.

Pepo. A berry with a leathery rind; derived from an inferior ovary; use often restricted to the fruit of the Cucurbitaceae.

Berry. A multiseeded indehiscent fruit in which the pericarp is fleshy throughout, as in the tomato.

Pome. A fleshy indehiscent fruit derived from an inferior ovary surrounded by an adnate hypanthium, as in the apple.

Hesperidium. A fleshy indehiscent fruit with conspicuous septations lined with succulent hairs; the fruit of the citrus group.

Accessory. A false fruit, as in the strawberry, in which the bulk of the fleshy portion is derived from receptacle rather than gynoecium.

Aggregate. A false fruit type in which the separate carpels of an apocarpous gynoecium collectively appear to form a fruit.

Syconium. A vase-like structure with an opening at its apex and whose interior wall is lined with tiny flowers.

Multiple. A type of false fruit in which several true fruits from separate flowers coalesce to produce a single structure that resembles a fruit, as in pineapple.

Hip. Vase-like leathery hypanthium containing several seed-like achenes; the false fruit of the rose.

ABBREVIATIONS USED IN THE CHEMICAL CONSTITUENTS SECTION

Following the names of each chemical constituent is an abbreviation indicating the part of the plant in which the constituent is present; a number is then followed indicating the amount of that constituent present. This value is listed in either parts per million (ppm) or in percentage (%). Some of these values have a wide range; this is because the amount of the constituent is based on the dry weight as well as the amount of moisture in the plant part in its natural state. The larger value is based on the dry weight and the smaller value on the natural moisture content of the part indicated. These values can also vary depending on such conditions as varieties, geographic location of production, method of production, maturity at harvesting, method of processing, and so forth.

Aer Aerial parts
An Anther
As Ash
Bd Bud
Bk Bark
Bu Bulb
Call Tiss Callus tissue
Cr Crown
Ct Coat
Cult Culture
Cx Calyx
Cy Cotyledon
Ct Coat
Em Embryo
EO Essential oil
Ep Epidermis
Fl Flower
Fr Fruit
Hu Hull
Ju Juice
Lf Leaf
Lx Latex
Pe Peel
Pc Pericarp
Pl Plant
Pu Pulp
Pn Panicle
Rh Rhizome
Rt Root
Sd Seed
Sh Shoot
St Stem
Tr Trunk
Tu Tuber
Tw Twig

Ppm	% Conversion	Ppm	% Conversion
10,000 ppm	1%	60,000 ppm	6%
20,000 ppm	2%	70,000 ppm	7%
30,000 ppm	3%	80,000 ppm	8%
40,000 ppm	4%	90,000 ppm	9%
50,000 ppm	5%	100,000 ppm	10%

2 | Abrus precatorius L.
Gaertn.

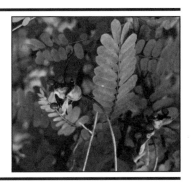

Common Names

Aainud-dik	India	Jequirity plant	Philippines
Aregllisse	West Indies	Jequirity	Taiwan
Benambo	Guinea-Bissau	Jequirity	India
Buck bean	Guyana	Jiquiriti	Brazil
Chanoti	Pakistan	Jumble bean	Virgin Islands
Chasm-I-kharosh	Pakistan	Jumble bean	Ivory Coast
Chirmu	Pakistan	Kalyani	India
Chunhati	India	Kikerewe	Tanzania
Crab's eye	Guam	Kolales halomtanto	Guam
Crab's eye	India	Koonch	India
Crab's eye	Nepal	Krikpe	Ivory Coast
Crab's eye	USA	Kunni	India
Crab's eye	Thailand	Laboma	Ivory Coast
Crab's stone	India	Latuwani	India
Damabo	Ivory Coast	Love bean	USA
Gaungchi	India	Lufyambo	East Africa
Gchi	India	Lyann legliz	Haiti
Ghongchi	India	Ma klam taanuu	Thailand
Ghumchi	India	Minimini	Mozambique
Ghun	India	Mishquina	Peru
Goassien	Ivory Coast	Miski miski	Peru
Guinea pea	India	Motipitipi	East Africa
Gunch	India	Moudie-bi-titi	Ivory Coast
Gunchi	Pakistan	Mwanga-la-nyuki	East Africa
Gundumani	India	Mwangaruchi	Tanzania
Gunja	India	Namugolokoma	Mozambique
Guri-ginja	India	Ndebie ni	Guinea
Gurivinda	India	Olho de pombo	Brazil
Gurje-tiga	India	Olinda	India
Habat al arus	Sudan	Ombulu	East Africa
Habat-elmlook	Sudan	Orututi	Tanzania
Indian licorice	India	Osito	East Africa
Indian licorice	Nigeria	Prayer bean	USA
Jequiriti bean	Taiwan	Precatory bean	USA

From: *Medicinal Plants of the World, vol. 1: Chemical Constituents, Traditional and Modern Medicinal Uses, 2nd ed.*
By: Ivan A. Ross © Humana Press Inc., Totowa, NJ

Rati gedi	Nepal	Saga	Indonesia
Rati	India	Saga saga	Philippines
Ratti	Pakistan	Sanga	Ivory Coast
Rosary bean	Pakistan	Sonkach	India
Rosary bean	USA	Sus	Egypt
Rosary pea	Egypt	Weglis	West Indies
Safed chirami	India		

BOTANICAL DESCRIPTION

A woody twinning plant of the LEGUMINOSAE family, with characteristic red and black seeds. The leaves are pinnate and glabrous, with many leaflets (12 or more) arranged in pairs. The leaflets are oblong, measuring 2.5-cm long and 1.5-cm wide. The plant bears orange-pink flowers, which occur as clusters in short racemes that are sometimes yellowish or reddish purple in color, small and typically pea-like. The plant produces short and stout brownish pods, which curl back on opening to reveal pendulous red and black seeds, 4 to 6 peas in a pod.

ORIGIN AND DISTRIBUTION

It grows wild in thickets, farms, and secondary clearings, and sometimes in hedges. It is most common in rather dry areas at low elevation throughout the tropics and subtropics.

TRADITIONAL MEDICINAL USES

Afghanistan. Dried seeds are taken orally as an aphrodisiac[AP063].

Brazil. Leaves and stem are said to be toxic when eaten by cattle[AP041]. Water extract of dried leaves and root is taken orally as a nerve tonic[AP063].

Cambodia. Hot water extract of seeds is taken orally for malaria[AP047].

Central Africa. Root is chewed as a snake bite remedy[AP045]. Seeds are taken orally by several Central African tribes for intestinal worms and as an oral contraceptive. The effect of a single dose (200 mg) is said to be effective for 13 menstrual cycles[AP045].

East Africa. Decoction of the aerial parts is taken orally for gonorrhea. A decoction of the plant plus 3 or 4 seed pods is taken. Fresh leaf juice is taken orally for gonorrhea, bilharziasis, stomach troubles, and as an antiemetic. Powdered leaves are applied to cuts and swellings. Decoction of leaves is taken orally for chest pains. For inflamed eyes, steam of boiling leaves is used. Water extract of dried seeds is applied to the eyes for purulent eye infections; the seeds are macerated in the water[AP106]. Fresh root is chewed as an aphrodisiac[AP045,AP056].

Egypt. Seeds are taken orally with honey as an aphrodisiac[AP082].

Guam. Seeds are reported to be toxic; half of one seed is reported as lethal. Seed coat must be broken to be toxic. Symptoms include acute gastroenteritis with vomiting, nausea, and diarrhea, followed by dehydration, convulsions, and death[AP044].

Guinea-Bissau. Leaf pulp is taken orally by men as an aphrodisiac and by women to facilitate childbirth. Seeds taken orally are considered an aphrodisiac and abortive[AP002].

Haiti. Decoction of leaves is taken orally for coughs and flu[AP109].

India. Hot water extract of dried leaves and roots are applied to the eye for eye diseases[AP105]. Hot water extract of root is taken orally as an emmenagogue[AP003]. Root brew is taken orally to produce abortion[AP022,AP047]. Hot water extract of seeds is taken orally as an antifertility agent[AP003], as an abortifacient[AP013], and to prevent conception[AP022]. Seeds are used as a poultice in the vagina in Ayurvedic and Unani medicine as an abortifacient.

Seeds are boiled in milk and taken orally by males in Unani and Ayurvedic medicine as an aphrodisiac. It is claimed that the boiling destroys the toxic action of Abrin[AP047]. As birth control, one seed completely covered with Jaggary is swallowed during the menstrual period and is sufficient to prevent conception for 1 year[AP111]. Decoction of dried seeds is taken orally to induce abortion[AP062]. Hot water extract of dried seeds is taken orally as a sexual stimulant in the Unani system of medicine[AP084]. It is also taken for tuberculosis, painful swellings[AP104], and as an aphrodisiac and purgative[AP121]. Dried seed oil is taken orally as an abortifacient[AP124]. Plant juice is administered intravaginally to induce abortion[AP117].

Ivory Coast. Water extract of leaves and stem is taken orally by males as an aphrodisiac and by females to facilitate childbirth[AP036].

Jamaica. Decoction of dried leaves and root boiled in milk is used as a tonic[AP063].

Kenya. Fresh leaf juice is taken orally for coughs. Fresh leaves are taken orally for coughs[AP075].

Mozambique. Hot water extract of root is administered orally as an aphrodisiac[AP067].

Nepal. Seeds are taken orally as an aphrodisiac[AP001].

Nigeria. Hot water extract of fresh root is administered orally as an antimalarial and anticonvulsant[AP100].

Pakistan. Hot water extract of seeds is administered orally as an aphrodisiac. Seeds are used as a suppository for inducing abortion[AP027].

Sudan. Hot water extract of the plant is taken orally as an antifertility agent[AP093].

Taiwan. Decoction of dried root is taken orally to treat bronchitis and hepatitis[AP051].

Tanzania. Decoction of roots and leaf sap is taken orally for asthma and as an aphrodisiac[AP106].

Thailand. Leaves crushed with oil are used as a poultice as an anti-inflammatory[AP115].

Virgin Islands. Extract of seeds is taken orally for coughs[AP119].

West Africa. Decoction of dried roots is taken orally as an antiemetic, for bilharziasis, tapeworms, gonorrhea, chest pains and is also used as an aphrodisiac. For snake bites the root is chewed[AP106].

West Indies. Seeds are taken orally as an emetic, purgative, and anthelmintic[AP083].

CHEMICAL CONSTITUENTS

(ppm unless otherwise indicated)

Abrine: Sd 0.85%, Lf, St[AP103]
Abrasine: Rt[AP025,AP004]
Abrectorin: Sd[AP087]
Abridin, Sd[AP112]
Abrin: Sd 0.12%[AP021]
Abrin A: Sd[AP005], Ker 0.10%[AP094]
Abrin B: Sd[AP088], Ker 125[AP094]
Abrin C: Ker 175[AP094], Sd[AP005]
Abrin D: Ker 5[AP094]
Abrin I: Sd[AP049]
Abrin II: Sd[AP049]
Abrin III: Sd[AP049]
Abrulin: Sd[AP023]
Abruquinone A: Rt 0.025–0.45%[AP051]
Abruquinone B: Rt 0.045–1.15%[AP051]
Abruquinone C: Rt 0.5%[AP051]
Abruquinone D: Rt 0.03%[AP051]
Abruquinone E: Rt 0.02%[AP051]
Abruquinone F: Rt 0.01%[AP051]
Abrus agglutinin: Kr 0.1%[AP094]
Abrus agglutinin APA-I: Sd[AP049]
Abrus agglutinin APA-II: Sd[AP049]
Abrus precatorius agglutinin: Sd[AP085]
Abrus precatorius alkaloid A: Sd[A08649]
Abrus precatorius lectin: Sd[AP077]
Abrus precatorius plant growth inhibitor: Sd[AP017]
Abrusgenic acid-methanol-solvate: Rt 0.0166%[AP101]
Abrusin: Sd 48.9[AP076]
Abrusin-2'-0-apioside: Sd 0.58%[AP076]
Abruslactone A: Rt, St[AP096], Lf 83–200[AP068], Rt 0.27%[AP101]
Abrusoside A: Lf 0.03%[AP078,AP072]
Abrusoside B: Lf 0.025%[AP072]
Abrusoside C: Lf 0.037%[AP072]
Abrusoside D: Lf 0.053%[AP072]
Abrussic acid: Pl[AP130]

Alanine: Sd[AP130]
Amyrin, alpha: Sd[AP009]
Amyrin, beta: Sd[AP035]
Anthocyanins: Sd[AP131]
Arabinose: St, Lf, Sd, Rt[AP097]
Arachidic acid: Sd oil 19.2%[AP061]
Arachidyl alcohol: Sd[AP035]
Aspartic acid: Sd[AP016,AP034]
Behenic acid: Sd oil 13.4%[AP061]
Brassicasterol: Sd[AP035]
Callistephin: Sd Ct[AP024]
Campesterol: Sd[AP050]
Centaureidin, demethoxy 7-O-beta-D-rutinoside: Sd[AP087]
Cholanic acid, 5-beta: Sd[AP026]
Cholesterol: Sd[AP035]
Choline: Sd, Rt 4.0%, Lf, St[AP008]
Chrysanthemin: Sd Ct[AP024]
Cycloartenol: Sd[AP035]
Cysteine: Sd[AP034]
Cystine: Sd[AP016]
Decan-1-ol: Sd[AP035]
Delphin: Sd Ct[AP024]
Delphinidin glycoside: Sd[AP123]
Delphinidin, (para-coumaroyl-galloyl) glucoside: Sd[AP095]
Delphinidin-3-sambubioside: Sd[AP095]
Docos-13-enoic acid: Sd[AP035]
Docosadienoic acid: Sd oil[AP037,AP038]
Docosan-1-ol: Sd[AP035]
Docosane, N: Sd[AP035]
Docosatetraenoic acid: Sd oil[AP037]
Docosatrienoic acid: Sd oil[AP037]
Docosenoic acid: Sd oil[AP037,AP038]
Dodecan-1-ol: Sd[AP035]
Dotriacontane, N: Sd[AP035]
Eicos-11-enoic acid: Sd[AP035]
Eicosadienoic acid: Sd oil[AP037,AP038]
Eicosenoic acid: Sd oil[AP037,AP038]
Eicosane, N: Sd[AP035]
Eicosatrienoic acid: Sd oil[AP037,AP038]
Elaidic alcohol: Sd[AP035]
Galactose: St, Rt, Sd, Lf[AP097]
Galacturonic acid: Sd[AP016]
Gallic acid: Sd[AP031]
Glucuronic acid: Sd[AP016]
Glutamic acid: Sd[AP034]
Glutamine: Sd[AP034]
Glycine: Sd[AP034]
Glycyrrhizin: Lf 9.0%[AP092], Rt 1.25%
Hederagenin: Sd 7.3[AP076]
Hemiphloin: Lf 83.3[AP068]

Heneicosan-1-ol: Sd[AP035]
Heneicosane,7,9,15-trimethyl: Sd[AP050]
Heneicosane,N: Sd[AP035]
Heptacosan-1-ol: Sd[AP035]
Heptadecan-1-ol: Sd[AP035]
Hexacosane,N: Sd[AP035]
Hexacosan-1-ol: Sd[AP035]
Hexadec-9-enoic acid: Sd[AP035]
Hexadecane,N: Sd[AP035]
Hexadecan-1-ol: Sd[AP035]
Hexadecenoic acid: Sd oil[AP037,AP038]
Hypaphorine: Sd, Lf, Rt[AP008], St[AP103]
Inositol, D monomethyl ether: Lf[AP128]
Kaikasaponin III: Sd 147.3[AP076]
Lauric acid: Sd oil[AP040]
Lectin (*Abrus precatorius*): Sd[AP054,AP055]
Leucine: Sd[AP016]
Lignoceric acid: Sd[AP035], Sd oil[AP037,AP038]
Linoleic acid: Sd oil[AP040]
Linolenic acid: Sd oil 0.5%[AP061]
Luteolin: Sd[AP087]
Lysine: Sd[AP034]
Montanyl alcohol: Lf[AP035]
Myricyl alcohol: Lf[A15248]
Myristic acid: Sd oil[AP037,AP038,AP040]
Nonacosane, N: Sd[AP035]
Nonadecan-1-ol: Sd[AP035]
Octacosan-1-ol: Sd[AP035]
Octacosane, N: Sd[AP035]
Octadeca-9,12-dienoic acid: Sd[AP035]
Octadecadienoic acid: Sd oil[AP037,AP038]
Octadecatrienoic acid: Sd oil[AP037,AP038]
Octadecane, N: Sd[AP035]
Octadecenoic acid: Sd oil[AP037,AP038]
Octanoic acid: Sd[AP035]
Oleic acid: Sd oil[AP061,AP035,AP040]
Orientin, iso: Sd[AP087]
Orientin: Sd[AP087]
P-Sterone: Sd[AP007]
Palmitic acid: Sd oil 15.8%[AP061]
Pelargonidin-3,5-diglucoside: Sd Ct[AP024]
Pentacosan-1-ol: Sd[AP035]
Pentacosane, N: Sd[AP035]
Pentacosanoic acid: Sd[AP050]
Pentadecan-1-ol: Sd[AP035]
Pentadecanoic acid: Sd oil[AP037,AP038]
Pentatriacontane, N: Sd[AP035]
Phenylalanine: Sd[AP034]
Pinitol: Lf[AP128]
Polysaccharide: Rt[AP129]
Precasine: Rt[AP025,AP004]
Precatorine: Rt 11.0%, Lf, St, Sd 11.0%[AP008]

Precol: Rt[AP025]
Rhamnose: Sd[AP016]
Serine: Sd[AP034,AP016]
Sitosterol, beta: Sd[AP043,AP050,AP035]
Sophoradiol: Sd 737[AP076]
Sophoradiol-22-0-acetate: Sd 31[AP076]
Squalene: Sd[AP035]
Stearic acid: Sd oil 4.9%[AP061]
Stigamsterol: Sd[AP043]
Tetracos-15-enoic acid: Sd[AP035]
Tetracosan-1-ol: Sd[AP035]
Tetracosane, N: Sd[AP035]
Tetradecan-1-ol: Sd[AP035]
Tetradecanoic acid: Sd[AP035]
Tetratriacontane, N: Sd[AP035]
Triacosan-1-ol: Sd[AP035]
Triacontane, N: Sd[AP035]
Tricosane, N: Sd[AP035]
Tridecan-1-ol: Sd[AP035]
Trigonelline: Sd[AP091], Rt, St, Lf [AP103]
Tritriacontan-1-ol: Sd[AP035]
Tritriacontane, N: Sd[AP035]
Tryptophan, N-N-dimethyl metho-cation methyl ester: Sd[AP008]
Tryptophan, trimethyl: Sd 684[AP076]
Tyrosine: Sd[AP016]
Undecan-1-ol: Sd[AP035]
Ursolic acid: Sd[AP009]
Valine: Sd[AP009,AP016]
Xylose: St, Rt, Sd, Lf [AP097]

PHARMACOLOGICAL ACTIVITIES AND CLINICAL TRIALS

Abortifacient effect. Chloroform/methanol extract of seeds, administered subcutaneously to rats at a dose of 50.0 mg/animal, was inactive. Water extract of dried seeds, administered intragastrically to pregnant rats at a dose of 125.0 mg/kg, was active[AP116]. Ethanol (95%) extract of seeds, administered orally at a dose of 200.0 mg/kg, was inactive on pregnant hamsters and active on pregnant rats[AP127]. Petroleum ether extract of seeds, administered orally to rats, was inactive[AP120].

Agglutinin activity. Water extract of fresh seeds, in cell culture at a concentration of 2.0 microliters/ml, was active on human lymphocytes[AP125].

Alkaline phosphatase inhibition. Petroleum ether extract of seed oil, administered orally, was active on the uterus of rats[AP108].

Analgesic activity. Ethanol/water (1:1) extract of the aerial parts, administered intraperitoneally to mice at a dose of 500.0 mg/kg, was inactive vs tail pressure method[AP118].

Anthelmintic activity. Water extract of dried seeds produced weak activity on *Caenorhabditis elegans*, LC$_{50}$ 15.8 mg/ml[AP064]. Extract of stem and root was active on schistosomules of the trematode *Schistosoma mansoni* and cystercoids of the cestode *Hymenolepis diminuta*, in vitro[AP134].

Antibacterial activity. Ethanol/water (1:1) extract of the aerial parts, at a concentration of 25.0 mcg/ml on agar plate, was inactive on *Bacillus subtilis*, *Escherichia coli*, *Salmonella typhosa*, *Staphylococcus aureus* and *Agrobacterium tumefaciens*[AP118]. Ether extract of seeds, on agar plate, was active on *Staphylococcus aureus*. The ethanol (95%) extract was active on *Escherichia coli* and *Staphylococcus aureus*[AP031].

Anticonvulsant activity. Ethanol (70%) extract of fresh root, administered intraperitoneally to mice of both sexes at variable dosage levels, was active vs metrazole-induced convulsions and inactive vs strychnine-induced convulsions[AP100]. Ethanol/water (1:1) extract of the aerial parts, administered to mice intraperitoneally at a dose of 500.0 mg/kg, was inactive vs electroshock-induced convulsions[AP118].

Antidiarrheal activity. Chromatographic fraction of dried seeds, administered intragastrically to rats at a dose of 10.0 mg/kg, was active vs castor oil-induced diarrhea[AP080].

Antiestrogenic effect. Ethanol (95%) extract of root, administered orally to mice at a dose of 10.0 mg/kg, was active[AP015].

Antifertility effect. Chloroform/methanol extract of seeds, administered subcutaneously to female rats at a dose of 50.0 mg/animal, was active[AP081]. Ethanol (80%)

extract of seeds, administered orally and subcutaneously to female rats at a dose of 1.0 mg/animal, was inactive[AP053]. Ethanol (95%) and water extracts of seeds, administered orally to mice, were inactive, and petroleum ether extract was active[AP006]. Ethanol (95%), water and petroleum ether extracts of leaves, administered orally to female mice, were inactive[AP006]. Ethanol extract of seeds, administered intragastrically to male rats at a dose of 100.0 mg/kg for 60 days, was active. There was a significant decrease in the number of pregnant females[AP069]. Ethanol/water (1:1) extract of dried seeds, administered by gastric intubation to male rats at a dose of 250.0 mg/kg, was active. No pregnancies were reported for the 20 females paired with 10 males treated for 60 days; mating probably occurred in all cases, but this is not entirely clear. Pregnancies were again reported after withdrawal of treatment[AP110]. Hot water extract of dried plant, administered orally to human females at a dose of 0.28 gm/person, was active. The extract was administered as a mixture of *Embelia ribes* (fruit), *Piper longum* (fruit), *Ferula assafoetida*, *Piper betele*, *Polianthes tuberosa* and *Abrus precatorius*. One dose was taken, starting from the second day of menstruation, twice daily for 20 days. Sexual intercourse was avoided during the dosing period. The treatment is claimed effective for 4 months. The biological activity has been patented[AP086]. Seed oil, administered orally to female mice at a dose of 25.0 mg/animal, to female mice, and to rats at a dose 150.0 mg/animal, was active. No control animal was used[AP015].

Antifungal activity. Ethanol/water (1:1) extract of the aerial parts, at a concentration of 25.0 mcg/ml on agar plate, was inactive on *Microsporum canis*, *Trichophyton mentagrophytes*, and *Aspergillus niger*[AP118].

Antigonadotropin effect. Ethanol (95%) extract of dried seeds, administered by gastric intubation to mice at a dose of 150.0 mg/kg, was active[AP107].

Anti-implantation effect. Chloroform/methanol (2:1) extract of seeds, administered subcutaneously to pregnant rats at a dose of 50.0 mg/animal, was active[AP081]. Ethanol (95%) extract of root, administered orally to rats at a dose of 100.0 mg/kg, was active[AP015]. Ethanol (95%) extract of seeds, administered orally to rats and hamsters at a dose of 200.0 mg/kg, was inactive[AP127]. Water extract of seeds, administered orally to rats, was inactive, and the petroleum ether extract was active. Ethanol (95%), water and petroleum ether extracts of leaves, administered orally to female rats, were inactive[AP006].

Anti-inflammatory activity. Ethanol/water (1:1) extract of the aerial parts, administered orally to rats at a dose of 500.0 mg/kg, was inactive vs carrageenin-induced pedal edema. Animals were dosed 1 hour before carrageenin injections[AP118]. Triterpenoid saponins isolated from the aerial parts, exhibited anti-inflammatory activity using the croton oil ear model. The acetates indicated greater inhibition than the parent compounds[AP133].

Antimolluscicidal effect. Forty and 80% of the 24 hour LC_{50} of abrin and glycyrrhizin produced a significant decrease in the levels of protein, free amino acid, DNA, and RNA in the nervous tissue of *Lymnaea acuminata*. Abrin produced a significant reduction in phospholipid levels and a simultaneous increase in the rate of lipid peroxidation in the treated snails[AP137].

Antispasmodic activity. Chromatographic fraction (a gel filtration fraction from a methanol-water (1:1) extract) of seeds, at a concentration of 0.2 mg/ml, was active on the uterus of rats vs PGE-2-, ACh-, oxytocin- and epinephrine-induced contractions[AP099]. Ethanol (95%) extract of dried leaves, at a concentration of 1.0 mg/ml, was active on the phrenic nerve-diaphragm of rats vs nerve stimulation. The inhibition was potentiated by D-tubocurarine but reversed by physostigmine. Results significant at $P < 0.001$ level. At a concentration of 4.0 mg/ml, the extract was active vs direct muscle stimulation. At 1.0 mg/ml, it was active on toad rectus abdominus muscle vs ACh-induced contractions. Water and hot water extracts of dried leaves, at a concentration of 6.72 mg/ml, were inactive on phrenic nerve-diaphragm of rats vs nerve stimulation and direct muscle stimulation. At concentrations of 16.8 and 16.72 mg/ml, respectively, the extracts were inactive on toad rectus abdominus muscle vs ACh-induced contractions. Petroleum ether extract, at concentrations of 19.2 and 48.0 mg/ml, were inactive on rat phrenic nerve-diaphragm vs nerve stimulation and direct muscle stimulation and on toad rectus abdominus muscle vs ACh-induced contractions, respectively[AP102]. Ethanol/water (1:1) extract of the aerial parts was inactive on guinea pig ileum vs ACh- and histamine-induced spasms[AP118].

Antispermatogenic effect. Ethanol extract of seeds, administered intragastrically to male rats at a dose of 100.0 mg/kg for 60 days, was inactive[AP069]. Ethanol/water (1:1) extract of dried seeds, administered by gastric intubation to rats at a dose of 250.0 mg/kg, was active. Although no significant histologic changes in the testes were reported, sperm concentration was reported to be significantly decreased in both cauda epididymis and testes after dosing for 60 days[AP110]. Sterol fraction of dried seeds administered intramuscularly to rats was active. Testicular lesions marked by the cessation of spermatogenesis and a significant reduction in the diameter of the seminiferous tubules were also noted[AP089].

Antitumor activity. Ethanol (95%) extract of dried leaves, administered intraperitoneally to mice at dose of 100.0 mg/kg was inactive on Sarcoma 180 (ASC) [AP074]. Water extract of seeds, administered intraperitoneally to mice at a dose of 5.0 mcg/kg was active on Sarcoma (Yoshida solid and ASC). A dose of 20.0 mcg/kg administered subcutaneously was inactive on Sarcoma (Yoshida ASC)[AP012]. Protein fraction of seeds, administered intraperitoneally to rats, was active on Sarcoma (Yoshida ASC)[AP019]. Agglutinin protein, crystallized at room temperature with polyethylene glycol 8000 as the precipitant from the seeds, produced a high antitumor activity[AP135].

Antiviral activity. Ethanol/water (1:1) extract of the aerial parts at a concentration of 50.0 mcg/ml in cell culture was inactive on Ranikhet virus and Vaccinia virus[AP118]. Water and methanol extracts of dried seeds in cell culture were inactive on virus-HLTV-1. $IC_{100} > 77.0$ and > 40.0 mcg/ml, respectively, were observed. Activity was not observed below the cytotoxic doses[AP065].

Antiyeast activity. Dried seeds at a concentration of 1.0% on agar plate were active on *Cryptococcus neoformans*[AP122]. Ethanol/water (1:1) extract of the aerial parts at a concentration of 25.0 mcg/ml on agar plate was inactive on *Candida albicans* and *Cryptococcus neoformans*[AP118].

CNS depressant activity. Ethanol (70%) extract of fresh root, administered intraperitoneally to mice of both sexes at variable dosage levels, was active[AP100].

Contraceptive and/or interceptive effect. Petroleum ether extract of seed oil, administered orally to rats, was active[AP108].

Cytotoxic activity. Ethanol (95%) extract of dried stem, in cell culture, was inactive on CA-9KB, $ED_{50} > 30.0$ mcg/ml[AP098]. Water and methanol extracts of dried seeds, in cell culture, produced weak activity on cells MT-4, $IC_{100} > 77.0$, and > 40.0 mcg/ml, respectively[AP065]. Water extract of seeds, in cell culture, produced strong activity on Sarcoma Yoshida ASC, ED_{50} 0.004 mcg/ml[AP029]. Water extract of seeds, in cell culture, was active on CA-9KB, ED_{50} < 20.0 mcg/ml[AP126]. Water extract of seeds was active on the testes of *Poecilocera picta*[AP039].

Death. Hot water extract of dried leaves, administered intravenously to chicken, was active at a dose of 20.0 mg/kg and caused spastic paralysis and death within 24 hours[AP102]. Seeds taken orally by male human adults were active. Twenty beans mixed with water in a blender and drunk produced death in 2 days. Symptoms included vomiting of blood, pain in eyes, and burning ears[AP046].

Diuretic activity. Ethanol/water (1:1) extract of the aerial parts, administered intraperitoneally to male rats at a dose of 250.0 mg/kg, was inactive. Saline-loaded animals were used. Urine was collected for 4 hours post-drug[AP118].

Embryotoxic effect. Ethanol (95%) extract of seeds, administered orally to pregnant hamsters and rats at doses of 200.0 mg/kg, was inactive[AP127]. Petroleum ether extract, administered orally to rats at a dose of 150.0 mg/kg, was inactive[AP120]. Water extract of dried seeds, administered intragastrically to pregnant rats at a dose of 125.0 mg/kg, was inactive[AP062].

Estrous cycle disruption effect. Seeds, administered orally to female rats at doses of 0.05, 0.5, and 5.0 mg/animal, were inactive[AP066]. Chloroform/methanol (2:1) extract of seeds, administered subcutaneously to rats at a dose of 1.0 mg/animal, was active[AP053]. Seeds, administered by gastric intubation to rats at doses of 10.0, 5.0, and 2.0 gm/kg, were active; 80, 50, and 25%, respectively, of the rats depicted extensive leukocytic smears, but with no significant effect on uterine weight[AP090].

Hemagglutinin activity. Water extract of seeds was active on the red blood cells of ant (leafcutter), buffalo, cat, chicken, dog, duckling, guinea pig, horse, human adult (blood groups A, B, and O), lamb, mice, pigeon, rabbit, rat, and ox; weakly active

on cow and ewe and inactive on goat[AP032,AP033].

Hypoglycemic activity. Ethanol/water (1:1) extract of the aerial parts, administered orally to rats at a dose of 250.0 mg/kg, was inactive. Less than a 30% drop in blood sugar level was observed[AP118].

Hypothermic activity. Ethanol/water (1:1) extract of the aerial parts, administered intraperitoneally to mice at a dose of 500.0 mg/kg, was inactive[AP118].

Inotropic effect positive. Hot water extract of dried entire plant, at a concentration of 320.0 microliters, was inactive on guinea pig atria[AP079].

Insect sterility induction. Petroleum ether extract of dried seeds, applied externally at a concentration of 1.0 microliter, was active on *Dysdercus cingulatus*. The extract was active in males alone. The saline extract produced weak activity in both males and females[AP071].

Insecticide activity. Acetone extract of dried root was inactive on *Culex quinquefasciatus*. Acetone extract of dried stem, at low concentration, was inactive on *Culex quinquefasciatus*[AP048]. Seeds, at a concentration of 10.0%, produced weak activity on *Musca domestica*. The activity was less than that of 0.25% DDT[AP030].

Intestinal fluid retention effect. Chromatographic fraction of dried seeds, administered intragastrically to rats at a dose of 10.0 mg/kg, was active on the small intestine vs PGE_2-induced enteropooling. Effect assayed 30 minutes after oral dose of PGE_2[AP080].

Intestinal motility inhibition. Chromatographic fraction of dried seeds, administered intragastrically to rats at a dose of 10.0 mg/kg, was active. Effect was not as great as that of an equal amount of atropine[AP080].

Luteal suppressant effect. Chloroform/methanol (2:1) extract of seeds, administered subcutaneously to rats at a dose of 50.0 mg/animal, was active[AP081].

Microglial cell markers. Lectin from the plant has been used to glycohistochemically identify the microglial cells activation in autopic brain samples from Alzheimer's disease subjects[AP138].

Mitogenic activity. Water extract of fresh seeds, in cell culture at a concentration of 2.0 microliters/ml, was inactive on human lymphocytes[AP125].

Mutagenic activity. Methanol (75%) extract of dried leaves, at a concentration of 10.0 mg/ml on agar plate, was inactive on *Salmonella typhimurium* TM677[AP072].

Neuromuscular blocking activity. Ethanol (95%) extract of dried leaves, at a concentration of 0.5 mcg/ml, was active on phrenic nerve-diaphragm[AP102].

Protease (HIV) inhibition. Water and methanol extracts of dried seeds were inactive, IC_{50} > 500 mcg/ml[AP057].

Reverse transcriptase inhibition. Water and methanol extracts of commercial sample of seeds, in cell culture, were inactive on virus-avian myeloblastosis, IC_{50} > 1000 mg/ml[AP058].

Semen coagulation. Ethanol/water (1:1) extract of the aerial parts, at a concentration of 2.0%, was inactive on rat semen[AP118].

Smooth muscle stimulant activity. Chromatographic fraction (gel filtration 4–9 of a methanol-water (1:1) extract of seeds, at a concentration of 0.2 mg/ml, was active on guinea pig ileum; a concentration of 0.5 mg/ml, was active on the stomach of rats[AP099]. Seed oil, at a concentration of 1.8 mcg/ml, was active on the ileum of guinea pigs[AP113].

Spermicidal effect. Ethanol extract of seeds, administered intragastrically to male rats at a dose of 100.0 mg/kg for 60 days, was active. Impaired sperm motility and structural abnormalities of sperm were observed. Sperm ATPase level was decreased[AP069]. Ethanol/water (1:1) extract of dried seeds was active on the sperm of rats. There was a decrease in motility when sperm was mixed with the extract. When administered by gastric intubation, at a dose of 250.0 mg/kg, there was a large decrease in motility of sperm from the cauda epididymis of the rats given the extract for 60 days[AP110]. Ethanol/water (1:1) extract of the aerial parts, at a concentration of 2.0%, was inactive on the sperm of rats[AP118]. Methanol extract of dried seeds was active on the sperm of human adults, IC_{50} 2.29 mg/ml[AP114].

Taste aversion. Butanol extract, at a concentration of 10.0 mg/ml; ethanol (80%) extract, at a concentration of 2.0 mg/ml; water extract, at a concentration of 10.0 mg/ml of dried leaves, in the drinking water of gerbils, were active. The ether and petroleum ether extracts, at concentrations of 5.0 mg/ml, were inactive[AP073].

Teratogenic activity. Water extract of dried seeds, administered intragastrically to pregnant rats at a dose of 125.0 mg/kg, was active[AP062,AP116].

Toxic effect (general). Seeds, administered orally to horses at a dose of 15.0 gm, were active. Tolerance developed when small, incrementally-increased doses were given[AP010]. Seeds, at a concentration of 0.5% of diet in chicken, were active. Chickens were fed a mixture of *Abrus precatorius* seeds and *Cassia senna* fruit. Toxicity included catarrhal enteritis, hepatocellular necrosis, reduced weight, and anemia[AP059]. Ethanol (95%) extract of seeds, administered subcutaneously to male mice at a dose of 500.0 mg/kg, was active. One hundred percent mortality was observed within 48–49 hours[AP028]. Seeds, administered orally to human adults, were active. Severe gastroenteritis, multiple serosal hemorrhages, swelling and inflammation of the Peyer's patches, swelling and inflammation of retroperitoneal lymph nodes, focal necrosis in the liver and kidneys, retinal hemorrhages early in course of intoxication, nausea, vomiting, diarrhea, dehydration, convulsions, and collapse are possible symptoms. Symptoms may begin after delay of up to several days and may persist for as long as 10–11 days. Death in children has been reported from eating 1 or more seeds[AP020]. Two children who chewed seeds became irrational, had tetany, flushing of skin, widely dilated pupils, and appeared to hallucinate. Treatment with neostigmine and barbiturates was successful[AP042]. Seeds, administered subcutaneously to male mice at a dose of 0.90 gm/kg, were active. Forty-four deaths were observed in 5–21 hours[AP028]. Seeds administered orally to cows at a dose of 0.09 gm/kg were active. Death was observed in 1 of 44 animals. Methanol (75%) extract of dried leaves, administered intragastrically to mice at a dose of 2.0 gm/kg, was inactive[AP072]. Leaf and stem, administered orally to cows at a dose of 15.4 gm/kg, was inactive[AP041]. Seeds, in the ration of livestock, were active; nitrate poisoning was observed[AP060]. Beans, ingested by human adult, produced pulmonary edema and hypertension[AP132].

Toxicity assessment. Ethanol/water (1:1) extract of the aerial parts, administered intraperitoneally to mice, produced $LD_{50} >$ 1.0 gm/kg[AP119]. Ethanol (95%) extract of dried leaves, administered intravenously to chicken, produced LD_{50} 12 mg/kg[AP102]. Water extract of seeds, administered subcutaneously to female guinea pigs, produced LD_{50} less than 0.40 mg/kg[AP028]. When administered orally to guinea pigs, mice, rabbits, and rats LD_{50} 0.299 gm/kg, 6.638 gm/kg, 48.7 mg/kg and 2.711 gm/kg, respectively, were observed[AP018]. Toxicity of Abrus to goats has been evaluated. Doses of 2, 1, or 0.5 gm/kg/day by stomach tube produced death between days 2 and 5 for those given 2 or 1 gm/kg. One goat that received 0.5 gm died on day 32, and the other was killed on day 33. The main signs of poisoning include inappetence, bloody diarrhea, dyspnea, dehydration, loss of condition, and recumbence. *Abrus agglutinin*, from the

plant is less lethal than abrina in mice, LD_{50} is 5 mg/kg vs 20 microgram/kg body weight[AP136].

Toxicity. Fatal incidents have been reported following ingestion of well-chewed seeds of *Abrus precatorius*. Because of its hard seed coat, it can pass through the gastrointestinal tract undigested and remain harmless. The unripe seed has a soft and easily broken seed coat and is thus more dangerous. It has been reported that poisoning has been experienced through a finger prick when stringing the seed. Symptoms may develop after a few hours to several days after ingestion. They include severe gastroenteritis with pronounced nausea and vomiting. Mydriasis will occur, as well, as muscular weakness, tachycardia, cold sweat, and trembling. There is no known physiological antidote. The treatment is essentially symptomatic. Since there is a long latent period associated with abrin poisoning, little value can be placed on induction of emesis or gastric lavage; these measures are useful only if ingestion has just occurred. Bismuth trisilicate may be given during poisoning by *Abrus precatorius* to reduce the degree of gastrointestinal damage. If the emesis and/or diarrhea become excessive, replacement fluids and electrolytes are advocated. If hemorrhage occurs, blood transfusion may be necessary.

Uterine relaxation effect. Chromatographic fraction (a gel filtration fraction from a methanol/water [1:1] fraction) of seeds, at a concentration of 1.1 mg/ml, was active on the uterus of rats[AP099].

Uterine stimulant effect. Chromatographic fraction (gel filtration fractions 4–9 of a methanol/water [1:1] extract) of seeds, at a concentration of 0.2 mg/ml, was active on the uteri of pregnant and nonpregnant rats[AP099]. Ethanol (95%) extract of dried seed oil, administered intravenously to guinea pigs at a dose of 1000 mcg/ml, produced weak activity[AP124]. Seed oil, at a concentration of 3.6 mg, was active on the uteri of guinea pigs and rats. The action was blocked by indomethacin but not by atropine[AP113]. Water extract of seeds was active on the uterus of guinea pig[AP013].

REFERENCES

AP001   Suwal, P. N. Medicinal plants of Nepal. Ministry of Forests, Department of Medicinal Plants, Thapathali, Kathmandu, Nepal, 1970.

AP002   Alvaro Viera, R. Subsidio Para O Estudo Da Flora Medicinal Da Guinea Portuguesa. Agencia-Geral Do Ultramar, Lisboa, 1959.

AP003   Malhi, B. S. and V. P. Trivedi. Vegetable antifertility drugs of India. Q J Crude Drug Res 1972; 12: 19–22.

AP004   Willaman, J. J. and H. L. Li. Alkaloid-bearing plants and their contained alkaloids, Lloydia 1970; 33S: 1–286.

AP005   Wei, C. H., F. C. Hartman, P. Pfuderer and W. K. Yang. Purification and characterization of two major toxic proteins from the seeds of Abrus precatorius. J Biol Chem 1974; 249: 3061-3067.

AP006   Bhaduri, B., C. R. Ghose, A. N. Bose, B. K. Moza and U. P. Basu. Antifertility Activity of some Medicinal Plants. Indian J Exp Biol 1968; 6: 252,253.

AP007   Ahmad, K. and A. F. M. Rahman. P-Sterone, A keto steroid from Abrus precatorius. Pak J Biol Agr Sci 1965; 8: 218.

AP008   Ghosal, S. and S. K. Dutta. Alakloids of Abrus precatorius. Phytochemistry 1971; 10: 195.

AP009   Maiti, P., S. Mukherjea and A. Chatterjee. Chemical examination of seeds of Abrus precatorius. J Indian Acad Forensic Sci 1970; 9: 64.

AP010   Simpson, K. S. and P. C. Banerjee. Cases of poisoning in the horse with Ratti seeds (Abrus precatorius) by oral administration. Indian J Vet Sci Anim Husb 1932; 2: 59.

AP011   Tung, Y. C. and M. C. Liau. Studies on the chemical components of the seed of Abrus precatorius. Taiwan I Hsueh Huitsa Chih 1960; 59: 868.

AP012   Subba Reddy, V. V. and M. Sirsi. Effects of Abrus precatorius on experimental tumors. Cancer Res 1969; 29: 1447–1451.

AP013   Hikino, H., K. Aota and T. Takemoto. Structure and absolute configuration of cyperotundone. Chem Pharm Bull 1966; 14: 890.

AP014   Desai, R. V. and E. N. Rupawala. Antifertility activity of the steroidal oil of the seed of Abrus precatorius. Indian J Pharmacy 1967; 29: 235–237.

AP015   Agarwal, S. S., N. Ghatak and R. B. Arora. Antifertility activity of the roots of Abrus precatorius. Pharmacol Res Commun 1970; 2: 159–164.

AP016   Zaidi, Z. H., B. S. Sdiqui and Z. Naim. Chemical investigations of seeds of Abrus precatorius. Pak J Sci Ind Res 1971; 14: 350.

AP017   Anderson, J. D., N. Mandava and C. R. Gunn. Plant growth inhibitor from Abrus precatorius seeds. Plant Physiol 1972; 49: 1024.

AP018   Genest, K., A. Lavalle and E. Nera. Comparative acute toxicity of Abrus precatorius and Ormosia seeds in animals. Arzneim-Forsch 1971; 21: 888.

AP019   Lalithakumari, H., V. V. S. Reddy, G. R. Rao and M. Sirsi. Purification of proteins from Abrus precatorius and their biological properties. Indian J Biochem Biophys 1971; 8: 321.

AP020   Hart, M. Hazards to health. Jequirity-bean poisoning. New England J Med 1963; 268: 885.

AP021   Lin, J. Y., L. L. Lei and T. C. Tung. Purification of abrin from Abrus precatorius (Leguminosae). Taiwan I Hsueh Hui Tsa Chih 1969; 68: 518.

AP022   Das, S. K. Medicinal, Economic and useful plants of India. Bally seed store, West Bengal, 1955.

AP023   Hameed, A. K., M. A. Hasmi and M. I. Khan. Abrus precatorius. I. Isolation and toxic properties of abrulin, A protein fraction from the seeds. Pak J Sci Ind Res 1961; 4: 53.

AP024   Heines, V. A study of pigments in seed coat of Abrus precatiorius. Trans Ky Acad Sci 1971; 32: 1.

AP025   Khaleqe, A., M. Aminuddin and S. A. U. Mulk. Investigations of Abrus precatorius. L. Constituents of dry root. Pak C S I R Bull Monogr 1966; 3: 203.

AP026 Mandava, N., J. D. Anderson, S. R. Dutky and M. J. Thompson. Novel occurrence of 5-Beta cholanic acid in plants: Isolation from jequirity bean seeds (*Abrus precatorius*). **Steroids** 1974; 23: 357–361.

AP027 Baquar, S. R. and M. Tasnif. Medicinal plants of Southern West Pakistan. **Pak P C S I R Bull Monogr** 1967; 3.

AP028 Niyogi, S. K. and F. Rieders. Toxicity studies with fractions from *Abrus precatorius* seed kernels. **Toxicon** 1969; 7: 211.

AP029 Tomita, M., T. Kurokawa, K. Onozaki, T. Osawa, Y. Sakurai and T. Ukita. The surface structure of murine ascites tumors 11. Difference in cytotoxicity of various phytoagglutinins toward Yoshida Sarcoma cells in vitro. **Int J Cancer** 1972; 10: 602.

AP030 Mameesh, M. S., L. M. El-Hakim and A. Hassan. Reproductive failure in female rats fed the fruit or seed of *Jatropha curcas*. **Planta Med** 1963; 11: 98.

AP031 Desai, V. B. and M. Sirsi. Antimicrobial activity of *Abrus precatorius*. **Indian J Pharmacy** 1966; 28: 164.

AP032 Misra, D. S., R. P. Sharma and B. K. Soni. Toxic and haemagglutinating properties of *Abrus precatorius*. **Indian J Exp Biol** 1966; 4: 161.

AP033 Khan, A. H., B. Gul and M. A. Rahman. The interactions of the erythrocytes of various species with agglutinins of *Abrus precatorius*. **J Immunol** 1966; 96: 554.

AP034 Riaz, M. and A. H. Khan. Studies on *Abrus precatorius* lll. Free Amino acids of jequirity seeds. **Pak J Sci Res** 1964; 16: 99.

AP035 Lefar, M. S., D. Firestone, E. C. Coleman and N. Brown. Lipids from the seeds of *Abrus precatorius*. **J Pharm Sci** 1968; 57: 1442.

AP036 Kerharo, J. and A. Bouquet. Plantes Medicinales et Toxiques de La Cote-D'Ivoire - Haute-Volta. Vigot Freres, Paris, 1950; 297pp.

AP037 Khan, A. H., Q. Khalio and S. S. Ali. Studies on the seed oil of *Abrus precatorius*. l. Composition of total fatty acids. **Pak J Sci Ind Res** 1970; 13: 388.

AP038 Khan, A. H., Q. Khalio and S. S. Ali. Studies on the seed oil of *Abrus precatorius*. l. Composition of the lipid classes. **Pak J Sci Ind Res** 1970; 13: 391.

AP039 Desai, V. B., M. Sirsi, M. Shankarappa and A. R. Kasturibai. Studies on the toxicity of *Abrus precatorius* 1. Effect of aqueous extracts of seeds on mitosis and meiosis in grasshopper (*Poecilocera picta*). **Indian J Exp Biol** 1966; 4: 164.

AP040 Derbsey, M. and F. Busson. The lipids of certain West African species. **Oleagineux** 1968; 23: 191.

AP041 Canella, C. F. C., C. H. Tokarnia and J. Dobereiner. Experiments with plants supposedly toxic to cattle in Northeastern Brazil, with negative results. **Pesqui Agropecu Brasil Ser Vet** 1966; 1: 345–352.

AP042 Gunsolus, J. M. Toxicity of Jequirity beans. **Journal Amer Med Assoc** 1955; 157: 779.

AP044 Inman, N. Notes on some poisonous plants of Guam. **Micronesica** 1967; 3: 55.

AP045 Watt, J. M. and M. G. Breyer-Brandwijk. The medicinal and poisonous plants of Southern and Eastern Africa. 2nd Ed, E. S. Livingstone, Ltd., London, 1962.

AP046 Buchanan, E. Grove man dies after eating rosary beans. **Miami Herald** April 18, 1976. Miami, Fla USA.

AP047 Burkhill, I. H. Dictionary of the economic products of the Malay peninsula. Ministry of Agriculture and Cooperatives, Kuala Lumpur, Malaysia. Vol. 1, 1966.

AP043 Gupta, N. C., B. Singh and D. S. Bhakuni. Steroids and triterpenes from *Alangium lamarckii*, *Allamanda cathartica*, *Abrus precatorius* and *Holoptelea integrifolia*. **Phytochemistry** 1969; 8: 791–792.

AP048 Hartzell, A. and F. Wilcoxon. A survey of plant products for insecticidal properties. **Contr Boyce Thompson Inst** 1941; 12: 127–141.

AP049 Hegde, R., T. K. Maiti and S. K. Podder. Purification and characterization of three toxins and two agglutinins from *Abrus precatorius* seed by using lactamyl-sepharose affinity chromatography. **Anal Biochem** 1991; 194(1): 101–109.

AP050   Bhaumik, H. L. Hydrocarbons, fatty acids, triterpenoid and sterols in the seeds of Abrus precatorius. **Sci Cult** 1987; 53(1): 23–24.

AP051   Chukuo, S., S. C. Chen, L. H. Chen, J. B. Wu, J. P. Wang and C. M. Teng. Potent antiplatelet, antiinflammatory and antiallergic isoflavanquinones from the roots of Abrus precatorius. **Planta Med** 1995; 61 4: 307–312.

AP052   Lupi, A., F. Delle Monache, G. B. Marini-Bettolo, D. L. B. Costa and I. L. D'Albuquerque. Abruquinones: New natural isoflavanquinones. **Gazz Chim Ital** 1979; 109: 9–12.

AP053   Samad, F., A. Mukhtar, Z. A. Jan and Z. U. Khan. Effect of alcohol extract of Ratti seeds (Abrus precatorius) on the reproduction of female rats. **J Math Sci** 1974; 12: 157.

AP054   Wei, C. H., C. Koh, P. Pfuderer and J. R. Einstein. Purification, properties and crystallographic data for a principal nontoxic lectin from seeds of Abrus precatorius. **J Biol Chem** 1975; 250: 4790.

AP055   Roy, J., S. Som, and A. Sen. Isolation, purification, and some properties of a lectin and abrin from Abrus precatorius. **Arch Biochem Biophys** 1976; 174: 359.

AP056   Kokwaro, J. O. Medicinal plants of East Africa. East Afr Literature Bureau, Niarobi, 1976.

AP057   Kusumoto, I. T., N. Kakiuchi, M. Hattori, T. Namba, S. Sutardjo and K. Shimotohno. Screening of some Indonesian Medicinal plants for inhibitory effects on HIV-1 Protease. **Shoyahugaku Zasshi** 1992; 46(2): 190–193.

AP058   Kusumoto, I. T., I. Shimada, N. Kakiuchi, M. Hattori, T. Namba and S. Supriyatna. Inhibitory effect of Indonesian plant extracts on reverse transcriptase of an RNA tumour virus (1). **Phytother Res** 1992; 6(5): 241–244.

AP059   Omer, S. A., F. H. Ibrahim, S. A. Khalid and S. E. I. Adam. Toxicological interactions of Abrus precatorius and Cassia senna in the diet of Lohmann broiler chicks. **Vet Hum Toxicol** 1992; 34(4): 310–313.

AP060   Apul, B. S. and J. K. Mali. Poisoning of livestock by some toxic plants. **Progressive Farming** 1982; 6,7.

AP061   Begum, S. Chemical investigation of white seeded variety of Abrus precatorius Linn. **Pak J Sci Ind Res** 193; 35(7/8): 270–271.

AP062   Nath, D., N. Sethi, R. K. Singh and A. K. Jain. Commonly used Indian abortifacient plants with special reference to their teratologic effects in rats. **J Ethnopharmacol** 1992; 36(2): 147–154.

AP063   Elisabetsky, E., W. Figueiro and G. Oliveria. Traditional Amazonian nerve tonics as antidepressant agents. Chaunochiton kappleri. A case study. **J Herbs Spices Med Plants** 1992; 1 (1/2): 125–162.

AP064   Ibrahim, A. M. Anthelmintic activity of some Sudanese Medicinal Plants. **Phytother Res** 1992; 6(3): 155–157.

AP065   Otake, T., H. Mori, M. Morimoto, N. Ueba, S. Sutardio, I. Kusumoto, M. Hattori and T. Namba. Screening of Indonesian plant extracts for anti-human immunodeficiency virus-Type 1 (HIV-1) activity. **Phytother Res** 1995; 9(1): 6–10.

AP066   Munsho, S. R., T. A. Shetye and R. K. Nair. Antifertility activity of three indigenous plant preparations. **Planta Med** 1977; 31: 73–75.

AP067   Amico, A. Medicinal plants of Southern Zambesia. **Fitoterapia** 1977; 48: 101–139.

AP068   Amnuoypol, S., C. Chaichantypyuth and R. Bavovada. Chemical constituents in the leaves of Abrus precatorius L. **Thai J Pharm Sci** 1986; 11(4): 197–203.

AP069   Rao, M. V. Antifertility effects of alcoholic seeds extract of Abrus precatorius Linn. in male albino rats. **Acta Eur Fertil** 1987; 18(3): 217–220.

AP070   Markham, K. R., J. W. Wallace, Y. Niranjan Babu, V. Krishnamurty and M. Gopala Rao. 8-C-Glucosyl-scutellarein 6,7-dimethyl ether and its 2"-0-apioside from Abrus precatorius. **Phytochemistry** 1989; 28(1): 299–301.

AP071   Satyanarayana, K. and K. Sukumar. Phytosterilants to control the cotton bug, *Dysdercus cingulatus* F. **Curr Sci** 1988; 57(16): 918–919.

AP072   Choi, Y. H., R. A. Hussain, J. M. Pezzuto, A. D. Kinghorn and J. F. Morton. Abrososides A-D, four novel sweet-tasting triterpene glycosides from the leaves of *Abrus precatorius*. **J Nat Prod** 1989; 52(5): 1118–1127.

AP073   Jakinovich Jr, W., C. Moon, Y. H. Choi and A. D. Kinghorn. Evaluation of plant extracts for sweetness using the Mongolian gerbil. **J Nat Prod** 1990; 53(1): 190–195.

AP074   Itokawa, H., F. Hirayama, S. Tsuruoka, K. Mizuno, K. Takeya and A. Nitta. Screening test for antitumor activity of crude drugs (III). Studies on antitumor activity of Indonesian Medicinal Plants. **Shoyakugaku Zasshi** 1990; 44(1): 58–62.

AP075   Johns, T., J. O. Kokwaro and E. K. Kimanani. Herbal remedies of the Luo of Siaya District, Kenya. Establishing quantitative criteria for consensus. **Econ Bot** 1990; 44(3): 369–381.

AP076   Kinjo, J., K. Matsumoto, M. Inoue, T. Takeshita and T. Nohara. A new sapogenol and other constituents in abri semen, the seeds of *Abrus precatorius* L. 1. **Chem Pharm Bull** 1991; 39(1): 116–119.

AP077   Chatterjee, B. P., N. Sarkar and A. S. Rao. Serological and chemical investigations of the anomeric configuration of the sugar units in the D-galacto-D-mannan of fenugreek (*Trigonella foenum-gracum*) seed. **Carbohydr Res** 1982; 104(2): 348–353.

AP078   Choi, Y. H., A. D. Kinghorn, X. B. Shi, H. Zhang and B. K. Teo. Abrusoside A: A new type of highly sweet triterpene glycoside. **Chem Commun** 1989; 1989: 887–888.

AP079   Carbajal, D., A. Casaco, L. Arruzazabala, R. Gonzalez and V. Fuentes. Pharmacological screening of plant decoctions commonly used in Cuban folk medicine. **J Ethnopharmacol** 1991; 33(1/2): 21–24.

AP080   Nwodo, O. F. C. and E. O. Alumanah. Studies on *Abrus precatorius* seeds. II. Antidiarrhoeal activity. **J Ethnopharmacol** 1991; 31(3): 395–398.

AP081   Zia-Ul-Haque, A., M. H. Qazi and M. E. Hamdard. Studies on the antifertility properties of active components isolated from the seeds of *Abrus precatorius* Linn. 1. **Pakistan J Zool** 1983; 15(2): 129–139.

AP082   Salah Ahmed, M., G. Honda and W. Miki. Herb drugs and herbalists in the Middle East. Institute for the study of languages and cultures of Asia and Africa. Studia Culturae Islamicae No. 8, 1979; 1–208.

AP083   Ayensu, E. S. Medicinal plants of the West Indies. **Unpublished Manuscript** 1978; 110pp.

AP084   Issar, R. K. and A. H. Israili. Pharmacognostic studies of the Unani drug "Ghongchi-Safaid" (*Abrus precatorius* Linn. seeds). **J Res Indian Med Yoga Homeopathy** 1978; 13: 34–44.

AP085   Herrmann, M. S. and W. D. Behnke. Physical studies on three lectins from the seeds of *Abrus precatorius*. **Biochim Biophys Acta** 1980; 621: 43-52.

AP086   Das, P. C. Oral contraceptive (Long-acting). **Patent-Brit-1445599** 1976; 11pp.

AP087   Bhardwaj, D. K., M. S. Bisht and C. K. Mehta. Flavonoids from *Abrus precatorius*. **Phytochemistry** 1980; 19: 2040–2041.

AP088   Lin, L. J., T. C. Lee and T. C. Tung. Isolation of antitumor proteins Abrin A and Abrin B from *Abrus precatorius*. **Toxicon Suppl** 1979; 17: 103.

AP089   Anon. A Barefoot Doctors's Manual, Revised Edition, Cloudburst Press of America, 2116 Western Ave., Seattle, Washington, USA. (ISBN-0-88930-012-7) **Book** 1977.

AP090   Prakesh, A. O., R. B. Gupta and R. Mathur. Effect of oral doses of *Abrus precatorius* Linn. seeds on the oestrus cycle, body weight, uterine weight and cellular structures of uterus in albino rats. **Probe** 1980; 19: 286–292.

AP091   Karawya, M. S., S. El-Gengaihi, G. Wassel and N. Ibrahim. Phytochemical studies of *Abrus precatorius* alkaloids. **Herba hung** 1980; 19(3): 21–25.

AP092   Akinloye, B. A. and L. A. Adalumo. *Abrus precatorius* leaves - a source of glycyrrhizin. **Niger J Pharm** 1981; 12: 405.

AP093 Hussein Ayoub, S. M. and A. Baerheim-Suendsen. Medicinal and aromatic plants in the Sudan. Usage and exploration. **Fitoterapia** 1981; 52: 243–246.

AP094 Lin, J., T. Lee, S. Hu and T. Tung. Isolation of four isotoxic proteins and one agglutinin from jequirity bean (*Abrus precatorius*). **Toxicon** 1981; 19: 41–51.

AP095 Karawya, M. S., S. E. Gengaihi, G. Wassel and N. A. Ibrahim. Anthocyanins from the seeds of *Abrus precatorius*. **Fitoterapia** 1981; 52: 175–177.

AP096 Chang, H. M., T. C. Chiang and C. W. Mak. Isolation and structure elucidation of abruslactone A: A new oleanene-type triterpene from the roots and vines of *Abrus precatorius* L. **Chem Commun** 1982; 1982: 1197–1198.

AP097 Karawya, M. S., S. E. Gengaihi, G. Wassel and N. A. Ibrahim. Carbohydrates of *Abrus precatorius*. **Fitoterapia** 1981; 52: 179–181.

AP098 Hussein Ayoub, S. M. and D. G. I. Kingston. Screening of plants in Sudan folk medicine for anticancer activity. **Fitoterapia** 1982; 53: 119–123.

AP099 Nwodo, O. F. C. and J. H. Botting. Uterotonic activity of extracts of the seeds of *Abrus precatorius*. **Planta Med** 1983; 47(4): 230–233.

AP100 Adesina, S. K. Studies on some plants used as anticonvulsants in Amerindian and African traditional medicine. **Fitoterapia** 1982; 53: 147–162.

AP101 Chang, H. M., T. C. Chiang and C. W. Mak. New oleanene-type triterpenes from *Abrus precatorius* and x-ray crystal structire of abrusgenic acid-methanol 1:1 solvate. **Planta Med** 1983; 49(3): 165–169.

AP102 Wambebe, C. and S. L. Amosun. Some neuromuscular effects of the crude extracts of the leaves of *Abrus precatorius*. **J Ethnopharmacol** 1984; 11(1): 49–58.

AP103 Karawaya, M. S., S. El-Gangaihi, G. Wassel and N. Ibrahim. Phytochemical studies of *Abrus precatorius* alkaloids. **Herba Hung** 1980; 19(3): 21–25.

AP104 Arseculeratne, S. N., A. A. L. Gunatilaka and R. G. Panabokke. Studies on medicinal plants of Sri Lanka. Part 14. Toxicity of some traditional medicineal herbs. **J Ethnopharmacol** 1985; 13(3): 323–335.

AP105 Jain, S. P. and D. M. Verma. Medicinal plants in the Folk-lore of Northern Circle Dehradun Up India. **Nat Acad Sci Lett (India)** 1981; 4(7): 269–271.

AP106 Hedberg, I., O. Hedberg, P. J. Madati, K. E. Mshigeni, E. N. Mshiu and G. Samuelsson. Inventory of plants used in traditional medicine in Tanzania. Part III. Plants of the families Papilionaceae-Vitaceae. **J Ethnopharmacol** 1983; 9(2/3): 237–260.

AP107 Jadon, A. and R. Mathur. Effects of *Abrus precatorius* Linn. seed extract on biochemical constituents of male mice. **J Jiwaji Univ** 1984; 9(1): 100–103.

AP108 Das, P. C., A. K. Sarkar and S. Thakur. Studies on animals of a Herbo-Mineral compound for long acting contraction. **Fitoterapia** 1987; 58(4): 257–261.

AP109 Weniger, B., M. Rouzier, R. Daguilh, D. Henrys, J. H. Henrys and R. Anthon. Popular medicine of the Plateau of Haiti. 2. Ethnopharmacological inventory. **J Ethnopharmacol** 1986; 17(1): 13–30.

AP110 Sinha, R. Post-testicular antifertility effects of *Abrus precatorius* seed extract in albino rats. **J Ethnopharmacol** 1990; 28(2): 173–181.

AP111 Vedavathy, S., K. N. Rao, M. Rajaiah and N. Nagaraju. Folklore information from Rayalaseema region, Andhra Pradesh for family planning and birth control. **Int J Pharmacog** 1991; 29(2): 113–116.

AP112 Zia-Ul-Haque, A., M. H. Qazi and M. E. Hamdard. Studies on the antifertility properties of active components isolated from the seeds of *Abrus precatorius* Linn. ll. **Pak J Zool** 1983; 15(2): 141–146.

AP113 Nwodo, O. F. C. Studies on *Abrus precatorius* seeds. 1. Uterotonic activity of seed oil. **J Ethnopharmacol** 1991; 31(3): 391–394.

AP114 Ratnasooriya, W. D., A. S. Amarasekera, N. S. D. Perera and G. A. S. Premakumara. Sperm antimotility properties of a seed extract of *Abrus precatorius*. **J Ethnopharmacol** 1991; 33(1/2): 85–90.

AP115   Panthong, A., D. Kanjanapothi and W. C. Taylor. ethnobotanical review of medicinal plants from Thai traditional books, Part 1. Plants with antiinflammatory, anti-asthmatic and antihypertensive properties. **J Ethnopharmacol** 1986; 18(3): 213–228.

AP116   Sethi, N., D. Nath and R. K. Singh. Teratological aspects of *Abrus precatorius* seeds in rats. **Fitoterapia** 1990; 61(1): 61–63.

AP117   Chopra, R. N., R. L. Badhwar and S. Ghosh. Poisonous plants of India. Manager of Publications, Government of India Press, Calcutta. Volume 1, 1949.

AP118   Dhawan, B. N., G. K. Patnaik, R. P. Rastogi, K. K. Singh and J. S. Tandon. Screening of Indian plants for biological activity. VI. **Indian J Exp Biol** 1977; 15: 208–219.

AP119   Oakes, A. J. and M. P. Morris. The West Indian Weedwoman of the United States Virgin Islands. **Bull Hist Med** 1958; 32: 164.

AP120   Prakash, A. O. and R. Mathur. Screening of Indian plants for antifertility activity. **Indian J Exp Biol** 1976; 14: 623–626.

AP121   Chopra, R. N. Indigenous drugs of India. Their medical and economic aspects. The art press, Calcutta, India, 1933; 550.

AP122   Sirsi, M. In Vitro study of the inhibitory action of some chemotherapeutic agents on a freshly isolated strain of *Cryptococcus neoformans*. **Hindustan Antibiot Bull** 1963; 6(2): 39-40.

AP123   Krishnamoorthy, V. and T. R. Seshadri. Survey of anthocyanins from Indian sources: Part III. **J Sci Ind Res-B** 1962; 21: 591–593.

AP124   Jamwal, K. S. and K. K. Anand. Preliminary screening of some reputed abortifacient indigenous plants. **Indian J Pharm** 1962; 24: 218–220.

AP125   Krupe, M., W. Wirth, D. Nies and A. Ensgraber. Studies on the "Mitogenic" effect of hemoglutinating extracts of various plants on the human small lymphocytes in peripheral blood cultured in vitro. **Z Immunitatsforsch Allerg Klin Immunol** 1968; 135(1): 19–42.

AP125   Krupe, M., W. Wirth, D. Nies and A. Ensgraber. Studies on the "Mitogenic" effect of hemoglutinating extracts of various plants on the human small lymphocytes in peripheral blood cultured in vitro. **Z Immunitatsforsch Allerg Klin Immunol** 1968; 135(1): 19–42.

AP126   ANON. Unpublished data, National Cancer Institute. National Cancer Inst. Central Files 1976.

AP127   Popli, S. P. Screening of Indian indigenous plants for antifertility activity. Progress report on project 74219 (WHO), Dec. 20, 1977.

AP128   Ali, E. and A. Malek. Chemical investigations on *Abrus precatorius* Linn. (Beng. Kunch). **Sci Res III** 1966; 3: 141–145.

AP129   Haq, Q. N., A. Awal and M. Kiamuddin. Polysaccharides from the roots of *Abrus precatorius*. **Bangladesh J Sci Ind Res** 1973; 8: 47.

AP130   Glasby, J. H. Dictionary of Plants Containing Secondary Metabolites. Taylor and Francis, New York, 1991, 488 pp.

AP131   List, P. H. and L. Horhammer. Hager's Handbuch der Pharmazeutischen Praxis, Vols. 2–6, Springer-Verlag, Berlin. 1969–1979.

AP132   Fernando, C. Poisoning due to *Abrus precatorius* (jequirity bean). **Anaesthesia** 2001; 56(12): 1178–1180.

AP133   Anam, E. M. Anti-inflammatory activity of compounds isolated from the aerial parts of *Abrus precatorius*. **Phytomedicine** 2001; 8(1): 24–27

AP134   Molgaard, P., S. B. Nielsen, D. E. Rasmussen, R. B. Drummond, N. Makaza and J. Andreassen. Anthelmintic acreening of Zimbabwean plants traditionally used against schistosomiasis. **J Ethnopharmacol** 2001; 74(3): 257–264.

AP135   Panneerselvam K., S. C. lin, C. L. Liu, Y. C. Liaw, J. Y. Lin and T. H. Lu. Crystallization of agglutinin from the seeds of *Abrus precatorius*. Acta **Crystallogr D Biol Crystallogr** 2000; 56(Pt. 7): 898–899.

AP136   Liu, C. L., C. C. Tsai, S. C. lin, L. I. Wang, C. I. Hsu, M. J. Hwang and J. Y. Lin. Primary structure and function analysis of the *Abrus precatorius* agglutinin A chain by site-directed mutagenesis. Pro(199) Of amphiphilic alpha-helix H impairs protein synthesis inhibitory activity. **J Biol Chem** 2000; 275(3): 1897–1901.

AP137 Singh, S. and D. K. Singh. Effect of molluscicidal components of *Abrus precatorius*, *Argemone mexicana* and *Nerium indicum* on certain biochemical parameters of *Lymnaea acuminata*. **Phytother Res** 1999; 13(3): 210–213.

AP138 Zambenedetti, P., R. Giordano and P. Zatta. Histochemical localization of glycoconjugates on microglial cells in Alzheimer's disease brain samples by using *Abrus precatorius*, *Maackia amurensis*, *Momordica charantia*, and *Sambucus nigra* lectins. **Exp Neurol** 1998 153(1): 167–171.

AP139 Ohba, H., T. Toyokawa, S. Yasuada, T. Hoshino, K. Itoh and N. Yamasaki. Spectroscopic analysis of the cytoagglutinating activity of abrin-b isolated from *Abrus precatorius* seeds against leukemic cells. **Biosci Biotechnol Biochem** 1997; 61(4): 737–739.

3 | Allium sativum L

Gaertn.

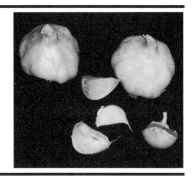

Common Names

Aglio	Italy	Kra thiam	Thailand
Aie	France	L'ail	West Indies
Ail	France	Lahsun	Fiji
Ail	Rodrigues Islands	Lahsun	India
Ail	Tunisia	Lai	Nicaragua
Ajo	Guatemala	Lai	West Indies
Ajo	Nicaragua	Lasan	Fiji
Ajo	Peru	Lasan	India
Akashneem	India	Lashun	India
Alubosa elewe	Nigeria	Lasun	Fiji
Banlasun	Nepal	Lasun	Nepal
Cebilhoums	France	Lasuna	India
Dasuan	China	Lay	Haiti
Dra thiam	Thailand	Lesun	Fiji
Garlic	Brazil	Majo	Mexico
Garlic	China	Onion	India
Garlic	Cuba	Poor man's treacle	Iran
Garlic	Europe	Rashun	India
Garlic	Guyana	Rason	India
Garlic	India	Sarimsak	Turkey
Garlic	Indonesia	Sarmisak	Turkey
Garlic	Iran	Seer	Iran
Garlic	Japan	Ta-suan	China
Garlic	Kuwait	Tellagaddalu	India
Garlic	Libya	Thom	Oman
Garlic	Mexico	Thoum	Jordan
Garlic	Nicaragua	Thum	Arabic countries
Garlic	Poland	Thum	Saudi Arabia
Garlic	Taiwan	Tum	Tunisia
Garlic	USA	Tuma	Morocco
Garlic	West Indies	Vellulli	India
Garlic clove	Nicaragua		

From: *Medicinal Plants of the World, vol. 1: Chemical Constituents, Traditional and Modern Medicinal Uses, 2nd ed.*
By: Ivan A. Ross © Humana Press Inc., Totowa, NJ

BOTANICAL DESCRIPTION

Garlic is an erect herb of the ALLIACEAE family, 30 to 60 cm tall. Bulb is on a disk-like stem, consisting of several segments (cloves), enclosed in a common membrane that is at the base of foliage leaves. Each clove consists of a protective cylindrical sheath and a small central bud. Leaf blade is linear, flat, and solid, 1 to 2.5 cm wide, and 30 to 60 cm long, having an acute apex. Leaf sheaths form a pseudostem. Inflorescence is umbellate, having smooth scape, round, solid coiled at first; sub-tended by membranous, long-beaked spathe, splitting on one side and remaining attachedto umbel. Small bulbils are produced in inflorescence; flowers are variable in number, and sometimes absent; they seldom open and may wither in bud. Flowers are on slender pedicels, consisting of perianth of 6 segments, about 4 to 6 mm long, pinkish; stamens: 6, anthers exerted; ovary superior, trilocular. Fruit is a small loculicidal capsule. Seeds are seldom, if ever, produced.

ORIGIN AND DISTRIBUTION

Garlic is indigenous to Asia. It is now found worldwide as a cultivated crop, which is usually grown at high altitudes.

TRADITIONAL MEDICINAL USES

Arabic countries. In Unani medicine, butanol extract of the dried bulb is administered by fumigation inhalation to pregnant women as an abortifacient. The extract is also used as an emmenagogue by fumigation inhalation and in the form of a pessary[AS318].

Argentina. Decoction of the dried bulb is taken orally against diarrhea, and to treat respiratory and urinary tract infections[AS116].

Brazil. Hot water extract of fresh bulb is taken orally to treat hypertension or induce diuresis[AS366].

China. Hot water extract of the bulb is taken orally to treat high blood pressure, and for amenorrhea[AS297].

East Asia. Hot water extract of bulb is taken orally as an aphrodisiac, anthelmintic and diuretic, and for asthma[AS440].

England. Hot water extract of dried bulb is taken orally for diabetes[AS197].

Ethiopia. The bulb is chewed with leaves of Ruta and seeds of *Nigella sativa* as a remedy for stomachache[AS287].

Europe. Butanol extract of the bulb is taken orally to protect against atherosclerosis risk factors[AS265].

Fiji. Fresh bulb, together with dried *Ferula assafoetida* and sugar, is taken orally to cleanse the new mother. Bulb, ground with ghee and sugar, is taken orally for dysentery. Fresh bulb juice, warmed with coconut oil, is dropped into the ear for earache[AS366].

Greece. Hot water extract of bulb is taken orally to protect against amoebae[AS026].

Guatemala. Hot water extract of dried bulb is used externally for ringworm, fungal diseases of the skin, and skin diseases and irritations, for leukorrhea and vaginitis, and infections of the skin and mucosa[AS411,AS230,AS405].

Haiti. Decoction of fresh bulb is taken orally for cutaneous infections; hot water extract is taken orally for malnutrition; the juice is taken orally for bronchitis, and butanol extract is taken orally for pneumonia[AS388].

India. Fresh bulb juice is taken orally as an abortifacient. Ten grams of *Momordica tuberosa* root, 5 grams of *Calotropis gigantea* stem bark, a few Brassica (species) seeds and a few cloves of *Allium sativum* are pound together and the juice extracted. Two to 3 tablespoons of extract produces abortion within 12 hours. To relieve dysmenorrhea, paving the way for effective conception in future menstrual cycles, a paste made of *Mucuna pruriens*, *Pygaeopremna herbacea*, *Tephrosia purpurea* and *Gardenia turgida* roots, plus a few cloves of *Allium sativum*, is given orally. Twenty grams of the paste is given on the third day of menstruation[AS353]. Hot water extract of bulb is taken orally as an emmenagogue[AS018] and anthelmintic[AS449]. Ten grams of *Cocconia indica* leaves are pound with 14 peppers and 14 pieces of bulb to make enough for 9 pills and given 1 per day for 9 days to treat rabies[AS081]. For scabies, Piper betel leaves pound with small quantities of sulfur, camphor, pepper, and garlic are roasted in sesame oil and applied to the skin. For leukorrhagia, garlic bulb is mixed with leaves of *Ziziphus mauritania*, pepper and salt and taken with buttermilk[AS081]. Hot water extract of dried bulb, mixed with an equal amount of honey, is taken once daily for 3 days to treat whooping cough[AS314]. Hot water extract of dried seeds is taken orally as an emmenagogue[AS395]. Infusion of the entire plant, along with sugar, is taken orally to treat fever[AS081].

Indonesia. Hot water extract of bulb, in a mixture with wild herbs, the slough of a snake and vinegar, is taken orally as an abortifacient[AS052].

Italy. Fresh bulb is taken orally for gastronomic purposes[AS435]. Hot water extract of dried bulb is used externally for inflammations, as a cicatrizing agent, and to treat insect bites. The extract is taken orally as an anthelmintic and hypotensive agent[AS435].

Jamaica. Hot water extract of bulb is taken orally as an emmenagogue[AS015].

Japan. Bulb is taken orally to treat hypertension[AS297]. Fresh bulb is taken orally as a food[AS176]. Water extract of fresh bulb is used externally to promote hair growth[AS316].

Kuwait. Bulb is taken orally to regulate menstruation[AS147].

Malaysia. Hot water extract of bulb is taken orally by females after childbirth[AS034].

Mexico. Decoction of dried bulb, *Allium cepa* and *Pimpinella anisum* is administered orally to newborn infants[AS346]. Hot water extract of bulb is taken orally to induce abortion[AS016]. Hot infusion, sweetened with honey, is taken orally to aid expulsion of placenta[AS019]. Bulb, crushed with leaves of *Clematis dioica*, is taken orally to treat catarrh[AS337]. A clove of garlic is inserted in the anus to reduce fever[AS437]. Hot water extract of fresh bulb is taken orally to speed labor, as an abortifacient and for rheumatism; the decoction is taken orally to facilitate childbirth[AS358].

Nepal. Hot water extract of dried bulbs is taken orally as a sedative and for fever[AS335].

Nigeria. Dried entire plant, soaked in juice of *Citrus aurantifolia* and a pinch of copper sulfate, is administered orally to children to treat convulsions. The mixture is left for 4 days in a bottle. Only a small quantity is to be given; excess results in vomiting or runny stool. To treat yellow fever, 1 to 2 handfuls of leaflets, ground with 1 small bulb of *Allium sativum*, is taken orally with "Pap"[AS067]. Fresh bulb is taken orally as a tonic, antirheumatic, antipyretic, hypotensive and analgesic[AS315].

Pakistan. Hot water extract of dried bulb is taken orally as a carminative, expectorant and febrifuge[AS360].

Peru. Hot water extract of fresh bulb is taken orally as a vermifuge, febrifuge, diuretic, antiscorbutic, anti-inflammatory for respiratory pathways, catarrh and arteriosclerosis, and externally as an antiseptic and disinfectant[AS405].

Saudi Arabia. Hot water extract of dried bulb is taken orally as a diuretic and for diabetes, rheumatism, pyrexia, intestinal worms, colic, flatulence and menstrual suppression, and mixed with sour milk, for stomach pain[AS362]. Hot water extract of fresh bulb is taken orally for diabetes, rheumatism, pyrexia, intestinal worms, colic, flatulence, menstrual suppression, hepatitis, piles, dysentery, tuberculosis, rheumatism, colic, facial paralysis, hypertension, diabetes and bronchitis, and as an aphrodisiac[AS205].

South Africa. Bulb is taken orally as an aphrodisiac[AS031].

South Korea. Hot water extract of dried rhizome is taken orally as an abortifacient and emmenagogue[AS361].

Sweden. Fresh bulb is applied to excoriations and erosions resulting from scratching dry skin[AS166].

Thailand. Decoction of fresh bulb is taken orally as an anti-inflammatory, and the crushed bulb is used as a poultice on inflamed joints[AS464]. Hot water extract of dried bulb is used externally for treating wounds and toothache, and for leprosy, and taken orally for epilepsy and chest pain[AS254].

Tunisia. Hot water extract of dried bulb is taken orally as a hypotensive and vermifuge[AS343].

USA. Butanol extract of bulb is taken orally as an aphrodisiac. The preparation is said to contain *Allium sativum* (25%), *Capsicum annuum* (50%), and *Purus saccharum* (25%). The propriety product is called "Pseudo love stimulant" and is used by both sexes[AS260]. Dried bulb is taken orally as an antihypertensive, vermifuge, and is also used against infection. Externally, the extract is used as a treatment of sinusitis and coryza[AS229]. Fresh bulb is taken orally to treat infectious diseases, lung diseases and tuberculosis, and as a blood purifier and stimulant. The bulb, applied to the feet, is used against diarrhea and fever[AS483].

West Indies. Clove tea is used for intestinal worms. Hot water extract of the bulb is taken orally for hypertension, and butanol extract is rubbed on the abdomen to facilitate parturition. Essential oil is taken orally as an antispasmodic, antimicrobial, diuretic, antiasthmatic and emmenagogue[AS262].

Yugoslavia. Hot water extract of fresh bulb is taken orally for diabetes[AS278].

CHEMICAL CONSTITUENTS

(ppm unless otherwise indicated)

1,2-(Prop-2-enyl)-disulfane: Bu[AS281]
1,2-Dimercaptocyclopentane: Bu[AS002]
1,2-Epithiopropane: Bu 0.1–1.66[AS002]
1,3-Dithiane: Bu 0.08–3[AS002]
1-Hexanol: Bu[AS001]
1-Methyl-2-(prop-2-enyl)-disulfane: Bu[AS281]
1-Methyl-3-(prop-2-enyl)-trisulfane: Bu[AS281]
2,5-Dimethyl-tetrahydrothiophene: Bu 0.6[AS002]
24-Methylene-cycloartenol: Pl[AS003]
2-Methylbenzaldehyde: Bu[AS002]
2-Propen-1-ol: Bu 0.1–121[AS002]
2-Propenyl L-cysteine sulfoxide: Bu[AS132]
2-Propenyl-1-propenyl disulfide: EO[AS175]
2-Vinyl-1,3-dithiene: Bu 2–29[AS333]
3,5-Diethyl-1,2,4-trithiolane: Bu 0.15–43[AS002]
3-Methyl-2-cyclopentene-1-thione: Bu 0.16–1.6[AS002]
3-Vinyl-4(H)-1-2 dithiin: Bu[AS152,AS157]
5-Butyl cysteine sulfoxide: Bu[AS487]
Acyl anthocyanin: Lf[AS047]
Adenosine: Bu[AS207]
Ajoene,cis: Bu[AS157]
Ajoene: Bu[AS156]
Alanine: Bu 0.132–0.3168%[AS004]
Allicin: Bu 0.15–2.78%[AS451,AS154]
Alliin: Bu 0.5–1.3%[AS049,AS424]
Alliinase: Bu 411[AS243]
Allin: Bu[AS427]
Allisatin: Pl[AS489]
Allistatin-1: Bu[AS489]
Allistatin-2: Bu[AS489]
Allium fructan K-1: Bu[AS092]
Allium fructan K-2: Bu[AS092]
Allium fructan K-3: Bu[AS092]
Allium fructan K-4: Bu[AS092]
Allium fructan K-5: Bu[AS092]
Allium fructan K-6: Bu[AS092]
Allium fructan K-7: Bu[AS092]
Allium fructan K-8: Bu[AS092]
Allium sativum D-galactan: Bu[AS148]
Allixin: Bu[AS007]
Allyl disulfide: Bu[AS375]
Allyl methyl disulfide: Bu[AS071], EO[AS158]
Allyl methyl sulfide: Bu[AS071], EO[AS158]
Allyl methyl trisulfide: Bu[AS152], EO[AS298]
Allyl trisulfide: Bu[AS071]
Alpha-prostaglandin-F-1: Bu[AS172]
Alpha-prostaglandin-F-2: Bu[AS172]
Alpha-tocopherol: Bu[AS285]
Aluminum: Bu 52[AS005]
Aniline: Bu 10[AS002]
Arachidonic acid: Bu[AS365]
Arginine: Bu 0.634–1.5216%[AS002]

Ascorbic acid: Bu[AS153], Fl 440–3,793, Lf 390–2,868 , Sh 420–1,883[AS006]

Aspartic acid: Bu 0.489–1.1736%[AS004], Lf[AS259]

Beta carotene: Bu 0–0.17[AS005], Fl 0.6–5, Lf 9–68, Sh 2–9[AS006]

Beta sitosterol: Pl[AS003]

Beta tocopherol: Bu[AS003]

Biotin: Bu 22 mcg/g[AS453,AS476]

Caffeic acid: Bu[AS308]

Chlorophyll: Bu[AS153]

Chromium: Bu 2.5–15[AS005]

Cycloalliin: Bu[AS204]

Cysteine: Lf[AS259]

Degalactotigonin: Rt 400[AS198]

Deoxy alliin: Bu[AS066]

Diallyl heptasulfide: Bu[AS070]

Diallyl hexasulfide: Bu[AS070]

Diallyl pentasulfide: Bu[AS095]

Diallyl sulfide: Bu 2–99[AS002]

Diallyl tetrasulfide: Bu[AS157]

Diallyl trisulfide: Bu 10–1,061[AS002]

Digalactosyl diglyceride: Bu[AS365]

Dimethyl ajoene: Bu[AS040,AS432]

Dimethyl difuran: Bu 5–30[AS002]

Dimethyl disulfide: Bu 0.6–2.5[AS002]

Dimethyl sulfide: EO[AS479]

Dimethyl trisulfide: Bu 0.8–19[AS002]

Eicosapentaenoic acid: Bu[AS365]

Eruboside B: Bu 13[AS425]

Essential oils: Bu 600–3,600[AS007]

Foliacin: Bu 1[AS004]

Fructose: Bu[AS325,AS285]

Gamma glutamyl phenyl alanine: Bu[AS471, AS474]

Gamma-L-glutamyl-L-phenylalanine: Bu 63.2[AS041]

Gamma-L-glutamyl-S-(2-carboxy-1-propyl)-cysteineglycine: Pl[AS008]

Gamma-L-glutamyl-S-allyl-cysteine: Bu[AS469,AS472]

Gamma-L-glutamyl-S-allyl-mercapto-cysteine: Bu[AS470]

Gamma-L-glutamyl-S-beta-carboxy-beta-methyl-ethyl-cysteinyl-glycine: Bu[AS474]

Gamma-L-glutamyl-S-methyl-L-cysteine-sulfoxide: Bu[AS471]

Gamma-L-glutamyl-S-propyl-L-cysteine: Bu[AS474]

Gibberellin-A-3: Bu[AS323]

Gibberellin-A-7: Bu[AS323]

Gitonin: Rt 300[AS198]

Glucose: Bu[AS325,AS285]

Glutamic acid: Bu 0.805–1.932%[AS004]

Glutathione: Bu[AS204]

Glycine: Bu 0.2–0.48%[AS004]

Guanosine: Bu[AS214]

Hexa-1,5-dienyl-trisulfide: Bu[AS333]

Hexokinase: Bu[AS288]

Histidine: Bu 0.113–0.2712%[AS004]

Isoleucine: Bu 0.217–0.521%[AS004]

Kaempferol: Pl[AS003]

Leucine: Bu 0.31–0.74%[AS004]

Linolenic acid: Pl[AS003]

Lysine: Bu 0.273–0.655%[AS004]

Magnesium: Bu 240–1,210[AS004,AS005]

Methyl ajoene: Bu[AS040,AS432]

Methyl allyl thiosulfinate: Bu[AS040]

Monogalactosyl diglyceride: Bu[AS365]

Myrosinase: Bu[AS009]

N-alpha-(1-deoxy-D-fructos-1-yl)-L-arginine: Bu 2.1-2.4 mmol/L[AS537]

Nicotinic acid: Bu 0.48 mg/100 gm[AS013]

Oleanolic acid: Pl[AS003]

Oleic acid: Pl[AS003]

Ornithine: Lf[AS259]

Phenylalanine: Bu 0.183–0.439%[AS004]

Phloroglucinol: Pl[AS003]

Phosphatidyl choline: Bu[AS321]

Phosphatidyl ethanolamine: Bu, Lf[AS365]

Phosphatidyl inositol: Bu[AS321]

Phosphatidyl serine: Bu[AS321]

P-Hydroxybenzoic acid: Pl[AS003]

Phytic acid: Pl[AS003]

Proline: Bu 0.10–0.24%[AS004]

Prop-2-enyl-disulfane: Bu[AS281]

Propene: Bu 0.01–6[AS002]

Propenethiol: Bu 1–41[AS002]

Prostaglandin-A-1: Bu[AS172]

Prostaglandin-A-2: Bu[AS172]

Prostaglandin-B-1: Bu[AS172]

Prostaglandin-B-2: Bu[AS172]

Prostaglandin-E-1: Bu[AS172]

Prostaglandin-E-2: Bu[AS172]

Protodegalactotigonin: Bu 10[AS198]

Protoeruboside-B: Bu 100[AS171]

Pseudoscoridinine-A: Bu[AS488]

Pseudoscoridinine-B: Bu[AS488]

Quercetin: Bu 200[AS473]

Quercetin-3-O-beta-D-glucoside: Pl[AS003]

Raffinose: Bu[AS285,AS092]

Rutin: Pl[AS003]

S-(2-carboxy-propyl)-glutathione: Bu 92.5[AS192]

S-allo-mercapto cysteine: Bu 2[AS470]
S-allyl cysteine sulfoxide: Bu[AS064], Cal Tiss[AS168]
S-allyl cysteine: Bu 10[AS478]
Sativoside-B-1: Bu 30[AS198]
Sativoside-R-1: Rt 500[AS198]
Sativoside-R-2: Rt 300[AS198]
Scordine: Bu 250[AS461]
Scordinin-A: Bu 3.9%[AS492]
Scordinin-A-1: Bu 67–30,000[AS460,AS462]
Scordinin-A-2: Bu 250–8,000[AS460,AS462]
Scordinin-A-3: Bu 333[AS460]
Scordinin-B: Bu 800[AS462]
Scorodose: Bu[AS325]
Selenium: Bu 16[AS005]
Serine: Bu 1,900–4,560[AS004]
S-ethyl cysteine sulfoxide: Bu[AS006,AS487]
Silicon: Bu[AS005]
S-methyl cysteine sulfoxide: Bu, Cal Tiss[AS168]
S-methyl cysteine: Bu[AS487]
S-methyl L-cysteine sulfoxide: Bu[AS132]
S-N-butyl cysteine sulfoxide: Bu[AS006]
S-propyl cysteine sulfoxide: Bu[AS168]
Stigmasterol: Pl[AS003]
Succinic acid: Pl[AS003]
Sucrose: Bu[AS325,AS092]
Taurine: Pl[AS003]
Thiamacornine: Bu[AS327]
Thiamamidine: Bu[AS327]
Threonine: Bu 1,570–3,768[AS004]
Tin: Bu 6[AS005]
Trans-1-propenyl methyl disulfide: Bu[AS093]
Trans-ajoene: Bu 268[AS164,AS157]
Trans-cis ajoene: Bu[AS152]
Trans-S-(propen-1-yl)(+)cysteine sulfoxide: Bu[AS481]
Trans-S-(propenyl-1-yl)-cysteine-disulfide: Bu[AS481]
Tryptophan: Bu 660–1,584[AS004]
Tyrosine: Bu 810–1,944[AS004]
Valine: Bu 2,910–6,984[AS004]
Zinc: Bu 15.3[AS004]

PHARMACOLOGICAL ACTIVITIES AND CLINICAL TRIALS

Abortifacient effect. Ethanol (95%) extract of seeds, at doses of 150.0 and 200.0 mg/kg, and petroleum ether extract at a dose of 100.0 mg/kg, administered orally to female rats, were inactive[AS438].

Acetylcholinesterase inhibition. Essential oil of dried bulb was active on *Macaronesia fortunata* and *Musca domestica*[AS485].

Acid phosphatase inhibition. Butanol extract of dried bulb, administered intragastrically to rats at a dose of 0.5 gm/kg, was active vs isoprenaline-induced tissue necrosis of heart, liver and pancreas[AS189].

ACTH-induction. Ethyl acetate and ethanol (95%) extracts of dried bulb, administered intramuscularly to rabbits at doses of 20.0 mg/animal daily for 4 days, were active[AS447].

Adenosine deaminase inhibition. Fresh bulb and sap, at concentration of 10.0 mcg, was inactive. Sap, at a concentration of 10.0 microliters, was active[AS429]. Water extract of dried bulb, at a concentration of 10.0 mcg/ml in cell culture, was active on aortic-endothelium[AS139].

Adherence inhibition (bacteria to host cells). Water extract of fresh bulb, in cell culture at a concentration of 0.4%, was active on *Candida albicans*, adherence to buccal epithelial cells pre-incubated with compound, and 0.1% (adherence to buccal epithelial cells after oral rinse was measured). A concentration of 0.8% was inactive vs L-cysteine, mercaptoethanol or glutathione antagonistic effect[AS200].

Aflatoxin production inhibition. Water extract of fresh bulb, at a concentration of 1.0 mg/ml, was active on *Aspergillus flavus*. Aflatoxin B-1 production was inhibited 60.35%. The extract was also active when administered intragastrically to ducklings at a dose of 2.5 mg vs aflatoxin B-1 hepatotoxicity. Enzyme was measured in serum[AS063].

AIDS therapeutic effect. Fresh bulb taken orally by human adults at variable dosage levels was active. Five grams of fresh bulb was taken daily for the first 6 weeks and 10 gm daily for the second 6 weeks. Diarrhea, genital herpes, candidiasis, and pansinusitus with recurrent fever improved in AIDS patients[AS199].

Alanine aminotransferase stimulation. Water extract of fresh bulb, administered intragastrically to rats at variable dosage levels, was inactive. Essential oil, administered intragastrically to rats at a dose of 0.067 mg/gm, was active[AS210].

Alanine aminotransferase inhibition. Seed essential oil, administered intragastrically to rats at a dose of 56.9 micromols, was active[AS408].

Alkaline phosphatase stimulation. Butanol extract of the dried bulb, in the ration of rats at a dose of 6.7% of the diet, was active vs cadmium toxicity[AS344]. Water extract of the fresh bulb, in the ration of rabbits at a dose of 1.0 gm/kg, was active vs cholesterol-loaded animals[AS422].

Alkaline phosphatase inhibition. Essential oil, administered intragastrically to rats at a concentration of 0.067 mg/gm, was active. The rats were fasted for 24 hours[AS210].

Allergenic activity. Ethyl acetate, ethanol (95%), and water extracts of bulbs, applied externally to human adults, were active[AS261]. Butanol extract of fresh bulb, applied externally to human adults, was active. Garlic was used as a wet dressing for itchy dry skin and erosions caused by scratching. Afterwards, dermatitis became worse and spread. After corticosteroid treatment, the eczema disappeared. The patient had slight anemia, leukopenia, and elevated total serum IgE[AS166].

Alpha-amylase inhibition. Water extract of bulbs was active[AS258].

Aminolevulinic (delta) acid dehydrase inhibition. Water extract of dried bulb, at a concentration of 0.1 millimols, was active on human blood[AS375].

Analgesic activity. Ethanol (70%) extract of fresh bulb, administered intraperitoneally to mice of both sexes at variable dosage levels, was active[AS315].

Angiotensin-converting enzyme inhibition. Lyophilized extract of fresh bulbs, at a concentration of 0.3 mg/ml, was inactive. Lyophilized extract of fresh leaves, at a concentration of 0.3 mg/ml, was active. 30% inhibition was produced[AS432].

Anthelmintic activity. Butanol extract of dried bulbs, administered by gastric intubation to mice at a dose of 200.0 mg/kg on days 1–5, was active on *Aspiculurus tetraptera*[AS490]. Dried bulb, administered by gastric intubation to ducks and geese infected with hymenolepis, produced weak activity[AS448]. Essential oil, administered intragastrically to mice at a dose of 0.025 ml/kg on days 1–5, was inactive on *Aspiculurus tetraptera*[AS490]. Fresh bulbs in the drinking water and hexane extracts were active on carp (*Capillaria obsignata*) at a dose 200.0 mg/liter dosing twice daily on days 1–3[AS174]. Saline extract of the fresh bulb, at a concentration of 5.0%, was active on *Anisakis* species larvae[AS141]. Water and methanol extracts of the dried bulb, on agar plate at a concentration of 10.0 mg/ml, produced weak activity on *Toxacara canis*[AS236].

Antiaging activity. Water extract of the dried bulb, in cell culture at a concentration of 100.0 mcg/ml, increased the lifespan of leuk-P388(ARA-C) cells in culture[AS114].

Antiallergenic activity. Water extract of fresh bulb, in cell culture at a concentration of 100.0 microliters/ml, was active on leuk-RBL 2H3 vs biotinylated anti-DNP IgE/avidin-induced beta-hexosaminidase release[AS176].

Antiamoebic activity. Essential oil, in broth culture at a concentration of 2.0 microliters/ml, was active on *Entamoeba histolytica*[AS135]. Fresh bulb juice, in broth culture at a concentration of 25.0 mcg/ml, was active on *Entamoeba histolytica*[AS180].

Antiarrhythmic activity. Dried bulb, in the ration of rats at a concentration of 1.0% of the diet for 10 weeks, decreased coronary artery ligation reperfusion-induced arrhythmias[AS073].

Antiascariasis activity. Ethanol (95%) extract of the bulb, applied externally, was active on earthworms. Paralysis occurred in 12 hours with death of 50% of the worms[AS046]. Water extract, applied externally to earthworms at a concentration of 10.0 mg/ml, produced strong activity[AS030].

Antiatherosclerotic activity. Butanol extract of dried bulb, taken orally by human adults, prevented the total rise in serum cholesterol, B-lipoprotein cholesterol, B-lipoprotein and serum triglycerides in patients with alimentary lipemia[AS332]. Dried bulb, in the ration of castrated rams at a concentration of 5% of the diet, produced weak activity[AS118]. Water extract of the fresh bulb, in the ration of rabbits at a dose of 1.0 gm/kg, was active vs cholesterol-loaded animals[AS422].

Antibacterial activity. Essential oil, on agar plate, was active on *Erwina amylovora*, MIC 112.5 mg/liter[AS233]. Amino acid fraction in cream form, extract in ointment, essential oil in wound-healing powder, and essential oil in gel of dried bulb, on agar plate, were active on *Escherichia coli, Klebsiella pneumonia, Proteus vulgaris* and *Shigella sonnei*[AS253]. Ethanol (95%) extract was active on *Escherichia coli, Salmonella typhosa, Shigella sonnei,* and *Staphylococcus aureus*[AS249]. Water extract was active on *Bacillus mycoides, Escherichia coli, Klebsiella pneumonia, Proteus vulgaris, Salmonella typhosa, Shigella sonnei* and *Staphylococcus aureus*[AS246]. Aqueous high speed supernatant, on agar plate at a concentration of 0.2 ml, was active on *Escherichia coli, Proteus mirabilis, Proteus vulgaris, Pseudomonas aeruginosa, Staphylococcus aureus* and *Klebsiella* species[AS351]. Bulb juice, in broth culture, was active on *Candida parapsilosis.* Thirty-eight millimeter zone of inhibition was produced[AS150]. Butanol, water, and hot water extracts of fresh bulb, on agar plate at variable concentrations, was active on *Bacillus subtilis* H-17(Rec+), M-45(Rec-)[AS336]. Decoction of the dried bulb, on agar plate, was active on *Pseudomonas aeruginosa*[AS116]. Hot water

extract, at a concentration of 62.5 mg/ml, was active on *Staphylococcus aureus*, and inactive on *Escherichia coli*[AS098]. Dried bulb, on agar plate, was active on *Xanthomonas campestris*[AS389]. Dried bulb, on agar plate at a concentration of 0.20 gm/plate, produced strong activity on *Escherichia coli* and *Bacillus subtilis*[AS368]. Essential oil of dried bulb, administered intradermally to rabbits, prevented Staphylococcal infections[AS468]. Essential oil of dried bulb, on agar plate, was active on *Klebsiella pneumonia, Proteus vulgaris* and *Pseudomonas aeruginosa*[AS253]. Fresh bulb juice, on agar plate undiluted, was active on *Bacillus subtilis, Pseudomonas aeruginosa* and *Salmonella typhosa*[AS475]. Fresh bulb juice, undiluted on agar plate, produced weak activity on *Streptococcus aureus* and *Escherichia coli*[AS465]. Fresh bulb and chloroform extract, on agar plate, were inactive on *Escherichia coli* and *Staphylococcus aureus*, MIC 7.5 and 6.0 mg/ml, respectively. Water extract, at a concentration of 30.0 microliters/disk on agar plate, was active on *E. coli, Shigella dysenteriae* 1, *Shigella flexneri* and *Shigella sonnei*. A dose of 1.5 ml/kg of fresh bulb, administered intragastrically to rabbits, was active on *Shigella flexneri*[AS228]. Fresh bulb juice, undiluted on agar plate, was active on *Proteus vulgaris*[AS454]. Fresh corn sap, on agar plate, was active on several Gram-negative organisms[AS319]. Fresh essential oil, undiluted on agar plate, was active on *Pseudomonas aeruginosa* and *Staphylococcus aureus*, and inactive on *Bacillus cereus* and *Escherichia coli*[AS317]. Infusion of the fresh bulb, in broth culture, was active on *Staphylococcus aureus*, MIC 10.0 mcg/ml; *Clostridium paraputrificum* and *Propionibacter acnes*, MIC 3.9 mg/ml; *Bacteroides vulgaris* and *Bifidobacterium longum*, MIC 7.8 mg/ml; inactive on *Clostridium perfringens, Bacteroides fragilis, Eubacterium limosum, Propionibacterium intermedium, Acinetobacter calcoaceticus,* and *Staphylococcus aureus* 25923, MIC 15.6 mg/ml; *Eubacterium nucleatum* and *E.*

lentum, MIC 31.3 mg/ml; *Bacteroides melaninogenicus* and *Peptostreptococcus productus*, MIC 62.5 mg/ml; *Citrobacter freundii* and *Serratia marcescens*, MIC 625.0 mcg/ml; *Pseudomonas aeruginosa* and *Streptococcus faecalis*, MIC >625 mcg/ml. The petroleum ether extract was inactive on *Clostridium paraputrificum*, MIC 156.0 mcg/ml; *Bifidobacterium longum*, MIC 312.0 mcg/ml; *Propionibacterium acnes*, MIC 78.0 mcg/ml and *S. aureus*, MIC 625 mcg/ml[AS177]. Leaf essential oil, on agar plate, was inactive on *Bacillus cereus*, *E. coli*, *Pseudomonas aeruginosa*, and *Staphylococcus aureus*[AS397]. Dried oleoresin, in broth culture at a concentration of 5.0 gm/liter, produced weak activity on *Staphylococcus aureus*[AS401]. Chloroform extract of dried bulb contained at least 2 active elements. One was chloroform soluble and had an antiseptic action, a slight tonic effect on the isolated frog heart, a slight hypertensive effect on etherized cats, and a paralyzing effect on isolated rabbit intestine. The chloroform-insoluble fraction had no antiseptic effect, no action on isolated frog heart, a strongly hypotensive effect on etherized cats, and a tonic effect on isolated rabbit intestine[AS459]. Powdered dried bulb, in broth culture at a concentration of 5.0 gm/liter, was inactive on *Staphylococcus aureus*[AS401]. Tincture of the dried bulb, on agar plate at a concentration of 30.0 microliters/disk (10 gm plant material in 100 ml ethanol), was active on *Escherichia coli*, *Pseudomonas aeruginosa*, and *Staphylococcus aureus*[AS405]. Water extract of the bulb, in broth culture at a concentration of 1.0%, was active on *Clostridium perfringens*[AS276]. Water extract, on agar plate, was active on *Escherichia coli*, *Pasteurella multocida*, *Proteus* species, *Providencia* species, *Staphylococcus aureus* and *Streptococcus faecalis*, and inactive on *Pseudomonas aeruginosa*. A dose of 1.0 ml/animal, administered orally to chicken, produced a reduction in intestinal tract bacteria[AS242]. Water extract of bulb, in

broth culture, was active on *Staphylococcus aureus*. The extract, administered intraperitoneally to mice, was inactive on *Staphylococcus aureus*. On agar plate, it was active on *Erwinia carotovora* and *Erwinia herbicola*[AS043]. Water extract of the bulb, on agar plate at a concentration of 1–10, was active on *Escherichia coli*. Complete inhibition of several enterotoxigenic strains of the test organisms was observed[AS307]. Water extract of the dried bulb, on agar plate, was active on *Streptococcus sanguis*, *Escherichia coli*, *Serratia marcescens*, *Lactobacillus odontolyticus*, *Streptococcus milleri*, *Streptococcus mutans*; weakly active on *Bacillus cereus*, *Enterobacter cloacae*, *Staphylococcus aureus*, *Streptococcus hominis* and inactive on *Pseudomonas aeruginosa*[AS324]. Water extract of fresh bulb was active on *E. coli* and *Micrococcus luteus*[AS143]. Fresh garlic powder, at a concentration of 1% solution, was effective on *Escherichia coli* 0–157. The powder from fresh garlic was more effective than that from aged garlic. The antiabcterial activity was lso shown against the methicillin-resistant *Staphylococcus aureus*, *Salmonella enteritidis*, and *Candida albicans*[AS550].

Anticarcinogenic effect. Bulb, administered orally to rats at a dose of 250 mg/kg 3 times a week, effectively suppressed 4-nitroquinoline 1-oxide-induced tongue carcinogenesis as revealed by the absence of carcinomas in the initiation phase and their reduced incidence in the post-initiation phase. There was a reduction in lipid peroxidation in the tumor tissue accompanied by a significant increase in the levels of reduced glutathione, glutathione peroxidase and glutathione S-transferase[AS512]. S-allylcysteine (SAC) and S-allylmercaptocysteine (SAMC), evaluated for their effects on proliferation and cell cycle progression in the human cancer cell lines, SW-480 and HT-29, inhibited the growth of both cell lines. SAMC also induced apoptosis that was associated with an increase in caspase3-lke activity. The effects were accompanied by induction of JUN kinase activity and a marked increase in dendogenous levels or reduce glutathione[AS540]. Garlic, administered orally to diethylnitrosoamine-induced hepato-carcinogenic male Wistar rats, produced a significant reduction in the number (50% reduction) and area (48% reduction) of glutathione S-transferase placental form positive foci compared with the control group of animals receiving water. Histopathological examination of rat livers using H & E staining indicated that there was no significant difference between the control and garlic treated groups in granularity and vacuolation of the cytoplasm[AS546]. Diallyl sulfide and diallyl disulfide, evaluated on p53-wild type H460 and p53-null type h1299 non small cell lung cancer cells, produced a significant number of cells in apoptotic state as measured by acridine orange staining. However, there was not a significant induction of apoptotic cells by MTT assay. Diallyl disulfide was more effective in inducing apoptosis on the cells[AS548].

Anticardiotoxic effect. Water extract of aged bulbs, administered intraperitoneally to mice at a dose of 0.05 ml/animal 6 times weekly, was active. Widening of GRS and lengthening of PR intervals induced by doxorubicin were diminished in treated animals. Doxorubicin-induced histologic changes were prevented by the treatment[AS119].

Anticholinergic activity. Water extract of dried bulb was inactive on the frog skeletal muscle and guinea pig small intestine vs ACh-induced contractions[AS251].

Anticlastogenic activity. Flower head juice, administered intragastrically to mice at a dose of 25.0 ml/kg, was active on bone marrow cells vs mitomycin C-, dimethylnitrosamine-, and tetracycline-induced micronuclei[AS117].

Anticonvulsant activity. Ethanol (70%) extract of the fresh bulb, administered intraperitoneally to mice of both sexes at variable dosage levels, was active vs metrazole-induced convulsions, and inactive vs strychnine-induced convulsions[AS315].

Anticrustacean activity. Ethanol (95%) extract of dried bulb was inactive on *Artemia salina*. The assay system was intended to predict for antitumor activity[AS060].

Anticytotoxic activity. Water extract of the bulb, administered intragastrically to mice at a dose of 100.0 mg/kg, was active vs arsenic-induced bone marrow cytotoxicity. Treatment with the extract reduced the chromosome breaks and cell damage induced by arsenic[AS080].

Antidiarrheal activity. Essential oil, administered orally to mice at a concentration of 0.01 ml/gm, was active vs castor oil-induced diarrhea[AS161].

Antiedema activity. Methanol extract of the bulb, applied externally to mice at a dose of 2.0 mg/ear, was active vs 12-0-tetradecan-oylphorbol-13-acetate (TPA)-induced ear inflammation. Inhibition ratio (IR) was 32[AS079].

Antiestrogenic effect. Water extract of the fresh bulb, administered intraperitoneally to female mice at a dose of 500.0 mg/day, was inactive[AS431].

Antifatigue activity. Ethanol (95%) extract of the bulb, administered intragastrically to mice at a dose of 125.0 mg/kg, was active. The dose had no effect after 1 session of rope climbing stress, but it prevented decline in performance, which was noted in controls after 2 weeks of repeated stress[AS165].

Antifilarial activity. Fresh bulb was active on *Setaria digitata*, LC_{100} 600 ppm[AS222].

Antifungal activity. Essential oil, on agar plate, was active on *Lenzites trabea*, *Lentinus lepideus* and *Polyporus versicolor*[AS032]. Bulb essential oil, on agar plate at a concentration of 10.0%/disk, was active on *Geotrichum candidum*, *Candida lipolytica*, *Rhodotorula rubra* and *Saccharomyces* cerevisiae, and inactive on *Brettanomyces anomalus*. One percent/disk was active on *Kloeckera apiculata*, *Kluyveromyces fragilis*, *Pichia membranaefaciens*, and *Torulopsis glabrata*. Strong activity was produced on *Debaryomyces hansenii*, *Hansenula anomala*, *Lodderomyces elongisporus* and *Metschnikowia pulcherrima*[AS334]. Bulb juice, applied externally to rabbits at a concentration of 10% for 10 days after typical fungal-induced lesions appear, was active on *Microsporum canis*[AS300]. Essential oil of the dried bulb, on agar plate, was active on *Trichophyton rubrum*[AS253]. Essential oil of the dried bulb, on agar plate, was active on *Epidermophyton floccosum*, *Microsporum gypseum* and *Trichophyton rubrum* (11% oil in gel was used). The water extract, at a concentration of 0.625%, was active on *Trichoderma* species and *Trichophyton mentagrophytes*; a concentration of 1.25% was active on *Aspergillus niger* and *Epidermophyton floccosum*, and inactive on *Aspergillus flavus*, *Basidiobolum meristosporus* strain T1, T2, T3, T4, T5 and T6, and *Trichophyton rubrum*; weak activity was produced on *Aspergillus fumigatus*, *Curvularia* species, and *Fusarium* species[AS254]. Juice, at a concentration of 0.25%, was active on *Trichophyton mentagrophytes*. A concentration 0.5% was active on *Trichophyton rubrum*[AS255]; 2.0% was active on *Alternaria alternata*, *Ceratocystis paradoxa*, *Fusarium solani*, *Geotrichum candidum*, *Melanconium fuligineum*, *Myrothecium roridum*, *Phytophthora* species, *Phytium aphanidermatum*, *Rhizopus microsporus*, *Sclerotium rolfsii*, *Thanatephorus cucumeris*, *Tricholoma crassum*, *Ustilago maydis*, and *Volvariella volvacea*; 4.0% was active on *Colletotrichum denatium*[AS252]; 1.25% was active on *Microsporum gypseum* and *Trichophyton violaceum*; 2.5% active on *Epidermophyton floccosum*, *Microsporum canis*, *Trichophyton mentagrophytes*, and *Trichophyton rubrum*[AS250]. Essential oil, on agar plate, was active on *Botryotrichum keratinophilum*, *Malbranchea aurantiaca* and

Nannizzia incurvata[AS184]. Ethanol/water (1:1) extract of the dried bulb, on agar plate at concentrations of 417.0 and 500.0 mg/ml (expressed as dry weight of bulb), were active on *Penicillium digitatum*, and inactive on *Aspergillus fumigatus*, *Aspergillus niger*, *Botrytis cinerea*, *Rhizopus nigricans*, *Trichophyton mentagrophytes* and *Fusarium oxysporum*[AS414,AS382]. Fresh bulb, on agar plate, was inactive on *Trichophyton andouinii*, *T. mentagrophytes*, *T. rubrum*, *T. schoenleini* and *T. tonsurans*, MIC 1000 mcg/ml; *Aspergillus fumigatus*, MIC 2000 mcg/ml and *Microsporum canis*, MIC 500 mcg/ml[AS420]. Fresh bulb, undiluted on agar plate, was active on *Nannizzia fulva*, *N. gypsea* and *N. incurvata*[AS374]. Water extract of the fresh bulb, at a concentration of 1.0 mcg/ml, inhibited growth in *Aspergillus flavus*[AS063]. The extract was active when applied externally at a dose of 20.0% twice daily for 15 days to a buffalo with dermatophytosis caused by *T. verrucosum*; twice daily for 10 days to a calf with dermatophytosis; twice daily for 10 days to a dog with dermatophytosis caused by *M. canis* and twice daily for 10–20 days to 6 patients with dermatophytosis caused by *T. rubrum*, and *T. mentagrophytes*[AS356]. A concentration of 10.0% was active on *Trichoconiella padwickii*[AS190]. Fresh essential oil, undiluted on agar plate, was inactive on *Penicillium cyclopium*, *Trichoderma viride* and *Aspergillus aegyptiacus*[AS317]. Hot water extract of the dried bulb, in broth culture at a concentration of 1.0 ml, was active on *Epidermophyton floccosum*, *Microsporum canis* and *Trichophyton mentagrophytes* vars. algodonosa and granulare[AS230]. Leaf essential oil, on agar plate, produced strong activity on *Aspergillus aegyptiacus*, *Penicillum cyclopium* and *Trichoderma viride*[AS397]. Water extract of the bulb, on agar plate at a concentration of 5.0 mg/ml, was active on *Fusarium oxysporum* F. Sp. Lycopersici[AS410]. Water extract of the dried bulb, in broth culture, was active on *Fusarium moniliforme*. A decrease in nitrate and dimethylnitrosamine formation of the fungus was observed[AS367]. Water extract of the fresh bulb, at a concentration of 0.01 microliters/disk, was equivocal on *Epidermophyton floccosum*; inactive on *Trichophyton soudanense*. A concentration of 6.67 mcg/disk was inactive on *Trichophyton erinacei* and *T. verrucosum*. The extract was active on *T. semii*, *Microsporum audouini*, *Trichophyton mentagrophytes*, *Microsporum canis*, *T. rubrum* and *T. violaceum*, IC_{50} 6.67 microliters/disk[AS131]. Water extract of the fresh bulb, on agar plate at a concentration of 5.0 mg/ml, was active on *Epidermophyton floccosum*, *Microsporum audouini*, *M. canis*, *M. gypseum*, *Trichophyton concentricum*, and several plant pathogenic fungi[AS463]. Water extract of fresh leaves, on agar plate at a concentration of 1:1 (one gram of dried leaves in 1.0 ml of water), was active on *Fusarium oxysporum*[AS121]. Strong activity was produced on *Ustilago maydis* and *U. nuda*[AS350]. Water extract of the bulb, in broth culture, was active on *Aspergillus fumigatus*, *Aspergillus flavus*, *Rhizopus rhizopodiformis*, *Aspergillus niger* and *Mucor pusillus*, and weak activity on *Rhizopus arrhizus*[AS245].

Antigout activity. Water extract of the bulb, administered by gastric intubation to rats at a dose of 100.0 mg/kg, was active. Daily dosing for 10 days to typhoid Bacillus-sheep RBC-stimulated animals showed the antibody titer to be significantly inhibited[AS310].

Antihematopoetic activity. Dried bulb, administered by gastric intubation to rats at a dose of 3.10 mg/kg, was equivocal. There was a slight decrease in erythrocyte and hemoglobin levels in female rats; a much smaller decrease was seen in male rats. At a dose of 10.0 mg/kg, administered for 3 months, there was a slight decrease in erythrocyte and hemoglobin levels[AS371].

Antihepatotoxic activity. Butanol extract of the bulb, administered intragastrically to mice at a dose of 100.0 mg/kg, was active vs CCl_4-induced hepatotoxicity. Conjugated diene levels, thiobarbituric acid levels, hepatic triglycerides content and hepatic lipid content were decreased[AS404]. Essential oil, of the dried bulb in cell culture (rat liver cells) at concentrations of 0.01 and 1.0 mg/ml, was active vs CCl_4-, and galactosamine-induced hepatotoxicity. Results significant at $P < 0.01$ and $P < 0.001$ levels, respectively[AS369]. Ethanol (20%) extract of fresh bulb, administered by gastric intubation to mice at a dose of 100.0 mg/kg, was inactive vs paracetamol- and carbon tetrachloride-induced hepatotoxicity[AS215]. Methanol-insoluble fraction of the fresh bulb, turmeric, asafoetida, cumin, ellagic acid, butylated hydroxy toluene and butylated hydroxy anisole, administered intragastrically to ducklings at a dose of 10.0 mg/animal, was active vs aflatoxin B-1-induced hepatotoxicity[AS115]. Garlic oil, as similar to N-acetylcysteine, has shown to eliminate electrophilic intermediates and free radicals through conjugation and reduction reactions. It protects the liver from toxic doses of acetaminophen. The clearance of the toxic metabolites of the acetaminophen from the liver occurs much faster with immediate treatment with garlic oil[AS501].

Antihistamine activity. Water extract of dried bulb was active on guinea pig small intestine vs histamine-induced contractions[AS251].

Antihyperglycemic activity. Garlicin, administered by intravenous drip at a dose of 60 mg/day for 10 days, markedly lowered the plasma endothelin and blood sugar levels in patients with hyperglycemia[AS521].

Antihypercholesterolemic activity. Bulb, in the ration of 16 week-old male rats at concentrations of 2.0 and 4.0% of the diet, was active in cholesterol-loaded and lard-fed animals. Results significant at $P < 0.05$

level[AS301]. Bulb, in the ration of rabbits at variable concentrations, in a feeding study for 52–82 days, was active vs cholesterol-loaded animals[AS036]. Bulb, taken orally by human adults at variable dosage levels, was active[AS297]. Bulb, administered by gastric intubation to dogs, was active[AS304], and when administered orally to male human adults, at a dose of 25.0 gm/person, was active[AS274]. Butanol extract, taken orally by human adults of both sexes at a dose of 1.35 gm/person daily for 100 days, was active[AS271]. Ten healthy subjects below the age of 40 took Butanol extract of fresh bulb orally. They were submitted to a 12-hour fast before receiving the test material. A fatty meal consisting of 100 gm butterfat on 4 slices of bread was given to each subject fresh; as well as boiled garlic were administered in the study. Garlic appeared to prevent an increase in serum cholesterol statistical data in the report indicating significant results[AS263]. Water extract of fresh bulb, in the ration of rabbits at a dose of 1.0 gm/kg, was active[AS422]. Butanol extract of fresh bulb, administered by gastric intubation and in the ration of rats at concentrations of 2.0% of the diet for 4 weeks, was active[AS306]; ethanol (95%) extract was inactive[AS392] vs cholesterol-loaded animals. Dried bulb, in the ration of castrated rams at a concentration of 5.0% of the diet, was active[AS118]. Essential oil, administered by gastric intubation to rabbits at variable dosage levels, was active vs cholesterol-loaded animals[AS129]. In a randomized placebo-controlled double-blind study of the efficacy of garlic powder on cholesterol level, 68 volunteers took powdered bulb at a dose of 600.0 mg/person. Average cholesterol fell from 223 to 214 mg/dl[AS129]. Dried bulb, in the ration of rats at a concentration of 2.0% of the diet, was active vs high-fat diet-induced hypercholesterolemia[AS113]. Dried bulb, taken orally at a dose of 198.0 mg/person, 3 doses in 34 human adults, was inac-

tive. A dose of 450.0 mg/person, 3 doses in 51 human adults, was inactive[AS377]; 600.0 mg/person for 4 weeks was active[AS183]. Dried bulb, taken orally by human adults twice daily for 15 days in a group of 10 hyperlipemic subjects, was active[AS303]. After garlic therapy of dried bulb (2 capsules 3 times daily after meals for 12 weeks), serum cholesterol levels were brought down within the normal range in 26 out of 37 patients. The extract also lowered plasma fibrinogen levels, prolonged coagulation time and enhanced fibrinolytic activity in some of the patients[AS303]. Essential oil, in the ration of male rabbit at doses of 0.25, 0.50, and 1.0 gm/animal, was active vs cholesterol-fed animals[AS256]. Essential oil, administered by gastric intubation to rabbits at a dose of 250.0 mg/kg 6 days per week for 4–12 weeks, was active vs cholesterol-loaded animals[AS355]. Essential oil, taken orally by human adults of both sexes at a dose equivalent to 1.0 gm/kg of raw garlic daily for 3 months, was active[AS272]. Essential oil, administered by gastric intubation to rats at a dose of 100.0 mg/kg for 60 days, was active. Results significant at $P < 0.01$ level vs ethanol-induced hyperglycemia[AS359]. When taken orally by human adults of both sexes at a dose of 0.25 mg/kg, the dose was active. In a study with 62 patients with coronary heart disease and high serum cholesterol levels and 20 healthy individuals as a control group, garlic oil was consumed daily for 10 months[AS289]. Ether extract of the fresh bulb, administered intragastrically to rats at a dose of 100.0 mg/kg, was active vs streptozotocin-induced hyperglycemia. High-fat diet was used[AS379]. Fixed oil, in the ration of male rats at a dose of 100.0 mg/kg, was active. Simultaneous feeding of unsaturated oil from the plant material with a high-sucrose diet, significantly reduced serum and tissue cholesterol levels, and a small but significant tissue-protein reducing effect was also observed[AS299]. Freeze-dried bulb, in the ration of female rats at concentrations of 0.5, 1.0, and 2.0% of the diet, was active. Animals were fed a cholesterol-high diet for 6–8 weeks[AS291]. Essential oil, at a concentration of 0.13% of the diet of female rats, was active vs cholesterol-loaded animals, results significant at $P < 0.001$ level[AS341]. Fresh bulbs, in the ration of male rats at a concentration of 5.0% of the diet, were active. Animals were fed a ration of 1% cholesterol plus 46.8% sucrose and 5% garlic[AS273]. Powdered dried bulb, taken orally by human adults of both sexes at a dose of 900.0 mg/day, was inactive in a double-blind, randomized crossover study on 30 subjects with mild to moderate hypercholesterolemia[AS133]. Water extract of fresh bulb, administered by gastric intubation to rabbits at a dose of 10.0 gm/animal (dry weight of plant) daily for 5 days, was active vs cholesterol-loaded animals[AS458].

Antihyperglycemic activity. Butanol extract of bulbs, taken orally by human adults of both sexes at a dose of 1.35 gm/person daily for 100 days, was active[AS271]. Chloroform extract of bulbs, administered orally to rabbits, was active vs glucose-primed animals. Activity was 79.4% that of tolbutamide[AS053]. Decoction of fresh bulb, administered intragastrically to mice at a dose of 0.5 ml/animal, was inactive vs alloxan-induced hyperglycemia. A 25% aqueous extract was used. Maximal change in blood sugar was 6.2%[AS202]. Dried bulb, taken orally by human adults at a dose of 350.0 mg/person twice daily, was inactive[AS170]. Ethanol (95%) extract of the bulb, administered by gastric intubation to rabbits, produced weak activity, and petroleum ether extract was active vs alloxan- and epinephrine-induced hyperglycemia[AS285]. Ether extract of the fresh bulb, administered intragastrically to rats at a dose of 100.0 mg/kg, was active vs streptozotocin-induced hyperglycemia[AS379]. Fresh bulb, in the ration of male rats at a concentration of 5.0% of

the diet, was active. Animals were fed a ration of 1% cholesterol plus 46.8% sucrose and 5% garlic. Significant reduction of serum glucose but increased serum insulin and liver glycogen appeared to be associated with an increase of insulin level[AS273]. Hot water extract of the dried bulb, administered by gastric intubation to mice at a dose of 0.5 ml (25% extract), was inactive vs alloxan-induced hyperglycemia[AS362]. Hot water extract of the fresh bulb, in the ration of mice at a dose of 6.25% of the diet, was inactive vs streptozotocin-induced hyperglycemia[AS213]. Water extract of bulb, administered orally to rats, was active vs alloxan-treated animals. There was a 20% decrease in blood glucose[AS045]. Water extract of fresh bulb, administered intragastrically to rats at a dose of 0.07 gm/animal for 30 days, was active vs inhibition of the formation of polyols in diabetic rat lens[AS186]. Fresh bulb juice, administered intragastrically to rabbits at a dose of 25.0 gm/animal (dry weight of plant material), was active vs glucose-induced hyperglycemia[AS038]. Aged garlic, administered orally to stress induced hyperglycemic mice using the immobilization stress model for 16 hours per day for 2 consecutive days, prevented adrenal hypertrophy, hyperglycemia and elevation of corticosterone, but did not alter serum insulin level[AS553].

Antihyperlipemic activity. Bulb, in the ration of 16 week-old male rats, at a concentration of 2.0 and 4.0% of the diet, was active in cholesterol-loaded and lard fed animals, results significant at $P < 0.05$ level[AS301]. Bulb, taken orally by male adults at a dose of 25.0 gm/person, was active[AS274]. Dried bulb, taken orally at a dose of 198.0 mg/person, 3 doses in 34 human adults, was inactive. A dose of 450.0 mg/person, 3 doses in 51 human adults, was inactive[AS377]; 600.0 mg/person for 4 weeks was active[AS183]. Dried bulb, taken orally by human adults twice daily for 15 days in a group of 10 hyperlipemic subjects, was active[AS309]. Water extract of dried bulb, administered orally to rabbits at a dose of 3.3 gm/kg daily for 2 months, was active on sucrose loaded animals (10 gm/kg/day). Statistical data indicated significant results[AS279]. Saponin fraction of the dried bulb, taken orally by human adults at a dose of 50.0 gm/person, was active[AS407]. Dried garlic preparations, given to 30 patients of primary hyperlipoproteinemia orally at a dose of 700 mg/day, were inactive. Serum cholesterol and triglycerides were not significantly reduced[AS396]. Essential oil, administered by gastric intubation to rabbit at a dose of 250.0 mg/kg 6 days per week for 4 to 12 weeks, was active vs cholesterol-loaded animals[AS355]. The essential oil, taken orally by human adults of both sexes at a dose equivalent to 1.0 gm/kg of raw garlic daily for 3 months, was active[AS272]. Essential oil, administered by gastric intubation to rat at a dose of 100.0 mg/kg for 60 days, was active. The effects were measured in liver, results significant at $P < 0.01$ level vs ethanol-induced hyperglycemia[AS354]. Fixed oil, in the ration of male rats at a dose of 100.0 mg/kg, was active. Simultaneous feeding of unsaturated oil from the plant material with a high sucrose diet significantly reduced serum and tissue lipids, and a small but significant tissue-protein reducing effect was also observed[AS299]. Fresh bulb, in the ration of male rats at a concentration of 5.0% of the diet, was active. Animals were fed a ration of 1% cholesterol plus 46.8% sucrose and 5% garlic[AS273]. Pollen, taken orally by human adults of both sexes at a dose of 900.0 mg/day, was inactive in a double-blind, randomized crossover study on 30 subjects with mild to moderate hypercholesterolemia[AS133]. Water extract, in the drinking water of rats at a dose of 1.0 gm/ml, was active[AS390].

Antihypertensive activity. Bulb, taken orally by human adults at variable dosage levels, was active[AS297]. Fresh bulbs, administered by gastric intubation to dogs and orally to human adults at variable concentrations, were active[AS036]. Butanol extract of bulbs, taken orally by human adults of both sexes at a dose of 1.35 gm/person daily for 100 days, was active[AS271]. Dried bulbs, taken orally by human adults at a dose of 2.4 gm/person, produced decrease in diastolic pressure 5–14 hours after dosing in 9 patients with essential hypertension[AS089]. Ethanol (95%) extract of bulb, administered orally to 25 patients with hypertension, was active[AS012]. Ethanol (95%) extract of fresh bulb, in the ration of rats at a dose of 8.0 ml/animal, was inactive. Extraction was made at 0°C; 4 ml of the extract was fed for 3 weeks, then salt was added and the dose increased to 8 ml. Salt did not affect blood pressure in the spontaneously hypertensive animals[AS188]. Fresh bulbs, taken orally by human adults, were active. Analysis of random, controlled studies lasting at least 4 weeks included 415 subjects, showed significant decreases in both systolic and diastolic pressures[AS112].

Antihypertriglyceridemic effect. Bulbs, in the ration of rats at a dose of 2.0% of the diet, was active vs high-fat diet induced hypertriglyceridemia[AS113]. Dried bulbs, taken orally by human adults at a dose of 900.0 mg/day, was active. Twenty-four volunteers with reduced HDL-cholesterol levels and hypertriglyceridemia were used in the 6-week study. Triglycerides levels were reduced up to 35% and HDL cholesterol levels increased[AS073]. Ether extract of the fresh bulb, administered intragastrically to rats at a dose of 100.0 mg/kg, was active. High fat diet was used[AS379]. Outer skin fiber, in the ration of male rats at a dose of 236.6 gm/day, was active. Water extract of fresh bulb was active[AS237].

Antihypotensive activity. Water extract of fresh bulb, administered intravenously to rabbit at a dose of 500.0 mg/kg, was active vs arachidonate-, and rat tail-solubilized-collagen-induced thrombocytopenia, hypotension and increased TXB2 levels. The extract inhibits histopathological changes in lung and liver[AS059]. Intravenous infusion was also active vs arachidonate-induced hypotension[AS428].

Antihypothermic activity. Ethanol (95%) extract of bulbs, administered intragastrically to mice at a dose of 250.0 gm/kg, was active vs 3 weeks of cold stress[AS165].

Anti-inflammatory activity. Bulbs, taken orally by 30 patients with different rheumatic conditions, was active[AS294]. Ethanol/water (1:1) extract of bulbs, administered intraperitoneally to rats, was active vs carrageenin-induced pedal edema[AS025]. Water extract, administered orally to rats at a dose of 2.0 gm/kg, produced weak activity vs granuloma pouch and formalin-induced pedal edema[AS021]. Dried bulbs, taken orally by human adults at variable dosage levels, were active. Ethanol (80%) extract of dried bulb, administered to male rats by gastric intubation at a dose of 100.0 mg/kg, was active vs carrageenin-induced pedal edema. A 23% inhibition of edema was observed. Seed oil, administered intragastrically to rats at a dose of 0.0025 ml/kg, was active vs formaldehyde-induced arthritis[AS408].

Anti-ischemic effect. Bulb, in a preparation containing nicotinic acid, was administered intragastrically to rats at a dose of 5.0 gm/kg daily for 7 days. During the last 2, isoproterenol was also given. Isoproterenol-induced ischemic effects on the heart were prevented[AS226]. Powdered dried bulb, in the ration of rats at a concentration of 1.0% of the diet for 10 days, reduced coronary artery ligation-induced infarct size[AS073].

Antileukemic activity. Garlic oil, incubated in human promyelocytic leukemia cells, HL-60 at a concentration of 20 microgram/ml, produced a marked suppression of HL-60 proliferation. The suppression was almost identical with those obtained by all-

trans-retinoic acid or dimethyl sulfoxide used as positive controls. The oil induced the generation of nitroblue tetrazolium-reducing activity, and about 20% of the HL-60 cells became nitroblue tetrazolium positive. CD11b, another marker of the differentiation of the cells, was also significantly induced by the oil[AS544].

Antimicrobial activity. Garlic oil, and 4 diallyl sulphides occurring naturally in these oils were tested on *Staphylococcus aureus*, methicillin-resistant *S. aureus*, 3 Candida species, and 3 Aspergillus species, indicated the magnitude of activity of the 4 sulphides followed the order diallyl tetrasulphide > diallyl trisulphide > diallyl disulphide > and diallyl monosulphide, suggesting that the disulphide bonds are an important factor in determining the antimicrobial activities[AS509].

Antimitotic effect. Diallyl disulfide, a major compound in garlic, was tested on colon neoplastic lesions in vivo and colon tumor cell growth in vitro. Using human colon adenocarcinoma HT-29 Glc(−/+) cell line, a subpopulation of tumoral cells with markedly different characteristics in terms of metablic capacities, adhesion properties, and distribution in the cell cycle phases was identified. After 1 to 2 days of treatment with 100 microM of diallyl disulfide, the HT-29 cells were largely released into the culture medium. The released cells accumulated in the G(2)/M phase were characterized by a 5-fold reduction in cell capacity for de novo protein synthesis[AS506].

Antimutagenic activity. Dried bulb, on agar plate at a concentration of 12.5 mg/plate, was active on *Salmonella typhimurium* TA100, vs aflatoxin B-1-induced mutagenesis. Metabolic activation was required for activity[AS415]. Fresh bulb in buffer, on agar plate a concentration of 14.75 mg/plate, was inactive on *E. coli* WP2 TRP(−) induced by UV. A concentration of 7.38 mg/plate was active on *E. coli* WP2 TRP (−) UVR (−) and *E. coli* WP2 TRP (−). Methanol extract of the fresh bulb, on agar plate, was active on *Salmonella typhimurium* TA98 and TA100[AS240]. Water extract of the fresh bulb, at a concentration of 0.8 microliters/ml, was active on Hepatoma-AH109A vs gamma-ray-induced mutation. A concentration of 1.0 mg/plate was inactive on *Salmonella typhimurium* TA100, vs 1,2-epoxy-3,3,3-trichloropropane-induced mutation. A concentration of 10.0 mcg/plate was inactive on *S. typhimurium* TA 100 vs sodium azide-induced mutation. A concentration of 100.0 mcg/plate was active on *S. typhimurium* TA 102 vs gamma-ray-induced mutation. Concentration of 3.0 mcg/plate was active on *S. typhimurium* TA 100 vs adriamycin-induced mutation. A concentration of 5.0 mcg/plate was inactive on *S. typhimurium* TA 100 and TA 98 vs 2-nitrofluorene-induced mutation. A concentration of 50.0 microliters/ml was active on *S. typhimurium* TA 102 vs cumene hydroperoxide-, T-butyl hydroperoxide-, hydrogen peroxide-, mitomycin C-, and streptomycin- induced mutations, and on TA 100 vs N-methyl-N- nitrosoguanidine-induced mutation[AS187].

Antimycobacterial activity. Bulb, taken orally at variable dosage levels by a group of 55 patients, was active on *Mycobacterium tuberculosis*[AS297]. Juice of the bulb, on agar plate, produced strong activity on M. *tuberculosis*[AS017]. Chloroform and water extracts of fresh bulbs, on agar plate at concentration of 1.0 mg/ml, produced weak activity on *Mycobacterium avium*[AS094]. Dried bulb, in broth culture, was active on *Mycobacterium tuberculosis* and *Mycobacterium intracellular*, MIC 1.72 and 2.29 mg/ml respectively. No synergy between garlic extract and any of 4 antituberculosis drugs (Isonazid, streptomycin, ethambutal, and rifampin) was observed[AS393]. Essential oil of the fresh bulb, on agar plate and when administered intraperitoneally to guinea pigs, was active on *Mycobacterium tuber-culosis*[AS086]. Ethanol (95%) extract of the bulb, on agar plate, was inactive on *Mycobacterium tuberculosis*[AS436].

Antineoplastic effect. Oil and water-soluble allyl sulfur compounds from garlic have been found to possess antitumorigenic properties. The property inceases as exposure increases both in vitro and in vivo. The ability of these compounds to suppress proliferation is associated with a depression in cell cycle progression and the induction of apoptosis. The depression in cell division coincides with an increase in the percentage of cell blocked in the G(2)/M phase of the cell cycle[AS528].

Antinephrotic activity. Garlic, administered orally to rats with acute and chronic nephrotic syndrome (NS) induced by apuromycin aminonucleoside, was unable to modify proteinuria in either acute or chronic NS, and hypercholesterolemia and hypertriglyceridemia in acute NS rats. The treatment diminished significantly total-cholesterol, LDL-cholesterol and triglycerides, but not HDL-cholesterol in chronic NS. Garlic induced no change in the percentage of sclerotic glomeruli in chronic NS and a significant decrease on the percentage of sclerotic area of the glomeruli[AS545].

Antioxidant activity. Ethanol/water (1:1) extract of aged bulbs at a concentration of 0.15% produced 30.7% inhibition of low-level chemiluminescence[AS123]. Fresh bulb at a concentration of 1.0% was active. The effect was seen at 120° F[AS144]. Hot water extract of aged bulbs, at a concentration of 2.0 mg/ml, was active vs hydrogen peroxide-induced LDH release and lipid peroxidation[AS128]. Powdered dried bulbs was able to reduce radicals generated by Fenton reaction. There were also marked quenching effects on radicals present in cigarette smoke[AS124]. Resin of dried bulb, at a concentration of 0.06%, was inactive. Lard was used as a substrate in the antioxidant activity test. Water extract of the dried bulbs, at a concentration of 10.0 mcg/ml, was active against photo-induced and superoxide radical mediated autoxidation of luminol. Photochemiluminescence method of detection was employed[AS125]. A concentration of 100.0 mcg/ml was active when tested in respect to the Cu2+-initiated oxidation of low-density lipoprotein. The extract showed dose-related oxidation-inhibiting effects. Garlic homogenate, administered orally to Wistar albino rats (150–200 gms) of either sex 6 days/week for 30 days at doses of 125, 250, 500, 1000, and 2000 mg/kg, produced dose-dependent augmented endogenous antioxidant effect, which has important direct cytoprotective effects on the heart, especially in the event of oxidant stress induced injury[AS499]. Fresh bulb homogenate, administered by gastric intubation to Wistar albino rats at doses of 250, 500, and 1000 mg/kg/day for 30 days, significantly reduced thiobarbituric acid reactive substances and glutathione peroxidase in the liver and kidneys. There was no change in catalase and reduced glutathione but superoxide dismutase increased significantly. The 500 and 1000 mg doses significantly reduced endogenous antioxidants with altering thiobarbituric acid reactive substances. The 1000 mg dose produced marked histopathological and ultrastructural changes in both liver and kidneys[AS511]. Diallyl sulfide, administered orally to mice at a dose of 200 mg/kg daily for 5 or 20 days after they were orally infected with *Trichinella spiralis* larvae, decreased thiobarbituric acid reactive substances and the agent did not have any effect on the total antioxidant status of blood in the Trichinella-infected mice[AS513]. Aged bulb as well as its components (S-allylcysteine and N-alpha-1(-deoxy-D-fructose-1-yl)-L-arginine (fructosyl arginine), inhibited the formation of dense erythrocytes in sickle cell anemia patients, in vitro[AS525]. Strong activity was found in the compound N-alpha-(1-deoxy-D-Fructos-1-yl)-L-arginine. The activity was comparable to that of ascorbic acid, scavenging hydrogen peroxide completely at 50 micromol/L and 37% at 10 micromol/L. Quantitative analysis using HPLC system revealed that the aged garlic extract contained 2.1–2.4 mmol/L, but none was detected in either raw or heated garlic juice. Further more it was shown that a minimum of 4 months of aging incubation was required for N-alpha-(1-deoxy-D-Fructos-1-yl)-L-arginine to be generated[AS537]. Bulbs, administered orally to rats at a concentration of 2% of the diet, decreased catalse activity and content, and catalase mRNA levels were unchanged in liver and kidneys. Catalase synthesis decreased and catalase degradation remained unchanged. In vivo H_2O_2 generation in kidneys and liver was markedly decreased in garlic-fed rats which could be due to a direct antioxidant effect of garlic[AS539]. Extract of garlic, administered orally to male Wistar rats for 5 consecutive days before intraperitoneal injection of N-methyl-N-nitro-N-nitrosoguanidine, enhanced lipid peroxidation in the stomach, liver and circulation of the treated rats. There was a significant decrease in glutathione and the activities of glutathione peroxidase, glutathione-S-transferase, and gamma glutamyl transpeptidase[AS552].

Antiproliferative effects. The bulb has shown to have significant antiproliferative actions on human cancers. Both hormone-responsive and hormone-unresponsive cell lines responded. The effects shown include induction of apoptosis, regulation of cell cycle progression and modification of pathways of signal transduction[AS529].

Antiprotozoan activity. Fresh bulb juice, undiluted in broth culture, was active on *Paramecium caudatum*[AS434]. Bulbs, administered orally to BALB/c mice at a dose of 20 mg/kg/day from day 30 after infection of leishmaniasis, for 2 weeks, was more effective than the usual antileishmanial drug in curing the infection. The treated mice developed Th1-type cytokine responses. In contrast, glucantime therapy led to a Th2-type response in the control group with a lower level of IL-2. However, a combination of garlic and glucantime treatment was more effective that either treatment alone, and resulted in a Th1-type response similar to that which developed with garlic treatment[AS541]. Whole garlic extract produced an IC_{50} at 24 hr of 0.3 mg/ml. Most of the components assayed were inhibitory to the organism, especially allyl alcohol and allyl mercaptan, with IC_{50} values of 7 microgram/ml and 37 microgram/ml, respectively. The surface topography and internal architecture of the organism changed during the incubation. Both whole garlic and allyl alcohol produced fragmentation of the disc and an overexpression of disc microribbons, internalization of flagella, vacuole formation and an increase in distended vesicles. Allyl mercaptan, however, only produced an increase in distended vesicles[AS543].

Antispasmodic activity. Butanol extract of the bulb, taken orally by 30 patients suffering from dyspepsia, gave moderate to full relief of major symptoms, i.e., abdominal distention and discomfort, belching and flatulence[AS290]. Water extract of the bulb, at a concentration of 1.0 mg/ml, was active on ureter[AS107]. Water extract of the dried bulb was active on the guinea pig small intestine. The biological activity was highly dose-dependent vs ACh-, barium- and histamine-induced contractions[AS251].

Antispermatogenic effect. Dried bulbs, administered by gastric intubation to male rats at a dose of 50.0 mg/animal daily for 45 and 70 days, caused spermatogenesis arrest at primary spermatocyte stage. The spermatogenesis arrest is claimed to be a secondary result of hypoglycemia-hypolipidemia[AS296]. Undiluted essential oil,

administered by inhalation to male rats, was inactive[AS443]. Water extract in the drinking water of mice, at a dose of 100.0 mg/kg, was inactive[AS431].

Antithiamine activity. Fresh bulb juice was active. The activity was heat stable[AS347].

Antithrombotic effect. Fresh bulb extract, administered intravenously to dogs at a dose of 1.0 ml/animal, was active. Cyclic flow reductions in an artificially stenosed coronary artery were inhibited by administration of the extract. This is attributed to inhibition of cyclic thrombus formation/embolization. Epinephrine reversed this effect[AS426]. Methyl allyltrisulfide, a component present in steam-distilled garlic oil, has been demonstrated to inhibit arachidonic acid cascade at the reaction site with PGH synthase. However, this enzyme catalyzes 2 successive reactions, from arachidonic acid to PGG2, and from PGG2 to PGH2. It was revealed that methyl allyltrisulfide inhibited the latter reaction[AS538].

Antitoxic activity. Butanol extract of the dried bulb, in the ration of rats at a dose of 6.7% of the diet, was active vs cadmium toxicity[AS344]. Dried bulb, in the ration of rats at a concentration of 6.7% of the diet for 10 weeks, was active vs methyl/mercury poisoning[AS383]. Dosing for 12 weeks lowered the effects of cadmium poisoning[AS363]. Butanol extract given for 12 weeks caused detoxication of phenylmercury poisoning[AS364]. Essential oil, administered by gastric intubation to rat at a dose of 100.0 mg/kg, was active. The dose prevented the ethanol-induced serum cholesterol and triglyceride rise, kidney and liver cholesterol accumulation, hepatic total lipid rise, and serum albumin reduction vs ethanol-induced hyperlipemia[AS354]. Fixed oil of the fresh bulb, in the ration of rats at a concentration of 1.5% of the diet, was active. The extract ameliorates pancreatic weight loss in animals on fructose and Cu-deficient diet[AS068]. Fresh bulb, administered intragastrically to mice at a dose of 100.0 mg/kg, was active. The frequency of chromosomal aberrations was significantly lower in animals maintained on crude plant extract during exposure to sodium arsenite, as compared to those treated with arsenite alone[AS109]. Ethanol (70%) extract of fresh bulbs, administered intraperitoneally to mice at a dose of 50.0 mg/kg, was active vs cyclophosphamide-induced toxicity, 77% ILS[AS417]. Butanol extract of dried bulbs, administered by gastric intubation to rats at a dose of 0.25 gm/kg, was active on liver, pancreas and heart vs isoprenaline-induced tissue necrosis[AS189].

Antitumor activity. Butanol extract of the dried bulb, in the ration of mice at a dose of 0.6 gm/day, was active on CA-Ehrlich-ascites. Results significant at $P < 0.001$ level[AS342]. Dried bulb, in the ration of mice, was active on Sarcoma 180 (solid). Ethanol (95%) extract of the bulb, administered intraperitoneally to rats at a dose of 50.0 mg/kg, produced weak activity on Sarcoma III(MTK)[AS028]. Fresh bulb, taken orally by human adults at variable dosage levels, was active. Interviews with 564 patients with stomach cancer and 1131 controls revealed a significant reduction in gastric cancer risk with increasing consumption of *Allium sativum*[AS173]. Whole plant, in the ration of female mice, produced complete inhibition of spontaneous leukemia in C3H mice[AS027]. Water extract of the bulb, administered intraperitoneally to mice at variable dosage levels, produced weak activity on CA-Ehrlich-Ascites[AS022], and on tumor system[AS297]. Water extract of the bulb, administered intravenously to mice, was active on Sarcoma 180(ASC)[AS014]. Water extract of the fresh bulb, administered intraperitoneally to mice at a dose of 50.0 mg/animal daily for 5 days, was active on CA-Ehrlich ascites, 17% ILS and Dalton's lymphoma, 9.1% ILS. Intragastric administration was active on CA-Ehrlich ascites,

41% ILS[AS211]. Essential oil, applied externally to female mice at a dose of 1.0 mg/animal, was active vs twice weekly 12-0-tetradecanoyl-phorbol-13-acetate-promotion (2 weeks) followed by mezerein promotion (2 weeks) followed by mezerein promotion (18 weeks). The dose, given with a second promoter, gave 24% decrease in incidence of papilloma[AS216]. Ethyl acetate extract of the fresh bulb, in cell culture at a concentration of 100.0 mcg/ml, was active on HELA cells, and a concentration of 5.0 mg/animal, administered externally to mice, was active vs 12-0-tetra-decanoyl-phorbol-13-acetate-induced tumor promotion[AS185]. The hot water extract, in cell culture, produced weak activity on RAJI cells vs phorbol myristate acetate-promoted expression of EB virus early antigen[AS078]. Fresh bulb was applied externally at a dose of 0.1 ml/animal, twice daily for 3 days every week before once per week application of DMBA, for 25 weeks. The incidence of tumors was decreased to 31.8% from 73.9% vs DMBA-induced carcinogenesis[AS223]. Water extract of the fresh bulb, applied externally to mice at a concentration of 200.0 microliters/animal, was active vs DMBA and croton oil treatment[AS211]. Fresh bulb, in the ration of Syrian hamsters at a dose of 10.0% of the diet, was active vs DMBA-induced carcinogenesis[AS218]. Hot water extract of the fresh bulb, applied externally to mice at a dose of 1.0 mg/animal, was active. Phorbol myristate acetate followed by dose of compound 30 minutes later. This promotion regime is repeated 3 times weekly for 47–60 weeks vs DMBA-induced carcinogenesis[AS412]. Aqueous extract, injected at the site of tumor transplantation of day 1 for 3 weeks and into established tumors for 5 weeks in combination with or without gene therapy using a replication-defective adenoviral vector containing a herpes simplex virus thymidine kinase gene under the transitional control of Rous sarcoma virus promoter plus ganciclovir, demonstrated a statistically significant reduction in incidence of transitional cell carcinoma. The extract combined with gene therapy had significant additive antitumor effects on transitional cell carcinoma[AS519]. Aqueous extract of the bulb, administered daily for 1 week, significantly augment splenic natural killer cells in vivo in generating cytotoxicity against YAC tumor targets[AS520]. Diallyl disulfide, administered orally to nude mice, resulted in a dose-dependent and significant inhibition of the growth of H-ras oncogene transformed NIH 3T3 cells implanted in the mice. The effect was apparent in terms of delay in the appearance of measurable tumors, tumor volume and tumor weight. On the other had, the growth of H-ras oncogene transformed tumors was not inhibited by dipropyl disulfide, a naturally occurring saturated analog of dially disulfide. The level of membrane-associated p21(H-ras) were markedly lower in the tumors of daillyl disulfide-treated mice than those of controls[AS531].

Antitussive activity. Fresh bulb, taken orally by human adults at variable dosage levels, was active[AS039]. Lyophilized extract of the dried bulb, inhaled by children at a dose of 1.0%, was effective against respiratory tract diseases[AS382].

Antiulcer activity. Fresh bulb, taken orally by human adults at variable dosage levels, was active[AS039].

Antiviral activity. Commercial sample of the bulb, in cell culture at a concentration of 0.15 mg/ml, was active on Herpes Simplex 1 virus, Influenza virus B (Lee), Coxsackie B1 virus and HELA cells. Results significant at $P < 0.001$ level[AS381]. Dried bulb, in cell culture, was active on Cytomegalovirus[AS083]. Fresh bulb pulp, in cell culture at a concentration of 1000 mg/ml, produced weak activity on Herpes Simplex 1 and 2 viruses, Parainfluenza virus 3, Vaccina virus Elstree and vesicular stomatitis virus[AS066].

Antiyeast activity. Amino acid fraction of dried bulb in ream form, 11% essential oil in gel, essential oil in wound healing powder, ethanol/chloroform (25%) extract on agar plate, and water extract, at a concentration of 0.313% in broth culture, were active on Candida albicans[AS253,AS254]. Juice, on agar plate at a concentration of 0.333%, was active on Candida guilliermondii, C. parapsilosis, C. tropicalis, C. albicans, C. stellatoidea, and C. krusei[AS247]. A concentration of 2.0% was active on Saccharomyces cerevisiae[AS252]. Concentrations of 0.0625, 0.125, and 0.25% in broth culture were active on Candida albicans, Candida krusei, Candida tropicalis, Cryptococcus neoformans, Candida parapsilosis, Candida stellatoidea, Cryptococcus albidus, Candida glabrata, and Candida guilliermondii[AS255]. A fresh extract of garlic, administered orally to human volunteers at a dose of 10–25 ml/person, produced weak activity. At intervals, serum and urine were collected and assayed for antifungal activity. The maximum tolerance dose of the extract was determined to be 25 ml, larger amounts produced severe burning sensations in the stomach and esophagus, and vomiting. After oral ingestion of the extract, anticandidal and anticryptococcal activities were detected in undiluted serum 0.5 and 1 hour after ingestion. No activity was found at comparable times in the urine. It was concluded that oral garlic is of limited value in the therapy of human fungal infections[AS245]. Dried oleoresin, on agar plate at a concentration of 500.0 ppm, was active on Debaryomyces hansenii vs ascospore production and Rhodotorula rubra vs pseudomycelium production; inactive on Candida lipolytica, Hansenula anomala, Lodderomyces elongisporus, Saccharomyces cerevisiae and Torulopsis glabrata vs pseudomycelium and ascospore production. In broth culture, a concentration of 50.0 ppm was active on Debaryomyces hansenii and Hansenula *anomala*, and at 500.0 ppm was active on *R. rubra* and *S. cerevisiae* vs biomass production. It was inactive on *Candida lipolytica*, *Kloeckera apiculata*, *Lodderomyces elongisporus* and *Torulopsis glabrata* vs biomass production[AS399]. Essential oil of dried bulb, on agar plate, was active on *Candida albicans*[AS253]. Essential oil, undiluted on agar plate, was active on *Candida albicans* and *C. monosa*[AS270]. Ethyl acetate extract of fresh bulb, on agar plate, was active on *Cryptococcus neoformans*, MIC 6.1 mcg/ml[AS127]. Water extract, on agar plate at a concentration of 5.0 mg/ml, was active on *Candida parapsilosis* and *C. tropicalis*, and inactive on *C. albicans*[AS191]. Water extract, administered intragastrically to mice at a dose of 0.5 ml/animal, produced weak activity on *Cryptococcus neoformans*[AS191]. Fresh bulb juice, undiluted on agar plate, was active on *Candida albicans*[AS465]. Fresh bulb, on agar plate, was inactive on *Candida stellatoide*, MIC 1000 mcg/ml and *C. albicans*, MIC 470.0 mcg/ml. Chloroform extract was inactive on *C. albicans*, MIC > 6.0 mg/ml[AS420]. Water extract, in broth culture, was active on *C. pseudotropicalis*, *C. tropicalis* and *C. albicans*, MIC 0.8 mg/ml[AS169]. Tincture of dried bulb, on agar plate at a concentration of 30.0 microliters/disk (10 gm plant material in 100 ml ethanol), was active on *Candida albicans*[AS405]. Methanol/water (1:1) extract of dried bulb, on agar plate, was active on *Candida albicans*[AS411]. Water extract of dried bulb, on agar plate, produced weak activity on *Candida albicans* and *Saccharomyces cerevisiae*[AS324]. Water extract of fresh bulb, in cell culture, was active on *Candida albicans*, MIC 0.8 mg/ml[AS200]. Water extract of fresh bulb, undiluted, was active on *Candida albicans*, *C. guilliermondii*, *C. krushei*, *C. parapsilosis*, *C. stellatoidea*, and *C. tropicalis*[AS163]. Water extract and chromatographic fraction of bulb, on agar plate, was active on *Candida albicans*[AS151]. Undiluted bulb juice, on agar plate, was active on

Trichosporum capitatum and *Candida pseudotropicalis*, 39 mm zone of inhibition; *Candida rugosa*, *Candida stellatoidea*, *Candida tropicalis* and *Candida krusei*, 40 mm zone of inhibition; *Cryptococcus neoformans*, *Cryptococcus laurentii*, *Rhodotorula rubra*, and *Trichosporon pullulans*, 37 mm zone of inhibition; *Cryptococcus terreus*, *Cryptococcus uniguttulatus* and *Candida albicans*, 36 mm zone of inhibition; *Candida guilliermondii* and *Candida tenuis*, 38 mm zone of inhibition; *Torulopsis glabrata*, 43 mm zone of inhibition; *Torulopsis candida* and *Torulopsis inconspicua*, 45 mm zone of inhibition[AS150]. Ethanol/water (1:1) extract of dried bulb, on agar plate at concentrations of 417.0 and 500.0 mg/ml (expressed as dry weight of bulb), was inactive on *Candida albicans* and *Saccharomyces pastorianus*[AS382].

Apoptosis induction. Ajoene significantly enhanced the activation of caspase-3 in both chemotherapeutic drugs cytarabine- and fludarabine-treated KGI human myeloid leukemia CD-34-positive-resistant cells. A dose of 40 microM of ajoene alone significantly reduced the bcl-2-expression from 239.5 ± 1.5 in control cultures to only 22.0 ± 4.0 in ajoene-treated cultures. Bcl-2-expression could not be detected in fludarabine plus ajoene-treated cultures[AS500].

Arichidonate metabolism inhibition. Ethanol (95%) extract, at a concentration of 40.0 mcg/ml, and water extract at a concentration of 20.0 microliters, in cell culture, were active on platelets[AS208].

Ascaricidal activity. Ether and ethanol (20%) extracts of bulb were active on *Ascaris lumbricoides*[AS457].

Aspartate aminotransferase induction. Essential oil, administered intragastrically to rats at a dose of 0.067 mg/gm, was active. Water extract of fresh bulbs, administered intragastrically to rats at a dose of 0.02 ml/gm, was active[AS210].

Atherosclerotic effect. The aged garlic extract, kyolic, was administered to rabbits fed a 1% cholesterol-enriched diet for 6 weeks at a dose of 800 ml/kg body weight. There was no reduction in plasma cholesterol but there was a 64% reduction of the surface area of the thoracic aorta covered by fatty streaks and significantly reduced aortic arch cholesterol. The extract also significantly inhibited by approximatley 50% of the development of thickened, lipid-filled lesions in preformed neointimas produced by Fogarty 2F balloon catheter injury of the right carotid artery in the cholesterol-fed rabbits. In vitro studies indicated that kyolic completely prevented vascular smooth muscle phenotypic change from contractile, high volume fraction of filament (V(v)myo) state, and inhibited proliferation of smooth muscle cells in the synthetic state with a 50% effective dose of 0.2%. Kyolic slightly inhibited the accumulation of lipid in cultured macrophages but not smooth muscle, and had no effect on the expression of adhesion molecules on the surface of the endothelium or the adherence of leukocytes[AS533].

ATP-ase (Na+/K+) inhibition. Aqueous (dialyzed) fraction of fresh bulb, at a concentration of 0.49 units, was active on the skin of toad. The extract was applied to the inner (serosal) surface of the skin. One unit of activity had the effect of 1 micromolar amiloride[AS225].

ATPase stimulation. Water extract of fresh bulb, at a concentration of 5.0 mg/ml, was active[AS257].

Bacterial stimulant activity. Dried oleoresin, in broth culture, was inactive on *Lactobacillus plantarum*. Fresh bulb, in broth culture at a concentration of 1.0 gm/liter, was active on *Lactobacillus plantarum*. Powdered dried bulb, in broth culture at a concentration of 5.0 gm/liter, was active on *Lactobacillus plantarum*[AS401].

Barbiturate potentiation. Ethanol (95%) extract of bulb, administered intraperitoneally to male mice at a dose of 500.0 mg/kg, was inactive[AS268].

Blood system effects. Butanol extract of fresh bulb, taken orally by human adults at a dose of 25.0 mg/day, was active. An 87-year-old man presented with paralysis of the lower extremities. A spinal mass proved to be a spontaneous spinal epidural hematoma. The hematoma was removed and the patient recovered adequately. The hematoma was attributed to the man's high consumption of garlic (4 cloves/day), as no other potential causes were found. Bleeding time during surgery was 11 minutes (3 minutes normal) and prothrombin time was 12.3 seconds[AS221].

Blood viscosity decrease. Dried bulbs were taken orally by 120 volunteers with a "probably increased thrombocyte aggregation", at a dose of 800.0 mg/person continued for 4 weeks in double-blind and placebo-controlled study. Plasma viscosity decreased by 3.2% vs control[AS419].

Body weight loss inhibition. Butanol extract of dried bulb, administered intragastrically to rats at a dose of 1.0 gm/kg, was active[AS189].

Bradycardia activity. Oven-dried bulb, administered to dog by gastric intubation at a dose of 15.0 mg/kg, was active. The action returned to normal after 15 minutes[AS418]. Water extract of dried leaves, administered intravenously to cats and rats at a dose of 5–20 mg/kg, produced weak activity[AS352].

Carcinogenesis inhibition. Dried bulb, in the ration of rats at a concentration of 2.0% of the diet, was active. Rats were fed the treatment diet for 20 weeks. The tumor incidence decreased from 85% to 40%, and the total number of tumors decreased from 41 to 18. In addition, the binding of DMBA to DNA decreased significantly vs carcinogenesis induced by 7,12-dimethylbenz-(a)anthracene[AS062]. Ethanol (20%) extract of 6 or 7 dried cloves, taken orally by 16 human adults daily for 3 months, was inactive[AS102]. Essential oil, applied externally to mice at a dose of 0.01 mg/animal, was active vs phorbol myristate acetate-induced carcinogenesis of mice skin[AS357]. Ethanol (95%) extract of dried bulb, in the drinking water of rats at a dose of 3.0 mg/ml for 9 weeks, was inactive. Hepatocarcinogenesis was induced by diethylnitrosamine[AS108]. Fresh bulb, administered intragastrically to mice at a dose of 400.0 mg/kg dosed 2 weeks before and 4 weeks following application of carcinogen, was active vs 3-methylcholanthrene-induced carcinogenesis in the uterine cervix[AS201]. Essential oil of fresh bulb, applied externally to mice at a dose of 100.0 microliters/animal, was active vs benzo(a)pyrene-induced skin carcinogenesis. Ten percent garlic oil in acetone and croton oil was also applied[AS181]. Fresh bulb, administered intragastrically to toad at a dose of 0.1 ml, was active vs aflatoxin B1-induced carcinogenesis (lung and kidney). Garlic oil, 0.1 ml dissolved in 1 ml of corn oil was administered for 4 months. The tumor incident decreased to 9%, which was originally 19% without the treatment. A dose of 20.0 mg/day was active vs aflatoxin B1-induced carcinogenesis (lung and kidney). Fresh garlic was administered for 4 months. The tumor incident decreased to 3%, which was originally 19% without the garlic treatment[AS103]. Fresh bulb, administered orally to hamsters at a dose of 0.5%/animal, was active. The extract was painted on the mucosa 3 times/week for 3 weeks. Eleven weeks later, DMBA (0.5%) was painted for 10 weeks. Six weeks later, animals were sacrificed. Controls were painted with extract for 30 weeks. Mineral oil was used as vehicle for the extract vs DMBA-induced carcinogenesis[AS217]. Powdered fresh bulb, in the ration of rats at a dose of 20.0 gm/kg, was active. Tumor incidence was reduced from 84% to 56%. Tumor incidence in rats fed selenium-enriched *Allium sativum* were reduced from 92% to 36% vs DMBA-induced carcinogenesis[AS055]. Water extract

of fresh bulb, administered by cheek pouch in mice, was active vs 7,12-dimethylbenz(A)anthracene-induced carcinogenesis[AS238].

Cardiotonic activity. Chloroform extract of dried bulb, contained at least 2 active elements. One was chloroform soluble and had an antiseptic action, a slight tonic effect on the isolated frog heart, a slight hypertensive effect on etherized cats and a paralyzing effect on the isolated rabbit intestine. The chloroform-insoluble fraction had no antiseptic effect, no action on the isolated frog heart, a strongly hypotensive effect on etherized cats and a tonic effect on the isolated rabbit intestine[AS459]. Garlicin, administered by intravenous drip at a dose of 60 mg/day for 10 days, showed that the total effective rate in improving symptoms and electrocardiogram after garlicin treatment was 82%. Nitroglycerine administered in 21 cases of the control group produced an effective rate of 62%[AS521].

Cardiotoxic activity. Essential oil of dried bulbs, administered intragastrically to rats at a dose of 2.0 gm/kg for 30 days, was active. Animals were maintained on normal diet while given the essential oil, then observed for 30 days. ECG showed flattened T-wave and depressed ST segment during the dosing period. The changes persisted after garlic withdrawal, indicating possible permanent coronary ischemic damage in 8 of 10 animals[AS400]. Ether extract of dried bulb was active on the frog heart. Effect is not reversed by norepinephrine and only partially reversed by caffeine or atropine[AS037].

Cardiovascular effects. Water extract of dried leaves, administered intravenously to cats and rats at a dose of 5–20 mg/kg, did not produced any appreciable alteration of ECG pattern[AS352].

Carminative activity. Dried bulb, taken orally at a dose of 0.64 gm/person, was active. In a series of 29 patients complaining of heaviness after eating, belching, gas colic, flatulence and nausea, 2 garlic tablets were given twice daily (after lunch and dinner) for a period of 2 weeks. A clinical investigation of dehydrated garlic showed this comparative to be highly effective for relief of heaviness after eating (epigastric and abdominal distress), belching, flatulence, gas colic, and nausea. Satisfactory therapeutic results were obtained in cases of flatulent dyspepsia, nervous dyspepsia and other gastric neuroses. Roentgenographically, a comparison of films with and without the medication showed that dehydrated garlic has a sedative effect on the stomach and intestines, relaxes spasms, retards hyperperistalsis, and disperses accumulation of gas. It is believed that these studies explained the carminative action of garlic as caused by unidentified principles that have been designated as gastroenteric allichalcone. Since dehydrated garlic tablets are safe for long continued use, they may be indicated in a wide variety of functional disturbances of the stomach and intestines[AS452].

Carnithine acetyl-coenzyme A transferase induction. Methanol extract of fresh bulb, in cell culture at a concentration 0.5 mg/ml, was active on rat hepatocytes[AS239].

Catecholamine-releasing effect. Fixed oil of fresh bulb, administered intragastrically to rabbit, was active vs cholesterol-fed animals[AS406].

Cell proliferation inhibition. Water extract of bulbs, in cell culture, was active on Morris hematoma[AS357]. Water extract of dried bulb, in cell culture at a concentration of 100.0 mcg/ml, was active on LEUK-P388(ARA-C). Cells transformed by SV-40 were more sensitive[AS114].

Chemopreventitive effect. Aged garlic extract (AGE), administered as 2% of the standard diet, depressed the absorption of fluorescein isothiocyanate-labeled dextran (FD-4) co-administered with the antitumor drugs methotrexate and 5-fluorouracil. FD-

4 absorption was increased in the antitumor drug-treated rats fed the diet without AGE[AS627]. Garlic juice, administered orally at a dose of 1.0 gm/kg simultaneously with 20 mg/kg methylmercury choride on day 7 of gestation, depressed the toxicity of methyl mercury chloride. There was a 10% decrease in maternal death rate, and 6.9% and 31.3% in pre- and post-implantation loss respectively[AS554].

Choleretic activity. Water extract of fresh bulb, in the ration of rats at a dose of 2%, was active[AS392].

Cholesterol acyltransferase inhibition. Water extract of dried bulb, in cell culture at a concentration of 1000 mcg/ml, was active on hepatocytes[AS232]. Water extract of fresh bulb, at a dose of 1.0 gm/kg in the ration of rabbit, was active[AS422].

Cholesterol inhibition. Plant, in the ration of rabbits, was active[AS051]. Unripe fruit juice, administered orally to cholesterol-fed male rabbits, was active[AS050]. Water extract of dried bulb, at a concentration of 20.0 microliters/insect, was active on *Lohita grandis*[AS372].

Cholesterol level decrease. Dried garlic, taken by human adults of both sexes at a dose of 200.0 mg/person, was active. Garlic-ginkgo combination tablets produced improvement in cholesterol, with no concurrent dietary or exercise changes[AS130]. Garlic powder, adminsitered orally to rats on a 2% cholesterol diet for 6 weeks, produced a significant reduction in the serum cholesterol levels compared with the group on high cholesterol diet without garlic powder[AS534].

Cholesterol synthesis inhibition. Chloroform and chloroform/acetone extracts of fresh bulbs, at concentrations of 166.0 mcg/ml, were active on liver homogenates. Synthesis was inhibited 52.1% and 44.4%, respectively[AS058]. Fresh bulb, in cell culture, was active on Hepatoma-HEP-G-2, IC_{50} 35.0 mcg/ml, and on rat hepatocytes, IC_{50}

90.0 mcg/ml. This inhibition was exerted at the level of hydroxymethylglutaryl-Co A reductase (HMG-Co A reductase) as indicated by direct enzymatic measurements and the absence of inhibition[AS088]. Water extract, in cell culture, was active on hepatocytes[AS232]. Water, methanol, and petroleum ether extracts of dried bulb, at concentrations of 50.0 gm/liter, were active on rat hepatocytes[AS113]. Eleven water-soluble and 6 lipid-solubel compounds of garlic were evaluated for inhibitory potential on cholesterogenesis in primary rat hepatocytes. Among the water-soluble compounds, A-allyl cysteine, S-ethyl cysteine, and S-propyl cysteine inhibited [2-14C]acetate incorporation into cholesterol in a concentration-dependent manner, achieving 42–55% maximal inhibition. Gamma-glutamyl-S-allyl cysteine, gamma-glutamyl-S-methyl cysteine, and gamma-glutamyl-S-propyl cysteine were less potent, producing only 16 to 29% inhibitions. Aliin, S-allyl-N-acetyl cysteine, S-allylsulfonyl alanine, and S-methyl cysteine had no effect on cholesterol synthesis. Of the lipid-soluble compounds, diallyl disulfide, diallyl trisulfide, and dipropyl disulfide depressed cholesterol synthesis by 10–25% at low concentrations (0.5 mmol/L or less), and abolish the synthesis at high concentrations (1.0 mmol/L or more). Diallyl sulfide, dipropyl sulfide, and methyl allyl sulfide inhibited [2–14C] acetate incorporation into cholesterol only at high concentrations. The complete depression of cholesterol synthesis by diallyl disulfide, diallyl trisulfide and dipropyl disulfide was associated with cytotoxicity as indicated by marked increase in cellular LDH release. There was no apparent increase in LDH secretion by the water-soluble compounds except S-allyl mercaptocysteine, which also abolished cholesterol synthesis[AS549].

Cholesterol-7-alpha-hydroxylase inhibition. Methanol extract of fresh bulbs, in the ration of pigs at a concentration of 3.15 gm/kg of diet for 29 days, was active. Hepatic enzymes assayed, and 40% inhibition was observed[AS178]. Water extract of bulbs, in the ration of chicken of both sexes at a concentration of 6.0% of the diet for 3 weeks, was active[AS322]. Water extract of dried bulb, in cell culture at a concentration of 1000 mcg/ml, was active on hepatocytes[AS232].

Cholinesterase inhibition. Water extract of fresh bulbs, at a concentration of 5.0 mg/ml, was active[AS257].

Chromosome aberration induction. Water extract of fresh bulb, administered intragastrically to mice at a dose of 100.0 mg/kg daily for 7 days, was active on bone marrow[AS084]. Water extract of the fresh bulb, administered intragastrically to mice at a dose of 100.0 mg/kg, was active on bone marrow cells vs sodium arsenite-, mitomycin- and cyclophosphamide-induced aberration[AS084].

Chronotropic effect (negative). Water extract of fresh bulbs, at a concentration of 0.1 mcg/kg, was active on the rat atria. When administered intravenously to dogs at a dose of 67.2 mg/kg, it was active[AS082].

Chronotrophic effect (positive). Essential oil of the dried bulb, administered intragastrically to rats at a dose of 2.0 gm/kg, was active during treatment and returned to normal after withdrawal. Animals maintained on normal diet were given essential oil for 30 days, then observed for 30 days[AS400]. Ethanol/water (1:1) extract of fresh bulb, administered by gastric intubation to rats at a dose of 40.0 ml/kg, was inactive[AS366]. Fresh bulb juice, administered intravenously to rats at a dose of 0.5 ml/animal, was active. There was a slight decrease in the P-R interval of the ECG[AS349].

Citrate lyase stimulation. Methanol extract of the fresh bulb, in the ration of pigs at a concentration of 3.15 gm/kg of diet for 29 days, was active. Hepatic enzymes were assayed[AS178].

CNS depressant activity. Ethanol (70%) extract of the fresh bulb, administered intraperitoneally to mice of both sexes at variable dosage levels, was active[AS315]. Ethanol (95%) extract of the bulb, administered intraperitoneally to male mice at a dose of 500.0 mg/kg, was inactive[AS268].

Coagulant activity. Essential oil, administered by gastric intubation to male rabbits at a dose of 1.0 gm/kg for 3 months, was active. Increased coagulation time was observed. Results significant at $P < 0.001$ level. Water extract of fresh bulb was active[AS237].

Common cold prevention. Allicin-containing garlic capsule, adminsterd daily for 12 weekds during the cold season, significantly prevented attack by the common cold. One hundred forty-six volunteers were randomized to receive a placebo or the allicin capsule. The active treatment group had significantly fewer colds than the placebo group (24 vs 65, $P < 0.001$)[AS504].

Conditioned avoidance response increased. Ethanol (95%) extract of the bulb, administered intragastrically to mice at a dose of 250.0 mg/kg, was active vs alcohol-induced deficits in acquisition and performance of "step-through" test[AS165].

Corticosteroid type activity. Ethyl acetate extract of the fresh bulb, administered intramuscularly to rats daily for 4 days, produced up to 4 times the normal 24 hour 17-keto steroid elimination[AS464].

Cyclo-oxygenase inhibition. Methanol extract of the dried bulb, at variable concentrations, was inactive vs ADP-, arachidonic acid-, epinephrine-, and thrombin-induced aggregation[AS333]. Chloroform extract of the bulb, administered to ewes at variable dosage levels, produced weak activity on platelets[AS301]. Chloroform and chloroform-acetone extracts of fresh bulb were active, IC_{50} 0.88 and 0.42 mcg/ml, respectively[AS432]. Fresh bulb was active vs DMBA-induced carcinogenesis[AS412]. The ether-soluble frac-

tion of methanol extract of the fresh bulb, at a concentration of 100.0 mcg/ml, produced 50% inhibition on rat platelets, and the ether-insoluble fraction produced 5% inhibition[AS087].

Cytochrome B-5 reductase inhibition. Water extract of the fresh bulb was active on liver microsomes[AS430].

Cytochrome C reductase inhibition. Methanol extract of fresh bulb, in cell culture at a concentration of 1.0 mg/ml, was inactive on rat hepatocytes[AS239].

Cytochrome oxidase induction. Essential oil of the dried bulb was inactive on *Macaronesia fortunata* and *Musca domestica*[AS485].

Cytochrome oxidase inhibition. Essential oil of the dried bulb was inactive on *Macaronesia fortunata* and *Musca domestica*[AS485].

Cytochrome P-450 inhibition. Water extract of the fresh bulb was active on liver microsomes[AS480]. Extracts of fresh garlic exhibited an inhibitory effect on cytochrome P450 mediated metabolism of a marker substrate. With the extracts tested, garlic had very low to moderate P-gp interaction as compared with the positive control verapamil[AS507].

Cytotoxic activity. Acetone extract of the dried bulb, at a concentration of 5.0% by the cylinder plate method, was equivocal on CA-Ehrlich-Ascites, 21 mm inhibition. Ether extract produced weak activity, 40 mm inhibition; water extract, equivocal, 20 mm inhibition; methanol extract, weak activity, 40 mm inhibition[AS441]. Ethanol (90%) extract of the dried bulb, in cell culture at a concentration of 0.5 mg/ml, was active on human lymphocytes; Vero cells, ED_{50} 0.155 mg/ml; Chinese hamster ovary cells (CHO), ED_{50} 0.275 mg/ml; and Dalton's Lymphoma, ED_{50} 0.5 mg/ml[AS160]. Ethanol (95%) extract of the fresh bulb, administered intragastrically to mice at a dose of 500.0 mg/kg, produced weak activity. The animals were dosed for 5 days followed by sacrifice of the animals and examination of marrow cells[AS205]. Fresh bulb, at a concentration of 200.0 mg/ml, was active on the rat liver. On perfusion through a liver preparation, diallyl disulfide and allyl mercaptan were the metabolites of garlic extract. Allicin did not appear in perfusate unless the concentration of extract became toxic[AS061]. Fresh bulb pulp, in cell culture at a concentration of 11.0 mg/ml, was active on HELA cells, and 3.5 mg/ml active on Vero cells[AS066]. Protein fraction of dried bulb, in cell culture at a concentration of 10.0 mcg/ml, was active on human lymphocytes; 5.0 mcg/ml active on LEUK-K562 and melanoma-M14, cytotoxicity was enhanced with IL-2[AS099]. Water extract of dried bulb, in cell culture at a concentration of 500.0 mcg/ml, produced weak activity on CA-Mammary-Microalveolar[AS227], and Fibroblast-Human-Lung-MRC-5[AS083]. Water extract of freeze-dried bulb, in cell culture, was inactive on LEUK-P815. Tumor toxic activity was evaluated by culturing mastocytoma P815 cells with macrophage cells and measuring the incorporation of ^{3}H-thimidine radioactivity. Allyl mercaptan, diallyl sulfide, diallyl trisulfide, steamed-distilled garlic oil, and vinyl-dithiin oil of garlic, at doses of 5, 25, 50, 125, 250, and 500 microgram/ml each, incubated in Hep-G2 cells, produced no significant cytotoxic effect in any group at concentrations up to 250 microgram/L. At concentrations above 250 microgram/L, the cell viability decreased drastically in all groups compared to control. At 25 microgram/L, for 4 hours, [^{3}H]acetate incorporation into cholesterol was significantly inhibited. The secretion of cholesterol into the medium was also significantly decreased in all groups except for vinyl-dithiin oil. The treatment had no effect on either [^{3}H]acetate incorporation into fatty acids or [^{3}H]glycerol incorporation into triglyceride or phospholipid[AS547].

Death. Essential oil, applied externally to mice at a dose of 10.0 mg/animal, was active[AS357].

Dermatitis producing effect. Butanol extract of fresh bulbs, applied topically to human adults, was active in 34 patients who developed contact dermatitis after exposure to *Allium sativum*[AS075]. Dried bulb, taken orally by male human adults in a double-blind oral provocation test to garlic tablets, was active[AS122]. Fresh bulb, applied externally to 3 males presented with bulbous eruptions on the arms and legs, was active. Questioning 2 of the subjects revealed that they had repeatedly rubbed crushed garlic onto the affected areas in hopes of inducing dermatitis in order to elude their military assignments[AS413].

Desmutagenic activity. Aqueous high speed supernatant of fresh fruit juice, at a concentration of 0.5 ml/plate on agar plate, was inactive on *Salmonella typhimurium* TA98 vs mutagenicity of L-tryptophan pyrolysis products. The assay was done in the presence of S9 mix[AS380].

Diuretic activity. Ethanol/water (1:1) extract of fresh bulbs (5 parts plant material in 100 parts ethanol/water), administered intragastrically to rats at a dose of 40.0 ml/kg, was active[AS167]. Oven-dried bulbs, administered by gastric intubation to dog at a dose of 10.0 mg/kg, was active[AS418]. Water extract of dried bulb, administered intragastrically to rats at a dose of 5.0 gm/kg, was inactive[AS193]. Purified fraction of the bulb, administered intravenously to anaesthesized dogs at a dose of 6 microgram/kg, produced a significant biphasic and natriuretic response, which reached a maximum at 180 min after injection. Chloride followed the natriuretic profile; potassium ions did not. No changes were observed in arterial blood pressure or in the electrocardiogram. The purified extract also induced an inhibitory dose-dependent effect on kidney Na, K-ATPase[AS551].

DNA protective effect. Diallyl sulfide and diallyl disulfide, applied in vitro to primary rat hepatocytes at doses of 0.5 and 2 mM and 0.5 and 1 mM, respectively, damaged by aflatoxin B1, significantly decreased DNA damage[AS515].

DNA repair induction. Water extract of the fresh bulb, at a concentration of 20.0 microliters/ml, was active[AS187].

DNA synthesis inhibition. Ethanol (90%) extract of dried bulb, at a concentration of 1.0 mg/ml, was active[AS160].

DNA-binding inhibition. Dried bulb, in the ration of rats at a concentration of 1.0%, water extract, at a concentration of 0.75%, and ethanol (95%) extract, at a concentration of 0.015% of the diet for 2 weeks prior to DMBA exposure, were active vs dimethyl-bene[A]anthracene binding to mammary cell DNA[AS090].

Dopamine-beta-hydroxylase stimulation. Fixed oil of fresh bulb, administered intragastrically to rabbit at a dose of 5.0 mg/kg, was active[AS406].

Early antigen viral induction inhibition. Dried bulb, in cell culture, was active on Cytomegalovirus[AS083].

Embryotoxic effect. Ethanol (95%) extract of seeds, at doses of 150.0 and 200.0 mg/kg, and petroleum ether extract, at a dose of 100.0 mg/kg, administered orally to female rats[AS438]; and a dose of 150.0 mg/kg administered by gastric intubation to pregnant rats, were inactive[AS305].

Enzyme effects. Ethanol (95%) extract of dried bulb, administered by gastric intubation to male rats at a dose of 100.0 mg/kg for 25 days, was active. Adipose tissue triglyceride lipase increased. Results significant at $P < 0.01$ level[AS340].

Estrogenic effect. Bulb juice, administered orally to immature rats at a dose of 10.0 ml/kg, produced weak activity. Ethanol (95%) extract of dried bulb, administered subcutaneously to ovariectomized rats at a dose of 2.0 mg/animal was active[AS446]. Water extract of fresh bulb, administered intraperitoneally to female mice at a dose of 500.0 mg/day, was inactive[AS431]. Water extract of

the bulb, administered subcutaneously to infant mice, was active[AS439].

Ethanol elimination increased. Ethanol (95%) extract of the bulb, administered intragastrically to mice at a dose of 125.0 mg/kg, was active. It lowered blood alcohol levels relative to controls when administered simultaneously with alcohol, but not 30 minutes before alcohol[AS165].

Ethoxycoumarin deethylase inhibition. Water extract of the fresh bulb was active on liver microsomes[AS430].

Fatty acid content decrease. Powdered, dried bulb, in the ration of rats at a concentration of 1.0% of the diet for 10 weeks, did not alter fatty acid composition of myocardial membrane[AS073].

Fatty acid synthase inhibition. Water extract of the bulb, in the ration of chicken of both sexes at a concentration of 6.0% of the diet for 3 weeks, was active on hepatocytes[AS322]. Water extract of the dried bulb, in cell culture at a concentration of 1000 mcg/ml, was active on hepatocytes[AS232].

Fatty acid synthase stimulation. Methanol extract of fresh bulb, in the ration of pigs at a concentration of 3.15 gm/kg of the diet for 29 days, was active. Hepatic enzymes were assayed[AS178].

Fatty acid synthesis inhibition. Water, methanol, and petroleum ether extracts of dried bulb, at concentrations of 50.0 gm/liter, were active on rat hepatocytes. If oleate was present, incorporation of labeled glycerol into triglycerides and phospholipids was not inhibited[AS113].

Fibrinolytic activity. Butanol extract of the dried bulb, taken orally by human adults, was active in the blood of patients with alimentary lipemia. Juice, in the ration of rabbits, was active[AS332]. Dried bulb, taken orally by human adults at a dose of 300.0 mg/person 3 times daily for 2 weeks by 7 healthy males, increased specific tissue plasminogen activator[AS077]. Dried bulb, taken orally by human adults at a dose of 600.0 mg/person for 4 weeks, was active[AS183]. Essential oil of bulb, administered by gastric intubation to male rabbits at a dose of 1.0 gm/kg for 3 months, caused a decrease in fibrinolytic activity. Results significant at $P < 0.001$ level[AS339]. The ether extract, administered by gastric intubation to rats in a feeding study at doses of 2–4 gm crude garlic daily for three weeks, was active[AS293]. Essential oil, taken orally by human adults of both sexes at a dose equivalent to 1.0 gm/kg of raw garlic daily for 3 months, was active[AS272]. The essential oil, taken orally, was also active in 30 patients with myocardial infarct and 10 normal (controls)[AS149]. Fresh bulb, taken orally by human adults at a dose of 0.5 gm/kg, was active. The study was conducted with 20 patients with ischemic heart disease. Fibrinolytic activity increased by 72% within six hours after administration and persisted for 12 hours[AS312]. Butanol extract of fresh bulb taken orally by human adults[AS266] and water extract in the ration of rabbit[AS422], at doses of 1.0 gm/kg, were active. Fried bulb, taken orally by human adults at a dose of 0.5 gm/kg, was active in 20 patients with ischemic heart disease. Fibrinolytic activity increased by 63% within 6 hours after administration and persisted for 12 hours[AS312]. Water extract of the fresh bulb was active[AS237].

Food consumption reduction. Dried bulb, together with *Panax ginseng* and Vitamin B1, administered by gastric intubation to rats at a dose 10.0 ml/kg for 3 months, was equivocal. Food consumption was lowered after 2–5 weeks, however, body weight gain was good[AS371].

Fungal stimulant. Butanol extract of fresh bulb, on agar plate at variable concentrations, was inactive on *Bacillus subtilis* M-45(Rec-)[AS336]. Dried bulb juice, on agar plate at a concentration of 2.0%, was active on *Absidia spinosa*, *Drechslera maydis*, *Pleurotus ostreatus* and *Sordaria fimicola*[AS252].

Gastric antisecretory activity. Dried bulb, taken orally by human adults, was inactive[AS491].

Gastric inhibitory polypeptide stimulation. Bulb, in the ration of rabbits and rats, was active vs cholesterol-loaded animals[AS295].

Gastric mucosal exfoliant activity. Water extract of fresh bulb, administered to human adults by gastric intubation at a dose of 0.75 gm/person, was active[AS219]. Dehydrated raw garlic powder (RGP), dehydrated boiled garlic powder (BGP), and aged garlic extract (AGE) was administered by endoscopic air-powered delivery system directly into the stomach. Among the 3 preparations, RGP produced severe damage, including erosion. BGP aslo produced reddening of the mucosa, whereas AGE did not produce any undesirable effects. Direct administration of pulverized enteric-coated products caused reddening of the mucosa. When an enteric-coated tablet was administered orally, it caused loss of epithelial cells at the top of crypts in the ileum[AS522].

Gastric secretory stimulation. Dried bulb, taken orally by human adults, was inactive[AS491].

Genotoxicity activity. Bulbs, administered by gastric intubation to mice at doses of 2.5 and 5.0 gm/kg, were inactive on bone marrow cells[AS329].

Germ tube growth inhibition. Water extract of the fresh bulb, in cell culture at a concentration of 0.4 mg/ml, was active on *Candida albicans*[AS200].

Glucose utilization stimulation. Protein fraction of the bulb, at a concentration of 100.0 mcg/ml, was active on macrophages[AS394].

Glucose-6-phosphate dehydrogenase inhibition. Bulbs, in the ration of 4-month old male rats at concentrations of 2.0 and 4.0% of the diet, was active in cholesterol-loaded and lard fed animals. Results significant at $P < 0.05$ level[AS301]. Methanol extract of fresh bulb, in the ration of pigs at a concentration of 3.15 gm/kg of the diet for 29 days, was active. Hepatic enzymes were assayed[AS178]. Dried bulb, in the ration of male rats at a concentration of 5.0% of the diet, was active[AS118]. Fixed oil of fresh bulb, in the ration of rats at a concentration of 1.5% of the diet, was active. The extract ameliorated increased in enzyme activity seen in animals fed fructose and Cu-adequate diet[AS068].

Glucose-6-phosphate dehydrogenase stimulation. Butanol extract of dried bulb, administered intragastrically to rats at a dose of 0.5 gm/kg, was active on heart, liver and pancreas vs isoprenaline-induced tissue necrosis[AS189].

Glutamate dehydrogenase stimulation. Methanol extract of the fresh bulb, in cell culture at a concentration of 1.0 mg/ml, was inactive on rat hepatocytes[AS239].

Glutamate oxaloacetate inhibition. Water extract of fresh bulbs, at a concentration of 10.0 mg/ml, was active[AS257].

Glutamate oxaloacetate transaminase inhibition. Essential oil and ether extract of dried bulb, administered by gastric intubation to rats at a dose of 5.0 mg/kg for 3 days, was active vs galactosamine-induced toxicity[AS369].

Glutamate oxaloacetate transaminase stimulation. Essential oil of dried bulb, administered orally to rats at a dose of 5.0 mg/kg for 3 days, produced weak activity. The ether extract was inactive[AS369].

Glutamate pyruvate inhibition. Water extract of the fresh bulb, at a concentration of 5.0 mg/ml, was active[AS257].

Glutamate pyruvate transaminase inhibition. Essential oil and ether extract of dried bulb, in cell culture at a concentration of 1.0 mg/ml, were inactive on rat hepatocytes. Essential oil, administered by gastric intubation to rats at a dose of 5.0 mg/kg for 3 days, was inactive. Ether extract, administered orally at a dose of 5.0 mg/kg for 3 days, was active vs galactosamine-induced toxicity[AS369].

Glutathione peroxidase inhibition. Lyophilized extract of fresh bulb, in the ration of chicken at a concentration of 2.0% of the diet, was active[AS057].

Glutathione peroxidase stimulation. Butanol extract of dried bulb, at a concentration of 13.0 mcg/ml, was active on rat liver microsomes. Juice, administered by gastric intubation to rats at a dose of 5.0% of the diet for 25 days, was active in liver[AS378]. Dried bulb, in the ration of castrated rams at a concentration of 5.0% of the diet, was active[AS118].

Glutathione reductase stimulation. Dried bulb, in the ration of male rats at a concentration of 5.0% of the diet, was active[AS118].

Glutathione transferase induction. Dried bulb, in the ration of male rats at a concentration of 5.0% of the diet, was active[AS118].

Glutathione-S-transferase induction. Dried bulb, in the ration of rats at a concentration of 2.0% of the diet, was active. Glutathione-S-transferase levels were 42% greater in rats fed the supplemented diet[AS062]. Dried bulb juice, in the drinking water of rats at a dose of 5.0% of the diet for 25 days, was active in liver[AS378].

Glutathione-S-transferase inhibition. Butanol extract of dried bulb, at a concentration of 8.0 mcg/ml, was active on rat liver microsomes[AS378].

GRAS status. Approved as a Generally Recognized As Safe flavoring agent by the United States of America Food and Drug Administration in 1976 (Sect. 582.10)[AS048].

Hair stimulant effect. Decoction of dried bulb, in a mixture with *Polygonum multiflorum*, *Allium sativum*, *Zingiber officinale*, *Panax ginseng*, *Carthamus tinctorius*, *Platycodon grandiflorum*, *Biota orientalis*, *Ligusticum wallichii*, *Salvia miltiorrhiza*, *Angelica sinensis*, and *Tetrapanax papyrifera* stimulated hair growth. The biological activity has been patented[AS065]. Decoction of fresh bulb, together with extracts of *Polygonum multiflorum*, *Thuja orientalis*, *Zingiber officinale*, *Ligusticum wallichii*, *Salvia miltiorrhiza*, *Angelica sinensis*, *Carthamus* *tinctorius* and *Tetrapanax* species, was active. The biological activity reported has been patented[AS069]. Fresh bulb juice, applied topically to male mice at a concentration of 0.1 ml/liter, was inactive[AS316].

Hematopoietic activity. Fixed oil of fresh bulb, in the ration of rats at a concentration of 1.5% of the diet, was active. The extract ameliorates decrease in hematocrit in animals on fructose and Cu-deficient diet[AS068].

Hepatotoxic activity. Dried bulb juice, in the drinking water of rats at a dose of 5.0% of the diet for 25 days, was inactive[AS378].

Histamine release inhibition. Ethanol (75%) extract of fixed oil, in cell culture, was active on human basophils. The biological activity has been patented[AS138].

HMG-CO-A inhibition. Water extract of bulb, in the ration of chicken of both sexes, at a concentration of 6.0% of the diet for 3 weeks, was active on the hepatocytes[AS322].

HMG-CO-A reductase inhibition. Water extract of dried bulb, in cell culture at a concentration of 50.0 mcg/ml, was active on hepatocytes[AS232]. Methanol extract of fresh bulb, in the ration of pigs at a concentration of 3.15 gm/kg of the diet for 29 days, was active. Hepatic enzymes were assayed and 40% inhibition was observed[AS178].

Hypercholesterolemic activity. Bulb, taken orally by human adults, was active. Cholesterol levels were elevated in subjects on moderate or heavy amounts of onion, 50–100 gm, and garlic, 5–10 gm[AS111]. Dried bulb, taken orally by human adults at a dose of 350.0 mg/person twice daily, was inactive[AS170]. Essential oil of dried bulb, administered intragastrically to rats at a dose of 2.0 gm/kg, was active. Animals were maintained on normal diet and given essential oil for 30 days, then observed for 30 days. Fixed oil of fresh bulb, in the ration of rat at a concentration of 1.5% of the diet, was active. The extract was effective in animals fed fructose and Cu-deficient diet[AS068].

Hyperlipidemic activity. Dried bulb, taken orally by human adults at a dose of 350.0 mg/person twice daily, was inactive[AS254].

Hypertensive activity. Ethanol (95%) extract of bulb, administered to dogs and rats by injection at variable dosage levels, were active[AS445]. Chloroform extract of dried bulb, administered intravenously to cats, produced weak activity. The alcoholic extract contained at least 2 active elements. One was chloroform-soluble and had an antiseptic action, a slight tonic effect on isolated frog heart, a slight hypertensive effect on etherized cats, and a paralyzing effect on isolated rabbit intestine. The chloroform-insoluble fraction had no antiseptic effect, no action on isolated frog heart, a strongly hypotensive effect on etherized cats and a tonic effect on isolated rabbit intestine[AS459].

Hypertriglyceridemic activity. Dried bulb, taken orally by 24 human adults with reduced HDL cholesterol levels and hypertriglyceridemia at a dose of 900.0 mg/day for 6 weeks, reduced triglyceride levels up to 35% and HDL cholesterol levels increased[AS072].

Hyperuremic activity. Essential oil, administered intragastrically to rats after fasting for 24 hours at a dose of 0.067 mg/gm, was active[AS210]. Water extract of fresh bulb, administered intragastrically to rats at variable dosage levels, was active[AS493].

Hypocholesterolemic activity. Dried bulb, administered by gastric intubation to male rats at a dose of 50.0 mg/animal daily for 70 days, was active. Results significant at $P < 0.001$ level[AS296]. When administered for 45 days the dose was also active. Results significant at $P < 0.05$ level[AS296]. Dried bulb, in the ration of rats at variable concentrations for 41 days, was active. Essential oil, taken orally by human adults at a dose of 0.25 ml/person daily for 1–2 months, was inactive[AS311]. Essential oil, taken orally by human adults of both sexes at a dose of 0.25 mg/kg, was active. The study was conducted with 20 subjects having a normal serum cholesterol level. Garlic oil was consumed daily for 10 months[AS289]. Ether extract of bulb, administered by gastric intubation to rats in a feeding study at doses of 2–4 gm crude garlic daily for three days, was inactive[AS298]. Water extract of bulb, taken orally by human adults at a dose of 0.5 ml/kg, was active[AS146]. Fresh bulb, taken orally by human adults at a dose of 4.0 ml/days, was active[AS212]. Methanol extract of fresh bulb, in the ration of pigs at a concentration of 3.15 gm/kg of the diet for 29 days, was active. Serum total cholesterol plus LDL cholesterol decreased, and HDL cholesterol was anomalously high after 29 days of feeding. Lyophilized extract of fresh bulb, in the ration of chicken at a concentration of 2.0% of the diet, was active[AS057]. Powdered fresh bulb, taken orally by human adults at a dose of 800.0 mg/day, was active on 221 hypercholesterolemic patients given treatment for a total of 16 weeks. Serum cholesterol levels dropped 12%[AS220]. Water extract of bulb, in the ration of chicken of both sexes at a concentration of 6.0% of the diet for 3 weeks, was active[AS322]. Water extract of fresh bulb, taken orally by human adults with normal blood serum cholesterol levels at a dose of 50.0 gm/person, was inactive[AS331]. Fresh bulb, taken orally by 25 healthy male adults (18–35 years) at a dose of 10.0 gm/person daily for 2 months, was active[AS269]. Garlic powder tablets with 9.6 mg allicin-releasing potential or matching placebo tablets were administered to mild to moderate hypercholesterolemic patients. After 12 weeks, the garlic supplement group had a significant reduction in total cholesterol (TC, 0.36 mmol/L) and LDL-cholesterol (LDL-C, 0.44 mmol/L) while the placebo group had a non-significant increase in TC (0.13 mmol/L) and LDL-C (0.18 mmol/L). HDL-cholesterol was significantly increased in the placebo group (0.09 mmol/L), compared to the garlic group (0.02 mmol/L). There

was no significant difference in triglycerides or in LDL/HDL ratio between the groups[AS510]. Raw and frozen garlic fractions, administered orally to rats, produced a decrease in plasma total cholesterol. This effect was higher in rats fed raw fractions. LDL decreased significantly with respect to the hypercholesterolemic group in all groups treated; however, an increase in HDL was found in those treated with the frozen fraction. The liver:body weight ratio decreased in all treated groups. The relaxing effect of acetylcholine was enhanced in arteries contracted with norepinephrine[AS535]. Lipid-soluble sulfur compounds (diallyl sulfide, diallyl disulfide, diallyl trisulfide, diporpyl sulfide and dipropyl trisulfide) at lower concentrations (0.05–0.5 mol/L) slightly inhibited cholesterol synthesis (10–15%) but became highly cytotoxic at high concentrations (1.0–4.0 mol/L). The water-soluble compounds, except S-allylmercaptocysteine, were not cytotoxic, judging from the release of cellular lactate dehydrogenase into the culture medium. Taken together, the results of our studies indicated that the cholesterol-lowering effects of garlic extract, such as aged garlic extract, stem in part from the inhibition of hepatic cholesterol synthesis by water-soluble sulfur compounds, especially S-allycysteine[AS536].

Hypoglycemic activity. Bulb, in the ration of 16-week-old male rats at concentrations of 2.0 and 4.0% of the diet, was active in cholesterol-loaded and lard-fed animals. Results significant at $P < 0.05$ level[AS301]. Dried bulb, administered by gastric intubation to male rats at a dose of 50.0 mg/animal for 45 and 70 days, was active. Results significant at $P < 0.001$ level. Water extract of dried bulb, administered orally to rabbits at a dose of 3.3 gm/kg daily for 2 months, was active on sucrose-loaded animals (10 gm/kg/day). Statistical report indicated significant results[AS279]. Dried bulb, taken orally by 120 human adults with "probably increased thrombocyte aggregation," at a dose of 800.0 mg/person for 4 weeks in a double-blind and placebo-controlled study, was active. Average blood glucose fell by 11.6% vs control[AS419]. Essential oil, taken orally by human adults at a dose of 0.25 ml/person daily for 1–2 months, was inactive[AS311]. Essential oil, administered intragastrically to rats, was active[AS074]. Ethanol (95%) extract of bulb, administered by gastric intubation, produced weak activity and petroleum ether extract was active[AS285]. Ether extract of bulb, administered by gastric intubation to rats in a feeding study at doses of 2–4 gm crude garlic daily for 3 days, was inactive[AS293]. Garlic, in a herb-drug interaction, produced changes in the pharmacokinetic variables of paracetamol, decreases blood concentrations or warfarin and produces hypoglycemia when taken with chlorpropamide[AS503].

Hypolipemic activity. Dried bulb, administered by gastric intubation to male rats at a dose of 50.0 mg/animal for 45 days, was inactive, and active when administered for 70 days. Results significant at $P < 0.05$ level[AS296]. Dried bulb, in the ration of rabbits, prevented a rise in the levels of serum cholesterol for up to 60 days[AS332]. Essential oil, administered by gastric intubation to rats at a dose of 100.0 mg/kg for 60 days, was active. The effects were measured in the liver. Results significant at $P < 0.01$ level vs ethanol-induced hyperlipemia[AS354]. Ethanol (95%) extract of dried bulb, administered by gastric intubation to male rats at a dose of 100.0 mg/kg for 25 days, was active[AS340]. Fresh bulb, taken orally by human adults at a dose of 4.0 ml/day, was active[AS212]. Methanol extract of fresh bulb, in the ration of pigs at a concentration of 3.15 gm/kg of diet, was active[AS178].

Hypotensive activity. Dried bulb, taken orally by 120 human adults with "probably increased thrombocyte aggregation" at a dose of 800.0 mg/person for 4 weeks in a double-blind and placebo-controlled study, was active. Average diastolic pressure fell by 9.5% vs control[AS419]. Essential oil, administered per rectum in human adults at a dose of 180.0 mg/person, was active. The dose was given in conjunction with mistletoe, milfoil, horsetail, amylocaine, and chlorophyll. The biological activity has been patented[AS482]. Ethanol (95%) extract of bulb, administered to dogs and rabbits by injection at variable dosage levels, was active[AS445]. Ethanol (95%) and water extracts of bulb, administered intravenously to dogs, guinea pigs and rabbits, were active[AS450]. Ethanol/water (1:1) extract, of fresh bulb, administered by gastric intubation to rats at a dose of 40.0 ml/kg, was active. Results significant at $P < 0.05$ level[AS366]. Ether extract of dried bulb, administered intravenously to rabbits at a dose of 4–8 ml/animal, was active[AS037]. Chloroform extract of dried bulb, administered intravenously to cats, was active. The alcoholic extract contained at least 2 active elements. One was chloroform-soluble, and had an antiseptic action, a slight tonic effect on the isolated frog heart, a slight hypertensive effect on etherized cats, and a paralyzing effect on the isolated rabbit intestine. The chloroform-insoluble fraction had no antiseptic effect, no action on the isolated frog heart, a strongly hypotensive effect on etherized cats and a tonic effect on the isolated rabbit intestine[AS459]. Oven-dried bulb, administered by gastric intubation to dogs at a dose of 15.0 mg/kg, was active. Gradual decrease was observed[AS418]. Water extract of dried leaves, administered intravenously to cats and rats at a dose of 5–20 mg/kg, produced weak activity[AS352]. Water extract of bulb, administered intravenously to cats at a dose of 0.05 gm/kg, was active[AS036]. Water extract of fresh bulb, administered intravenously to dogs at a dose of 67.2 mg/kg, was active[AS082].

Hypotriglyceridemic activity. Lyophilized extract of fresh bulb, in the ration of chicken at a dose of 2.0% of the ration, was inactive[AS057]. Powdered fresh bulb, at a dose of 800.0 mg/days taken orally by 219 hypertriglyceridemic patients given the treatment for a total of 16 weeks, was active. Serum triglyceride levels fell a total of 17%[AS220]. Powdered fresh bulb, in the ration of rats at a concentration of 0.8% of the diet, was active[AS140].

Immunomodulatory activtiy. Aged garlic extract (AGE) was evaluated on various kinds of models on immune functions. In the immunoglobulin IgE-mediated allergic model, AGE significantly decreased the antigen-specific ear swelling induced by picryl chloride ointment to the ear and intravenous administration of antitrinitrophenyl antibody. In the transplanted carcinoma cell model, AGE significantly inhibited the growth of Sarcoma-180 (allogenic) and LL/2 lung carcinoma (syngenic) cells transplanted into mice, concomitantly, increases in natural killer and killer activities of spleen cells observed in Sarcoma-180 bearing mice administered AGE. In the psychological stress model, AGE significantly prevented the decrease in spleen weight and restored the reduction of anti-SRBC hemolytic plaque-forming cells caused by the electrical stress[AS526].

Immunosuppressant activity. Hot water extract of bulb, administered intraperitoneally to rats, was active[AS286]. Lyophilized extract of freeze-dried bulb, in the ration of mice at a concentration of 4.0% of the diet, was active vs UVB-induced suppression of contact hypersensitivity to oxazolone and cis-urocainic acid (topical)-induced suppression of contact hypersensitivity to dinitrofluorobenzene[AS104].

Inotropic effect (negative). Water extract of fresh bulb, at a concentration of 0.1 mcg/ml, was active on rat atrium[AS082].

Inotropic effect (positive). Essential oil of dried bulb, administered intragastrically to rats at a dose of 2.0 gm/kg, was active and returned to normal after garlic withdrawal. Animals were maintained on normal diet and given the dose for 30 days[AS400]. Fresh bulb juice, administered intravenously to rat at a dose of 0.1 ml/animal, increased the amplitude of P wave and the ventricular complex QRS of ECG. The activity was highly dose-dependent[AS349].

Insect attractant activity. Butanol extract of fresh bulb, undiluted, produced weak activity on *Delia antiqua*[AS155].

Insecticide activity. Dried bulb, at a concentration of 1.0%, was active. One month after treatment, moisture, ash, fiber, fat, protein and carbohydrate level remained unaffected[AS097]. A concentration of 2.0% produced weak activity on *Trogoderma granarium* in maize stored for 6 months. After 6 months, changes in nutritional composition were proportional to insect damage[AS097]. Essential oil of the dried bulb was active on *Macaronesia fortunata* and *Musca domestica*[AS485]. Dried bulb was active on *Pericallia ricini* and *Spodoptera litura* larvae[AS056]. The eggs of Aedes aegypti hatched in deionized water undergo complete fracture near the anterior poles producing free shell caps. In contrast, eggs placed in 6% reconstituted Kyolic garlic extract are only partially fractured, display attached shell caps, and the larvae remained trapped within the shells. No larvae were observed in garlic extract suggesting the embryos wer disabled before they could escape from their shells as viable larvae[AS517].

Insulin induction. Dried bulb, taken orally by human adults at a dose of 350.0 mg/person twice daily, was inactive[AS254]. Hot water extract of fresh bulb, in the ration of mice at a dose of 6.25% of the diet, was inactive vs streptozotocin-induced hyperglycemia[AS213].

Insulin level increase. Fixed oil of fresh bulb, in the ration of rats at a concentration of 1.5% of the diet, was active. The extract ameliorates a decrease in insulin levels in animals fed fructose and Cu-deficient diet[AS068].

Insulin release inhibition. Essential oil, administered intragastrically to rats, was active[AS074].

Interleukin induction. Water extract of freeze-dried bulb was inactive, IL-1 activity was measured by the IL-1 dependent growth of a T-helper cell line[AS224].

Interleukin-1 formation stimulation. Water extract of fresh bulb, in cell culture at a concentration of 0.4 mg/ml, was active on lymphocytes. Thiosulfonate fraction, at a concentration of 1.6 mg/ml, was inactive[AS110].

Interleukin-4 formation stimulation. Water extract of fresh bulb, in cell culture at a concentration of 0.4 mg/ml, was active on lymphocytes. Thiosulfonate fraction, at a concentration of 1.6 mg/ml, was active[AS110].

Intestinal motility inhibition. Essential oil, administered orally to mouse at a dose of 0.01 ml/gm, was active. Gastrointestinal transit of charcoal meal was reduced[AS161].

Lactate dehydrogenase stimulation. Essential oil, administered intragastrically to rats at a concentration of 0.067 mg/gm after fasting for 24 hours, was active[AS210]. Water extract of fresh bulb, administered intragastrically to rats at variable dosage levels, was active[AS493].

Lactate dehydrogenase-X inhibition. Water extract of fresh bulb, at a concentration of 10.0 mg/ml, was active[AS257].

Larvicidal activity. Decoction of dried stem, at a concentration of 100.0 ppm, produced weak activity on *Aedes fluviatilis*[AS085]. Petroleum ether extract of essential oil, at variable concentrations, was active on culex, pipens-quinquefasciatus 1st instar larvae[AS494].

Lipase inhibition. Water extract of fresh bulb, in the ration of rabbits at a dose of 1.0 gm/kg, was active vs cholesterol-loaded animals[AS422].

Lipid metabolism effects. Fresh garlic was taken orally by 9 human adults with hyperlipidemia at a dose of 14 gm/day for 5 months. The serum triglyceride levels were lowered and the high-density lipoprotein levels were increased[AS159]. Ethanol (95%) extract of fresh bulb, in the ration of rats at a dose of 8.0 ml/animal, was active. Extraction was made at 0 °C. Four milliliters of the extract was fed for 3 weeks, then salt was added and the dose increased to 8 ml. Salt did not affect blood pressure in the spontaneously hypertensive animals; linoleic acid increased and arachidonic acid decreased[AS188].

Lipid peroxidation effect. Essential oil of dried bulb, in cell culture at a concentration of 0.01 mg/ml, was active on rat liver microsomes. Results significant at $P < 0.01$ level[AS369]. Ethanol (20%) extract of fresh bulb, at a concentration of 20.0 microcuries/ml, was active. Formation of fluorescent substances was measured as an index of lipid peroxidation. At a concentration of 40.0 microcuries/ml, strong activity was produced. Thiobarbituric acid was assayed to determine peroxidation[AS196]. Hot water extract of fresh bulb produced weak activity vs T-butyl hydroperoxide/heme-induced luminol enhanced chemiluminescence[AS078]. Powdered fresh bulb, at a concentration of 5.0 mg/ml, inhibited lipid peroxidation by 45%[AS421]. Water extract of aged bulb, administered intraperitoneally to mice at a dose of 0.05 ml/animal, was active vs doxorubicin-induced lipid peroxidation[AS119]. Water extract of fresh bulb was active[AS430]. Aged garlic extract (AGE) significantly prevented the decrease of erythrocyte deformability induced by lipid peroxidation in a dose-dependent manner. The addition of AGE significantly inhibited an increase in thiobarbituric acid-reactive substances and hemolysis rate and pevented the loss of intraerythrocytic ATP and 2,3-diphosphoglycerate in oxidized erythrocytes. Moreover, AGE siginficantly suppressed not only the hemolysis rate induced by peroxidation but also hemolysis due to nonperoxidation[AS532].

Lipid synthesis stimulation. Water extract of fresh bulb was active[AS237].

Lipopolysaccharide degradation. Garlic juice, 30% hydrogen peroxide, and 1:1 garlic juice/3% hydrogen peroxide were tested on the degradation of lipopolysaccharide (LPS). The most powerful, hydrogen peroxide, degraded LPS by fractionization of phosphoryl in position 1 from lipid A. the next powerful, garlic juice, bound LPS molecule and influenced its effect besides LPS hydrolysis[AS502].

Lipoxygenase inhibition. Ether extract of fresh bulb, in cell culture, was active[AS206]. Methanol extract of dried bulb, at variable concentrations, was inactive vs ADP-, arachidonic-, epinephrine- and thrombin-induced aggregation[AS333]. Essential oil of fresh bulb was active, IC_{50} 15.0 mcg/ml[AS195]. The ether-insoluble fraction of methanol extract of fresh bulb, at concentration 100.0 mcg/ml, produced 44% inhibition on rat platelets and the ether-soluble fraction produced 5% inhibition[AS087]. Ethanol (75%) extract of fixed oil was active on guinea pig polymorphonuclear leukocytes. The biological activity has been patented [AS138]. Chloroform and chloroform/acetone extracts of fresh bulb were active, IC_{50} 2.95 and 0.51 mcg/ml respectively[AS432].

Longevity prolongation. Ethanol (95%) extract of aged bulb, in the ration of senescence accelerated mice(SAM P8) and senescence resistant strain(SAM R1) at a dose of 2.0% of the diet, was active[AS134].

Macrophage cytotoxicity enhancement. Protein fraction of bulb, at a concentration of 100.0 mcg/ml, was active[AS394].

Malate dehydrogenase inhibition. Bulb, in the ration of 16-weeks-old male rats at concentrations of 2.0 and 4.0% of the diet, was active in cholesterol-loaded and lard fed animals. Results significant at $P < 0.05$ level[AS301].

Malic enzyme stimulation. Methanol extract of fresh bulb, in the ration of pigs at a concentration of 3.15 gm/kg of the diet for 29 days, was active. Hepatic enzymes were assayed[AS178].

Malondialdehyde inhibition. Water extract of fresh bulb, at a concentration of 4.0%, was active vs hydrogen peroxide-induced malondialdehyde formation[AS187].

Membrane fluidity increase. Ethanol (20%) extract of fresh bulb, at a concentration of 20.0 mg/ml, was active. Fluidity was measured by fluorescence anisotropy of DPH[AS196].

Memory retention improvement. Ethanol (95%) extract of aged bulb, in the ration of senescence-accelerated mice (SAM P8 and SAM R1) at a dose of 2.0% of the diet, was active[AS134].

Miscellaneous effects. Fixed oil of fresh bulb, administered subcutaneously to cat, was active on spinal dorsal horn cells[AS105]. Fresh bulb was taken orally by a total of 100 females and males in Helsinki who were interviewed to evaluate beliefs, attitudes and norms concerning the consumption of garlic. In a subsequent postal questionnaire, the annoyance related to the smell of garlic, compared with other social odors, was also measured. The most frequent beliefs about garlic pertained to its good taste, unpleasant smell, and healthiness. Users and non-users showed distinctly different belief patterns. Sweat and alcohol were considered the most annoying social odors, and garlic and perfume/aftershave the least so. The Fishbein-Ajen model, in which individual beliefs and there evaluations, as well as subjective norms, were used as predictors explained 30–35% of the variation of the reported consumption and intention to use garlic. The predictive power of the model rose 56–62% when past behavior was included as a third independent variable. Although the predictive power of attitudes was greater than that of subjective norms, the latter were also significant predictors. Thus, use of garlic is a somewhat unusual form of food-related behavior in that both attitudes and normative factors control it[AS101]. Ginseng soaked in fresh bulb juice is used to facilitate the release of the active ingredients from the ginseng. The extract was free of bitter taste. The biological activity has been patented[AS244].

Mitogenic activity. Protein fraction of bulb, at variable concentrations, was active on mice splenocytes[AS394].

Mutagenic activity. Butanol extract of fresh bulb, on agar plate at variable concentrations, was inactive on *Bacillus subtilis* H-17(Rec+). Water and hot water extracts, at concentrations of 0.5 ml/disk on agar plate, were inactive on *B. subtilis* H-17(Rec+) and M-45(Rec–)[AS336]. Ethanol (95%) extract of dried bulb, at a concentration of 10.0 mg/plate on agar plate, was inactive on *Salmonella typhimurium* TA98 and TA102[AS060]. Ethanol (95%) extract of fresh bulb, administered intragastrically to mice at a dose of 500.0 mg/kg daily for 5 days followed by sacrificing the animals and examination of marrow cells, was active[AS205]. Fresh bulb, in buffer at concentrations of 14.75 and 7.38 mg/plate on agar plate, was inactive on *E. coli* WP2 TRP(–) and *E. coli* WP2 TRP(–) UVR(–)[AS194]. Fresh bulb, on agar plate at a concentration of 1.2 mg/plate, was active on *Salmonella typhimurium* TA1535 and TA1538, and inactive on TA98. A concentration of 2.4 mg/plate was active on *S. typhimurium* TA1537. Essential oil of fresh bulb, at a concentration of 5.0 picoliters/plate, was active on *Micrococcus flavus*[AS495]. Tincture of bulb, on agar plate at a concentration of 160.0 microliters/disk, was inactive on *Salmonella typhimurium* TA98 and TA100. Metabolic activation had no effect on the results[AS496]. Water extract of fresh bulb, at a concentration of 100.0 mcg/ml, was inactive on *S. typhimurium* TA102[AS187].

Natriuretic activity. Oven-dried bulbs, administered by gastric intubation to dog at a dose of 10.0 mg/kg, was active[AS418]. Water extract of dried bulb, administered intragastrically to rats at a dose of 5.0 gm/kg, was inactive[AS193].

Natural killer cell enhancement. Water extract of fresh bulb, in cell culture at a concentration of 0.4 mg/ml, was inactive on lymphocytes; thiosulfinate fraction at a concentration of 0.2 mg/ml was active[AS110]. Fresh bulb, taken orally by human adults at variable dosage levels, was active. Five grams were taken daily for the first 6 weeks and 10 gm taken daily for the second 6 weeks. Diarrhea, genital herpes, candidiasis and pansinusitus with recurrent fever improved in AIDS patients[AS199].

Neurotropic effects. Aged garlic extract was active on cultured fetal rat hippocampal neurons. Genes differentially expressed by the addition of the extract in primary cultured hippocampal neurons were screened using mRNA differential display. Four cDNA clones were significantly enhanced at their transcriptional level. Quantitative reverse transcription-polymerase chain reaction as well as dot-blot hybridization combined with reverse transcription-polymerase chain reaction, confirmed that the transcription from these 4 genes was elevated at least twofold, particularly the mRNA of one that was identified as an alpha 2-microglobulin-related protein (alpha 2MRP) gene. Transcription of this gene was increased > 20 times 72 hours after the addition of the extract. Induction of the alpha 2MRP gene expression occurred within 24 hours after addition of the extract[AS523].

Neutrophil migration effect. Neutrophils and/or human umbilical endothelial cells were pre-treated with garlic extract using moderate, high and low concentrations. Moderate plasma concentrations of garlic extract inhibited neutrophil migration through endothelial cell monolayer (ECM) significantly when both cell types were treated. Treating either neutrophils of ECM alone produced significant reductions in migratory rate. Treatment of both cell types had an additive effect[AS498].

Nitric oxide synthesis stimulation. Cell culture, at a concentration of 25.0 mg/ml, was active on placenta and platelets; the activity is highly dose-dependent. Bulb, taken orally by human adults at a dose of 4.0 gm/person, was active on platelets[AS137].

Norepinephrine level increase. Powdered, fresh bulb, in the ration of rats at a concentration of 0.8% of the diet, was active. Interscapular brown adipose tissue was increased[AS140].

Oxidative phosphorylation inhibition. Essential oil of dried bulb was inactive on *Macaronesia fortunata* and *Musca domestica*[AS485].

Oxidative phosphorylation stimulation. Essential oil of dried bulb was inactive on *Macaronesia fortunata* and *Musca domestica*[AS485].

Peroxisomal fatty acyl-coenzyme A oxidase induction. Methanol extract of fresh bulb, in cell culture at a concentration of 0.5 mg/ml, was active on the rat hepatocytes[AS239].

Phagocytosis stimulation. Essential oil of dried bulb, administered intradermally to mice, was active[AS468]. Protein fraction of bulb, administered intraperitoneally to mice at a dose of 5.0 mg/kg, was active vs clearance of colloidal carbon[AS394].

Pharmacokinetic study. Essential oil was administered per rectum in human adults, at a dose of 180 mg/person together with mistletoe, milfoil, horsetail, amylocaine and chlorophyll. The suppository was well absorbed through the rectal mucosa[AS482].

Phorbol ester antagonist. Essential oil, applied externally to female mice at a dose of 5.0 mg/animal, was active. The dose was applied 1 hour before application of 12-O-tetradecanoyl-phorbol-13-acetate. The rate of DNA synthesis 16 hours later was decreased by 55% vs DMBA-induced carcinogenesis[AS216]. Fresh bulb was active vs phorbol myristate acetate-induced decrease in glutathione peroxidase, and stimulation of ornithine decarboxylase vs DMBA-induced carcinogenesis[AS412].

Phosphogluconate dehydrogenase stimulation. Methanol extract of fresh bulb, in the ration of pigs at a concentration of 3.15 gm/kg of diet for 29 days, was active. Hepatic enzymes were assayed[AS178].

Phospholipase inhibition. Water extract of fresh bulb, at a concentration of 20.0 microliters, was active on cat platelets[AS208].

Plant germination inhibition. Water extract of dried leaves, at a concentration of 500.0 gm/liter, was active after 6 days exposure of *Cuscuta reflexa* seeds[AS497]. Water extract of dried stem, at a concentration of 500.0 gm/liter, was active on *Cuscuta reflexa* seeds after 6 days of exposure to the extract[AS497].

Plant growth inhibition. Water extract of dried leaves, at a concentration of 500.0 gm/liter, was active after 6 days exposure of *Cuscuta reflexa* seedling. Length, weight and dry weight were measured[AS497]. Water extract of dried stem, at a concentration of 500.0 gm/liter, produced weak activity on *Cuscuta reflexa* after 6 days of exposure to the extract. Seedling length, weight and dry weight were measured[AS497].

Plant pollen tube elongation inhibition. Fresh tuber, at a concentration of 0.4 gm/well, was active vs *Camellia sinensis* pollen[AS398].

Plasminogen activation stimulation. Dried bulb, taken orally by human adults at a dose of 600.0 mg/person for 4 weeks, was active vs streptokinase activated plasminogen[AS183]. The essential oil and water extract of fresh bulb were inactive[AS313].

Platelet adhesion inhibition. Essential oil, at a concentration of 1:2, was active[AS384]. Essential oil of bulb, administered by gastric intubation to male rabbits at a dose of 1.0 gm/kg for 3 months, was active. Results significant to $P < 0.001$ level[AS339]. A concentration of 7.20% was active. When foreign material comes in contact with blood, protein is immediately adsorbed onto its surface. Thus, the effect of garlic oil vs controls of phosphoryl choline and stearic acid on protein adsorption onto polyether urethane urea was studied. In the presence of garlic oil, more albumins and less fibrinogen were adsorbed than in the presence of controls. Since platelets adhere to fibrinogen, this protein-adsorption phenomenon affected the results of the platelet-aggregation experiments[AS179]. Essential oil, at a concentration of 2.5 mcg, was active on adult human platelets vs ADP-, collagen-, and epinephrine-induced aggregation[AS330].

Platelet aggregation inhibition. Alcohol extract of fresh bulb, in cell culture at a concentration of 0.01%, was active vs epinephrine-induced aggregation. A concentration of 0.1% was active vs ADP-induced aggregation[AS137]. Butanol extract of fresh bulb, taken orally by a patient who suffered a spontaneous spinal epidural hematoma at a dose of 2000 mg/day, was active[AS221]. Water extract of fresh bulb, in cell culture at a concentration of 0.01%, was active vs ADP- and epinephrine-induced aggregation[AS137]. A concentration of 10.0 microliters was active vs collagen-, epinephrine-, ADP-, and arachidonic acid-induced aggregation[AS209] and a concentration of 15.0 microliters was active vs ADP- and arachidonic acid-induced aggregation[AS203]. Butanol extract of dried tuber, at a con-centration of 11%, was active on human platelets vs ADP-induced aggregation[AS214]. Chloroform extract of bulb, at variable dosage levels, was active on rabbit and human adult platelets. The inhibition of platelet aggregation was produced by blocking thromboxane synthesis[AS267]. Chloroform extract of fresh bulb, at a concentration of 60.0 mcg/ml, was active, 86.57% inhibition was observed vs PAF-induced aggregation and 99.89% inhibition vs ADP-induced aggregation. Chlo-

roform/acetone extract was active with 24.70% inhibition vs PAF-induced aggregation, and 35.55% inhibition vs ADP-induced inhibition[AS432]. Dried bulb, taken orally by 120 human adults with "probably increased thrombocyte aggregation," at a dose of 800.0 mg/person for 4 weeks in a double-blind and placebo-controlled study, was active[AS419]. Methanol extract, at variable concentrations, was active vs ADP-, arachidonic acid, epinephrine-and thrombin-induced aggregation[AS333]. Powdered, dried bulb, taken orally by a 72-year-old man with platelet dysfunction, was active[AS142]. Dried bulb, taken orally by human adults at a dose of 300.0 mg/person 3 times daily for 2 weeks to 7 healthy males, was active vs ADP- and collagen-induced aggregation[AS077]. Dried bulb, taken orally by human adults at a dose of 600.0 mg/person for 4 weeks, was inactive vs ADP- and collagen-induced aggregation[AS183]. A dose of 800.0 mg/day was active[AS096]. Essential oil, at a concentration of 10.30 mcg/ml, was active on adult human platelet vs ADP-induced aggregation. There was induction of a redistribution of the products of the lipoxygenase pathway. At a concentration of 30–60 mcg/ml there was complete suppression of the formation of all oxygenase products vs ADP-induced aggregation[AS292]. The essential oil produced weak activity on rabbit platelets vs ADP-induced platelet aggregation[AS282]. Ethanol/chloroform (25%) extract of fresh bulb was active vs epinephrine-induced aggregation[AS237]. Fixed oil was active vs arachidonic acid-induced aggregation[AS136]. Fresh bulb, taken orally by human adults of both sexes at a dose of 10.0 gm/person, was active[AS284]. Water extract of bulb, in cell culture was active vs collagen-induced aggregation, IC_{50} 460.0 mcg/ml[AS433]. Water extract of fresh bulb, at a concentration of 1.1%, was active[AS162]. Water extract of fresh bulb, at a concentration of 5.0 microliters, was active vs ADP-, collagen, arachidonate-, calcium ionophore A23187 and epinephrine-induced platelet aggregation[AS208]. Water extract of fresh bulb was active vs ADP or arachidonic acid-induced platelet aggregation[AS280]. Water extract of fresh bulb, administered intravenously to rabbit at a dose of 500.0 mg/kg, was active vs arachidonate-induced thrombocytopenia, hypotension and increased TXB2 levels. The extract inhibits histopathologic changes in the lung and liver[AS059].

Platelet aggregation stimulation. Water extract of fresh bulb was active[AS237].

Platelet constituent release. Methanol extract of dried bulb, at variable concentrations, was inactive. There was no degranulation, difference in ultrastructure, cell shape, distribution of granules or microtubule structures in the treated platelets when compared to controls[AS333].

Platelet stimulant. Water extract of fresh bulb, administered by intravenous infusion to rabbits at a dose of 500.0 mg/kg, was active vs arachidonate-induced platelet count decrease[AS428].

Pro-oxidant activity. Fresh bulb, at a concentration of 1.0%, was inactive. The effect was seen at 140°F. Peroxides were assayed in peanut oil[AS144].

Prostaglandin inhibition. Water extract of fresh bulb, administered by intravenous infusion to rabbits at a dose of 500.0 mg/kg, was active vs arachidonate, and collagen induced 6-keto-prostaglandin-F-alpha synthesis[AS428]. Water extract of fresh bulb, in cell culture, was active on platelets[AS203]. Water extract of bulb, at a concentration of 12.5 mg/ml, was active[AS107].

Prostatitic effect. S-allylmercaptocysteine, evaluated in himan prostatic carcinome cells (LNCaP), significantly decreased prostate specific antigen. Pre-exposure of LNCaP cells to S-allylmercaptocysteine resulted in enhanced rate of testosterone disappearance from the culture medium at 6 hr and at 48 hr compared to media from cells not previously exposed the S-allylmercaptocysteine. In lysates of S-allylmercaptocysteine–treated LNCaP cells, the rate of testosterone catabolism was twice that from phosphate buffered saline-treated cells[AS542].

Prothrombin time decrease. Dried bulb, taken orally by human adults at a dose of 198.0 mg/person, 3 doses in 34 subjects and a dose of 450.0 mg/person, 3 doses in 51 subjects, were inactive[AS377]. Ether extract of bulb, administered by gastric intubation to rats in a feeding study at doses of 2–4 gm crude garlic daily for 3 weeks, was inactive[AS293].

Prothrombin time increase. Dried bulb, taken orally by human adults at a dose of 198.0 mg/person, 3 doses in 34 subjects and a dose of 450.0 mg/person, 3 doses in 51 subjects, were inactive[AS377]. Butanol extract of fresh bulb, taken orally by human adults at a dose of 25.0 mg/day, was active[AS221]. Essential oil, administered intragastrically to rats at a dose of 50.0 mg/day, was active vs streptozotocin-induced hyperglycemia[AS076].

Radical scavenging effect. Powdered fresh bulb, at a concentration of 90.0 mg/ml, was active[AS421].

Salidiuretic effect. Water extract of dried bulb, administered intragastrically to rats at a dose of 5.0 gm/kg, was inactive[AS193].

Sclerosing effect. Chloroform extract, at a concentration of 138.0 mcg/ml, and ethanol (95%) extract, at a concentration 53.0 mcg/ml of fresh bulb, in cell culture, was active on vein vs ADP-, epinephrine-, and arachidonic acid-induced aggregation[AS206].

Senescence ameliorative effect. S-allylcysteine, administered orally to senescence-accelerated prone P8 mice at a dose of 40 mg/kg for 8 months, had a significantly attenuated decrease in the conditioned avoidance response compared with those not give S-allylcysteine. In the elevated plus-maze test using senescence-accelerated prone P10 mice, the percentage of time spent on the open arm was greater compared with the senescence-resistant control mice. Chronic dietary treatment with 40 mg S-allylcysteine/kg decreased the time in the open arm in senescence-accelerated prone P10 mice[AS524].

Sensitization (skin). Powdered bulb, applied topically to human adults at a concentration of 10.0%, was inactive[AS091].

Sickle cell dehydration inhibition. Aged garlic extract, at a concentration of 6 mg/ml, inhibited in vitro dehydration of sickle red blood cells to 30% of the control level[AS518].

Smooth muscle relaxant activity. Ethanol (95%) extract of bulb was active on rabbit intestine[AS445]. Ethanol (95%) extract of fresh bulb, at a concentration of 0.016 mg/ml, was active on rat colon[AS182]. Ethanol/chloroform (25%) extract of fresh bulb, at a concentration of 0.002 mg/ml, was active on rat fundus (stomach) vs ACh- and PGE-induced contractions[AS338]. Ether extract of dried bulb was active on rabbit intestine[AS037]. Fresh bulb juice, at a concentration of 0.5 ml/unit, was active on guinea pig ileum and rabbit jejunum. Juice, in amounts of 0.005–0.5 ml, inhibited ventricular contractions in rabbit[AS235]. Water extract of dried bulb, at a concentration of 0.04 gm/ml, was active on the guinea pig small intestine[AS251].

Smooth muscle stimulant activity. Ethanol (95%) extract of fresh bulb, at a concentration of 0.016 mg/ml, was active on rat fundus (stomach)[AS182]. Fresh bulb juice, undiluted, was active on the rabbit intestine[AS454]. Chloroform extract of dried bulb contained at least 2 active elements. One was chloroform soluble and had an antiseptic action, a slight tonic effect on isolated frog heart, a slight hypertensive effect on etherized cats and a paralyzing effect on isolated rabbit intestine. The chloroform-insoluble fraction had no antiseptic effect, no action on isolated frog heart, a strongly hypotensive effect on etherized cats and a tonic effect on isolated rabbit intestine[AS459].

Water extract of dried bulb, at a concentration of 0.04 gm/ml, was active on guinea pig small intestine. The effect was blocked by atropine and antihistamine[AS251].

Snake venom prophylaxis. The therapeutic dose of 18 mg/kg of bulb, administered orally to rats daily for 10 days prior to the intamuscular injection of cobra venom, induced a prophylactic activity against the pathogenic effects of the venom in gastric and hepatic tissues. The dose had no serious side effects on the tissues[AS514].

Spasmogenic activity. Ether extract of dried bulb, administered intravenously to rats at a dose of 20.0 ml/animal, was active[AS037].

Spasmolytic activity. Fresh bulb juice, at a concentration of 0.5 ml/unit, was active on guinea pig and rabbit aorta vs norepinephrine-induced contractions, and on rabbit trachealis muscle vs ACh- and histamine-induced contractions[AS235]. Water extract of fresh bulb was active on rat aorta vs norepinephrine-induced contractions, ED_{50} 5.28 mg/ml[AS120].

Spermicidal effect. Essential oil was active on the guinea pig and rat sperm[AS448].

Spontaneous activity reduction. Water extract of dried bulb, at a concentration of 20.0%, was active on the frog stomach[AS251].

Spontaneous activity stimulation. Ethanol (95%) extract of bulb, administered intragastrically to mice at a dose of 250.0 mg/kg, was active. The extract inhibited decrease in spontaneous motor activity induced by oscillation stress[AS165].

Stability. Garlic and its lipid- or water-soluble components have many pharmacological properties; however it have been demonstrated that heating has a negative influence on these beneficial effects. As little as 60 seconds of microwave heating or 45 min over heating can block the ability of garlic to inhibit in vivo binding of mammary carcinogen [7,12-dimethylbenzene-(a)anthracene metabolites to rat mammary epithelial cell DNA. Allowing crushed garlic to stand for 10 min before microwave heating for 60 seconds prevented the total loss of anticarcinogenic activity[AS530].

Succinate dehydrogenase stimulation. Butanol extract of dried bulb, administered intragastrically to rats at a dose of 0.5 gm/kg, was active on heart, liver and pancreas vs isoprenaline-induced tissue necrosis[AS189].

Superoxide dismutase inhibition. Lyophilized extract of fresh bulb, in the ration of chicken at a concentration of 2.0% of the ration, was active. Cu-Zn superoxide dismutase activity was inhibited[AS057].

Superoxide inhibition. Lyophilized extract of fresh bulb, in the ration of chicken at a concentration of 2.0% of the diet, was active[AS057].

Sympathomimetic activity. Water extract of dried leaves, administered intravenously to cats at a dose of 5–20 mg/kg, had no effect on the contractile response of the cat nictating membrane evoked by preganglionic cervical sympathetic nerve stimulation[AS352].

Tachycardia activity. Ether extract of dried bulb, administered intravenously to rabbits at a dose of 10.0 ml/animal, was active[AS037].

Testosterone release stimulation. Ethanol (95%) extract of dried bulb, administered by gastric intubation to male rats at a dose of 100.0 mg/kg for 25 days, was active. Results significant at $P < 0.001$ level[AS340]. Rats, fed an experimental diet with protein levels with or without 0.8 gm/100 gm garlic powder for 28 days, produced significantly higher testosterone levels in the testis and significantly lower plasma cortisterone concentrations than those fed diets without garlic powder[AS505].

Thrombin inhibition. Essential oil, administered intragastrically to rats at a dose of 50.0 mg/day, was active vs streptozotocin-induced hyperglycemia[AS076].

Thrombocytopenic activity. Ether extract of bulb, administered by gastric intubation to rats in a feeding study at doses of 2–4 gm crude garlic daily for 3 weeks, was active[AS293].

Thromboplastin time increase. Essential oil, administered intragastrically to rats at a dose of 50.0 mg/day, was active vs streptozotocin-induced hyperglycemia. Kaolin activated partial thromboplastin time was assayed[AS076].

Thromboxane B-2 synthesis inhibition. Chloroform extract of bulb, at variable dosage levels, was active on rabbit and human platelets vs incubation with labeled arachidonic acid. Blocking thromboxane synthesis produced inhibition of platelet aggregation[AS267]. Ether and water extracts of fresh bulb, in cell culture, were active on platelets[AS206]. Water extract of fresh bulb, administered intravenously to rabbits at a dose of 500.0 mg/kg, was active vs arachidonate- and rat tail solubilized collagen-induced thrombocytopenia, hypotension and increased TXB2 levels, and vs arachidonate- and collagen-induced thromboxane B-2 synthesis. The extract inhibits histopathological changes in the lung and liver[AS428]. Water extract of fresh bulb, in cell culture, was active on platelets[AS203]. Water extract of fresh bulb was active[AS280].

Thyroxine level increase. Fixed oil of fresh bulb, in the ration of rat at a concentration of 1.5% of the diet, was active. The extract ameliorated T4 decrease in animals fed a fructose and Cu-deficient diet[AS068].

Toxic effect (general). Butanol extract of fresh bulb, taken orally by human adults, was active. Two cases were reported of increased normalized ratio results previously stabilized to warfarin. Increases were attributed to ingestion of garlic products, since there were no other changes in medication and habits in either case. One patient had started taking garlic pearls, the other, garlic tablets, but in both cases, clotting times were roughly doubled. It was warned that this could be a potentially serious interaction. Dried bulb juice, in the drinking water of rats at a dose of 5.0% of the diet for 25 days, was inactive[AS378]. Dried bulb, taken orally by human adults at a dose of 350.0 mg/person twice daily, was inactive[AS170]. Dried bulb, together with *Panax ginseng* and Vitamin B1, administered by gastric intubation to rats of both sexes at a dose of 10.0 ml/kg for up to 3 months, was equivocal. Food consumption was decreased, but there was no change in body weight gain. Erythrocyte and hemoglobin levels were slightly low. There were no histopathological changes seen in the liver, stomach, pancreas, lung, heart, kidney, spleen, thymus, bone marrow, ovary, testis, thyroid and adrenal. No other toxic symptoms were noted[AS371]. When administered by gastric intubation, dried bulb was inactive. Rats received from 0.3 to 10 ml/kg for 3 to 6 months. Body weight gain and urinary measurements were normal. There was a slight though inconsistent decrease in erythrocyte and hemoglobin levels, and slight enlargement of the spleen in high dose rats. There were no histopathological changes seen in the spleen, liver, stomach, pancreas, lung, heart, kidney, thymus, ovary, testis, adrenal and thyroid[AS370]. Essential oil of dried bulb, administered to rabbits at a dose of 0.755 ml/kg, was active. The toxicity produced is described as "excitostupefactive" [AS466]. Ethanol (95%) extract of dried bulb, administered by gastric intubation to rats at variable dosage levels, was inactive[AS459]. Ether extract of bulb, administered by gastric intubation to rats in a feeding study at doses of 2–4 gm crude garlic daily for 3 weeks, was inactive. No histopathological lesions of heart, kidney, adrenals, liver, spleen or thyroid could be seen on autopsy[AS293]. Fresh bulb, applied externally to a 17-month-old human infant was presented with burns on both feet derived from a garlic plaster that was improperly applied. A mixture of more than 50% garlic cloves plus petroleum jelly had been applied to the feet for 8 hours. Blisters were found on the dorsal surfaces of both feet, extending to the skin over the arches. There was a diffuse erythema around the blisters. Burns were diagnosed as second-degree burns and covered 4% of the body surface. The burns healed in 2 weeks with topical silver and sulfadiazine[AS234]. Butanol extract of fresh bulb, taken orally by human adults at a dose of 25.0 mg/day, was active. An 87-year-old man was presented with paralysis of the lower extremities. A spinal mass proved to be a spontaneous spinal epidural hematoma. The hematoma was removed and the patient recovered adequately. The hematoma was attributed to the man's high consumption of garlic (4 cloves/day), as no other potential causes were found. Bleeding time during surgery was 11 minutes (3 minutes normal) and prothrombin time was 12.3 seconds[AS221]. Fresh bulb, inhaled by 3 cases of occupational asthma and rhinitis, was active[AS100]. Fresh bulb juice, administered intravenously to rats at a dose of 1.0 ml/animal, was inactive[AS349]. Seed oil, administered intraperitoneally to rat at a dose of 0.5 ml/kg, was inactive[AS408]. Garlic extract, adminsitered orally to female rats at a dose of 5 mg per kg body weight daily for 6 weeks concomitantly with lead acetate, significantly reduced lead concentration indicating the potential therapeutic activity of garlic against lead[AS508].

Toxicity assessment (quantitative). Dried bulb, administered by gastric intubation and subcutaneously to rats of both sexes, produced $LD_{50} > 30.0$ ml/kg. When administered intraperitoneally to female rats, produced LD_{50} 13.86 ml/kg, and to males, LD_{50} 13.09 ml/kg[AS370,AS371]. Essential oil, administered intragastrically to rats fasted for 24 hours at a dose of 0.1 mg/gm, was active[AS493].

Triglyceride synthesis inhibition. S-allyl cysteine and S-propyl cysteine, incubated at 0.05 and 4.0 mmol/L, respectively, with cultured hepatocytes, decreased [2-14C]acetate incorporation into triglyceride in a concentration-dependent fashion achieving a maximal inhibition at 4.0 mmol/L of 43 and 51%, respectively[AS516].

Tumor promoting effect. Hot water extract of fresh bulb, applied externally to mice at a dose of 1.0 mg/animal, was inactive. The dose was applied 3 times weekly for 49–60 weeks after tumor initiation vs DMBA-induced carcinogenesis[AS412].

Tumor promotion inhibition. Methanol extract of fresh root, in cell culture at a concentration of 200.0 mcg, was inactive on EBV vs 12-0-hexadecanoylphorbol-13-acetate-induced EBV activation[AS402]. Water and methanol extracts of fresh sprouts, in cell culture at concentrations of 200.0 mcg, produced weak activity on EBV vs 12-hexadecanoylphorbol-13-acetate-induced EBV activation[AS402].

Ulcerogenic activity. Ether extract of bulb, administered by gastric intubation to rats in a feeding study at doses of 2–4 gm crude garlic daily for 3 weeks, was active[AS293].

Uterine stimulant effect. Ethanol (95%) extract of bulb, at a concentration of 2.0 mg, was active on the nonpregnant guinea pig uterus. There was an increase in tone and peristalsis. The same effect as 0.001 IU of pituitrin was produced. The extract was also active on the nonpregnant human uterus[AS010, AS011]. Ethanol (95%) extract of dried bulb, at a concentration of 4–10 mg, was active on nonpregnant guinea pig uterus[AS444]. Water extract of bulb, at a concentration of 50.0 mg/ml, produced weak activity. The dose was equivalent to 0.003 IU of oxytocin[AS020]. Water extract of bulb was active on the nonpregnant uterus and produced strong activity on the pregnant uterus of mice and rats[AS029].

Vasodilator activity. Dried bulb, taken orally by human adults at a dose of 900.0 mg/person in a randomized placebo-controlled double-blind crossover study, showed significant increase in skin capillary perfusion 5 hours after administration[AS423]. Water extract of fresh bulb was active[AS237].

WBC stimulant. Fresh bulb juice, administered intraperitoneally to mice, increased neutrophil accumulation 82%, ED_{50} 0.07 ml/animal[AS054].

WBC-macrophage stimulant. Water extract of freeze-dried bulb, at a concentration of 20.0 mcg/ml, was active. Nitrite formation was used as an index of the macrophage stimulating activity to screen effective foods[AS224].

Weight gain inhibition. Powdered, fresh bulb, in the ration of rats at a concentration of 0.8% of the diet, was active[AS140].

Weight increase. Ethanol (95%) extract of bulb, administered intragastrically to mice at a dose of 250.0 mg/kg, was active vs 3 weeks of cold stress. Weight gain was faster than in controls[AS165].

Wound healing acceleration. Plant, applied externally to human adults, was active. Perforated eardrums were healed in 18 cases[AS145].

REFERENCES

AS001 **J Agri Food Chemistry** 1992; Vol. 40.

AS002 **J Agri Food Chemistry** 1992; Vol. 37.

AS003 Stitt, P. A. Why George Should Eat Broccoli. Dougherty Co., Milwaukee, WI. 1990; 399 pp.

AS004 USDA Agricultural Handbook No. 8 and sequels; strictly nutritional data.

AS005 Pedersen, M. Nutritional Herbology. Pederson Publishing, Bountiful, UT 1987; 377 pp.

AS006 Wasuwat, S., M. Mokhasmith, P. Wannissorn, C. Sankamnoed and P. Bamphenwatana. Research and development on water-soluble, natural garlic concentrated powder (garlic natura). **Abstr 10th Conference of Science and Technology** 1984; 220–221.

AS007 Kodera, Y., H. Matsuura S. Yoshida, T. Sumida, Y. Itakura, T. Fuwa and H. Nishino. Allixin, a stress compound from garlic. **Chem Pharm Bull** 1989; 37(6): 1656–1658.

AS008   Glasby, J. H. Dictionary of Plants Containing Secondary Metabolites. Taylor and Francis, New York, 1991; 488 pp.

AS009   List, P. H. and L. Horhammer. Hager's Handbuck der Pharmazeutischen Praxis. Vols 2–6, Springer-Verlag, Berlin, 1969–1979.

AS010   Lorenzo Velasquez, B., B. Sanchez, F. Murias and C. Dominguez Mijan. Garlic extract as an oxtocic substance. **Arch Inst Farmacol Exp** 1958; 10: 10–14.

AS011   Mateo Tinao, M. and R. Calvo Terren. Actions of *Allium sativum* (Garlic) and combinations on uterine motility. **Arch Inst Farmacol Exp** 1955; 8: 127.

AS012   Podolsky, E. The hypotensive properties of *Allium sativum*. **Ill Med J** 1938; 74: 176.

AS013   Rolleri, F. Occurrence of nicotinic acid and nicotinamide in curative plants. **Arch Pharm** 1943; 281: 118.

AS014   Weisberger, A. S. and J. Pensky. Tumor-inhibiting effects derived from an active principle of garlic (*Allium sativum*). **Science** 1957; 126: 1112.

AS015   Asprey, G. F. and P. Thornton. Medicinal Plants of Jamaica Part I. **West Indian Med J** 1953; 2(4): 233–252.

AS016   Steggerda, M. and B. Korsch. Remedies for diseases as prescribed by Maya Indian herb-doctors. **Bull Hist Med** 1943; 13: 54.

AS017   Fitzpatrick, F. K. Plant substances active against *Mycobacterium tuberculosis*. **Antibiot Chemother** 1954; 4: 528.

AS018   Saha, J. C., E. C. Savini and S. Kasinathan. Ecbolic properties of Indian medicinal plants: Part I. **Indian J Med Res** 1961; 49: 130–151.

AS019   Shattuck, G. C. The Peninsula of Yucatan: Medical, Biological, Meteorological and Sociological Studies. 1933.

AS020   Saha, J. C. and S. Kasinathan. Ecbolic properties of Indian medicinal plants: Part II. **Indian J Med Res** 1961; 49: 1094–1098.

AS021   Prasad, D. N., S. K. Bhattacharya and P. K. Das. A study of antinflammatory activity of some indigenous drugs in albino rats. **Indian J Med Res** 1966; 54: 582.

AS022   Di Paolo, J. and C. Carruthers. The effect of allicin from garlic on tumor growth. **Cancer Res** 1960; 20: 431.

AS023   Ibragimov, F. I. and V. S. Ibragimov. Principal remedies of Chinese medicine. Foreign Technology Div, Air Force Systems Command, Wright-Patterson Air Force Base, 1964.

AS024   Jochle, W. Menses-inducing drugs: Their role in antique, medieval and renaissance gynecology and birth control. **Contraception** 1974; 10: 425–439.

AS025   Bhakuni, O. S., M. L. Dhar, M. M. Dhar, B. N. Dhawan and B. N. Mehrotra. Screening of Indian plants for biological activity: Part II. **Indian J Exp Biol** 1969; 7: 250–262.

AS026   Lawrendiadis, G. Contribution to the knowledge of the medicinal plants of Greece. **Planta Med** 1961; 9: 164.

AS027   Kroning, F. Garlic as an inhibitor for spontaneous tumors in mice. **Acta Unio Intern Contra Cancrum** 1964; 20: 855.

AS028   Kimura, Y. and K. Yamamoto. Cytological effect of chemicals on tumors. XXIII: Influence of crude extracts from garlic and some related species on MTK-Sarcoma III. **Gann** 1964; 55: 325.

AS029   Sharaf, A. Food plants as a possible factor in fertility control. **Qual Plant Mater Veg** 1969; 17: 153.

AS030   Krishnakumari, M. K. and S. K. Majumder. Bioassay of piperazine and some plant products with earthworms. **J Sci Ind Res-C** 1960; 19: 202.

AS031   Watt, J. M. and M. G. Breyer-Brandwijk. The Medicinal and Poisonous Plants of Southern and Eastern Africa, 2nd Edition. **South African Inst Med Research** 1962.

AS032   Maruzzella, J. C., D. Scrandis, J. B. Scrandis and G. Grabon. Action of odoriferous organic chemicals and essential oils on wood-destroying fungi. **Plant Dis Rept** 1960; 44: 789.

AS033   Maruzzella, J. C. and J. Balter. The action of essential oils on phytopathogenic fungi. **Plant Dis Rept** 1959; 43: 1143–1147.

AS034   Burkill, I. H. Dictionary of the Economic Products of the Malay Peninsula: Vol. I. **Ministry of Agriculture and Cooperatives, Kuala Lumpur** 1966.

AS035   Walter-Levy, L. and R. Strauss. Inorganic deposits in plants. **C R Acad Sci** 1954; 239: 897.

AS036 Petkov, V. Pharmacological and clinical studies of garlic. **Dtsch Apoth Ztg** 1966; 51: 1861–1867.

AS037 Uemori, T. Pharmacological investigation of *Allium sativum*. **Nippon Yakurigaku Zasshi** 1929; 9(1): 21–26.

AS038 Jain, R. C., C. R. Vyas and O. P. Mahatma. Hypoglycemic action of onion and garlic. **Lancet** 1973; 1491.

AS039 Stein, D. and M. H. Kotin. Clinical studies with *Allium sativum* (garlic). **New York Physician** 1937.

AS040 Sendl, A. and H. Wagner. Isolation and identification of homologues of ajoene and alliin from bulb-extracts of *Allium ursinum*. **Planta Med** 1991; 57(4): 361–362.

AS041 Mutsch-Eckner, M., B. Meier, A. D. Wright and O. Sticher. Gamma-glutamyl peptides from *Allium sativum* bulbs. **Phytochemistry** 1992; 31(7):2389–2391.

AS042 Kaku, H., I. J. Goldstein, E. J. M. Van Damme and W. J. Peumans. New mannose-specific lectins from garlic (*Allium sativum*) and ramsons (*Allium ursinum*) bulbs. **Carbohydr Res** 1992; 229(2): 347–353.

AS043 Lund, B. M. and G. D. Lyon. Detection of inhibitors of *Erwinia carotovora* and *E. herbicola* on thin-layer chromatograms. **J Chromatogr** 1975; 110: 193.

AS044 Fletcher, R. D., B. Parker and M. Hassett. Inhibition of coagulase activity and growth of *Staphylococcus aureus* by garlic extracts. **Folia Microbiol** 1974; 19: 494.

AS045 Jain, R. C. and C. R. Vyas. Garlic in alloxan-induced diabetic rabbits. **Amer J Clin Nutr** 1975; 28: 684.

AS046 Kaleysa Raj, R. Screening of indigenous plants for anthelmintic action against human *Ascaris lumbricoides*: Part II. **Indian J Physiol Pharmacol** 1975; 19: 47–49.

AS047 Du, C. T. and F. J. Francis. Anthocyanins from garlic (*Allium sativum*). **J Food Sci** 1975; 40: 1101.

AS048 GRAS status of foods and food additives. **Fed Regist** 1976; 41: 38644.

AS049 Uchida, Y., T. Takahashi and N. Sato. The characteristics of the antibacterial activity of garlic. **Jap J Antibiot** 1975; 28: 638.

AS050 Sharma, K. K., N. K. Chowdhury and A. L. Sharma. Long term effect of onion on experimentally induced hypercholesteremia and consequently decreased fibrinolytic activity in rabbits. **Indian J Med Res** 1975; 64: 1629.

AS051 Jain, R. C. Onion and garlic in experimental cholesterol induced atherosclerosis. **Indian J Med Res** 1976; 64: 1509.

AS052 Devereux, G. A study of abortion in primitive societies. The Julian Press, 1976.

AS053 Gupta, R. K. and S. Gupta. Purification of the hypoglycemic principle of onion. **IRCS Libr Compend** 1976; 4: 410.

AS054 Yamazaki, M. and T. Nishimura. Induction of neutrophil accumulation by vegetable juice. Biosci Biotech Biochem 1992; 56(1): 150–151.

AS055 Ip, C., D. J. Lisk and G. S. Stoewsand. Mammary cancer prevention by regular garlic and selenium-enriched garlic. **Nutr Cancer** 1992; 17(3): 279–286.

AS056 Rajendran, B. and M. Gopalan. Note on the insecticidal properties of certain plant extracts. **Indian J Agr Sci** 1979; 49: 295–297.

AS057 Sklan, D., Y. N. Berner and H. D. Rabinowitch. The effect of dietary onion and garlic on hepatic lipid concentrations and activity of antioxidative enzymes in chicks. **J Nutr Biochem** 1992; 3(7): 322–325.

AS058 Sendl, A., M. Schliack, R. Loser, F. Stanislaus and H. Wagner. Inhibition of cholesterol synthesis in vitro by extracts and isolated compounds prepared from garlic and wild garlic. **Atherosclerosis** 1992; 94(1): 79–85.

AS059 Alnaqeeb, M. A., M. Ali, M. Thomson, S. H. Khater, S. A. Gomes and J. M. Al-Hassan. Histopathological evidence of protective action of garlic against collagen and archidonic acid toxicity in rabbits. **Prostaglandins Leukotrienes Essent Fatty Acids** 1992; 46(4): 301–306.

AS060 Mahmoud, I., A. Alkofahi and A. Abdelaziz. Mutagenic and toxic activities of several spices and some Jordanian medicinal plants. **Int J Pharmacog** 1992; 30(2): 81–85.

AS061   Egen-Schwind, C., R. Eckard and F. H. Kemper. Metabolism of garlic constituents in the isolated perfused rat liver. **Planta Med** 1992; 58(4): 301–305.

AS062   Liu, J. Z., R. I. Lin and J. A. Milner. Inhibition of 7,12-dimethylbenz-[A]athracene-induced mammary tumors and DNA adduct by garlic powder. **Carcinogenesis** 1992; 13(10): 1847–1851.

AS063   Bilgrami, K. S., K. K. Sinha and A. K. Sinha. Inhibition of aflatoxin production and growth of *Aspergillus flavus* by eugenol and onion and garlic extracts. **Indian J Med Res** 1992; 96(34): 171–175.

AS064   Sheela, C. G. and K. T. Augusti. Antidiabetic effects of S-allyl cysteine sulphoxide isolated from garlic (*Allium sativum* Linn.). **Indian J Exp Biol** 1992; 30(6): 523–526.

AS065   Huang, M. F., W. J. Hang and Q. Zhong. Hair growth stimulating preparations containing medicinal plant extracts. **Patent-Faming Zhuanli Shening Gongkai Shuomingshu** 1990; 1,043,624: 6 pp.

AS066   Weber, N. D., D. O. Anderson, J. A. North, B. K. Murray, L. D. Lawson and B. G. Hughes. In vitro virucidal effects of *Allium sativum* (garlic) extract and compounds. **Planta Med** 1992; 58(5): 417–423.

AS067   Bhat, R. B., E. O. Eterjere and V. T. Oladipo. Ethnobotanical studies from Central Nigeria. **Econ Bot** 1990; 44(3): 382–390.

AS068   Fields, M., C. G. Lewis and M. D. Lure. Garlic oil extract ameliorates the severity of copper deficiency. **J Amer Coll Nutr** 1992; 11(3): 334–339.

AS069   Huang, M. F., W. J. Hang and Q. Zhong. Hair growth stimulating preparations containing medicinal plant extracts. **Patent-Faming Zhuanli Shenqing Gongkai Shuomingshu** 1990; 1,043,624: 6pp.

AS070   Horie, T., S. Awazu, Y. Itakura and T. Fuwa. Identified diallyl polysulfides from an aged garlic extract which protects the membranes from lipid peroxidation. **Planta Med** 1992; 58(5): 468–469.

AS071   Weinberg, D. S., M. L. Manier, M. D. Richardson and F. G. Haibach. Identification and quantification of organo-sulfur compliance markers in a garlic extract. J Agr **Food Chem** 1993; 41(1): 37–41.

AS072   Rotzsch, W., F. Rassoulf and A. Walper. Postprandial lipaemia under treatment with *Allium sativum*/controlled double-blind study in health volunteers with reduced HDL2-Cholesterol levels. **Arzneim-Forsch** 1992; 42(10): 1223–1227.

AS073   Isensee, H., B. Rietz and R. Jacob. Cardioprotective actions of garlic (*Allium sativum*). **Arzneim-Forsch** 1993; 43(2): 94–98.

AS074   Venmadhi, S. and T. Devaki. Studies on some liver enzymes in rats ingesting ethanol and treated with garlic oil. **Med Sci Res** 1992; 20(20): 729–731.

AS075   McFadden, J. P., I. R. White and R. J. G. Rycroft. Allergic contact dermatitis from garlic. **Contact Dermatitis** 1992; 27(5): 333–334.

AS076   Adoga, G. I. and C. O. Ohaeri. Effect of garlic oil on prothrombin, thrombin and partial thromboplastin times in streptozotocin-induced diabetic rats. **Med Sci Res** 1991; 19: 407–408.

AS077   Legnani, C., M. Frascaro, G. Guazzaloca, S. Ludovici, G. Cesarano and S. Coccheri. Effects of a dried garlic preparation on fibrinolysis and platelet aggregation in health subjects. **Arzneim-Forsch** 1993; 43(2): 119–121.

AS078   Maeda, H., T. Katsuki, T. Akaike and R. Yasutake. High correlation between lipid peroxide radical and tumor-promoter effect: Suppression of tumor promotion in the Epstein-Barr virus/B-lymphocyte. **Jap J Cancer Res** 1992; 83(9): 923–928.

AS079   Yasukawa, K., A. Yamaguchi, J. Arita, S. Sakurai, A. Ikeda and M. Takido. Inhibitory effect of edible plant extracts on 12-0-tetradecanoylphorbol-13-acetate-induced ear oedema in mice. **Phytother Res** 1993; 7(2): 185–189.

AS080   Roychoudhury, A., T. Das, A. Sharma and G. Talukder. Use of crude extract of garlic (*Allium sativum* L.) in reducing cytotoxic effects of arsenic in mouse bone marrow. **Phytother Res** 1993; 7(2): 163–166.

AS081 Reddy, M. B., K. R. Reddy and M. N. Reddy. A survey of plant crude drugs of Anantapur district, Andhra Pradesh, India. **Int J Crude Drug Res** 1989; 27(3): 145–155.

AS082 Martin, N., L. Bardisa, C. Pantoja, R. Roman and M. Vargas. Experimental cardiovascular depressant effects of garlic (*Allium sativum*) dialysate. **J Ethnopharmacol** 1992; 37(2): 145–149.

AS083 Guo, N. L, D. P. Lu, G. Woods, E. Reed, G. Z. H. Zhou, L. B. Zhang and R. Waldman. Demonstration of the antiviral activity of garlic extract against human cytomegalovirus in vitro. **Chin Med J** 1993; 106(2): 93–96.

AS084 Das, T., A. Roychoudhury, A. Sharma and G. Talukder. Modification of clastogenicity of three known clastogens by garlic extract in mice in vivo. **Environ Molec Mutagen** 1993; 21(4): 383–388.

AS085 Consoli, R. A. G. B, N. M Mendes, J. P. Pereira, B. D. S. Santos and M. A. Lamounier. Properties of plant extracts against *Aedes fluviatilis* (Lutz) (Diptera: Culcidae) in the laboratory. **Mem Inst Oswaldo Cruz** 1988; 83(1): 87–93.

AS086 R. C. Jain. Antitubercular activity of garlic oil. **Indian Drugs** 1993; 30(2): 73–75.

AS087 Sekiya, K., T. Fushimi, T. Kanamori, N. Ishikawa, M. Itoh, M. Takita and T. Nakanishi. Regulation of arachidonic acid metabolism in platelets by vegetables. **Biosci Biotech Biochem** 1993; 57(4): 670–671.

AS088 Gebhart, R. Multiple inhibitory effects of garlic extracts on cholesterol biosynthesis in hepatocytes. **Lipids** 1993; 28(7): 613–619.

AS089 McMahon, F. G. and R. Vargas. Can garlic lower blood pressure? A pilot study. **Pharmacotherapy** 1993; 13(4): 406–407.

AS090 Amagase, H. and J. A. Milner. Impact of various sources of garlic and their constituents on 7,12-dimethylbenz-[A]anthracene binding to mammary cell DNA. **Carcinogenesis** 1993; 14(8): 1627–1631.

AS091 Meding, B. Skin symptoms among workers in a spice factory. **Contact Dermatitis** 1993; 29(4): 202–205.

AS092 Koch, H. P., W. Jager, U. Groh, J. E. Hovie, G. Plank, U. Sedlak and W. Praznik. Carbohydrates from garlic bulbs (*Allium sativum* L.) as inhibitors of adenosine deaminase enzyme activity. **Phytother Res** 1993; 7(5): 387–389.

AS093 Ohsumi, C., T. Hayashi, K. Kubota and A. Kobayashi. Volatile flavor compounds formed in an interspecific hybrid between onion and garlic. **J Agr Food Chem** 1993; 41(10): 1808–1810.

AS094 Deshpande, R. G., M. B. Khan, D. A. Bhat and R. G. Navalkar. Inhibition of *Mycobacterium avium* complex isolates from AIDS patients by garlic (*Allium sativum*). **J Antimicrob Chemother** 1993; 32(4): 623–626.

AS095 Jin, H. P., et al. Protective effect of diallyl sulfide, a natural extract of garlic, on mnng-induced damage of rat glandular stomach mucosa. **Chunghua Chung Liu Tsa Chih** 1990; 12(6): 429–431.

AS096 Kiesewetter, H., F. Jung, E. M. Jung, C. Mrowietz, J. Koscielny and E. Wenzel. Effect of garlic on platelet aggregation in patients with increased risk of juvenile ischaemic attack. **Eur J Clin Pharmacol** 1993; 45(4): 333–336.

AS097 Jood, S., A. C. Kapoor and R. Singh. Evaluation of some plant products against *Trogoderma granarium* everts in stored maize and their effects on nutritional composition and organoleptic characteristic of kernels. **J Agr Food Chem** 1993; 41(10): 1644–1648.

AS098 Anesini, C. and C. Perez. Screening of plants used in Argentine folk medicine for antimicrobial activity. **J Ethnopharmacol** 1993; 39(2): 119–128.

AS099 Morioka, N., L. L. Sze, D. L. Morton and R. F. Irie. A protein fraction from aged garlic extract enhances cytotoxicity and proliferation of human lymphocytes mediated by interleukin-2 and concanavalin A. **Cancer Immunol Immunother** 1993; 37(5): 316–322.

AS100 Seuri, M., A. Taivanen, P. Ruoppi and H. Tukiainen. Three cases of occupational asthma and rhinitis caused by garlic. **Clin Exp Allergy** 1993; 23(12): 1011–1014.

AS101 Rosin, S., H. Tuorila and A. Uutela. Garlic: a sensory pleasure or a social nuisance? **Appetite** 1992; 19: 133–143.

AS102 Gwilt, P. R., C. L. Lear, M. A. Tempero, D. D. Birt, A. C. Grandjean, R. W. Ruddon and D. L. Nagel. The effect of garlic extract on human metabolism of acetaminophen. **Cancer Epidemiol Biomarkers Prevention** 1994; 3(2): 155–160.

AS103 El-Mofty, M. M., S. A. Sakr, A. Essawy and H. S. A. Gawad. Preventive action of garlic on aflatoxin B1-induced carcinogenesis in the toad *Bufo regularis.* **Nutr Cancer** 1994; 21(1): 95–100.

AS104 Reeve, V. E., M. Bosnic, E. Rozinova and C. Boehm-Wilcox. A garlic extract protects from ultraviolet B (280–320 nm) radiation-induced suppression of contact hypersensitivity. **Photochem Photobiol** 1993; 58(6): 813–817.

AS105 Hong, S. K., S. D. Koh, H. K. Shin and K. S. Kim. Effects of garlic oil, garlic juice and allyl sulfide on the responsiveness of dorsal horn cell in the cat. **Hanyang Uidae Haksulchi** 1992; 12(2): 621–633.

AS106 Soni, K. B., A. Rajan and R. Kuttan. Reversal of aflatoxin-induced liver damage by turmeric and curcumin. **Cancer Lett** 1992; 66(2): 115–121.

AS107 Ali, M., M. Angelo-Khattar, A. Farid, R. A. H. Hassan and O. Thulesius. Aqueous extracts of garlic (*Allium sativum*) inhibit prostaglandin synthesis in the ovine ureter. **Prostagladins Leukotrienes Essent Fatty Acids** 1993; 49(5): 855–859.

AS108 Lee, Y. S. and J. J. Jang. Modifying effect of garlic and red pepper extracts on diethylnitrosamine-induced hepatocarcinogenesis. **Environ Mutagens Carcinog** 1991; 11(1):21–28.

AS109 Das, T., A. R. Choudhury, A. Sharma and G. Talkdr. Modification of cytotoxic effects of inorganic arsenic by a crude extract of *Allium sativum* L. in mice. **Int J Pharmacog** 1993; 31(4): 316–320.

AS110 Burger, R. A., R. P. Warren, L. D. Lawson and B. G. Hughes. Enhancement of in vitro human immune function by *Allium sativum* L. (garlic) fractions. **Int J Pharmacog** 1993; 31(3): 169–174.

AS111 Sogani, R. K. and K. Katoch. Correlation of serum cholesterol levels and incidence of myocardial infarction with dietary onion and garlic eating habits. **J Asso Phys Ind** 1981; 29(6): 443–446.

AS112 Silagy, C. A. and H. A. W. Neil. A meta-analysis of the effect of garlic on blood pressure. **J Hypertension** 1994; 12(4): 463–468.

AS113 Yeh, Y. Y. and S. M. Yeh. Garlic reduces plasma lipids by inhibiting hepatic cholesterol and triacylglycerol synthesis. **Lipids** 1994; 29(3): 189–193.

AS114 Svendsen, L., S. I. S. Rattan and B. F. C. Clark. Testing garlic for possible anti-aging effects on long-term growth characteristics, morphology and macromolecular synthesis of human fibroblasts. **J Ethnopharmacol** 1994; 43(2): 125–133.

AS115 Soni, K. B., A. Rajan and R. Kuttan. Inhibition of aflatoxin-induced liver damage in ducklings by food additives. **Mycotoxin Res** 1993; 9(1): 22–27.

AS116 Perez, C. and C. Anesini. Inhibition of *Pseudomonas aeruginosa* by Argentinean medicinal plants. **Fitoterapia** 1994; 65(2): 169–172.

AS117 Lim-Sylianco, C. Y., J. A. Concha, A. P. Jocano and C. M. Lim. Antimutagenic effects of eighteen Philippine plants. **Philippine J Sci** 1986; 115(4): 293–296.

AS118 Heinle, H. and E. Betz. Effects of dietary garlic supplementation in a rat model of atherosclerosis. **Arzneim-Forsch** 1994; 44(5); 614–617.

AS119 Kojima, R., Y. Toyama and S. T. Ohnishi. Protective effects of an aged garlic extract on *doxyrubicin*-induced cardiotoxicity in the mouse. **Nutr Cancer** 1994; 22(2): 163–173.

AS120 Ozturk, Y., S. Aydin, M. Kosar and K. H. C. Baser. Endothelium-dependent and independent effects of garlic on rat aorta. **J Ethnopharmacol** 1994; 44(2): 109–116.

AS121 Singh, J., A. K. Dubey and N. N. Tripathi. Antifungal activity of Mentha spicata. **Int J Pharmacog** 1994; 32(4): 314–319.

AS122 Burden, A. D., S. M. Wilkinson, M. H. Beck and R. J. G. Chalmers. Garlic-induced systemic contact dermatitis. **Contact Dermatitis** 1994; 30(5): 299–300.

AS123 Imai, J., N. Ide, S. Nagge, T. Moriguchi, H. Matsuura and Y. Itakura. Antioxidant and radical scavenging effects of aged garlic extract and its constituents. **Planta Med** 1994; 60(5): 417–420.

AS124 Torok, B., J. Belagyi, B. Rietz and R. Jacob. Effectiveness of garlic on the radical activity in radical generating systems. **Arzneim-Forsch** 1994; 44(5): 608–611.

AS125 Popov, I., A. Blumstein and G. Lewin. Antioxidant effects of aqueous garlic extract. **Arzneim-Forsch** 1994; 44(1): 602–604.

AS126 Canduela, V., I. Mongil, M. Carrascosa, S. Docio and P. Cagigas. Garlic: Always good for health? **Brit J Dermatol** 1995; 132(1): 161–162.

AS127 Davis, L. E., J. K. Shen and R. E. Royer. In vitro synergism of concentrated *Allium sativum* extract and amphotericin B against *Cryptococcus neoformans*. **Planta** Med 1994; 60(6): 546–549.

AS128 Yamasaki, T., L. Li and B. H. S. Lau. Garlic compounds protect vascular endothelial cells from hydrogen peroxide-induced oxidant injury. **Phytother Res** 1994; 8(7): 408–412.

AS129 Saradeth, T., S. Seidl, K. L. Resch and E. Ernst. Does garlic alter the lipid pattern in normal volunteers? **Phytomedicine** 1994; 1(3): 183–185.

AS130 Kenzelmann, R. and F. Kade. Limitation of the deterioration of lipid parameters by a standardized garlic-ginkgo combination product. A multicenter placebo-controlled double-blind study. **Arzneim-Forsch** 1993; 43(9): 978–981.

AS131 Venugopal, P. V. and T. V. Venugopal. Antidermatophytic activity of garlic (*Allium sativum*) in vitro. **Int J Dermatol** 1995; 34(4): 278–279.

AS132 Thomas, D. J. and K. L. Parkin. Quantification of alk(en)yl-L-cysteine sulfoxides and related amino acids in alliums by high-performance liquid chromatography. **J Agr Food Chem** 1994; 42(8): 1632–1638.

AS133 Simons, L. A., S. Balasubramaniam, M. Von Konigsmark, A. Parfitt, J. Simons and W. Peters. On the effect of garlic on plasma lipids and lipoproteins in mild hypercholesterolaemia. **Atherosclerosis** 1995; 113(2): 219–225.

AS134 Moriguchi, T., K. Takashina, P. J. Chu, H. Saito and N. Nishiyama. Prolongation of life span and improved learning in the senescence accelerated mouse produced by aged garlic extract. **Biol Pharm Bull** 1994; 17(12): 1589–1594.

AS135 DeBlasi, V., S. Debrot, P. A. Menoud, L. Gendre and J. Schowing. Amoebicidal effect of essential oils in vitro. **J Toxicol Clin Exp** 1990; 10(6): 361–373.

AS136 Ariga, T., T. Seki, K. Ando, S. Teramoto and H. Nishimura. Antiplatelet principle found in the essential oil of garlic (*Allium sativum* L.) and its inhibition mechanism. **Dev Food Eng Proc Int Congr Eng Food 6th** 1993; 2: 156–158.

AS137 Das, I., N. S. Khan and S. R. Sooranna. Potent activation of nitric oxide synthase by garlic: a basis for its therapeutic applications. **Current Med Res Opinion** 1995; 13(5): 257–263.

AS138 Lichtenstein, L. M. and W. C. Pickett. Treatment of allergies and inflammatory conditions. **Patent-Eur Pat Appl** 1985; 153,881: 21pp.

AS139 Melzig, M. F., E. Krouse and S. Franke. Inhibition of adenosine deaminase activity of aortic endothelial cells by extracts of garlic (*Allium sativum* L.). **Pharmazie** 1995; 50(5): 359–361.

AS140 Oi, Y., T. Kawada, K. Kitamura, F. Oyama, M. Nitta, Y. Kominato, S. Nishimura and K. Iwai. Garlic supplementation enhances norepinephrine secretion, growth of brown adipose tissue, and triglyceride catabolism in rats. **Nutr Biochem** 1995; 6(5): 250–255.

AS141 Kasuya, S., C. Goto and H. Ohtomo. Studies on prophylaxis against anisakiasis-A screening of killing effects of extracts from foods on the larvae. **Kansensh Ogaku Zasshi** 1988; 62(12): 1152–1156.

AS142   German, K., U. Kumar and H. N. Blackford. Garlic and the risk of turp bleeding. **Brit J Urol** 1995; 76(4): 512.

AS143   Akema, R., N. Okazaki and K. Takizawa. Antibacterial substance in commercial *Allium* plants. **Kanagawa-ken Eisei Kenkyusho Kenkyu Hokoku** 1987; 17: 39–40.

AS144   G. Gazzani. Anti- and pro-oxidant activity of some vegetables in the Mediterranean diet. **Riv Sci Aliment** 1994; 23(3): 413–420.

AS145   Hsu, W. C. Garlic slice in repairing eardrum perforation. **Chung Hua I Hsueh Tsa Chih** 1977; 3: 204.

AS146   Augusti, K. T. Hypocholesterolemic effect of garlic (*Allium sativum*). **Indian J Exp Biol** 1977; 15: 489.

AS147   Alami, R., A. Macksad and A. R. El-gindy. Medicinal Plants in Kuwait. Al-Assiriya Printing, 1976.

AS148   Das, N. N., A. Das and A. K. Mukherjee. Structure of the D-galactan isolated from garlic (*Allium sativum*) bulbs. **Carbohydr Res** 1977; 56: 337.

AS149   Bordia, A. K., H. K. Joshi, Y. K. Sanadhya and N. Bhu. Effect of essential oil of garlic on serum fibrinolytic activity in patients with coronary artery disease. **Atherosclerosis** 1977; 28: 155–159.

AS150   Moore, G. S. and R. D. Atkins. The fungicidal and fungistatic effects of an aqueous garlic extract on medically important yeast-like fungi. **Mycologia** 1977; 69: 341.

AS151   Barone, F. E. and M. R. Tansey. Isolation, purification, identification, synthesis, and kinetics of activity of the anticandidal component of *Allium sativum*, and a hypothesis for its mode of action. **Mycologia** 1977; 69: 793.

AS152   Block, E., S. Ahmad, M. K. Jain, R. W. Crecely, R. Apitz-Castro and M. R. Cruz. (E,E)-Ajoene: a potent antithrombotic agent from garlic. **J Amer Chem Soc** 1984; 106(26): 8295–8296.

AS153   Zhao, S. Q. and L. Wang. Transformation of the main components of garlic during low-temperature controlled-atmosphere storage. **Xibei Shifan Xueyuan Xuebao Ziran Kexueban** 1983; 1983(1): 70–79.

AS154   Miething, H. Allicin and oil in garlic bulbs — HPLC quantitative determi-

nation. **Dtsch Apoth Ztg** 1985; 125(41): 2049–2050.

AS155   Miller, J. R., M. O. Harris and J. A. Breznak. Search for potent attractants of onion flies. **J Chem Ecol** 1984; 10(10): 1477–1488.

AS156   Voigt, M. and E. Wolf. Garlic HPLC determination of garlic components in extracts, powder, and pharmaceuticals. **Dtsch Apoth Ztg** 1986; 126(12): 591–593.

AS157   Block, E., S. Ahmad, J. L. Catalfamo, M. K. Jain and R. Apitz-Castro. Antithrombotic organosulfur compounds from garlic: structural, mechanistic and synthetic studies. **J Amer Chem Soc** 1986; 108(22): 7045–7055.

AS158   Vernin, G., J. Metzger, D. Fraisse and C. Scharff. GC-MS (EI, PCI, NCI) computer analysis of volatile sulfur compounds in garlic essential oils. Application of the mass fragmentometry sim technique-1. **Planta Med** 1986; 1986(2): 96–101.

AS159   Nitiyanant, W., S. Wasuwat, S. Ploybutr and S. Tandhanand. Effect of the dried powder extract, water soluble of garlic (*Allium sativum*) on cholesterol, triglyceride and high density lipoprotein in the blood. **J Med Ass Thailand** 1987; 70(11): 646–648.

AS160   Unnikrishnan, M. C. and R. Kuttan. Cytotoxicity of extracts of spices to cultured cells. **Nutr Cancer** 1988; 11(4): 251–257.

AS161   Joshi, D. J., R. K. Dikshit and S. M. Mansuri. Gastrointestinal actions of garlic oil. **Phytother Res** 1987; 1(3): 140–141.

AS162   Mohammad, S. F. and S. C. Woodward. Characterization of a potent inhibitor of platelet aggregation and release reaction isolated from *Allium sativum* (garlic). **Thrombosis Res** 1986; 44(6): 793–806.

AS163   Phonphok, C. Y. Effects of garlic extract on growth of various *Candida* species. **J Natl Res Counc Thailand** 1983; 15: 53–65.

AS164   Kasuga, S., A. Kanesawa and S. Nakagawa. Extraction of ajoene from garlic for treatment of liver diseases.

Patent-Japan Kokai Tokkyo Koho 1988; 63 08,328: 5pp.

AS165 Takasugi, N., K. Kotoo, T. Fuwa and H. Saito. Effect of garlic on mice exposed to various stresses. **Oyo Yakuri Pharmacometrics** 1984; 28(6): 991–1002.

AS166 Bojs, G. and A. Svensson. Contact allergy to garlic used for wound healing. **Contact Dermatitis** 1988; 18(3): 179–181.

AS167 De a Ribeiro, R., F. Barros, M. Margarida, R. F. Melo, C. Muniz, S. Chieia, M. G. Wanderley, C. Gomes and G. Trolin. Acute diuretic effects in conscious rats produced by some medicinal plants used in the state of Sao Paulo, Brasil. **J Ethnopharmacol** 1988; 24(1): 19–29.

AS168 Lancaster, J. E., E. M. Dommisse and M. L. Shaw. Production of flavour precursors [S-alk(en)yl-L-cysteine sulphoxides] in photomixotrophic callus of garlic. **Phytochemistry** 1988; 27(7): 2123–2124.

AS169 Ghannoum, M. A. Studies on the anticandidal mode of action of *Allium sativum* (garlic). **J Gen Microbiol** 1988; 134(11): 2917–2924.

AS170 Sitprija, S., C. Plengvidhya, V. Kangkaya, S. Bhuvapanich and M. Tunkayoon. **J Med Ass Thailand Suppl** 1987; 70(2): 223–227.

AS171 Matsuura, H., T. Ushiroguchi, Y. Itakura, N. Hayashi and T. Fuwa. **Chem Pharm Bull** 1988; 36(9): 3659–3663.

AS172 Al-Nagdy, S. A., M. O. Abdel-Rahman and H. I. Heiba. Evidence for some prostaglandins in *Allium sativum* extracts. **Phytother Res** 1988; 2(4): 196–197.

AS173 You, W. C., W. J. Blot, Y. S. Chang, A. Ershow, Z. T. Yang, Q. An, J. F. Fraumeni, Jr. and T. G. Wang. *Allium* vegetable and reduced risk of stomach cancer. **J Nat Cancer Inst** 1989; 81(2): 162–164.

AS174 Pena, N., A. Auro and H. Sumano. A comparative trial of garlic, its extract and ammonium-potassium tartrate as anthelmintics in carp. **J Ethnopharmacol** 1988; 24(2/3): 199–203.

AS175 Pino, J., A. Rosado and A. Gonzalez. Volatile flower components of garlic essential oil. **Acta Aliment** 1991; 20 (3/4): 163–171.

AS176 Tanaka, Y., M. Kataoka, Y. Konishi, T. Nishmune and Y. Takagaki. Effects of vegetable foods on beta-hexosaminidase release from rat basophilic leukemia cells (RBL-2H3). **Jpn J Toxicol Environ Health** 1992; 38(5): 418–424.

AS177 Didry, N., M. Pinkas and L. Dubreuil. Antibacterial activity of species from the genus *Allium*. **Pharmazie** 1987; 42(10): 687–688.

AS178 Qureshi, A. A., T. D. Crenshaw, N. Abuirmeileh, D. M. Peterson and C. E. Elson. Influence of minor plant constituents on procine hepatic lipid metabolism. **Atherosclerosis** 1987; 64(2/3): 109–115.

AS179 Sharma, C. P. and M. C. Summy. Effects of garlic extracts and of three pure components isolated from it on human platelet aggregation, arachidonate metabolism, release reaction and platelet ultra-structure-comments. **Thrombosis Res** 1988; 52(5): 492–494.

AS180 Mirelman, D., D. Monheit and S. Varon. Inhibition of growth of *Entamoeba histolytica* by allicin, the active principle of garlic extract (*Allium sativum*). **J Infect Dis** 1987; 156(1): 243–244.

AS181 Sadhana, A. S., A. R. Rao, K. Kucheria and V. Bijani. Inihibitory action of garlic oil on the initiation of benzo[a]pyrene-induced skin carcinogenesis in mice. **Cancer Lett** 1988; 40(2): 193–197.

AS182 Rashid, A., M. Hussain and H. H. Khan. Bioassay for prostaglandin-like activity of garlic extract using isolated rat fundus strip and rat colon preparation. **J Pak Med Ass** 1986; 36(6): 138–141.

AS183 Harenburg, J., C. Giese and R. Zimmermann. Effect of dried garlic on blood coagulation, fibrinolysis, platelet aggregation and serum cholesterol levels in patients with hyperlipoproteinemia. **Atherosclerosis** 1988; 74(3): 247–249.

AS184 Singh, B. G. and S. C. Agrawal. Efficacy of odoriferous organic compounds on the growth of keratinophylic fungi. **Curr Sci** 1988; 57(14): 807–809.

AS185   Nishimo, H., A. Iwashima, Y. Itakura, H. Matsuura and T. Fuwa. Antitumor-promoting activity of garlic extracts. **Oncology** 1989; 46(4): 277–280.

AS186   Srivastava, V. K. and Z. Afao. Garlic extract inhibits accumulation of polyols and hydration in diabetic rat lens. **Curr Sci** 1989; 58(7): 376–377.

AS187   Knasmuller, S., R. DeMartin, G. Domjan and A. Szakmary. Studies on the antimutagenic activities of garlic extract. **Environ Molec Mutagen** 1989; 13(4): 357–365.

AS188   Kiviranta, J., K. Huovinen, T. Seppanen-Laakso, R. Hiltunen, H. Karppanen and M. Kilpelainen. Effects of onion and garlic extracts on spontaneously hypertensive rats. **Phytother Res** 1989; 3(4): 132–135.

AS189   Ciplea, A. G. and K. D. Richter. The protective effect of *Allium sativum* and crataegus on isoprenaline-induced tissue necroses in rats. **Arzneim-Forsch** 1988; 38(11): 1583–1592.

AS190   Shetty, S. A., H. S. Prakash and H. S. Shetty. Efficacy of certain plant extracts against seed-borne infection of *Trichoconiella padwickii* in paddy (*Oryza sativa*). **Can J Bot** 1989; 67(7): 1956–1958.

AS191   Louria, D. B., M. Lavenhar, T. Kaminski and R. H. K. Eng. Garlic (*Allium sativum*) in the treatment of experimental cryptococcosis. **J Med Vet Mycol** 1989; 27(4): 253–256.

AS192   Tsuboi, S., S. Kishimoto and S. Ohmori. S-(2-carboxypropyl)-glutathione in vegetables in *Liliflorae*. **J Agr Food Chem** 1989; 37(3): 611–615.

AS193   Tanira, M. O. M., A. M. Ageel and M. S. Al-Said. A study of some Saudi medicinal plants used as diuretics in traditional medicine. **Fitoterapia** 1989; 60(5): 443–447.

AS194   Zhang, Y. S., X. R. Chen and Y. N. Yu. Antimutagenic effect of garlic (*Allium sativum* L.) on 4NQO-induced mutagenesis in *Escherichia coli* WP2. **Mutat Res** 1989; 227(4): 215–219.

AS195   Belman, S., J. Soloman, A. Segal, E. Block and G. Barany. Inhibition of soybean lipoxygenase and mouse skin tumor promotion by onion and garlic components. **J Biochem Toxicol** 1989; 4(3): 151–160.

AS196   Horie, T., T. Murayama, T. Mishima, F. Itoh, Y. Minamide, T. Fuwa and S. Awazu. Protection of liver microsomal membranes from lipid peroxidation by garlic extract. **Planta Med** 1989; 55(6): 506–508.

AS197   Aslam, M. and I. H. Stockley. Interaction between curry ingredient (karela) and drug (chlorpropamide). **Lancet** 1979; 607.

AS198   Matsuura, H., T. Ushiroguchi, Y. Itakura and T. Fuwa. Further studies on steroidal glycosides from bulbs, roots and leaves of *Allium sativum* L. **Chem Pharm Bull** 1989; 37(10): 2741–2743.

AS199   Abdullah, T. H., D. V. Kirkpatrick and J. Carter. Enhancement of natural killer cell activity in AIDS with garlic. **Deutsche Z Onkol** 1989; 21(2): 52–53.

AS200   Ghannoum, M. A. Inhibition of *Candida* adhesion to buccal epithelial cells by an aqueous extract of *Allium sativum* (garlic). **J Appl Bacteriol** 1990; 68(2): 163–169.

AS201   Hussain, S. P., L. N. Jannu and A. R. Rao. Chemopreventive action of garlic on methylcholanthrene-induced carcinogenesis in the uterine cervix of mice. **Cancer Lett** 1990; 49(2): 175–180.

AS202   Mossa, J. S. A study on the crude antidiabetic drugs used in Arabian folk medicine. **Int J Crude Drug Res** 1985; 23(3): 137–145.

AS203   Srivastava, K. C. Aqueous extracts of onion, garlic and ginger inhibited platelet aggregation and alter arachidonic acid metabolism. **Biomed Biochem Acta** 1984; 43(8/9): 5335–5346.

AS204   Ueda, Y., M. Sakaguchi, K. Hirayama, R. Miyajima and A. Kimizuka. Characteristic flavor constituents in water extract of garlic. **Agr Biol Chem** 1990; 54(1): 163–169.

AS205   Shah, A. H., M. Tariq, A. M. Ageel and S. Qureshi. Cytological studies on some plants used in traditional Arab medicine. **Fitoterapia** 1989; 60(2): 171–173.

AS206   Srivastava, K. C. and U. Justesen. Isolation and effects of some garlic components on platelet aggregation and metabolism of arachidonic acid in human blood platelets. **Wien Klin Wochenschr** 1989; 101(8): 293–299.

AS207 Makheja, A. N. and J. M. Bailey. Antiplatelet constituents of garlic and onion. **Agents Actions** 1990; 29(3/4): 360–363.

AS208 Srivastava, K. C. Evidence for the mechanism by which garlic inhibits platelet aggregation. **Prostaglandins Leukotrienes Med** 1986; 22:313–321.

AS209 Srivastava, K. C. Effects of aqueous extracts of onion, garlic and ginger on platelet aggregation and metabolism of arachidonic acid in the blood vascular system: In vitro study. **Prostaglandins Leukotrienes Med** 1984; 13(2): 227–235.

AS210 Joseph, P. K. and C. S. Sundaresh. Serum urea and enzymes in rat on intragastric administration of garlic oil and garlic extracts. **Curr Sci** 1989; 58(24): 1409–1410.

AS211 Unnikrishnan, M. C. and R. Kutan. Tumour reducing and anticarcinogenic activity of selected spices. **Cancer Lett** 1990; 51(1): 85–89.

AS212 Lau, B. H. S., F. Lam and R. Wang-Cheng. Effect of an odor modified garlic preparation on blood lipids. **Nutr Res** 1987; 7:139–149.

AS213 Swanston-Flatt, S. K., C. Day, C. J. Bailey and P. R. Flatt. Traditional plant treatments for diabetes. Studies in normal and streptozotocin diabetic mice. **Diabetologia** 1990; 33(8): 462–464.

AS214 Okuyama, T., K. Fujita, S. Shibata, M. Hoson, T. Kawada, M. Masaki and N. Yamate. Effects of Chinese drugs "Xiebai" and "Dasuan" on human platelet aggregation (*Allium bakeri*, *A. sativum*). **Planta Med** 1989; 55(3): 242–244.

AS215 Nakagawa, S., S. Kasuga and H. Matsuura. Prevention of liver damage by aged garlic extract and its components in mice. **Phytother Res** 1989; 3(2): 50–53.

AS216 Perchellet, J. P., E. M. Perchellet and S. Belman. Inhibition of DMBA-induced mouse skin tumorigenesis by garlic oil and inhibition of two tumor-promotion stages by garlic and onion oils. **Nutr Cancer** 1990; 14(3/4): 183–193.

AS217 Meng, C. L. and K. W. Shyu. Inhibition of experimental carcinogenesis by painting with garlic extract. **Nutr Cancer** 1990; 14(3/4): 207–217.

AS218 Shyu, K. W. and C. L. Meng. The inhibitory effect of oral administration of garlic on experimental carcinogenesis in hamster buccal pouches by DMBA painting. **Proc Natl Sci Couc Part B Repub China** 1987; 11(2): 137–147.

AS219 Desai, H. G., R. H. Kalro and A. P. Choksi. Effect of ginger and garlic on DNA content of gastric aspirate. **Indian J Med Res [B]** 1990; 92(2): 139–141.

AS220 Mader, F. H. Treatment of hyperlipidaemia with garlic-powder tablets: Evidence from the German Assocation of General Practitioners' multicentric placebo-controlled double-blind study. **Arzneim-Forsch** 1990; 40(10): 1111–1116.

AS221 Rose, K. D., P. D. Croissant, C. F. Parliament and M. B. Levin. Spontaneous spinal epidural hematoma with associated platelet dysfunction from excessive garlic ingestion: a case report. **Neurosurgery** 1990; 26(5): 880–882.

AS222 Suresh, M and R. K. Rai. Cardol: The antifilarial principle from *Anacardium occidentale*. **Curr Sci** 1990; 59(9): 477–479.

AS223 Rao, A. R., A. S. Sadhana and H. C. Goel. Inhibition of skin tumors in DMBA-induced complete carcinogenesis system in mice by garlic (*Allium sativum*). **Indian J Exp Biol** 1990; 28(5): 405–408.

AS224 Miwa, M., Z. L. Kong, K. Shinohara and M. Watanabe. Macrophage stimulating activity of foods. **Agr Biol Chem** 1990; 54(7): 1863–1866.

AS225 Norris, B. C., C. V. Pantoja, L. C. H. Chiang, J. B. Concha, V. R. Neumann and D. V. Ferrada. Inhibitory effect of garlic (*Allium sativum*) on sodium transport in isolated toad skin. **J Ethnopharmacol** 1991; 31(3): 309–318.

AS226 Arora, R. B., T. Khanna, M. Imran and D. K. Balani. Effect of lipotab on myocardial infarction induced by isoproterenol. **Fitoterapia** 1990; 61(4): 356–358.

AS227 Sato, A. Studies on anti-tumor activity of crude drugs: I. The effects of aqueous extracts of some crude drugs in short-term screening test. **Yakugaku Zasshi** 1989; 109(6): 407–423.

AS228   Chowdhury, A. K. A, M. Ahsan, S. K. Islam and Z. U. Ahmed. Efficacy of aqueous extract of garlic and allicin in experimental shigellosis in rabbits. **Indian J Med Res [A]** 1991; 93(1): 33–36.

AS229   Giordano, J. and P. J. Levine. Botanical preparations used in Italian folk medicine: Possible pharmacological and chemical basis of effect. **Social Pharmacol** 1989; 3(1/2): 83–110.

AS230   Caceres, A., B. R. Lopez, M. A. Giron and H. Logemann. Plants used in Guatemala for the treatment of dermatophytic infections: I. Screening for antimycotic activity of 44 plant extracts. **J Ethnopharmacol** 1991; 31(3): 263–276.

AS231   Sunter, W. H. Warfarin and garlic. **Pharm J** 1991; 246(6640): 722.

AS232   Gebhardt, R. Inhibition of cholesterol biosynthesis by a water-soluble garlic extract in primary cultures of rat hepatocytes. **Arzneim-Forsch** 1991; 41(8): 800–804.

AS233   Scortichini, M. and M. P. Rossi. In vitro activity of some essential oils toward *Erwinia amylovora* (Burrill) Winslow, et al. **Acta Phytopathol Entomol Hung** 1989; 24(3/4): 421–423.

AS234   Parish, R. A., S. McIntire and D. M. Heimbach. Garlic burns: a naturopathic remedy gone awry. **Pediatric Emergency Care** 1988; 3(4): 258–260.

AS235   Aqel, M. B., M. N. Gharaibah and A. S. Salhab. Direct relaxant effects of garlic juice on smooth and cardiac muscles. **J Ethnopharmacol** 1991; 33(1/2): 13–19.

AS236   Kiuchi, F., N. Nakamura, N. Miyashita, S. Nishizawa, Y. Tsuda and K. Kondo. Nematocidal activity of some anthelmintics, traditional medicines and spices by a new assay method using larvae of *Toxocara canis*. **Shoyakugaku Zasshi** 1989; 43(4): 279–287.

AS237   Mansell, P and J. P. Reckless. Effects on serum lipids, blood pressure, coagulation, platelet aggregation and vasodilation. **Brit Med J** 1991; 303(6799): 379–380.

AS238   Meng, C. L. and K. W. Shyu. Inhibition of experimental carcinogenesis by painting with garlic extract. **Nutr Cancer** 1990; 14(3/4): 207–217.

AS239   Orellana, A., M. E. Kawada, M. N. Morales, L. Vargas and M. Bronfman. Induction of peroxisomal fatty acyl-coenzyme A transferase in primary cultures of rat hepatocytes by garlic extracts. **Toxicol Lett** 1992; 60(1): 11–17.

AS240   Kim, S. H., J. O. Kim, S. H. Lee, K. Y. Park, H. J. Park and H. Y. Chung. Antimutagenic compounds identified from the chloroform fraction of garlic (*Allium sativum*). **Hanguk Yongyang Siklyong Hakhoe Chi** 1991; 20(3): 253–259.

AS241   Misra, S. B. and S. N. Dixit. Antifungal spectrum of some plant extracts. **Geobios** 1977; 4(1): 29–30.

AS242   Sharma, V. D., M. S. Sethi, A. Kumar, and J. R. Rarotra. Antibacterial property of *Allium sativum*, in vivo and in vitro studies. **Indian J Exp Biol** 1977; 15: 466.

AS243   Kazaryan, R. A. and E. V. Goryachenkova. Allinase: Purification and physicochemical properties. **Biokhimiya** 1978; 43: 1905–1913.

AS244   Tonoda, A. Preparation of ginseng extracts. **Patent-Japan Kokai Tokkyo Koho** 1983; 58 29,713: 2 pp.

AS245   Caporaso, N., S. M. Smith and R. H. K. Eng. Antifungal activity in human urine and serum after ingestion of garlic (*Allium sativum*). **Antimicrob Agents Chemother** 1983; 23(5): 700–702.

AS246   Sangmahachai, K. Effect of onion and garlic extracts on the growth of certain bacteria. **Master Thesis** 1978; 88pp.

AS247   Wongcharoentham, B. Studies on the effect of garlic extract on the growth of *Candida*. **Undergraduate Special Project Report Fac Med** 1978; 35pp.

AS248   Mand, J. K., P. P. Gupta, G. L. Soni and R. Singh. Role of garlic (*Allium cepa*) in the reversal of atherosclerosis in rabbits. **Abstr 3rd Congress of the Federation of Asian and Oceanian Biochemists** 1983; 79.

AS249   Chaiyasothi, T. and V. Rueaksopaa. Antibacterial activity of some medicinal plants. **Undergraduate Special Project Report** 1975; 109pp.

AS250   Malaengpoothong, B. Studies on the antifungal activity of garlic extract.

Undergraduate Special Project Report Fac Med 1980; 31pp.

AS251 Poopipatpol, A. and U. Siriboonyarit. The effect of garlic water extract on smooth muscle. **Undergraduate Special Project Report** 1980; 51pp.

AS252 Soytong, K., V. Rakvidhvasastra and T. Sommartya. Effect of some medicinal plants on growth of fungi and potential in plant disease control. **1Abstr 11th Conference of Science and Technology** 1985; 361.

AS253 Anussorn-Nitisara, N. and A. M. Vudthludomlert. Modification of pharmaceutical preparation of garlics. **Abstr 10th Conference of Science and Technology** 1984; 241–242.

AS254 Imwidthaya, S., A. Plangpatanapanichya and P. Thasnakorn. Antifungal activity of garlic extract. **Bull Fac Med Tech Mahido Univ** 1978; 2(2): 67–77.

AS255 Ploddee, A. and R. Palakornkol. Antifungal activity of garlic. **Undergraduate Special Project Report** 1977; 23pp.

AS256 Jain, R. C. and D. B. Konar. Effect of garlic oil in experimental cholesterol atherosclerosis. **Atherosclerosis** 1978; 29: 125.

AS257 Bogin, E. and M. Abrams. The effect of garlic extract on the activity of some enzymes. **Food Cosmet Toxicol** 1976; 14: 417–419.

AS258 Suh, M. J. Effects of condiments upon alpha-amylase activity. **Hanguk Yongyang Hakhoe Chi** 1976; 9: 104.

AS259 Demkevich, L. I. Change in the amino acid composition of garlic leaves in the vegetation period. **Izv Vyssh Uchebn Zaved Pisch Tekhnol** 1978; 149.

AS260 Czajka, P., D. Pharm, J. Field, P. Novak and J. Kunnecke. Accidental aphrodisiac ingestion. **J Tenn Med Ass** 1978; 71: 747.

AS261 Van Ketel, W. G. and P. DeHann. Occupation eczema from garlic and onion. **Contact Dermatitis** 1978; 4: 53–54.

AS262 Ayensu, E. S. Medicinal Plants of the West Indies. **Unpublished manuscript** 1978; 110pp.

AS263 Sharma, K. K., A. L. Sharma, K. K. Dwived and P. K. Sharma. Effect of raw and boiled garlic on blood cholesterol in butter fat lupaemia. **Indian J Nutr Diet** 1976; 13: 7–10.

AS264 Tyrell, H. ...Or garlic. **Lancet** 1979; 1294A.

AS265 Slater, N. G. P. ...Or garlic. **Lancet** 1979; 1294A

AS266 Bordia, A. K. and H. K. Joshi. Garlic on fibrinolytic activity in cases on acute myocardial infarction. Part II. **J Ass Phys India** 1978; 26: 323–326.

AS267 Makheja, A. N., J. Y. Vanderhoek and J. M. Bailey. Inhibition of platelet aggregation and thromboxane synthesis by onion and garlic. **Lancet** 1979; 781.

AS268 Woo, W. S., K. H. Shin and I. C. Kim. The effects of irritating spices on drug metabolizing enzyme activity. Effects on hexobarbital hypnosis in mice. **Korean J Pharmacog** 1977; 8: 115–119.

AS269 Bhushan, S., S. P. Sharma, S. P. Singh, S. Agrawal, A. Indrayan and P. Seth. Effect of garlic on normal blood cholesterol level. **Indian J Physiol Pharmacol** 1979; 23: 211–214.

AS270 Petricic, J., M. Kupinic and B. Lulic. Garlic (*Allium sativum* L.) antifungal effect of some components of volatile oil. **Acta Pharm Jugoslav** 1978; 28: 41–43.

AS271 Raman, J. S., K. V. Srinivasamurthy, B. Padmarajarao. A compound of Lasuna (garlic) in the prevention and treatment of cardiovascular diseases. **J Nat Integrated Med Ass** 1978; 20: 225–227.

AS272 Bordia, A. K., S. K. Sanadhya, A. S. Rathore and N. Bhu. Essential oil of garlic on blood lipids and fibrinolytic activity in patients of coronary artery disease: Part I. **J Ass Phys India** 1978; 26: 327–331.

AS273 Chang, M. L. W. and M. A. Johnson. Effect of garlic on carbohydrate metabolism and lipid synthesis in rats. **J Nutr** 1980; 110: 931–936.

AS274 Sainani, G. S., D. B. Desai, N. H. Gorhe, D. V. Pise and P. G. Sainani. Effect of garlic and onion on important lipid and coagulation parameters in alimentary hyperlipaemia. **J Ass Phys India** 1979; 27: 57–64.

AS275 Arunachalam, K. Antimicrobial activity of garlic, onion and honey. **Geobios** 1980; 7(1): 46–47.

AS276 Mantis, A. J., P. A. Koidis and P. A. G. Karaioannoglou. Effect of garlic extract on food poisoning bacteria. **Lebensm Wiss Technol** 1979; 12: 330–332.

AS277 Jain, R. C. Effect of alcoholic extract of garlic in atherosclerosis. **Amer J Clin Nutr** 1978; 31: 1982–1983.

AS278 Tucakov, J. Ethnophytotherapy of diabetes. **Srp Arh Celok Lek** 1978; 106: 159–173.

AS279 Zacharias, N. T., K. L. Sebastian, B. Philip and K. T. Augusti. Hypoglycemic and hypolipidaemic effects of garlic in sucrose-fed rabbits. **Indian J Physiol Pharmacol** 1980; 24: 151–154.

AS280 Makheja, A. N., J. Y. Vanderhoek, R. W. Bryant and J. M. Bailey. Altered arachidonic acid metabolism in platelets inhibited by onion or garlic extracts. **Adv Prostaglandin Thromboxane Res** 1980; 6: 309–312.

AS281 Lang, Y. J. and K. Y. Cheng. Studies on the active principles of garlic. **Chung Ts'ao Yao** 1981; 12(1): 4–6.

AS282 Ariga, T. and S. Oshiba. Effects of the essential oil components of garlic cloves on rabbit platelet aggregation. **Igaku To Seibutsugaku** 1981; 102(4): 169–174.

AS283 Ariga, T. and S. Oshiba. Inhibition of human platelet aggregation by garlic oil and related substances. **Igaku To Seibutsugaku** 1981; 102(4): 175–180.

AS284 Boullin, D. J. Garlic as a platelet inhibitor. **Lancet** 1981; 776–777.

AS285 Osman, S. A. Chemical and biological studies of onion and garlic in an attempt to isolate a hypoglycaemic extract. **Abstr 4th Asian Symp Med Plants Spices** 1980; 117.

AS286 Godhwani, J. L. and J. B. Gupta. Modification of immunological response by garlic, guggal and turmeric: An experimental study in animals. **Abstr 13th Annual Conf Indian Pharmacol Soc** 1980; Abstr-12.

AS287 Kloos, H. Preliminary studies of medicinal plants and plant products in markets of Central Ethiopia. **Ethnomedicine** 1977; 4(1): 63–104.

AS288 Bhat, P. G. and T. N. Pattabiraman. Solubilization and purification of a particulate hexokinase from garlic (*Allium sativum*) bulbs. **Indian J Biochem Biophys** 1979; 16: 284–287.

AS289 Bordia, A. Effect of garlic on blood lipids in patients with coronary heart disease. **Amer J Clin Nutr** 1981; 34: 2100–2103.

AS290 Gurpratap, S. and K. Raghuvansh. Garlic in dyspepsia (a trial in 30 cases). **Antiseptic** 1981; 78: 197–200.

AS291 Kamanna, V. S. and N. Changrasekhara. Effect of garlic (*Allium sativum* Linn.) on serum lipoproteins and lipoprotein cholesterol levels in albino rats rendered hypercholesteremic by feeding cholesterol. **Lipids** 1982; 17(7): 483–488.

AS292 Vanderhoek, J. Y., A. N. Makheja and J. M. Bailey. Inhibition of fatty acid oxygenases by onion and garlic oils: Evidence for the mechanism by which these oils inhibit platelet aggregation. **Biochem Pharmacol** 1980; 29: 3169–3173.

AS293 Kumar, C. A., K. K. Saxena, C. Gupta, R. Gopal, R. C. Singh, S. Juneja, R. K. Srivastava and D. N. Prasad. Allium sativum: Effect of three weeks feeding in rats. **Indian J Pharmacol** 1981; 13: 91.

AS294 Amla, V., D. Singh, R. K. Raina and T. R. Sharma. Preliminary clinical evaluation of garlic capsule in chronic rheumatic disorders. **Indian J Pharmacol** 1981; 13: 64.

AS295 Kaur, J., S. Goyal, V. Bhasin, V. K. Kulshrestha and D. N. Prasad. Effect of C. *mukul*, A. *sativum* and A. *cepa* on coagulation and fibrinolysis in experimental atherosclerosis. **Indian J Pharmacol** 1981; 13(3): 90–91.

AS296 Dixit, V. P. and S. Joshi. Effects of chronic administration of garlic (*Allium sativum* Linn.) on testicular function. **Indian J Exp Biol** 1982; 20: 534–536.

AS297 Bolton, S., G. Null and W. M. Troetel. The medical uses of garlic: fact and fiction. **Amer Pharm NS** 1982; 22(8): 40–43.

AS298 Ariga, T. and S. Oshiba. Inhibition of platelet aggregation by garlic oil components: Separation and identification of an effective substance. **Igaku No Ayumi** 1981; 118: 859–862.

AS299 Adamu, I., P. K. Joseph and K. T. Augusti. Hypolipidemic action of onion and garlic unsaturated oils in sucrose-fed rats over a two-month period. **Experientia** 1982; 38: 899–901.

AS300 Prasad, G., V. D. Sharma and A. Kumar. Efficacy of garlic (*Allium sativum* L.) therapy against experimental dermatophytosis in rabbits. **Indian J Med Res** 1982; 75: 465–467.

AS301 Chi, M. S., E. T. Koh and T. J. Stewart. Effects of garlic on lipid metabolism in rats fed cholesterol or lard. **J Nutr** 1982; 112: 241–248.

AS302 Maroli, S. and S. Javale. Garlic (*Allium sativum*) as a common household remedy. **Pediatr Clin India** 1982; 17(2): 9–10.

AS303 Sainani, G. B., D. P. Bhalode, S. M. Natu, D. V. Pise and R. Kayerkar. Garlic pearls in cases of hyperlipidaemia (A report of a clinical trial). **Antiseptic** 1982; 79: 201–204.

AS304 Das, S. N., A. K. Pramanik, S. K. Mitra and B. N. Mukherjee. Effect of garlic pearls (ranbaxy) on blood cholesterol level in normal dogs. **Indian Vet J** 1982; 59: 937–938.

AS305 Prakash, A. O., R. B. Gupta and R. Mathur. Effect of oral administration of forty-two indigenous plant extracts on early and late pregnancy in albino rats. **Probe** 1978; 17(4): 315–323.

AS306 Chi, M. S. Effects of garlic products on lipid metabolism in cholesterol-fed rats. **Proc Soc Exp Biol Med** 1982; 171: 174–178.

AS307 Kumar, A. and V. D. Sharma. Inhibitory effect of garlic (*Allium sativum*) on enterotoxigenic *Escherichia coli*. **Indian J Med Res** 1982; 76: 66–70.

AS308 Bekdairova, K. Z. Caffeic acid — Natural inhibitor of garlic bulb growth. **Izv Akad Nauk Kaz SSR** 1981; 4: 20–24.

AS309 Baldwa, V. S., P. C. Ranka, J. P. Rishi and R. R. Rai. Commiphora mukul (guggul), garlic extract and clofibrate in hypolipidaemic states. **Rajasthan Med J** 1981; 20(2): 73–76.

AS310 Godhwani, J. D., J. B. Gupta and A. P. Dadhich. Modification of immunological response by garlic, guggal and turmeric: an experimental study in albino rats. **Proc Indian Pharmacol Soc** 1980; Abstr 1–2.

AS311 Zaman, Q. A. M., H. Banoo, S. Choudhury and A. Khaleque. Effect of garlic oil on serum cholesterol and blood sugar levels in adult human volunteers in Bangladesh. **Bangladesh Med J** 1981; 10(1): 6–10.

AS312 Chutani, S. K. and A. Bordia. The effect of fried versus raw garlic on fibrinolytic activity in man. **Atherosclerosis** 1981; 38: 417–421.

AS313 Nagda, K. K., S. K. Ganeriwal, K. C. Nagda and A. M. Diwan. Effect of onion and garlic on blood coagulation and fibrinolysis in vitro. **Indian J Physiol Pharmacol** 1983; 27(2): 141–145.

AS314 Lal, S. D. and B. K. Yadav. Folk medicine of Kurukshetra district (Haryana), India. **Econ Bot** 1983; 37(3): 299–305.

AS315 Adesina, S. K. Studies on some plants used as anticonvulsants in Amerindian and African traditional medicine. **Fitoterapia** 1982; 53: 147–162.

AS316 Tanaka, S., M. Saito and M. Tabata. Bioassay of crude drugs for hair growth promoting activity in mice by a new simple method. **Planta Med Suppl** 1980; 40: 84–90.

AS317 Ross, S. A., N. E. El-Keltawi and S. E. Megalla. Antimicrobial activity of some Egyptian aromatic plants. **Fitoterapia** 1980; 51: 201–205.

AS318 Razzack, H. M. A. The concept of birth control in Unani medical literature. **Unpublished manuscript.** 1980; 64pp.

AS319 Srivastava, K. C., A. D. Perera and H. O. Saridakis. Bacteriostatic effects of garlic sap on Gram negative pathogenic bacteria — An in vitro study. **Lebensm Wiss Technol** 1982; 15(2): 74–76.

AS320 Foushee, D. B., J. Ruffin and U. Banerjee. Garlic as a natural agent for the treatment of hypertension: A preliminary report. **Cytobios** 1982; 34: 145–152.

AS321 Yang, K. Y. and H. S. Shin. Lipids and fatty acid composition of garlic (*Allium sativum* Linnaeus). **Hanguk Sikp'um Kwahakhoe Chi** 1982; 14(4): 388–393.

AS322 Qureshi, A. A., N. Abuirmeileh, Z. Z. Din, C. E. Elson and W. C. Burger. Inhibition of cholesterol and fatty acid biosynthesis in liver enzymes and chicken hepatocytes by polar fractions of garlic. **Lipids** 1983; 18(5): 343–348.

AS323   Rakhimbaev, I. R. and R. V. Ol'Shanskaya. Preliminary identification of natural gibberellins of garlic. **Izv Akad Nauk Kaz SSR Ser Biol** 1981; 2: 17–22.

AS324   Elnima, E. I., S. A. Ahmed, A. G. Mekkawi and J. S. Mossa. The antimicrobial activity of garlic and onion extracts. **Pharmazie** 1983; 38(11): 747–748.

AS325   Arime, M. and M. Deki. Components of sugars in garlic. **Kanzei Chuo Bunsekishoho** 1983; 23: 89–93.

AS326   Naito, S., N. Yamaguchi and Y. Yokoo. Studies on natural antioxidants: III. Fractionation of antioxidant activity from garlic extract. **Nippon Shokuhin Kogyo Gakkaishi** 1981; 28(9): 465–470.

AS327   Kominato, Y., S. Nishimura and K. Takeyama. Studies on biological active component in garlic (*Allium scorodoprasm* L. or *Allium sativum*): II. Thiamin-retaining effects of scordinin A, B mixture and antibacterial activities of the scordinin decomposition product. **Oyo Yakuri** 1976; 12: 571–577.

AS328   Stauffer, M. Germanium, a constituent in various medicinal plants. **Erfahrungsheilkunde** 1980; 29: 646–647.

AS329   Abraham, S. K. and P. C. Kesavan. Genotoxicity of garlic, turmeric and asafoetida in mice. **Mutat Res** 1984; 136(1): 85–88.

AS330   Bordia, A. Effect of garlic on human platelet aggregation in vitro. **Atherosclerosis** 1978; 30(4): 355–360.

AS331   Sharma, K. K. and S. P. Sharma. Effect of onion and garlic on serum cholesterol in normal subjects. **Mediscope** 1979; 22(7): 134–136.

AS332   Jain, R. C. and C. R. Vyas. Onion and garlic in atherosclerotic heart disease. **Medikon** 1977; 6(5): 12–14.

AS333   Castro, R. A., S. Cabrera, M. R. Cruz, E. Ledezma and M. K. Jain. Effects of garlic extract and of three pure components isolated from it on human platelet aggregation, arachidonate metabolism, release reaction and platelet ultrastructure. **Thromb Res** 1983; 32(2): 155–169.

AS334   Conner, D. E. and L. R. Beuchat. Effects of essential oils from plants on growth of food spoilage yeasts. **J Food Sci** 1984; 49(2): 429–434.

AS335   Lechner-Knecht, S. Sacred healing plants in Nepal. **Dtsch Apoth Ztg** 1982; 122: 2122–2129.

AS336   Ungsurungsie, M., O. Suthienkul and C. Paovalo. Mutagenicity screening of popular Thai spices. **Food Chem Toxicol** 1982; 20: 527–530.

AS337   Martinez, M. A. Medicinal plants used in a Totonac community of the Sierra Norte de Puebla: Tuzamapan de Galeana, Puebla, Mexico. **J Ethnopharmacol** 1984; 11(2): 203–221.

AS338   Gaffen, J. D., I. A. Tavares and A. Bennett. The effect of garlic extracts on contractions of rat gastric fundus and human platelet aggregation. **J Pharm Pharmacol** 1984; 36(4): 272–274.

AS339   Chauhan, L. S. J. Garg, H. K. Bedi, R. C. Gupta, B. S. Bomb and M. P. Agarwal. Effect of onion, garlic and clofibrate on coagulation and fibrinolytic activity of blood in cholesterol-fed rabbits. **Indian Med J** 1982; 76(10): 126–127.

AS340   Sodimu, O., P. K. Joseph and K. T. Augusti. Certain biochemical effects of garlic oil on rats maintained on high fat-high cholesterol diet. **Experientia** 1984; 40(1): 78–79.

AS341   Kamanna, V. S. and N. Changrasekhara. Hypocholestermic activity of different fractions of garlic. **Indian J Med Res** 1984; 79(4): 580–583.

AS342   Choy, Y. M., T. T. Kwok, K. P. Fung and C. Y. Lee. Effect of garlic, Chinese medicinal drugs and amino acids on growth of Erlich ascites tumor cells in mice. **Amer J Chin Med** 1983; 11(1/4) 69–73.

AS343   Boukef, K, H. R. Souissi and G. Balansard. Contribution to the study on plants used in traditional medicine in Tunisia. **Plant Med Phytother** 1982; 16(4): 260–279.

AS344   Kim, S. K., E. S. Bae and C. W. Cha. A study on the effect of garlic on the toxicity of cadmium in rats. **Koryo Taehakkyo Uikwa Taehak Nonmunjip** 1984; 21(1): 65–76.

AS345   Hsu, B. Recent progress in antineoplastic drug research in China (review). **Cancer Research in the People's Republic of China and the United States of America — Epidemiology, Causation and Approaches to Therapy** 1980; 235–250.

AS346 Cosminsky, S. Anthropology of Human Birth, Chapter 12. 1982: 233–252.

AS347 Rattanapanone, V. Antithiamin factor in fruits, mushrooms and spices. **Chiang Mai Med Bull** 1979; 18: 9–16.

AS348 Kanezawa, A., S. Nakagawa, H. Sumiyoshi, K. Masamoto, H. Harada, S. Nakagami, S. Date, A. Yokota, M. Nishikawa and T. Fuwa. General toxicity testing of a garlic extract preparation containing vitamins (kyoleopin). **Oyo Yakuri** 1984; 27(5): 909–929.

AS349 Tongia, S. K. Effects of intravenous garlic juice (*Allium sativum*) on rat electrocardiogram. **Indian J Physiol Pharmacol** 1984; 28(3): 250–252.

AS350 Singh, K. V. and R. K. Pathak. Effect of leaves extracts of some higher plants on spore germination of *Ustilago maydes* and *U. nuda*. **Fitoterapia** 1984; 55(5): 318–320.

AS351 Singh, K. V. and N. P. Shukla. Activity on multiple resistant bacteria of garlic (*Allium sativum*) extract. **Fitoterapia** 1984; 55(5): 313–315.

AS352 Ojewole, J. A. O., A. D. Adekile and O. O. Odebiyi. Pharmacological studies on a Nigerian herbal preparation: 1. Cardiovascular actions of cow's urine concoction (CUC) and its individual components. **Int J Crude Drug Res** 1982; 20: 71–85.

AS353 Hemadri, K. and S. Sasibhushana Rao. Antifertility, abortifacient and fertility promoting drugs from Dandakaranya. **Ancient Sci Life** 1983; 3(2): 103–107.

AS354 Bobboi, A., K. T. Augusti and P. K. Joseph. Hypolipidemic effects of onion oil and garlic oil in ethanol-fed rats. **Indian J Biochem Biophys** 1984; 21(3): 211–213.

AS355 Sarkar, A. R. and M. K. De. Some observations on the role of garlic in the treatment of experimental hyperlipidemia. **Cal Med J** 1983; 80(11/12): 157–161.

AS356 Prasad, G., V. D. Sharma, V. N. Rao and A. Kumar. Efficacy of garlic (*Allium sativum*) treatment against dermatophy-tosis in man and animals. **Indian Vet Med J** 1983; 7(3): 161–163.

AS357 Anon. More praise for onions and garlic. **Food Chem Toxicol** 1984; 22(11): 918.

AS358 Browner, C. H. Plants used for reproductive health in Oaxaca, Mexico. **Econ Bot** 1985; 39(4): 482–504.

AS359 Bobboi, A., K. T. Augusti and P. K. Joseph. Hypolipidemic effects of onion oil and garlic oil in ethanol-fed rats. **Indian J Biochem Biophys** 1984; 21(3): 211–213.

AS360 Said, M. Potential of herbal medicines in modern medical therapy. **Ancient Sci Life** 1984; 4(1): 36–47.

AS361 Woo, W. S., E. B. Lee, K. H. Shin, S. S. Kang and H. J. Chi. A review of research on plants for fertility regulation in Korea. **Korean J Pharmacog** 1981; 12(3): 153–170.

AS362 Mossa, J. S. A study on the crude antidiabetic drugs used in Arabian folk medicine. **Int J Crude Drug Res** 1985; 23(3): 137–145.

AS363 Lee, H. S., E. S. Bae and C. W. Cha. The effect of garlic on pathological damages of testis due to cadmium poisoning. **Koryo Taehakkyo Uikwa Taehak Nonmunjip** 1984; 21(3): 39–47.

AS364 Park, J. S. and C. W. Cha. A study on the effect of garlic on the toxicity of phenyl mercuric acetate in rats. **Koryo Taehakkyo Uikwa Taehak Nonmunjip** 1984; 21(3): 49–58.

AS365 Afzal, M., R. A. H. Hassan, A. A. El-Kazimi and R. M. A. Fattah. *Allium sativum* in the control of atherosclerosis. **Agr Biol Chem** 1985; 49(4): 1187–1188.

AS366 Singh, Y. N. Traditional medicine in Fiji: Some herbal folk cures used by Fiji Indians. **J Ethnopharmacol** 1986; 15(1): 57–88.

AS367 Liu, J., X. Lin, C. Li, X. Lin and S. Peng. The blocking effect of garlic on dimethylnitrosamine formation mediated by *Fusarium monoliforme*. **Shandong Yixueyuan Xuebao** 1985; 23(2): 31–34.

AS368 Inouye, S., H. Goi, K. Miyauchi, S. Muraki, M. Ogihara and Y. Iwanami. Inhibitory effect of volatile constituents of plants on the proliferation of bacteria — antibacterial activity of plant volatiles. **J Antibact Antifung Agents** 1983; 11(11); 609–615.

AS369   Hikino, H., M. Tohkin, Y. Kiso, T. Namiki, S. Nishimura and K. Takeyama. Antihepatotoxic actions of *Allium sativum* bulbs. **Planta Med** 1986; 3: 163–168.

AS370   Kanezawa, A., S. Nakagawa, H. Sumiyoshi, K. Masamoto, H. Harada, S. Nakagami, S. Date, A. Yokota, M. Nishikawa and T. Fuwa. General toxicity tests of garlic extract preparation-contained vitamins (kyoleopin). **Pharmacometrics** 1984; 27(5): 909–929.

AS371   Nakagawa, S., H. Sumiyoshi, K. Masamoto, A. Kanezawa, H. Harada, S. Nakagami, S. Date, A. Yokota, M. Nishikawa and T. Fuwa. Acute and subacute toxicity tests of a ginseng and garlic preparation containing vitamin B-1 (Leopin-five). **Pharmacometrics** 1984; 27(6): 1133–1150.

AS372   Mandal, S. and D. K. Choudhuri. Cholesterol metabolism in Lohita grandis gray (*Hemiptera: Pyrrhocoridae: Insecta*): Effect of corpora allatectomy and garlic extract. **Curr Sci** 1982; 51(7): 367–369.

AS373   Singh, V., A. Kumar and S. P. Singh. Effect of normal saline, potassium permanganate and garlic extract on healing of contaminated wound in buffalo calves. **Indian J Anim Sci** 1984; 54(1): 41–45.

AS374   Singh, K. V. and S. K. Deshmukh. Volatile consituents from members of Liliaceae and spore germination of *Microsporum gypseum* complexes. **Fitoterapia** 1984; 55(5): 297–299.

AS375   Lee, D. G., J. G. Min and C. W. Cha. A study on the effect of garlic in the inhibitory action of cadmium on aLAD activities in human blood in vitro. **Koryo Taehakkyo Uikwa Taehak Nonmunjip** 1985; 22(1): 135–141.

AS376   Khan, M. R. and N. Mahmood. A study of lipase activity of garlic. **J Nat Sci Math** 1984; 24(1): 75–82.

AS377   Luley, C., W. Lehmann-Leo, B. Moller, T. Martin and W. Schwartzkopff. Lack of efficacy of dried garlic in patients with hyper-lipoproteinemia. **Arzneim-Forsch** 1986; 36(4): 766–768.

AS378   Huh, K., J. M. Park and S. I. L. Lee. Effect of garlic on the hepatic glutathione s-transferase and glutathione peroxidase activity in rat. **Arch Pharm Res** 1985; 8(4): 197–203.

AS379   Farva, D., I. A. Goji, P. K. Joseph and K. T. Augusti. Effects of garlic oil on streptozotocin-diabetic rats maintained on normal and high-fat diets. **Indian J Biochem Biophys** 1986; 23: 24–27.

AS380   Morita, K., M. Hara and T. Kada. Studies on natural desmutagens: screening for vegetable and fruit factors active in inactivation of mutagenic pyrolysis products from amino acids. **Agr Biol Chem** 1978; 42(6): 1235–1238.

AS381   Tsai, Y., L. L. Cole, L. E. Davis, S. J. Lockwood, V. Simmons, G. C. Wild. Antiviral properties of garlic: In vitro effects on Influenza B, Herpes simplex and Coxsackie viruses. **Planta Med** 1985; 5: 460–461.

AS382   Alkiewicz, J. and B. Dabrowski. Investigations of application of a lyophilized extract from garlic (*Allium sativum* L.) in aerosol therapy of respiratory tract diseases in children. **Herba Pol** 1982; 28(3/4): 195–204.

AS382   Guerin, J. C. and H. P. Reveillere. Antifungal activity of plant extracts used in therapy: I. Study of 41 plant extracts against 9 fungi species. **Ann Pharm Fr** 1984; 42(6): 552–559.

AS383   Hwang, J., E. S. Bae and C. W. Cha. A study on the protective effect of Korean garlic on the albino rat, chronically exposed to methylmercury. **Koryo Taehakkyo Uikwa Taehak Nonmunjip** 1986; 23(1): 121–130.

AS384   Sharma, C. P. and N. V. Nirmala. Effects of garlic extract and of three pure components isolated from it on human platelet aggregation, arachidonate metabolism, release reaction and platelet ultra-structure — Comments. **Thromb Res** 1985; 37(3): 489–490.

AS385   Singhvi, S., K. C. Joshi, S. Hiran, S. Bhandari and L. K. Tambi. Effect of onion and garlic on blood lipids. **Rajasthan Med J** 1984; 23(1): 3–6.

AS386   Kiviranta, J, T. Seppanen, H. Karppanen, H. Huovinen and R.

Hiltunen. Effects of onion and garlic extracts of spontaneously hypertonic rats. **Pharm Weekbl (Sci Ed)** 1987; 9(4): 237.

AS387 Papageorgion, C., J. P. Corbet, F. M. Brandao, M. Pecegueiro and C. Benezia. Allergic contact dermatitis to garlic (*Allium sativum* L.): Identification of the allergens — the role of monodisulphides and trisulphides present in garlic. **Arch Dermatol Res** 1983; 275(4): 229–234.

AS388 Weniger, B., M. Rouzier, R. Daguilh, D. Henrys, J. H. Henrys and R. Anton. Popular medicine of the Central Plateau of Haiti: 2. Ethnopharmacological inventory. **J Ethnopharmacol** 1986; 17(1): 13–30.

AS389 Grainge, M., L. Berger and S. Ahmed. Effect of extracts of *Artabotrys uncinatus* and *Allium sativum* on *Xanthomonas campestris* pv. *Oryzae*. **Curr Sci** 1985; 54(2): 90.

AS390 Ikpeazu, O. V., K. T. Agusti and P. K. Joseph. Hypolipidemic effect of garlic extracts mixed with 3% ethanol in rats fed sucrose high-fat diet. **Indian J Biochem Biophys** 1987; 24(4): 252–253.

AS391 Mirhadi, S. A. and S. Singh. Effect of garlic extract on in vitro uptake of CA2+ and H_2PO_4 by matrix of sheep aorta. **Indian J Exp Biol** 1987; 25: 22–23.

AS392 Chi, M. S., E. T. Koh and T. J. Stewart. Effects of garlic on lipid metabolism in rats fed cholesterol or lard. **J Nutr** 1982; 112(2): 241–248.

AS393 Abbruzzese, M. R., E. C. Delaha and V. F. Garagusi. Absence of antimycobacterial synergism between garlic extract and antituberculosis drugs. **Diagn Microbiol Infect Dis** 1987; 8(2): 79–85.

AS394 Hirao, Y., I. Sumioka, S. Nakagami, M. Yamamoto, S. Hatono, S. Yoshida, T. Fuwa and S. Nakagawa. Activation of immunoresponder cells by the protein fraction from aged garlic extract. **Phytother Res** 1987; 1(4): 161–164.

AS395 Kamboj, V. P. A review of Indian medicinal plants with interceptive activity. **Indian J Med Res** 1988; 4: 336–355.

AS396 Plengvidhya, C., S. Chinayon, S. Sitprija, S. Pasatrat and M. Tankeyoon. Effects of spray-dried garlic preparation of primary hyperlipo-proteinemia. **J Med Ass Thailand** 1988; 71(5): 248–252.

AS397 El-Keltawi, N. E. M., S. E. Megalla and S. A. Ross. Antimicrobial activity of some Egyptian aromatic plants. **Herba Pol** 1980; 26(4): 245–250.

AS398 Iwanami, Y. Inhibiting effects of volatile constituents of plants on pollen growth. **Experientia** 1981; 37(12): 1280–1281.

AS399 Conner, D. E. and L. R. Beuchat. Inhibitory effects of plant oleoresins on yeast. **Interact Food Proc Int IUMS-ICFMH 12th Sym** 1984; 447–451.

AS400 Gupta, P. P., P. Khetrapal and C. L. Ghai. Effect of garlic on serum cholesterol and electrocardiogram of rabbit consuming normal diet. **Indian J Med Sci** 1987; 41(1): 6–11.

AS401 Nes, I. F., R. Skjelkvale, O. Olsvik and B. P. Berdal. The effect of natural spices and oleoresins on *Lactobacillus plantarum* and *Staphylococcus aureus*. **Microb Assoc Interact Food Proc Int IUMS-ICFMH 12th Sym** 1984; 435–440.

AS402 Koshimizu, K., H. Ohigashi, H. Tokuda, A. Kondo and K. Yamaguchi. Screening of edible plants against possible anti-tumor promoting activity. **Cancer Lett** 1988; 39(3); 247–257.

AS403 Ramirez, V. R., L. J. Mostacero, A. E. Garcia, C. F. Mejia, P. F. Pelaez, C. D. Medina and C. H. Miranda. Vegetales Empleados en Medicina Tradicional Norperuana. **Banco Agrario del Peru and NACL Univ Trujillo** 1988; 54pp.

AS404 Kagawa, K., H. Matsutaka, Y. Yamaguchi and C. Fukuhama. Garlic extract inhibits the enhanced peroxidation and production of lipids in carbon tetrachloride-induced liver injury. **Jap J Pharmacol** 1986; 42(1): 19–26.

AS405 Caceres, A., L. M. Giron, S. R. Alvarado and M. F. Torres. Screening of antimicrobial activity of plants popularly used in Guatemala for the treatment of dermatomucosal diseases. **J Ethnopharmacol** 1987; 20(3): 223–237.

AS406 Nityanand, S. and N. K. Kappor. Effect of hypocholesterolemic agents of plant origin on catecholamine bio-synthesis in normal and cholesterol-fed rabbits. **J Biosci** 1984; 6(3): 277–282.

AS407 Singhvi, S., K. C. Joshi, S. Hiran, S. Bhandari and L. K. Tambi. Effect of onion and garlic on blood lipids. **Rajasthan Med J** 1984; 23(1): 3–6.

AS408 Shah, S. A. and S. B. Vohora. Boron enhances anti-arthritic effects of garlic oil. **Fitoterapia** 1990; 61(2): 121–126.

AS409 Lau, B. H. S, P. P. Tadi and J. M. Tosk. *Allium sativum* (garlic) and cancer prevention. **Nutr Res** 1990; 10(8): 937–948.

AS410 Tariq, V. N. and A. C. Magee. Effect of volatiles from garlic bulb extract on *Fusarium oxysporum* F. sp. *Lycopersici*. *Mycol Res 1990; 94(5): 617–620.*

AS411 Giron, L. M., G. A. Aguilar, A. Caceres and G. L. Arroyo. Anticandidal activity of plants used for the treatment of vaginitis in Guatemala and clinical trial of a *Solanum nigrescens* preparation. **J Ethnopharmacol** 1988; 22(3): 307–313.

AS412 Belman, S., A. Sellakumar, M. C. Bosland, K. Savarese and R. D. Estensen. Papilloma and carcinoma production in DMBA-initiated, onion oil-promoted mouse skin. **Nutr Cancer** 1990; 14(2): 141–148.

AS413 Kaplan, B., M. Schaewach-Millet and S. Yorav. Factitial dermatitis induced by application of garlic. **Int J Dermatol** 1990; 29(1): 75–76.

AS414 Guerin, J. C. and H. P. Reveillere. Antifungal activity of plant extracts used in therapy: I. Study of 41 plant extracts against 9 fungi species. **Ann Pharm Fr** 1984; 42(6): 553–559.

AS415 Tadi, P. P., R. W. Teel and B. H. S. Lau. Organosulfur compounds of garlic modulate mutagenesis, metabolism and DNA binding of aflatoxin B1. **Nutr Cancer** 1991; 15(2): 87–95.

AS416 Lee, T. Y. and T. H. Lam. Contact dermatitis due to topical treatment with garlic in Hong Kong. **Contact Dermatitis** 1991; 24(3): 193–196.

AS417 Unnikrishnan, M. C., K. K. Soudamini and R. Kuttan. Chemoprotection of garlic extract toward cyclophospha-

mide toxicity in mice. **Nutr Cancer** 1990; 13(3): 201–207.

AS418 Pantoja, C. V., L. C. Chiange, B. C. Norris and J. B. Concha. Diuretic, natriuretic and hypotensive effects produced by *Allium sativum* (garlic) in anaesthetized dogs. **J Ethnopharmacol** 1991; 31(3): 325–331.

AS419 Kiesewetter, H., F. Jung, G. Pindur, E. M. Jung, C. Mrowietz and E. Wenzel. Effect of garlic on thrombocyte aggregation, microcirculation and other risk factors. **I J Clin Pharmcol Ther Tox** 1991; 29(4): 151–155.

AS420 Hughes, B. G. and L. D. Lawson. Antimicrobial effects of *Allium sativum* L. (garlic), *Allium ampeloprasum* L. (elephant garlic), *Allium cepa* L. (onion), garlic compounds and commercial garlic supplement products. **Phytother Res** 1991; 5(4): 154–158.

AS421 Kourounakis, P. N. and E. A. Rekka. Effect on active oxygen species of alliin and *Allium sativum* (garlic) powder. **Res Commun Chem Pathol Pharmacol** 1991; 74(2): 249–252.

AS422 Mirhadi, S. A., S. Singh and P. P. Gupta. Effect of garlic supplementation of cholesterol-rich diet on development of atherosclerosis in rabbits. **Indian J Exp Biol** 1991; 29(2): 162–168.

AS423 Jung, E. M., F. Jung, C. Mrowietz, H. Kiesewetter, G. Pindur and E. Wenzel. Influence of garlic powder on cutaneous microcirculation. **Arzneim-Forsch** 1991; 41(6): 626–630.

AS424 Brosche, T. and D. Platt. Garlic. **Brit Med J** 1991; 303(6805): 785.

AS425 Uda, N. Extraction of eruboside B from plants as an inhibitor of carcinogens. **Patent- Japan Kokai Tokkyo Koho** 1990; 02 243,631: 4 pp.

AS426 Deboer, L. W. V. and J. D. Folts. Garlic extract prevents acute platelet thrombus formation in stenosed canine coronary arteries. **Amer Heart J** 1989; 117(4): 973–975.

AS427 Batistic, M. A. Thin-layer chromatographic characterization of preparation from *Allium sativum* L. **Rev Inst Adolfo Lutz** 1989; 49(1): 5–10.

AS428 Ali, M., M. Thomson, M. A. Alnaqeeb, J. M. Al-Hassan, S. H. Khater and S. A. Gomes. Antithrombotic activity of garlic: Its inhibition of the synthesis of thromboxane-B2 during infusion of arachidonic acid and collagen in rabbits. **Prostaglandins Leukotrienes Essent Fatty Acids** 1990; 41(2): 95–99.

AS429 Koch, H. P., W. Jager, J. Hysek and B. Korpert. Garlic and onion extracts: In vitro inhibition of adenosine deaminase. **Phytother Res** 1992; 6(1): 50–52.

AS430 Oelkers, B., H. Diehl and H. Liebig. In vitro inhibition of cytochrome P-450 reductases from pig liver microsomes by garlic extracts. **Arzneim-Forsch** 1992; 42(2): 136–139.

AS431 Al-Bekairi, A. M., A. H. Shah and S. Qureshi. Effect of *Allium sativum* on epididymal spermatozoa, estradiol-treated mice and general toxicity. **J Ethnopharmacol** 1990; 29(2): 117–125.

AS432 Sendl, A., G. Elbl, B. Steinke, K. Redl, W. Breu and H. Wagner. Comparative pharmacological inverstigations of *Allium ursinum* and *Allium sativum*. **Planta Med** 1992; 58(1): 1–7.

AS433 Lawson, L. D., D. K. Ransom and B. G. Hughes. Inhibition of whole blood platelet-aggregation by compounds in garlic clove extracts and commercial garlic products. **Thrombosis Research** 1992; 65(2): 141–156.

AS434 Panthong, A., D. Kanjanapothi and W. C. Taylor. Ethnobotanical review of medicinal plants from Thai traditional books: Part 1. Plants with anti-inflammatory, antiasthmatic and antihypertensive properties. **J Ethnopharmacol** 1986; 18(3): 213–228.

AS435 Lokar, L. C. and L. Poldini. Herbal remedies in the traditional medicine of the Venezia Giulia region (Northeast Italy). **J Ethnopharmacol** 1988; 22(3): 231–239.

AS436 Mukerji, B. and S. K. Gupta. Indigenous drugs in experimental tuberculosis. **Chemotherapy Proc Symposium Lucknow** 1959; 90–.

AS437 Pennington, C. W. Medicinal plants utilized by the Pima Montanes of Chihuahua. **Amer Indigena** 1973; 33: 213–232.

AS438 Prakash, A. O. and R. Mathur. Screening of Indian plants for antifertility activity. **Indian J Exp Biol** 1976; 14: 623–626.

AS439 Bickoff, E. M. Estrogen-like substances in plants. **Physiology of Reproduction** 1963; 93–118.

AS440 Dragendorff, G. Die Heilpflanzen der Verschiedenen Volker und Zeiten, F. Enke, Stuttgart 1898; 885pp.

AS441 Ueki, H., M. Kaibara, M. Sakagawa and S. Hayashi. Antitumor activity of plant consituents I. **Yakugaku Zasshi** 1961; 81: 1641–1644.

AS442 Appleton, H. A. and M. R. Tansey. Inhibition of growth of zoopathogenic fungi by garlic extract. **Mycologia** 1975; 67: 882–885.

AS443 Tokin, I. B. The effect of phytonocides on spermatozoa and spermatogenesis in mammals. **Dokl Akad Nauk SSSR** 1953; 93: 567–568.

AS444 Lopez Sotomayor, M. A. Antagonism of *Allium sativum* and procaine in the uterus. **Arch Inst Farmacol Exp** 1958; 10: 27–33.

AS445 Velasquez, B. L., P. S. Garcia, C. D. Mijan and A. O. Hernando. Vascular effect of garlic extract: its mechanism of action. **Arch Inst Farmacol Exp** 1958; 10: 15–22.

AS446 Lorenzo Velazquez, B. and J. M. Orellana Rodriguez. Action of garlic, corticotropin and cortisone on vaginal estrus. **Arch Inst Farmacol Exp** 1955; 8: 5–9.

AS447 Lorezo Velazquez, B. and J. M. Orellana Rodriguez. Elimination of 17-Keto steroids following the action of garlic extract. **Arch Inst Farmacol Exp** 1955; 8: 10–22.

AS448 Vasil'ev, A. A. Therapy of ducks and geese in hymenolepidosis. **Veterinariya** 1957; 34(1): 43–46.

AS449 Chopra, R. N. Indigenous Drugs of India, Their Medical and Economic Aspects. The Art Press 1933; 550pp.

AS450 Sanfilippo, G. and G. Ottaviano. Pharmacological investigations on *Allium sativum*. I. General action II. Action on the arterial pressure and on the respiration. **Boll Soc Ital Biol Sper** 1944; 19: 156–158.

AS451 Cavallito, C. J. and J. H. Bailey. Allicin, the antibacterial principle of *Allium sativum*: 1. Isolation, physical properties and antibacterial effects. **J Amer Chem Soc** 1944; 66: 1950–1951.

AS452   Damrau, F. and E. A. Ferguson. The modus operandi of carminatives: the therapeutic value of garlic in functional gastrointestinal disorders. **Rev Gastroenterol** 1949; 16: 411–419.

AS453   Filippov, V. and M. Ii'ina. The state of biotin in plant material. **Dokl Akad Nauk SSSR** 1954; 95: 1267–1270.

AS454   Lehmann, F. A. Investigation of the pharmacology of *Allium sativum* (garlic). **Arch Exp Pathol Pharmakol** 1930; 147: 245–264.

AS455   Keck, K. and O. Hoffmann-Ostenhof. Constituents of garlic and their effects: III. The mutagenic action of garlic extracts. **Monatsh** 1956; 87: 240–242.

AS456   Thiersch, H. The effect of garlic on the experimental cholesterol arteriosclerosis of rabbits. **Z Ges Exp Med** 1936; 99: 473–477.

AS457   Rico, J. T. Antihelminthic properties of *Allium sativum*. **Compt Rend Soc Biol** 1926; 95: 1597–1599.

AS458   Tempel, K. H. Effect of garlic on experimental cholesterol atherosclerosis in rabbits. **Med Ernaehr** 1962; 3(9); 197–199.

AS459   Umbert de Torrescasana, E. Experimental studies of the pharmacology of the active principles of *Allium sativum* (garlic). **Rev Espan Fisiol** 1946; 2: 6–31.

AS460   Kominato, K. Scordinines A and B from garlic. **Patent- Japan** 1970; 70 12,876: 4pp.

AS461   Kominato, H. Scordine from garlic. **Patent- Japan** 1968; 71 14,918: 3pp.

AS462   Kominato, K and M. Kominato. Separation of scordinine A-1, A-2, and B from garlic. **Patent- Japan** 1972; 72 15,115: 4pp.

AS463   Tansy, M. R. and J. A. Appleton. Inhibition of fungal growth by garlic extract. **Mycologia** 1975; 67: 409–413.

AS464   Rodriguez, J. M. O. Elimination of 17-keto steroids activated by garlic extracts. **Anales Inst Farmcol Espan** 1956; 5: 85–109.

AS465   Tynecka, Z. and Z. Gos. Inhibitory action of garlic (*Allium sativum*) on growth and respiration of some microorganisms. **Acta Microbiol Pol Ser B** 1973; 5(1): 51–62.

AS466   Perrin, M., P. Dombray and M. Vlaikovitch. Experimental toxicity of garlic. **Compt Rend Soc Biol** 1924; 90: 1431–1432.

AS467   Carpenter, C. W. Antibacterial properties of yeasts, Fusarium species, onion and garlic. **Hawaiian Planters Record** 1945; 49: 41–67.

AS468   Kolodin, A. V. Effect of a preparation containing volatile fractions of garlic on some mechanisms of nonspecific immunity. **Sovrem Metody Issled** 1968; 1: 101–103.

AS469   Virtanen, A. I. and I. Mattila. Gamma-L-glutamyl-s-allyl-L-cysteine in garlic. **Suomen Kemistilehti** 1961; 34B(3): 44.

AS470   Sugii, M., T. Suzuki, S. Nagasawa and K. Kawashima. Isolation of Gamma-L-glutamyl-s-allylmercapto-L-cysteine and s-allylmercapto L-cysteine from garlic. **Chem Pharm Bull** 1964; 12(9): 1114–1115.

AS471   Suzuki, T., M. Sugii and T. Kakimoto. New gamma-glutamyl peptides in garlic. **Chem Pharm Bull** 1961; 9: 77–78.

AS472   Suzuki, T., M. Sugii and S. Nagasawa. Isolation of (-)-(s)-propenyl-L-cysteine from garlic. **Chem Pharm Bull** 1963; 11: 548–549.

AS473   Okajima, M. Consituents of the pigmented outer skin of onion bulbs. II. The separation of quercetin from the onion skin with aqueous alkaline solutions. **Sci Papers Inst Phys Chem Research** 1960; 54: 245–246.

AS474   Virtanen, A. I., M. Hatankaka and M. Berlin. Gamma-L-glutamyl-s-propylcysteine in garlic. **Suomen Kemistilehti** 1962; 35B(3): 52.

AS475   Abdou, I. A., A. A. Abou-Zeid, M. R. El-Sherbeeny and Z. H. Abou-el-Gheat. Antimicrobial activities of *Allium sativum, Allium cepa, Raphanus sativus, Capsicum frutescens, Eruca sativa, Allium kurrat* on bacteria. **Qual Plant Mater Veg** 1972; 22(1): 29–35.

AS476   Filippov, V. and M. Il'ina. The state of biotin in plant material. **Dokl Akad Naur SSSR** 1954; 95: 1267–1270.

AS477   Song, C. S., Y. S. Kim, D. J. Lee and C. C. Nam. A blood anticoagulant substance from garlic: II. Chemical analysis and studies on the biochemical and pharmocological effects. **Yonsei Med J** 1963; 4: 21–26.

AS478   Suzuki, T., M. Sugii, T. Kakimoto and N. Tsuboi. Isolation of (-) S-allyl-L-cysteine from garlic. **Chem Pharm Bull** 1961; 9: 251–252.

AS479   Schultz, O. E. and H. L. Mohrmann. Analysis of constituents of garlic (*Allium sativum*): II. Gas chromatography of garlic oil. **Pharmazie** 1965; 20(7): 441–447.

AS480   Atal, C. K. and J. K. Sethi. Occurrence of amino acids and alliin in the Indian Allium (garlics). **Curr Sci** 1961; 30: 338–340.

AS481   Granroth, B. Separation of *Allium* sufur amino acids and peptides by thin-layer electrophoresis and thin-layer chromatography. **Acta Chem Scand Ser A** 1968; 22(10): 3333–3335.

AS482   Szabason, A. Hypotensive suppository. **Patent-Belg** 1963; 631,712: 3pp.

AS483   Liebstein, A. M. Therapeutic effects of various food articles. **Amer Med** 1927; 33–38.

AS484   Seabrook, W. B. Adventures in Arabia Among the Bedouins, Druses, Whirling Dervishes & Yezidee Devil Worshippers. Blue Ribbon Book 1927; 99–105.

AS485   Bhatnagar-Thomas, P. L. and A. K. Pal. Insecticidal activity of garlic oil: II. Mode of action of the oil as a pesticide in *Musca domestic nebulo* and *Trogoderma granarium*. **J Food Sci Technol** 1974; 11(4): 153–158.

AS486   Echandi, R. J. An organoleptic and chemical investigation of the linguacheaceric properties of onion (*Allium cepa* L.) and garlic (*Allium sativum* L.). **Diss Abstr Int B** 1966; 26(10): 5632–5633.

AS487   Hoerhammer L., H. Wagner, M. Seitz, Z. J. Vejdelek. Evaluation of garlic preparations: I. Chromatographic studies of the actual components of *Allium sativum*. **Pharmazie** 1968; 23(8): 462–467.

AS488   Kominato, K. Separation and purification of metabolism regulators from natural products. **Patent-Japan** 1970; 18,679: 10pp.

AS489   Prasad, D. N., S. K. Bhattacharya, P. K. Das. A study of antiinflammatory activity of some indigenous drugs in albino rats. **Indian J Med Res** 1966; 54(6): 582–590.

AS490   Standen, O. D. Experimental chemotherapy of oxyuriasis. **Brit Med J** 1953; II: 757–758.

AS491   Kim, M. S. The effect of certain condiments on gastric secretion. **Korean Med J** 1933; 3: 115–118.

AS492   Kominato, K. and Y. Kominato. Silkworm attractant, scordinin A, from garlic. **Patent-Japan Kokai** 1973; 87,009: 3pp.

AS493   Joseph, P. K., K. R. Rao and C. S. Sundaresh. Toxic effects of garlic extract and garlic oil in rats. **Indian J Exp Biol** 1989; 27(11): 977–979.

AS494   Amonkar, S. V. and A. Banerji. Isolation and characteristization of larvicidal principle of garlic. **Science** 1971; 174: 1343–1344.

AS495   Sivaswamy, S. N., B. Balachandran, S. Balanehru and V. M. Sivaramakrishnan. Mutagenic activity of south Indian food items. **Indian J Exp Biol** 1991; 29(8): 730–737.

AS496   Schimmer, O., A. Kruger, H. Paulini and F. Haefele. An evaluation of 55 commercial plant extracts in the Ames mutagenicity test. **Pharmazie** 1994; 49(6): 448–451.

AS497   Chauhan, J. S., N. K. Singh and S. V. Singh. Screening of higher plants for specific herbicidal principle active against dodder, *Cuscuta reflexa* Roxb. **Indian J Exp Biol** 1989; 27(10): 877–884.

AS498   Hofbauer, R., M. Frass, B. Gmeiner, A. D. Kaye and E. A. Frost. Effects of garlic extract (*Allium sativum*) on neutrophil migration at the cellular level. **Heart Dis** 2001; 3(1): 14–17.

AS499   Banerjee, S. K., M. Maulik, S. C. Mancahanda, A. K. Dinda, S. K. Gupta and S. K. Maulik. Dose-dependent induction of endogenous antioxidants in rat heart by chronic administration of garlic. **Life Sci** 2002; 70(13): 1509–1518.

AS500   Ahmed, N., L. Laverick, J. Sammons, H. Zhang, D. J. Maslin and H. T. Hassan. Ajoene, a garlic-derived natural compound, enhances chemotherapy-induced apoptosis in human myeloid leukaemia CD4-positive resistant cells. **Anticancer Res** 2001; 21(5): 3519–3523.

AS501 Kalantari, H. and M. Salehi. The protective effect of garlic oil on hepatoxicity induced by acetaminophen in mice and comparison with N-acetylcysteine. **Saudi Med J** 2001; 22(12): 1080–1084.

AS502 Li, D., B. Jiao and Y. Zhu. Effect and mechanism of garlic juice and hydrogen peroxide on the degradation of lipopolysaccharide. **Zhonghua Kou Qiang Yi Xue Za Zhi** 2000; 35(5): 333–335.

AS503 Izzo, A. A. and E. Ernst. Interactions between herbal medicines and prescribed drugs: A systematic review. **Drugs** 2001; 61(15): 2163–2175.

AS504 Josling, P. Preventing the common cold with a garlic supplement: A double-blind, placebo-controlled survey. **Adv Ther** 2001; 18(4): 189–193.

AS505 Oi, Y., M. Imafuku, C. Shishido, Y. Kominato, S. Nishimura and K. Iwai. Garlic supplementation increases testicular testosterone and decreases plasma corticosterone in rats fed a high protein diet. **J Nutr** 2001; 131(8): 2150–2156.

AS506 Robert, V., B. Mouille, C. Mayuer, M. Michaud and F. Blachier. Effects of the garlic compound diallyl disulfide on the metabolism, adherence and cell cycle of HT-29 colon carcinoma cells: Evidence on sensitive and resistant sub-populations. **Carcinogenesis** 2001; 22(8): 1155–1161.

AS507 Foster, B. C., M. S. Foster, S. Vandenhock, A. Krantis, J. W. Budzinski, J. T. Arnason, K. D. Gallicano and S. Choudri. An in vitro evaluation of human cytochrome P450 3A4 and P-glycoprotein inhibition by garlic. **Pharm Pharm Sci** 2001; 4(2): 176–184.

AS508 Senapti, S. K., S. Dey, S. K. Dwivedi and D. Swarup. Effect of garlic (*Allium sativum* L.) extract on tissue lead level in rats. **Ethnopharmacol** 2001; 76(3): 229–232.

AS509 Tsao, S. M. and M. C. Yin. In-vitro antimicrobial activity of four diallyl sulphides occurring naturally in garlic and Chinese leek oils. **J Med Microbiol** 2001; 50(7): 646–649.

AS510 Kannar, D., N. Wattanapenpaiboon, G. S. Savige and M. L. Wahlqvist. Hypocholesterolemic effect of an enteric-coated garlic supplement. **J Am Coll Nutr** 2001; 20(3): 225–231.

AS511 Banerjee, S. K., M. Maulik, S. C. Manchanda, A. K. Dinda, T. K. Das and S. K. Maulik. Garlic-induced alteration in rat liver and kidney morphology and associated changes in endogenous antioxidant status. **Food Chem Toxicol** 2001; 39(8): 793–797.

AS512 Balasenthil, S., C. R. Ramachandran and S. Nagini. Prevention of 4-nitorquinoline 1-oxide-induced rat tongue carcinogenesis by garlic. **Fitoterapia** 2001; 72(5): 524–531.

AS513 Grudzinski, I. P., A. Frankiewicz-Jozko and J. Bany. Diallyl sulfide-a flavour component from garlic (*Allium sativum*) attenuates lipid peroxidation in mice infected with *Trichinella spiralis*. **Phytomedicine** 2001; 8(3): 174–177.

AS514 Rahmy, T. R. and K. Z. Hemmaid. Prophylactic action of garlic on the histological and histochemical patterns of hepatic and gastric tissues in rats injected with a snake venom. **Nat Toxins** 2001; 10(2): 137–165.

AS515 Sheen, L. Y., C. C. Wu, C. K. Lii and S. J. Tsai. Effect of diallyl sulfide and diallyl disulfide, the active principles of garlic, on the aflatoxin B(1)-induced DNA damage in primary rat hepatocytes. **Toxicol Lett** 2001; 122(1): 45–52.

AS516 Liu, L. and Y. Y. Yeh. Water-soluble organosulfur compounds of garlic inhibit fatty acid and triglyceride syntheses in cultured rat hepatocytes. **Lipids** 2001; 36(4): 395–400.

AS517 Jarial, M. S. Toxic effect of garlic extracts on the eggs of *Aedes aegypti* (Diptera: Culicidae): A scanning electron microscope study. **J Med Entomol** 2001; 38(3): 446–450.

AS518 Ohnishi, S. T., T. Onsishi and G. B. Ogunmola. Green tea extract and aged garlic extract inhibit anion transport and sickle cell dehydration in vitro. **Blood Cells Mol Dis** 2001; 27(1): 48–57.

AS519 Moon, D. G., J. Cheon, D. H. Yoon, H. S. Park, H. K. Kim, J. J. Kim and S. K. Koh. *Allium sativum* potentiates suicide gene therapy from murine transitional cell carcinoma. **Nutr Cancer** 2000; 38(1): 98–105.

AS520 Abuharfeil, N. M., M. Salim and S. Von Kleist. Augmentation of natural killer cell activity in vivo against tumour cells by some wild plants from Jordan. **Phytother Res** 2001; 15(2): 109–113.

AS521 Li, G., Z. Shi, H. Jia, J. Ju, X. Wang, Z. Xia, L. Qin, C. Ge, Y. Xu, L. Cheng, P. Chen and G. Yuan. A clinical investigation on garlicin injection for treatment of unstable angina pectoris and its actions on plasma endothelin and blood sugar levels. **J Tradit Chin Med** 2000; 20(4): 243–246.

AS522 Hoshino, T., N. Kashimoto an S. Kasuga. Effects of garlic preparations on the gastrointestinal mucosa. **J Nutr** 2001; 131(3s): 1109S–1113S.

AS523 Sumi, S., T. Tsuneyoshi, H. Matsuo and T. Yoshimatsu. Isolation and characterization of the genes up-regulated in isolated neurons by aged garlic extract (AGE). **J Nutr** 2001; 131(3s): 1096S–1099S.

AS524 Nishiyama, N., T. Moriguchi, N. Morihara and H. Saito. Ameliorative effect of S-allylcysteine, a major thioallyl constituent in aged garlic extract, on learning deficits in senescence-accelerated mice. **J Nutr** 2001; 131(3s): 1093S–1095S.

AS525 Ohnishi, S. T. and T. Ohnishi. In vitro effects of aged garlic extract and other nutritional supplements on sickle erythrocytes. **J Nutr** 2001; 131(3s): 1085S–1092S.

AS526 Kyo, E., N. Uda, S. Kasuga and Y. Itakura. Immunomodulatory effects of aged garlic extract. **J Nutr** 2001; 131(3s): 1075S–1079S.

AS527 Horie, T., S. Awazu, Y. Itakura and T. Fuwa. Alleviation by garlic of antitumor drug-induced damage to the intestine. **J Nutr** 2001; 131(3s): 1071S–1074S.

AS528 Knowles, L. M. and J. A. Milner. Possible mechanism by which allyl sulfides suppress neoplastic cell proliferation. **J Nutr** 2001; 131(3s): 1061S–1066S.

AS529 Pinto, J. T. and R. S. Rivlin. Antiproliferative effects of allium de-rivatives from garlic. **J Nutr** 2001; 131(3s): 1058S–1060S.

AS530 Song, K. and J. A. Milner. The influence of heating on the anticancer properties of garlic. **J Nutr** 2001; 131(3s): 1054S–1057S.

AS531 Singh, S. V. Impact of garlic organosulfides on p21(H-ras) processing. **J Nutr** 2001; 131(3s): 1046S–1048S.

AS532 Moriguchi, T., N. Takasugi and Y. Itakura. The effects of aged garlic extract on lipid peroxidation and the deformability of erythrocytes. **J Nutr** 2001; 131(3s): 1016S–9S.

AS533 Campbell, J. H., J. L. Efendy, N. J. Smith and G. R. Campbell. Molecular basis by which garlic suppresses atherosclerosis. **J Nutr** 2001; 131(3s): 1006S–1009S.

AS534 Ali, M., K. K. Al-Qattan, F. Al-Enezi, R. M. Khanafer and T. Mustafa. Effect of allicin from garlic powder on serum lipids and blood pressure in rats fed with a high cholesterol diet. **Prostaglandin Leukot Essent Fatty Acids** 2000; 62(4): 253–259.

AS535 Slowing, K., P. Ganado, M. Sanz, E. Ruiz and T. Tejerina. Study of garlic extracts and fractions on cholesterol plasma levels and vascular reactivity in cholesterol-fed rats. **J Nutr** 2001; 131(3s): 994S–999S.

AS536 Yeh, Y. Y. and L. Liu. Cholesterol-lowering effect of garlic extracts and organosulfur compounds: Human and animal studies. **J Nutr** 2001; 131(3s): 989S–993S.

AS537 Ryu, K., N. Ide, H. Matsuura and Y. Itakura. N alpha-(1-deoxy-D-fructos-1-yl)-L-arginine, and antioxidant compound identified in aged garlic extract. **J Nutr** 2001; 131(3s): 972S–976S.

AS538 Ariga, T., K. Tsuj, T. Seki, T. Moritomo and J. I. Yamamoto. Antithrombotic and antineoplastic effects of phyto-organosulfur compounds. **Biofactors** 2000; 13(1–4): 251–255.

AS539 Pedraza-Chaverri, J., M. D. Granados-Silvestri, O. N. Medina-Campos, P. D. Maldonado, I. M. Olivares-Corichi and M. E. Ibarra-Rubio. Post-transcriptional control of catalase expression in garlic-treated rats. **Mol Cell Biochem** 2001; 216(1–2): 9–19.

AS540   Shirin, H., J. T. Pinto, Y. Kawabata, J. W. Soh, T. Delohery, S. F. Moss, V. Murty, R. S. Rivlin, P. R. Holt and I. B. Weinstein. Antiproliferative effects of S-allylmercaptocysteine on colon cancer cells when tested alone or in combination with sulindac sulfide. **Cancer Res** 2001; 61(2): 725–731.

AS541   Ghazanfari, T., Z. M. Hassan, M. Ebtekar, A. Ahmadiani, G. Naderi and A. Azar. Garlic induces a shift in cytokine pattern in Leishmania major-infected BALB/c mice. **Scand J Immunol** 2000; 52(5): 491–495.

AS542   Pinto, J. T., C. Qiao, J. Xing, B. P. Suffoletto, K. B. Schubert, R. S. Rivlin R. F. Huryk, D. J. Bacich and W. D. Heston. Alterations of prostate biomarker expression and testosterone utilization in human LNCaP prostatic carcinoma cells by garlic-derived S-allylmercaptocysteine. **Prostate** 2000; 45(4): 304–314.

AS543   Harris, J. C., S. Plummer, M. P. Turner and D. Lloyd. The microaerophilic flagellate Giardia intestinalis: *Allium sativum* (garlic) is an effective antigiardial. **Microbiology** 2000; 146(12): 3119–3127.

AS544   Seki, T., K. Tsuji, Y. Hayato, T. Moritomo and T. Ariga. Garlic and onion oils inhibit proliferation and induce differentiation of HL-60 cells. **Cancer Lett** 2000; 160(1): 29–35.

AS545   Pedraza-Chaverri, J., O. N. Medina-Campos, M. A. Granados-Silvestre, P. D. Maldonado, I. M. Olivares-Corichi and R. Hernandez-Pando. Garlic ameliorates hyperlipidemia in chronic aminonucleoside nephrosis. **Mol Cell Biochem** 2000; 211(1–2): 69–77.

AS546   Samaranayake, M. D., S. M. Wickramasinghe, P. Angunawela, S. Jayasekera, S. Iwai and S. Fukushima. Inhibition of chemically induced liver carcinogenesis in Wistar rats by garlic (*Allium sativum*). **Phytother Res** 2000; 14(7): 564–567.

AS547   Cho, B. H. and S. Xu. Effects of allyl mercapatan and various allium-derived compounds on cholesterol synthesis and secretion on Hep-G2 cells. **Comp Biochem Physiol C Toxicol Pharmacol** 2000; 126(2): 195–201.

AS548   Hong, Y. S., Y. A. Ham, J. H. Choi and J. Kim. Effects of allyl sulfur compounds and garlic extract on the expression of Bcl-2, Bax, and p53 in non small cell lung cancer cell lines. **Exp Mol Med** 2000; 32(3): 127–134.

AS549   Liu, L. and Y. Y. Yeh. Inhibition of cholesterol biosynthesis by organosulfur compounds derived from garlic. **Lipids** 2000; 35(2): 197–203.

AS550   Sasaki, J., T. Kita, K. Ishita, H. Uchisawa and H. Matsue. Antibacterial activity of garlic powder against *Escherichia coli* O-157. **J Nutr Sci Vitaminol (Tokyo)** 1999; 45(6): 785–790.

AS551   Pantoja, C. V., N. T. Martin, B. C. Norris and C. M. Contreras. Purification and bioassays of a diuretic and natriuretic fraction from garlic (*Allium sativum*). **J Ethnopharmacol** 2000; 70(1): 35–40.

AS552   Arivazhagan, S., S. Balasenthil and S. Nagini. Modulatory effects of garlic and neem leaf extracts on N-methyl-N'-nitro-N-nitrosoguanidine (MNNG)-induced oxidative stress in Wistar rats. **Cell Biochem Funct** 2000; 18(1): 17–21.

AS553   Kasuga, S., M. Ushijima, N. Morihara, Y. Itakura and Y. Nakata. Effect of aged garlic extract (AGE) on hyperglycemia induced by immobilization stress in mice. **Nippon Yakurigaku Zasshi** 1999; 114(3): 191–197.

AS554   Lee, J. H., H. S. Kang and J. Roh. Protective effects of garlic juice against embryotoxicity of methylmercuric chloride administered to pregnant Fischer 344 rats. **Yonsei Med J** 1999; 40(5): 483–489.

4 | Aloe vera

(L.) Burm. f.

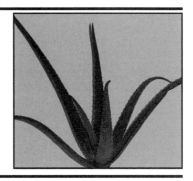

Common Names

'Awa'awa	Argentina	Grahakanya	India
Acibar	Argentina	Guarka-patha	India
Aloe	Argentina	Gwar-patha	India
Aloe	Bimini	Indian aloe	Nepal
Aloe cactus	Cook Islands	Kathazhai	India
Aloe	Rodrigues Islands	Korphad	India
Aloe	USA	Kumari	India
Aloe	Venezuela	Kumaro	India
Aloes	Argentina	Kunvar pata	India
Aloes	Trinidad	Kunwar	India
Aloes vrai	Tunisia	Laloi	Haiti
Aloes	West Indies	Laloi	India
Alovis	West Indies	Laluwe	Trinidad
Barbados aloe	USA	Laluwe	West Indies
Barbados aloe	India	Lo-hoei	Vietnam
Barbados aloe	Nepal	Lo-hoi	Vietnam
Barbados aloe	West Indies	Lou-houey	Vietnam
Bitter aloes	Guyana	Lu-chuy	Vietnam
Bunga raja raja	Malaysia	Manjikattali	India
Chirukattali	India	Mediterranean aloe	West Indies
Curacao aloe	West Indies	Murr sbarr	Tunisia
Dickwar	India	Musabar	India
Gawar	India	Panini	India
Ghai kunwar	India	Rapahoe	India
Ghai kunwrar	India	Sabar	Saudi Arabia
Ghee-kanwar	India	Saber	Jordan
Gheekuar	India	Sabila	Canary Islands
Ghikanvar	India	Sabila	Guatemala
Ghikuar	Pakistan	Sabila	Malaysia
Ghikumar	India	Sabila	Nicaragua
Ghikumari	India	Sabila	Puerto Rico
Ghikwar	India	Sabilla	Cuba
Ghiu kumari	Nepal	Sabilla	West Indies
Ghrit kumari	India	Sabr	Saudi Arabia
Ghrita kumari	India	Saqal	Oman

From: *Medicinal Plants of the World, vol. 1: Chemical Constituents, Traditional and Modern Medicinal Uses, 2nd ed.*
By: Ivan A. Ross © Humana Press Inc., Totowa, NJ

Savila	Mexico	Wan-hangchorakhe	Thailand
Savila	Peru	Yaa dam	Thailand
Savilla	Bolivia	Yadam	Thailand
Semper vivum	West Indies	Zabila	Canary Islands
Siang-tan	Vietnam	Zabila	Mexico
Sobbar	Jordan	Zabila	Panama
Tuna	Panama	Zabila	Venezuela
Waan haang charakhe	Thailand		

BOTANICAL DESCRIPTION

A short-stemmed succulent perennial herb of the LILIACEAE family, the succulent leaves are crowded on the top of their stems, spreading grayish green and glaucous; spotted when young, 20 to 50 cm long, 3 to 5 cm wide at the base, tapering gradually to the pointed tip, 1 to 2.5 cm thick; having spiny edges and bitter latex inside. Flowers are borne in cylindrical terminal racemes on central flower stalks, 5 to 100 cm high. The yellow perianth is divided into 6 lobes, about 2.5 cm long, with scattered bracts. Each flower has 6 protruding stamens and three-celled ovary with long style. Forms of the species vary in sizes of leaves and colors of flowers.

ORIGIN AND DISTRIBUTION

Aloe vera is native to North Africa, the Mediterranean region of southern Europe, and to the Canary Islands. It is now cultivated throughout the West Indies, tropical America, and the tropics in general.

TRADITIONAL MEDICINAL USES

Argentina. Hot water extract of leaves is taken orally to induce abortion and to facilitate menstruation[AV015].

Bimini. Leaf juice is used externally for skin irritations, cuts, boils and sunburn[AV095].

Bolivia. Fresh leaf juice is used as an analgesic topically for burns and wounds. Orally, the juice is used as a laxative[AV116].

Brazil. Fresh leaf juice is taken orally as an anthelmintic and febrifuge. Infusion of dried root is taken orally to treat colic[AV142].

Canary Islands. Fresh fruit juice (unripe) is taken orally as an antiasthmatic and purgative[AV141]. Infusion of fresh leaf juice is taken orally as a laxative, for dental caries, and as a teniafuge[AV124].

China. Hot water extract of leaf juice is taken orally as an emmenagogue[AV027].

Cook Islands. Fresh sap, in water, is taken orally regularly, to prevent high blood pressure, cancer and diabetes. Externally it is used to treat burns and cuts[AV045].

Cuba. Water extract of leaf pulp is taken as an emmenagogue[AV125].

Egypt. Fresh leaf juice, administered intravaginally, is a contraceptive before or after coitus. Data was obtained as a result of questioning 1200 puerperal women about their knowledge of birth control methods. 52.3% practiced a method, and 47.6% of these depend on indigenous methods and/or prolonged lactation[AV163].

England. Hot water extract of dried leaves with a mixture of *Zingiber officinale*, *Mentha phlegium* (essential oil), *Ipomoea purga*, *Glycyrrhiza glabra* and *Canella alba* is taken orally for amenorrhea[AV174].

Guatemala. Hot water extract of dried leaves is used externally for wounds, ulcers, bruises, sores, skin eruptions, erysipelas, dermatitis, inflammations, burns, abscesses, furuncles and scrofula[AV137].

Haiti. Hot water extract of dried leaves is taken orally as a purgative, for diabetes and intestinal worms[AV107].

India. Decoction of dried leaves is taken orally to induce abortion[AV035] and for sexual vitality[AV121]. The dried leaf juice is taken orally as an emmenagogue[AV131]. Decoction of root is taken orally for venereal disease and externally it is used to treat wounds[AV081]. Fresh fruit juice (unripe) is taken orally as a laxative, cathartic and for fevers[AV176]. Fresh leaves are crushed and applied locally for guinea worms[AV083]. Hot water extract of dried entire plant is taken orally as an emmenagogue, purgative, anthelmintic, and stomachic, for liver and spleen enlargement and piles. Hot water extract of fresh plant juice is taken orally for inflammation and amenorrhea[AV139]. The pulp of the plant is mixed together with salt and fermented sugar cane juice then taken orally to treat pain and inflammation of the body[AV048]. Hot water extract of leaf juice is taken orally as a cathartic; pregnant women should not use it[AV005]. Leaf pulp is taken orally regularly for 10 days by women to prevent conception[AV077]. Leaf juice is taken orally to treat viral jaundice. The juice is taken twice daily for 3 days[AV081].

Malaysia. Hot water extract of leaf juice is taken orally as a cholagogue and emmenagogue[AV017]. Hot water extract of leaves is taken orally as an emmenagogue[AV002].

Mexico. Fresh stem juice is taken orally for diabetes[AV031]. Infusion of dried leaves is taken orally to treat ulcers[AV036].

Nepal. Fresh leaf pulp is taken orally to relieve amenorrhea. 10–15 gm of leaf pulp is given with sugar or honey once a day[AV049]. Hot water extract of dried entire plant is taken orally as a purgative and to terminate pregnancy[AV102].

Panama. Fresh leaf, crushed with egg white, is taken orally as a laxative and demulcent. Sap is taken orally for stomach ulcers and externally for erysipelas and to treat swellings caused by injuries[AV098].

Peru. Hot water extract of fresh leaves is taken orally for asthma, as a purgative, and antivenin. Externally, the extract is used as an antiseptic for washing wounds[AV136].

Puerto Rico. Drink made from fresh leaf pulp of Aloe vera and fruit pulp of *Genipa americana* is a popular remedy for colds[AV118].

Saudi Arabia. Hot water extract of dried aerial parts is taken orally for liver complaints and piles, as an emetic and antipyretic, against tumors, for enlarged spleen, as a cooling agent and purgative, and for diabetes, skin diseases and asthma[AV140]. Hot water extract of dried leaves is taken orally for functional sterility, amenorrhea, piles, thermal burns, constipation, flatulence, intestinal worms and diabetes, to treat functional sterility, amenorrhea, constipation and piles. Externally the extract is used for burns[AV123].

South Korea. Hot water extract of whole dried plant is taken orally as a contraceptive, an abortifacient and emmenagogue. Use of the extract is contraindicated during pregnancy[AV122].

Switzerland. Hot water extract of the leaf is taken orally as an abortifacient[AV003].

Taiwan. Decoction of dried leaves is taken orally to treat hepatitis[AV085].

Thailand. Fresh leaf juice is used on burns[AV125]. Hot water extract of dried resin is taken orally as a cathartic[AV178].

Trinidad. Gum is taken orally as an abortifacient[AV026].

Tunisia. Hot water extract of the dried leaf is taken orally for diabetes, and to treat problems of venous circulation. Externally, the extract is used for eczema[AV119].

USA. Fresh leaf juice is taken orally for stomach ulcers, and externally to heal wounds[AV167]. Fluidextract of the leaf juice is taken orally as an emmenagogue[AV016]. Hot water extract of dried leaves is taken orally as a cathartic[AV177]. Hot water extract of gum is taken orally as an emmenagogue to promote and stimulate menstruation[AV157]. Water extract of leaves is used externally for insect bites, myopathies, arthritis, topical ulcers and other skin conditions[AV022]. Hot water extract is taken orally to increase menstrual flow; the extract should be avoided during pregnancy[AV053].

Venezuela. Bitter latex is taken orally as a laxative[AV014]. Hot water extract of leaves is taken orally as an emmenagogue[AV025].

Vietnam. Sap is taken orally as an emmenagogue[AV012].

West Indies. Gum is taken orally as an abortifacient[AV096]. Leaf juice is taken orally as an emmenagogue, anthelmintic and purgative[AV013]. Yellow latex from the epidermis is taken orally to prevent syphilis, as a purgative, to improve appetite, for intestinal worms, and to promote menstrual flow. Externally, split leaves are applied to wounds to promote healing[AV096].

CHEMICAL CONSTITUENTS
(ppm unless otherwise indicated)

1,8-Dihydroxyanthracene: Pl[AV151]
1-1-2-Triphenyl cyclopropane: Gel[AV037]
1-1-Bis-(2-hydroxy-3-5-dimethyl-phenyl)-2-methyl propane: Gel[AV037]
12-Methyl tridecanoic acid methyl ester: Gel[AV037]
13-Methyl pentadecanoic acid methyl ester: Gel[AV037]
14-Methyl pentadecanoic acid methyl ester: Gel[AV037]
15-Methyl hexadecanoic acid: Gel[AV037]
16-Methyl heptadecanoic acid methyl ester: Gel[AV037]
2(3H)-Benzothiazolone: Gel[AV037]
2-Methyl-2-phytyl-6-chromanol: Pl[AV151]
3-3'-Bis para methane: Gel[AV037]
4-4-Dimethyl-3-(2-4-5-trimethoxy-phenyl)pentanoic acid ethyl ester: Gel[AV037]
7-Hydroxyaloin: Pl[AV150]
7-Hydroxy-chromone: Pl[AV151]
8-Methyl-tocol: Pl[AV151]
8-Oleic acid methyl ester: Gel[AV037]
9-Propanoyl-methoxy-methyl phenanthrene: Gel[AV037]
Acemannan: Lf[AV182,AV194]
Alanine: Lf 177 micromols[AV187]
Aloctin I: Lf[AV212]
Aloctin II: Lf[AV212]
Alocutin A: Pl[AV151]
Aloe emodin anthranol: Pl[AV150]

Aloe emodin: Lf[AV197,AV186]
Aloe polypeptides (MW 4,000–70,000): Lf[AV183]
Aloe vera compound HM: Lf 7.5%[AV021]
Aloe vera compound LM: Lf 47.5%[AV021]
Aloeferon: Gel[AV195]
Aloemannan: Lf[AV214]
Aloenin: Pl[AV151]
Aloeride: Ju[AV202]
Aloesin: Lf[AV198]
Aloesone: Pl[AV150]
Aloetic acid: Pl[AV151]
Aloetin: Pl[AV151]
Aloetinic acid: Pl[AV152]
Aloin A,7-hydroxy-6'-0-para-coumaroyl: Lf[AV185]
Aloin B,7-hydroxy-6'-0-para-coumaroyl: Lf[AV185]
Aloin: Lf[AV074]
Aloinose: Pl[AV151]
Aloinoside-A: Pl[AV151]
Aloins: Pl 27–30%[AV151]
Alpha cellulose: Pl[AV151]
Aluminum: Lf 22[AV153]
Anthranol: Lf[AV197]
Anthraquinone glycoside: Pl[AV151]
Anthraquinones: Pl[AV151]
Anthrol: Pl[AV151]
Apoise: Pl[AV151]
Arabinan: Pl[AV151]
Arabinose: Lf[AV187]
Arachidic acid methyl ester: Gel[AV037]
Arachidonic acid: Aer[AV196]
Arginine: Lf[AV187]
Ascorbic acid: Lf 0.63%[AV153]
Asparagine: Lf 344 micromols[AV187]
Aspartic acid: Lf 237 micromols[AV187]
Barbaloin: Pl[AV120]
Behenic acid methyl ester: Gel[AV037]
Benzaldehyde,4-hydroxy-3-5-di-tert-butyl: Gel[AV037]
Benzylacetone: Pl[AV151]
Beta barbaloin: Lf[AV003]
Beta carotene: Pl 7.2.mcg/gm[AV179]
Beta sitosterol: Lf 148 micromols[AV187]
Calcium oxalate: Lf[AV179]
Campesterol: Lf 12.4 micromols[AV187]
Carbohydrates: Lf 89.6%[AV153]
Casanthranol-I: Pl[AV151]
Casanthranol-II: Pl[AV151]
Catalase: Pl[AV151]
Cholesterol: Lf 10.8 micromols[AV187], St EO 7.2 mcg/gm[AV179]

Choline salicyclate: Pl[AV151]
Choline: Pl[AV151]
Chromium: Lf[AV153]
Chrysamminic acid: Pl[AV151]
Chrysazin: Lf[AV148]
Chrysophanic acid: Pl[AV120]
Chrysophanol glycoside: Pl[AV151]
Chrysophanol: Pl[AV151]
Cobalt: Lf[AV153]
Coniferyl alcohol: Pl[AV151]
Coumarin acid, para: Lf[AV018]
Cycloeicosane: Gel[AV037]
Cysteine: Lf[AV138]
Cystine: Lf Ju[AV187]
Decyl cyclohexane: Gel[AV037]
Dehydro-abietal: Gel[AV037]
Dehydro-abietic acid methyl ester: Gel[AV037]
D-freidooleanan-3-one: Gel[AV037]
D-galactan: Pl[AV151]
D-galactose: Lf[AV191]
D-galactouronic acid: Pl[AV151]
D-glucitol: Pl[AV151]
D-glucose: Lf[AV191]
Di-(2-ethylhexyl)phthalate: Pl[AV151]
Dibutyl phthalate: Gel[AV037]
Diethylhexylphthalate: Pl[AV205]
Diheptyl phthalate: Gel[AV037]
Dioctyl phthalate: Gel[AV037]
D-mannose: Lf[AV191]
Dodecyl benzene: Gel[AV037]
Emodin: Pl[AV151]
Fat: Lf 8000[AV153]
Fiber: Lf 17.7%[AV153]
Formic acid: Pl[AV151]
Fructose: Lf, St, EO[AV179]
Galactan (Aloe vera): Lf Pu 0.01%[AV192]
Galactose: Lf[AV187]
Gluco-galacto mannan (Aloe vera): Lf[AV191]
Glucomannan (Aloe vera): Lf Pu[AV193]
Glucosamine: Pl[AV151]
Glucose: Lf 21.2 mmols[AV187]
Glutamic acid: Lf 294 micromols[AV187]
Glutamine: Lf[AV187]
Glycerol: Pl[AV151]
Glycine: Lf 67 micromols[AV187]
Hecogenin: Pl[AV151]
Heneicosanoic acid methyl ester: Gel[AV037]
Heptadec-1-ene: Gel[AV037]
Hexauronic acid: Pl[AV151]
Histidine: Lf[AV187]
Homonataloin: Pl[AV151]
Hydrocinnamic acid: Pl[AV151]

Hydroxy proline: Lf Ju[AV187]
Hydroxymethylanthraquinone: Pl[AV151]
Isobarbaloin: Pl[AV154]
Iso-citric acid: Lf[AV181]
Iso-leucine: Lf 65 micromols[AV154]
Kilocalories: Lf 2800[AV153]
L-asparagine: Pl[AV151]
Lauric acid methyl ester: Ge[AV037]
Lauric acid: Gel[AV037]
Leucine: Lf 53 micromols[AV187]
Lignin: Pl[AV151]
Linoleic acid ethyl ester: Gel[AV037]
Linoleic acid: Gel[AV037]
Lupeol: Lf 66.1 micromols[AV187]
Lysine: Lf 53 micromols[AV187]
Lysophosphatidyl inositol: Aer[AV196]
Magnesium: Lf 930[AV153]
Manganese: Lf 6[AV153]
Mannose: Lf 8.3 mmols[AV187]
Margaric acid methyl ester: Gel[AV037]
Margaric acid: Gel[AV037]
Mono-octyl phthalate: Gel[AV037]
M-protocatechuic aldehyde: Pl[AV151]
Mucilage (aloe vera): Lf[AV198]
Mucopolysaccharides: Pl[AV151]
Myristic acid methyl ester: Gel[AV037]
Myristic acid: Gel[AV037]
Nataloin: Pl[AV151]
N-docosane: Gel[AV037]
N-eicosane: Gel[AV037]
N-heneicosane: Gel[AV037]
N-heptadecane: Gel[AV037]
N-hexadecane: Gel[AV037]
Niacin: Lf 64[AV153]
N-nonadecane: Gel[AV037]
N-octadecane: Gel[AV037]
Nonadec-1-ene: Gel[AV037]
Nonadec-trans-5-ene: Gel[AV037]
Octadec-1-ene: Gel[AV037]
Octadec-7-enoic acid: Gel[AV037]
Octadeca-10-13-dienoic acid methyl ester:
    Gel[AV037]
Octadeca-6-9-dienoic acid methyl ester:
    Gel[AV037]
Octadeca-9-12-dienoic acid methyl ester:
    Gel[AV037]
Oleic acid ethyl ester: Gel[AV037]
Oleic acid methyl ester: Gel[AV196]
Oleic acid: Aer[AV196]
Oligosaccharide (aloe vera): Lf Pu[AV190]
Oxidase: Pl[AV151]
Palmitic acid ethyl ester: Gel[AV037]

Palmitic acid methyl ester: Gel[AV037]
Palmitic acid: Gel[AV037]
Palmitoleic acid methyl ester: Gel[AV037]
Palmitoleic acid: Gel[AV037]
Para coumaric acid: Lf[AV018,AV187]
P-coumaric acid: Pl[AV151]
Pectic acid: Pl[AV151]
Pentadecanoic acid: Gel[AV037]
Phosphatidic acid: Aer[AV196]
Phosphatidyl choline: Aer[AV196]
Phosphatidyl ethanolamine: Aer[AV196]
Phosphatidyl inositol: Aer[AV196]
Phosphatidyl serine: Aer[AV196]
Phosphorus: Lf 6-940[AV153]
Phytosterols: Pl[AV151]
P-Methoxybenzylacetone: Pl[AV151]
P-methoxy-hydrocinnamic acid: Pl[AV151]
Polyphenols: Pl[AV151]
Polysaccharide (Aloe vera): Lf[AV180,AV188,AV189]
Polyuronide: Pl[AV151]
Proline: Lf 29 micromols[AV187]
Protein: Lf Ju 2.5%[AV187]
Proteinase: Pl[AV151]
Pteroylglutamic acid: Pl[AV151]
Quinone: Pl[AV151]
Resin: Pl[AV155]
Rhamnose: Lf[AV187]
Rhein: Pl[AV151]
Riboflavin: Lf[AV153]
Sapogenin: Pl[AV151]
Saponins: Pl[AV155]
Selenium: Lf 23[AV153]
Serine: Lf 224 micromols[AV187]
Silicon: Lf 22[AV153]
Spingomyelin: Aer[AV196]
Stearic acid ethyl ester: Gel[AV037]
Stearic acid: Gel[AV037]
Stigmasterol: Aer[AV196]
Sulfoquinovosyl diglyceride: Aer[AV196]
Tetradecyl benzene: Gel[AV037]
Thiamin: Lf 0.8[AV153]
Threitol: Pl[AV151]
Threonine: Lf 123 micromols[AV187]
Tin: Lf 11[AV153]
Tricosanoic acid methyl ester: Gel[AV037]
Tridecyl benzene: Gel[AV037]
Trihydroxymethylanthraquinone: Pl[AV151]
Triolein: Aer[AV037]
Tyrosine: Lf 28 micromols[AV187]
Undecyl cyclohexane: Gel[AV037]
Uronic acid: Pl[AV151]

Valine: Lf 109 micromols[AV187]
Xylose: Lf[AV187]

PHARMACOLOGICAL ACTIVITIES AND CLINICAL TRIALS

Abortifacient effect. Ethanol (95%), water, and petroleum ether extracts of fresh leaves, administered orally to female rats at doses of 150.0, 150.0, and 100.0 mg/kg, respectively, were inactive[AV158].

Adjuvant activity. Aqueous (dialyzed) fraction of freeze-dried leaf juice, administered intraperitoneally to mice at variable dosage levels, was active[AV068].

Alkalinizing activity. Undiluted fresh leaf juice, applied externally on female adults with dermatitis caused by X-ray treatment, was active[AV161].

Analgesic activity. Ethanol (95%) extract of aerial parts, administered intragastrically to mice at a dose of 500.0 mg/kg, was active vs hot plate method[AV067]. Fresh leaf gel, at a concentration of 0.125% formulated into toothpaste that also contained sodium fluoride, was equivocal. Alleviation of root pain was not significantly greater in treatment group vs controls[AV042]. Fresh leaf pulp, used externally on patients with chronic and acute athletic injuries 3 times per week for 3 weeks, was active[AV066]. Water extract of dried leaf juice, administered intraperitoneally to rats at a dose of 250.0 mg/kg, was active vs tail flick response to radiant heat[AV117]. Water extract of fresh leaf juice, administered subcutaneously to mice at a dose of 100.0 mg/kg, was active. Decolorizing *Aloe vera* extract was given daily for 7 days to normal and diabetic test groups. The treated normal group showed a doubling of the time to pain response relative to untreated diabetics (13.7 vs 10.7 seconds) vs carrageenin-induced pedal edema and hot plate method[AV062].

Anesthetic activity (local). Undiluted fresh leaf juice was active as an analgesic for insect stings on human adults. The biological activity has been patented[AV099].

Anti-asthmatic activity. Fresh leaf extract, administered orally to human adults, was active[AV138].

Antibacterial activity. Chromatographic fraction of fresh leaves, on agar plate, was active on *Bacillus subtilis*[AV134]. Decoction of dried fruit, on agar plate, produced weak activity on *Streptococcus mutans*, MIC 62.5 mg/ml[AV070]. Dried entire plant juice, on agar plate, was active on *Proteus vulgaris* and *Pseudomonas aeruginosa*[AV120]. Ethanol (95%) and water extracts of leaves, on agar plate, were inactive on *Escherichia coli* and *Staphylococcus aureus*[AV020]. Fresh leaf juice, at a concentration of 1:50 on agar plate, was active on *Streptococcus pyogenes*, *Corynebacterium xerosis* and *Staphylococcus aureus*; and inactive on *Escherichia coli* and *Salmonella schottmuelleri*. The activity was lost quickly as the juice darkened in color. Whole leaf minus the juice, the leaf mesophyll and leaf epidermis was devoid of activity[AV156]. Tincture of dried leaves, at a concentration of 30.0 ml/disk (10 gm of leaves in 100 ml ethanol) on agar plate, was inactive on *Escherichia coli*, *Pseudomonas aeruginosa* and *Staphylococcus aureus*[AV137]. Undiluted fresh leaf juice, in broth culture, was active on *Bacillus subtilis*, *Enterobacter* species, *Escherichia coli*, *Serratia marcescens*, *Staphylococcus aureus*, *Streptococcus agalactiae*, and *Streptococcus pyogenes*, and inactive on *Klebsiella* species[AV101].

Antiburn effect. Dried entire plant juice, applied externally to guinea pigs, was active vs experimental burn[AV120]. Fresh undiluted leaf juice, applied externally to human adults of both sexes, was active. Three cases of burn caused by hot water and 2 cases of severe sunburn were treated[AV103]. Undiluted fresh leaf juice, applied externally to human adults of both sexes with X-ray-induced ulcers, was active[AV162]. Undiluted fresh leaf juice, applied topically to X-ray-induced,

acute third degree burns, was active[AV160]. Undiluted leaf gel, applied externally, was inactive. Twelve volunteers received UVB irradiation from a light pen at 2 sites on each arm. Aloe leaf gel was applied to 2 sites on 1 arm. Blood flow and redness of irradiated areas did not differ from controls at 6 and 24 hours post-burn[AV080]. Water extract of dried leaves, applied externally to third degree burns induced by X-rays on rats at a concentration of 10.0%, was active. The inner rind of the leaf was dried before being extracted[AV160].

Anticancer activity. Aloe-emodin, a hydroxyanthraquinone present in the leaves, has a specific in vitro and in vivo antineuroectodermal tumor activity. The growth of human neuroectodermal tumors was inhibited in mice with severe combined immunodeficiency without any appreciable toxic effects on the animals. The compound does not inhibit the proliferation of normal fibroblasts or that of hemopoietic progenitor cells. The cytotoxicity mechanism consists of the induction of apoptosis, whereas the selectivity against neuroectodermal tumor cells is found on a specific energy-dependent pathway of drug incorporation[AV208].

Antichemopreventive effects. Gel extract was evaluated using in vitro short-term screening methods associated with both initiation and promotion processes in carcinogenesis. In B[a]P-DNA adduct formation, 180 micrograms/ml of the extract inhibited B[a]P binding to DNA in mouse liver cells. Oxidative damage by 8-hydroxydeoxyguanosine was significantly decreased by the extract. In screening antitumor promoting effect, the extract significantly inhibited phorbol myristic acetate-induced ornithine decarboxylase activity in Balb/3T3 cells. In addition, the extract significantly inhibited phorbol myristic acetate-induced tyrosine kinase activity in human leukemic cells. Superoxide anion formation was also significantly inhibited[AV213].

Anticomplement activity. Aqueous (dialyzed) fraction of freeze-dried leaf juice, at a concentration of 300.0 mg/ml, was active on human serum. Inhibition of alternate pathway complement activity was observed. The effect resulted from depletion of complement factor 3[AV068]. Water extract and polysaccharide fraction of leaves were active in human serum[AV133]. Water extract of fresh leaves, at variable concentrations, was active[AV021].

Anticrustacean activity. Ethanol (95%) extract of dried plant juice was inactive on *Artemia salina*. The assay system was intended to predict for antitumor activity[AV029].

Antidiabetic effect. Leaf pulp and gel extracts, administered orally to non-diabetic, Type I and type II diabetic rats, were ineffective on lowering the blood sugar level in non-diabetic rats. The leaf pulp extract showed hypoglycemic activity on type I and type II rats. The effectiveness being enhanced for type II diabetes in comparison with glibenclamide. On the contrary, the leaf gel extract showed hyperglycemic activity on type II rats. It has been concluded from this study that the leaves devoid of the gel could be useful in the treatment of non-insulin dependent diabetes mellitus[AV201].

Antifertility effect. Ethanol (95%) and petroleum ether extracts of leaves, administered orally to female mice, were active. Positive data was reported, but they are of questionable significance to fertility regulation. Water extract was inactive. Ethanol (95%), water and petroleum ether extracts of root, administered orally to female mice, were inactive[AV006].

Antifungal activity. Anthraquinone fraction of fresh leaf juice, on agar plate, was active on *Trichophyton mentagrophytes*[AV043]. Dried juice from entire plant, applied externally to human adults, was active in treating trichophytiasis[AV120].

Antihypercholesterolemic activity. Hot water extract of dried leaf juice, administered intragastrically to rats at a dose of 0.5 gm/kg for 7 days, was active. A mixture of *Nigella sativa*, *Commiphora*, *Ferula assafoetida*, *Aloe vera*, and *Boswellia serrata* vs streptozotocin-induced hyperglycemia tested the effect[AV065].

Antihyperglycemic activity. Twenty-five percent aqueous extract of decoction and hot water extract of dried leaves, administered intragastrically to mice at a dose of 0.5 ml/animal, were inactive vs alloxan-induced hyperglycemia[AV123]. Chromatographic fraction of a commercial sample of leaves, administered intraperitoneally to mice at a dose of 5.0 mg/kg daily for 4 days, was active vs alloxan-induced hyperglycemia. Leaf exudate, administered intragastrically to mice at a dose of 500.0 mg/kg, was inactive. When administered twice daily for 4 days, the exudate was active vs alloxan-induced hyperglycemia[AV072]. Fresh leaf gel, administered intragastrically to male rats at a dose of 2.0 ml/kg, was inactive. The gel did not lower blood glucose in alloxan treated rats. Blood glucose rose with the treatment[AV044]. Fresh sap, administered intragastrically to mice at a dose of 1.0 gm/kg, was active vs alloxan-induced hyperglycemia[AV069]. When administered orally to 5 diabetic patients for 4–14 weeks, the sap was active[AV069]. Hot water extract of dried leaf juice, administered intragastrically to rats at a dose of 0.5 gm/kg for 7 days, was active. The effect was tested by a mixture of *Nigella sativa*, *Commiphora*, *Ferula assafoetida*, *Aloe vera*, and *Boswellia serrata* vs streptozotocin-induced hyperglycemia[AV065].

Anti-implantation effect. Ethanol (95%) and petroleum ether extracts of leaves, administered orally to female rats, were active. Positive data was reported, but they are of questionable significance to fertility regulation. The water extract was inactive[AV006]. Ethanol (95%) extract of leaf pulp, administered orally to female rats at a dose of 100.0 mg/kg, was inactive[AV009]. Ethanol (95%), water and petroleum ether extracts of root, administered orally to female mice, were inactive[AV006].

Anti-inflammatory activity. Water extract of fresh leaf juice, applied externally to mice at a concentration of 1.0%, was active. Decolorized Aloe vera extract was applied to the ear 30 minutes after the application of croton oil. The extract reduced ear swelling by 67% relative to controls[AV061]. The extract was also active in rats vs mustard-induced pedal edema. Inhibition of edema was greater with RNA and vitamin C added. When administered subcutaneously to rats at a dose of 10.0 mg/kg, the extract was active. Decolorized *Aloe vera* extract was given 1 day before induction of edema by plantar injection of 2% mustard solution. A 60% reduction of edema was seen in treated diabetic animals relative to untreated diabetics vs carrageenin-induced pedal edema. A dose of 400 mg/kg was inactive vs cotton pellet granuloma[AV058]. Ethanol (95%) extract of fresh leaf juice, applied externally on mice, was active vs croton oil-induced edema and carrageenin-induced pedal edema[AV043]. Ethanol/water (1:1) extract of leaf juice, applied externally to mice at a concentration of 5.0%, was active vs croton oil-induced edema[AV004]. Fresh leaf gel, administered intraperitoneally to male rats at a dose of 2.0 ml/kg, was active vs carrageenin-induced pedal edema[AV040]. Fresh leaf juice, administered by means of injection to 50 patients with first-third stage of parodontosis, yielded a satisfactory effect only in the first and second stages of the disease. The content of calcium elevated in the blood serum in parodontosis normalizes in the treatment with Aloe extract[AV175]. Fresh leaf juice, applied externally to female mice at a dose of 5.0%, was active vs croton oil-induced edema[AV073]. The decolorized extract, at a concentration of 1.0%, was active vs

croton oil-induced edema[AV079]. When administered subcutaneously to rats at a dose of 25.0 mg/kg, the extract was active vs mustard-induced pedal edema, 46% decrease in paw volume; when combined with 1.0 mg/kg hydrocortisone, 66% decrease in paw volume; 86% inhibition of edema for combination with 0.1% hydrocortisone vs croton oil-induced edema[AV079]. Ethanol/water (1:1) extract of fresh leaves, administered subcutaneously to mice at a dose of 150.0 mg/kg, was active vs croton oil-induced edema[AV148]. Fresh leaf pulp, administered via drinking water and intragastrically to rats at a dose of 100.0 mg/kg, were active vs croton oil-induced ear swelling. A time study showed that food grade *Aloe vera* administration reduced swelling to a large degree when used over a 21-day period as opposed to 7 or 14 days. Decolorized *Aloe vera* was inactive when administered through the drinking water as well as intragastrically. A dose of 150.0 mg/kg, administered subcutaneously to rats, was active vs gelatin, kaolin-, albumin-, carrageenin-, dextran-, and mustard-induced pedal edema[AV075]. Leaf juice, injected into mice at a dose of 10.0%, was active. Inflammation was introduced by the administration of air under the skin producing a pouch followed by administration of 1% carrageenin directly into the 7-day-old air pouch, which produced an inflammation characterized by an increase in mast cells and wall vascularity. After administration of the extract, vascularity was reduced by 50% and the number of mast cells was decreased by 48%[AV090]. Water extract of dried leaves, administered subcutaneously to male mice at a dose of 20.0 mg/kg, was active[AV076]. Water extract of fresh leaf gel (undiluted) was active when applied externally on human adults[AV149]. Fresh leaf gel, applied externally on mice at a dose of 300.0 mg/kg, was active[AV033].

Antileukemic effect. The effect of diethylhexylphthalate on apoptosis of human leukemic cell lines K562, HL60 and U937 was investigated for its pharmacological activity. At doses of 10 microgram/ml diethylhexylphthalate a significant antileukemic effect was observed for all of the cell lines, as measured by clonogenic assay. After treatment with 10 microgram/ml for 4 hours, agarose gel electrophoresis and flow cytometric analysis confirmed the occurrence of apoptosis. These results indicated that diethylhexylphthalate extracted from *Aloe vera* has a potent antileukemic effect, and thus represents a new type of pharmacological activity with respect to human leukemic cells[AV205].

Antileukopenic activity. Dried entire plant juice was active vs cobalt-60 or X-ray radiation[AV120].

Antimutagenic acitivity. Diethylhexylphthalate produce anti-mutagenic activity on *Salmonella typhimurium* mutation assay. The number of mutant colonies of *Salmonella typhimurium* strain TA98 upon exposure to AF-2 (0.2 microgram/plate) decreased in a concentration-dependent manner in the presence of different concentrations of diethylhexylphthalate. Concentrations of 100, 50, 10, 5, and 1 microgram/plate, reduced AF-2-induced mutagenicity at 91.5%, 89.0%, 80.0%, 77.5%, and 57.4%, respectively[AV206].

Antimycobacterial activity. Ethanol (95%) and water extracts of fresh leaves, in broth culture, was active on *Mycobacterium tuberculosis*[AV018]. Ethanol (95%) and water extracts, of leaves on agar plate, were inactive on *Mycobacterium tuberculosis*[AV020]. Ethyl acetate extract of dried leaves, on agar plate, was active on *Mycobacterium tuberculosis*[AV019].

Antipyretic activity. Ethanol (95%) extract of aerial parts, administered intragastrically to mice at a dose of 500.0 mg/kg, was active vs yeast-induced pyrexia[AV067].

Antitumor activity. Acid/water extract of dried leaves, administered subcutaneously to mice of both sexes at a dose of 0.005 gm/kg, and dried-leaf, administered as a powdered suspension at a dose of 1.0 gm/kg, were inactive on Sarcoma 37[AV177]. Dried juice from the entire plant, administered intraperitoneally to mice, was active on CA-Ehrlich-Ascites and Sarcoma 180 (solid)[AV120]. Leaf gel of dried gland (ink), administered intraperitoneally to male mice at doses of 10.0 and 50.0 mg/kg, were inactive on Sarcoma 180 (solid). The relative change in the tumor weight was not statistically significant[AV038].

Antiulcer activity. Aqueous slurry (homogenate) of dried exudate, administered by gastric intubation to rats at doses of 0.5 and 1 gm/kg, was inactive vs phenylbutazone-, cysteamine-, and reserpine-induce ulcers; the 500.0 mg/kg dose was inactive vs stress-induced ulcers. Aqueous slurry (homogenate) of fresh leaves, administered by gastric intubation to rats at a dose of 1.0 gm/kg, was inactive vs phenylbutazone- and cysteamine-induced ulcers; a dose of 0.5 gm/kg was inactive vs aspirin-, reserpine-, and stress-induced (restraint) ulcers[AV126]. Fresh leaf gel, administered intragastrically to male rats at a dose of 2.0 ml/kg, was inactive. The gel did not prevent ethanol-induced or cold-restraint gastric ulcers. Also, neither pre nor post-treatment accelerated healing of ulcers[AV044]. Fresh leaf pulp juice, administered intragastrically to rats at a dose of 2.0 ml/animal daily for 7 days after induction of lesions, was active vs stress-induced (restraint) ulcers and aspirin-induced ulcers[AV113]. Blended fresh leaf pulp, administered orally to rats at a dose of 2.0 ml/animal twice daily for 6 days, was active. Ulcer reduction of 50% relative to control was observed vs aspirin-induced ulcers[AV104]. Water extract of leaf pulp, administered orally to rats at a dose of 4.0 ml/animal, was active. Gastric ulcers were produced by forced immobilization. The effect was both prophylactic and therapeutic[AV023].

Antiviral activity (plant pathogens). Ethanol (95%) extract of dried leaves, in cell culture, was active on distortion ringspot, mild mosaic and ringspot viruses[AV152].

Antiviral activity. Aloe polymannose, a high mannose biological response modifier purified from the plant, was tested for activity in enhancing antibody titres against coxsackie virus B3 and coxsackie virus B3-induced myocarditis in murine models of the disease. Inoculation of mice with the polymannose over a range of 3 nontoxic doses and in varying schedules did not reduce virus titres in heart tissues or ameliorate virus-induced cardiopathological alterations during acute disease. However, the biological response modifier was found to significantly enhanced titres of anti-coxsackie virus-B3 antibodies produced during acute infection of 3 strains of mice with coxsackie virus-B3. Simultaneous intraperitoneal inoculation of the polymannose, at a dose of 0.5 mg/kg body weight per mouse with purified coxsackie virus-B3, significantly increased ELISA titres of anti-coxsackie virus-B3 antibodies and the proportion of mice with these titres, compared with similar parameters in mice inoculated only with coxsackie virus-B3. The data indicated that the polymannose can immunopotentiate antibody production against capsid protein epitopes of a nonenveloped picornvirus and suggest this biological response marker might be of benefit in enhancing antibody titres against other enteroviruses during a natural infection and poliovirus vaccine strains[AV207].

Antiviral activity. Anthraquinone fraction of fresh leaf juice, in cell culture, was active on herpes simplex virus (HSV) 1[AV043]. Methanol extract of dried leaves, applied externally, was active on HSV 1 and 2. The

biological activity reported has been patented[AV128].

Antiyeast activity. Ethanol (60%) extract of dried leaves, on agar plate, was inactive on *Candida albicans*[AV091]. Tincture (extract of 10 gm leaves in 100 ml ethanol), at a concentration of 30 microliters/disk on agar plate, was inactive[AV137]. Undiluted fresh leaf juice, in broth culture, was active on *Candida albicans*[AV101].

Aphthous stomatitis effect. An open study was performed with 31 pediatric outpatients; age 6-14 years, affected by mouth ulcers. For each case, data on case history and clinical profile, patterns of the lesion, presence of spontaneous or provoked pain were collected at baseline, and a bioadhesive patch ("Alovex patch") was administered on the basis of a daily regimen of not less than 3 patches for 4 days. Data on modification of the above-mentioned parameters, with patients and physicians opinion on the therapeutical efficacy, were collected during a control visit (4 days later). Moreover, by means of a daily diary, patients recorded information on the course of the symptoms during the 4 days and were also asked to compare the current treatment with other previous therapies. At the control visit 77% of the patients have shown a marked resolution of spontaneous pain, while in the other patients, pain was significantly decreased to a mild or moderate level. No one declared to suffer from severe pain. Also, provoked pain resulted to be significantly decreased after treatment. Global efficacy was judged positively, being the therapeutic effect in more than 80% of cases as evaluated by physicians and patients. A positive improvement of symptomatology started within the second day of treatment in 74% of the patients. The compliance (adhesive, acceptability and palatability) of the formulation was judged largely favorable in more than 90% of the patients. The results of the investigation underlined the efficacy and compliance of the patch for the treatment of aphtous stomatitis; also the limit of topical available therapies, linked to the "contact time", to develop their therapeutic action, seems not to be evinced on the basis of this investigation, so the application of this patch seems to be more easy and beneficial[AV209].

Arachidonate metabolism inhibition. Anthraquinone fraction of fresh leaf juice was active on calf skin[AV043].

ATP-ase (Na+/K+) inhibition. Anthraquinone fraction of fresh leaf juice increases permeability across colonic mucosa[AV043].

Bradykinin antagonist activity. Exudate of fresh leaf juice was active[AV043].

Bronchodilator activity. Hot water extract of dried leaves, administered intravenously to guinea pigs at a dose of 1.5 ml/animal, was inactive[AV086].

Burn wound effect. In a study comparing moist exposed burn ointment (containing aloe) with conventional management with respect to wound healing, antibacterial and analgesic effect, and hospital costs was investigated in 115 patients between the ages of 12 and 80 who had partial-thickness thermal burns covering less than 40% of body surface area. Fifty seven patients were assigned the moist exposed burn ointment and 58 patients to the conventional method. The latter group received twice-daily dressing changes; moist exposed patients received treatment every 4 hours. The patients were hospitalized until 75% of the body surface area had healed. Body surface area was determined by visual inspection and charted on Lund and Browder charts regularly. Wound healing rate, bacterial infection rate, pain score, and hospitalization costs were recorded. The median time to 75% healing was 17.0 and 20.0 days with the ointment and conventional, respectively. Bacterial infection rates were similar between the 2 groups. The ointment imparted greater analgesic effect in the first

5 days of therapy and reduced hospital cost by 8%. The ointment is as effective as the conventional management but is not the panacea for all burn wounds. The use of the ointment eases the management of face and neck burns and facilitates early institution of occupational therapy in hand burns. It confers better pain relief such that fewer opiates are used during the first 5 days after burn injury[AV218].

Cardiac depressant activity. Tincture of leaf juice produced weak activity in rabbit heart perfusion[AV004].

Cell attachment enhancement effect. Fresh leaf homogenates, in cell culture, was active vs human embryonic-lung cells and inactive vs CA-ME-180[AV135]. Fresh leaves were active on human lung cells and CA-cervical-squamous cells[AV170]. Leaf homogenate, in cell culture, was active on CA-ME-180 and human embryonic lung cells[AV135]. Leaf juice (commercial sample) was active on CA-cervical-squamous and human-lung cells[AV127]. Fresh leaf homogenate, in cell culture, was active vs human embryonic lung cells, and inactive vs CA-ME-180[AV135]. Fresh leaves were active on human lung cells and CA-cervical-squamous cells[AV127].

Cell proliferation stimulation. Water extract of fresh leaf gel, in cell culture at a concentration of 0.162 mcg/ml, was active on pheochromocytoma-rat-PC12 cells. A concentration of 0.325 mcg/ml was active on human fibroblast lung-HEL. The result was seen only in long-term culture[AV046].

Cell transformation inhibition. Freeze-dried gel, in cell culture, was active on C3H-10T1/2 cells vs methylcholantrene-induced transformation[AV037].

Chemomodulatory activity. Fresh leaf pulp extract, administered orally to mice at doses of 30 and 60 microliter/day for 14 days, was effective. The extract was examined on carcinogen-metabolizing phase-I and phase-II enzymes, antioxidant enzymes, glutathione content, lactate dehydrogenase, and lipid peroxidation in the liver. The modulatory effect of the extract was also examined in the lung, kidneys, and forestomach for the activities of glutathione S-transferase, DT-diophorose, superoxide dismutase, and catalase. The positive control mice were treated with butylated hydroxyanisole. Significant increases in the levels of acid soluble sulfydryl content, NADPH-cytochrome P450 reductase, NADH-cytochrome b5 reductase, glutathione S-transferase, DT-diaphorase, superoxide dismutase, catalase, glutathione peroxidase, and glutathione reductase were observed in the liver. The extract significantly reduced the levels of cytochrome P450 and cytochrome b5. Thus, the extract is clearly an inducer of phase-II enzyme system. Treatment with both doses produced a decrease in malondialdehyde formation and the activity of lactate dehydrogenase in the liver, suggesting its role in protection against prooxidant-induced membrane and cellular damage. The microsomal and cytosolic protein was significantly enhanced, indicating the possibility of its involvement in the induction of protein synthesis. BHA, an antioxidant compound, provided the authenticity of the assay protocol and response of animals against modulator. The extract was effective in inducing glutathione S-transferase, DT-diaphorase, superoxide dismutase, and catalase as measured in extrahepatic organs. Thus, besides the liver, the lung, kidney, and forestomach were also influenced favorably in order to detoxify reactive metabolites, including chemical carcinogens and drugs[AV204].

CNS depressant activity. Hot water extract of leaves, administered intraperitoneally to rabbits at a dose of 10.0 mg/kg, was active[AV114].

Conditioned taste aversion. Frozen stem and leaves, administered intragastrically to rats at a dose of 925.0 mg/kg, was inactive.

Administration of test substance was temporally paired with introduction of sodium saccharin solution. Consumption of saccharin solution 2 days after test was used to estimate aversiveness of the test substance[AV127].

Cosmetic activity. A mixture of *Aloe vera*, *Mentha piperita* extract and allantoin was active when applied externally on human adults. The biological activity has been patented[AV064].

Cytotoxic activity. Ethanol/water (1:1) extract of leaves, in cell culture, was inactive on CA-9KB, ED_{50} > 20.0 mcg/ml[AV011]. Ethanol/water (1:1) extract of the entire plant, in cell culture, was inactive on CA-9KB, ED_{50} >20.0 mcg/ml[AV007]. Leaf gel of dried gland (ink), in cell culture, produced weak activity on human colorectal cancer cell line SNU-C2A, IC_{50} 5.0 mg/ml and on human SNU-1 cells, IC_{50} 5.25 mg/ml[AV038].

Death. Ethanol (95%) extract of the aerial parts, administered intragastrically to mice at a dose of 3.0 gm/kg, was inactive[AV067].

Diarrhea induction and the effect of nitrous oxide. Leaf, administered orally to rats at a dose of 5 gm/kg and 20 gm/kg, produced diarrhea in 20% and 100% of the rats, respectively. Pretreatment with nitrous oxide synthase inhibitor N(G)-nitro-L-arginine methyl ester at a dose of 2.5–25 mg/kg reduced the diarrhea induced by 20 gm/kg of aloe 9 hours after its oral administration. It also reduced the increase in fecal water excretion. L-arginine, administered to rats pretreated with N(G)-nitro-L-arginine methyl ester (25 mg/kg) intraperitoneally at a dose of 1500 mg/kg, drastically reduced the effect of N(G)-nitro-L-arginine methyl ester on diarrhea and increase in fecal water excretion induced by 20 mg/kg of aloe. Given alone, L-arginine did not modify aloe-induced diarrhea. Basal Ca^{2+}-dependent nitrous oxide synthase activity in the rat colon was dose dependently inhibited by 0.1–20 gm/kg of aloe and by aloin (0.2–1 gm/kg), the active ingredient of aloe[AV216].

DNA synthesis inhibition. Chromatographic fraction of fresh leaf gel, in broth culture, was active on *Bacillus subtilis*[AV134].

Embryotoxic effect. Benzene, water, petroleum ether and ethanol (95%) extract, of leaves, administered orally to pregnant rats at doses of 100.0 mg/kg, were active. 50%, 85%, 37%, and 85% reduction in fertility, respectively, were observed. The chloroform extract was equivocal, 28% reduction in fertility[AV094]. Ethanol/water (1:1) extract, administered orally to female rats at a dose of 200.0 mg/kg, was active[AV159]. Ethanol (95%) extract of leaf pulp, administered orally to female rats at a dose of 100.0 mg/kg, was inactive[AV009]. Ethanol (95%), water and petroleum ether extracts of fresh leaves, administered orally to female rats at doses of 150.0, 150.0, and 100.0 mg/kg, respectively, were inactive[AV158]. Ethanol/water (1:1) extract of dried leaves, at a dose of 150.0 mg/kg, water extract at a dose of 125.0 mg/kg and benzene extract at a dose of 100.0 mg/kg, administered by gastric intubation to pregnant rats, were inactive[AV109]. Water extract of dried entire plant, administered intragastrically to pregnant rats at a dose of 125.0 mg/kg, was equivocal[AV063].

Emollient effect. Undiluted leaf juice, applied externally on human adults, was active[AV051].

Estrogenic effect. Leaf juice, administered orally to immature rats at a dose of 10.0 ml/kg, produced weak activity[AV052].

Glucose-6-phosphate dehydrogenase inhibition. Anthraquinone fraction of fresh leaf juice was active[AV043].

Hair conditioner. Water extract of dried leaves, applied externally on human adults at a concentration of 86.6%, was active[AV028].

Hair loss inhibition. Fresh leaf gel, applied externally to human adults at a concentration of 6.8 ml/day, was active. Biological activity has been patented[AV034].

Hair loss stimulant effect. Fresh leaf gel, applied externally to human adults at a concentration of 6.8 ml/day, was active. Biological activity has been patented[AV034]. Fresh, undiluted leaf juice, applied externally to human adults, was active. There was improvement of hair growth in patients with alopecia areata[AV173].

Hemagglutinin activity. A commercial sample of leaf juice was active[AV127]. Chromatographic fraction of fresh leaf gel was active on human red blood cells[AV047]. Fresh leaf homogenates was active[AV135]. Aloctin I and II, precipitated at 50% ammonium sulphate concentration from crude leaf pulp. Hemagglutinating activity was estimated visually by adding a 4% rabbit erythrocyte suspension to serial two-fold dilutions of the lectins in microtitration plates. None of the 20 sugars tested inhibited hemagglutinating activity of aloctin I up to a concentration of 500 mM. Aloctin II was inhibited by N-acetly-D-galactosamine at 250 mM concentration. Of 10 metal ions tested, only Al^{3+} salts were found to activated aloctin I and II. On the other hand, it was shown that neither lectin possessed any alpha and beta galactosidase or alpha and beta glucosidase activity[AV212].

Histamine release inhibition. Water extract of dried leaves was active on mast cells of rats, IC_{50} 0.14 mg/ml vs antigen-induced histamine release, and IC_{50} 0.92 mg/ml vs compound 48/80-induced histamine release[AV041].

Hypoglycemic activity. Fresh sap, administered intragastrically to mice at a dose of 1.0 gm/day for five days, was active[AV069]. Fresh stem juice, administered intragastrically to rabbits at a dose of 4.0 ml/kg, was active. Glucose levels were decreased 27.9%[AV031]. Polysaccharide fraction of dried whole plant was active on mice[AV054]. Polysaccharide fraction of fresh leaves, administered intraperitoneally to mice at a dose of 100.0 mg/kg, was active[AV055]. Polysaccharide fraction of fresh leaves, administered intraperitoneally to mice at a dose of 100.0 mg/kg, was active[AV138]. Polysaccharide fraction of fresh leaves, administered intraperitoneally to mice at a dose of 100.0 mg/kg, was active[AV055].

Hypolipemic activity. Hot water extract of dried leaf juice, administered intragastrically to rats at a dose of 0.5 gm/kg for 7 days, was active. The effect was tested by a mixture of *Nigella sativa*, *Commiphora*, *Ferula assafoetida*, *Aloe vera*, and *Boswellia serrata* vs streptozotocin-induced hyperglycemia[AV065].

Hypotensive activity. Tincture of leaf juice, administered intravenously to rabbits, was inactive[AV004].

Immunomodulatory activity. Acemannan, a major constituent of *Aloe vera* gel, was tested on dendritic cells, which are the most important accessory cells for the initiation of primary immune responses. Immature dendritic cells were generated from mouse bone marrow cells by culturing in a medium supplemented with GM-CSF and IL-4, and then stimulated with acemannan, sulfated acemannan, and LPS, respectively. Phenotypic analysis for the expression of class II MHC molecules and major co-stimulatory molecules such as B7-1, B7-2, CD40, and CD54 confirmed that acemannan could induce maturation of immature dendritic cells. Functional maturation of immature dendritic cells was supported by increased allogeneic mixed lymphocyte reaction and IL-12 production. The differentiation-inducing activity of acemannan was almost completely abolished by chemical sulfation[AV199].

Immunostimulatory activity. Lyophilized extract of leaves, applied externally on mice at a concentration of 1.67%, was active vs UV irradiation-induced suppression of contact hypersensitivity[AV151]. Aloeride, at 0.5 microgram/ml, increased NF-kappa B directed luciferase expression in THP-1 human monocytic cells to levels 50% of those achieved by maximal concentrations (10 microgram/ml) of LPS. Aloeride induced the expression of the mRNA encoding IL-beta and TNF-alpha to levels equal to those observed in cells maximally activated by LPS. Acemannan, at 200 microgram/ml in the macrophage assay, resulted in negligible NF-kappa B activation. Analysis of acemannan and aloeride, using size-exclusion chromatography, indicated that the low activity of acemannan is due to trace amounts of aloeride. Although aloeride comprises only 0.015% of the aloe juice dry weight, its potency for macrophage activation accounts fully for the activity of the crude juice[AV202].

Irritant activity. Water extract of dried leaves, applied externally to guinea pigs in a 6-week cutaneous irritation study at a concentration of 5.0%, was inactive[AV115].

Lectin activity. Chromatographic fraction of fresh leaf gel was active. The fraction bound to alpha-D-glucose and mannose sites[AV047].

Leukocyte migration inhibition. Decolorized extract of fresh leaves, administered subcutaneously to rats at a dose of 25.0 mg/kg, was active vs mustard-induced pedal edema, resulting in 64% reduction in migration and 84% reduction of migration for combination with 0.1 mg/kg hydrocortisone[AV079].

Metabolism. Aloemannan, administered orally and intravenously to mice at a dose of 120 mg/kg, indicated that aloemannan was metabolized in to smaller molecules that mainly accumulated in the kidneys. Aloemannan was catabolized by the human intestinal microflora to catabolites 1 and 2 with molecular weights of 30 and 10 KD, respectively[AV214].

Mitogenic activity. Chromatographic fraction of fresh leaf gel was active[AV047].

Molluscicidal activity. Aqueous slurry (homogenate) of fresh entire plant was inactive on *Lymnaea columella* and *Lymnaea cubensis*, LD_{100} >1000 ppm[AV106].

Mutagenic activity. Ethanol (95%) extract of dried plant juice, on agar plate at a concentration of 10.0 mg/plate, was inactive on *Salmonella typhimurium* TA98 and produced weak activity on *Salmonella typhimurium* TA102[AV029].

Neurotransmission effect. The effect of aloe extract on neurotransmission processes in crayfish neuromuscular junction was investigated. The concentration-response relationships of the extract on excitatory junctional potentials at the opener muscle of the dactyl in the first and second walking limbs were studied. Concentration-dependent depolarizations of the muscle fiber membrane resting potential, depression of excitatory junctional potential amplitudes and an increase in latency to onset of the of the excitatory junctional potential following electrical stimulation of the isolated excitatory axon in the meropodite were observed. The effects occurred with concentrations within 1%–10% (wt/vol) range. Effects of lower concentrations, ranging to a minimum of 0.01% were equivocal. The effects of the extract were at least partially, and in a majority of cases totally, reversible. Excitatory junctional potential reduced by the extract could be restored by increasing the nerve stimulation amplitude. This along with the latency increase suggests a depression of action potential generation and conduction. The results provide a preliminary characterization of the effects of he extract on the neurotransmission process and suggest that these effects may at least partially account for analgesic and antiinflammatory effects of aloe[AV211].

Ovulation inhibition effect. Ethanol/water (1:1) extract of leaves, administered orally to female rabbits at a dose of 100.0 mg/kg, was equivocal vs copper acetate-induced ovulation[AV159].

Oxygen radical inhibition. Water extract of fresh leaf juice, in cell culture, was active on polymorphonuclear leukocytes vs PMA-stimulated release. The effect was antagonized by Ca^{2+} ionophore[AV043].

Peptidyl transferase inhibition. Dried leaves, at a concentration of 10.0 mg, were active[AV074].

Peroxidase activity. Leaf extract and commercial gel, where it is notably stable, have been investigated for the relevant properties of peroxidase. In vitro, the activity is localized in the vascular system of inner aqueous leaf parenchyma. The acid optimum pH (5.0) for activity and the low KM for H_2O_2 (0.14 mM) suggested that, when topically applied, aloe peroxidase may scavenge H_2O_2 on the skin surface[AV203].

Phagocytosis inhibition. Aqueous (dialyzed) fraction of fresh leaves, at a concentration of 0.5 mg/ml, was inactive on polymorphonuclear leukocytes. Phagocytosis and intracellular killing of *Staphylococcus aureus* and *Candida albicans* were not inhibited[AV145].

Phagocytosis stimulation. Fresh leaf juice, at a concentration of 4.0 mg/ml, was active[AV138].

Phorbol ester antagonist. Aqueous (dialyzed) fraction of fresh leaves, at a concentration of 0.5 mg/ml, was active on polymorphonuclear leukocytes vs phorbol myristate acetate activation. Low M-R gel-extract-constituents were examined, and oxygen uptake and oxygen and hydrogen peroxide release were inhibited[AV145].

Hypersensitivity effect. Aloe oligosaccharides prevented suppression delayed-type hypersensitivity responses in vivo and reduced the amount of interleukin-10 observed in UV-irradiated murine epidermis. Aloe oligosaccharide also prevented suppression of immune responses to alloantigen in mice exposed to 30 kJ/m² UVB radiation. To assess the effect of the carbohydrates on keratinocytes, murine Pam212 cells were exposed to 300 Jm2 UVB radiation and treated for 1 hour with the oligosaccharides. The treatment reduced

IL-10 production by approximately 50% compared with the cells treated with UV radiation alone and completely blocked UV activated phosphorylation at SAPK/JNK protein but had no effect on p38 phosphorylation[AV217].

Plant germination inhibition. Water extract of dried leaves, at a concentration of 500.0 gm/liter, produced strong activity on *Cuscuta reflexa* seeds after 6 days of exposure to the extract. Water extract of dried stem, at a concentration of 500.0 gm/liter, was active on *Cuscuta reflexa* seeds after 6 days of exposure to the extract[AV089].

Plant growth inhibitor. Water extract of dried leaves, at a concentration of 500.0 gm/liter, was active on *Cuscuta reflexa* seedlings length; weight and dry weight were measured after 6 days of exposure to the extract. Water extract of the dried stem, at a concentration of 500.0 gm/liter, was active on *Cuscuta reflexa* seedlings after 6 days exposure to the extract. Seedling length, weight and dry weight were measured[AV089].

Polymorphonuclear leukocyte activation inhibition. Water extract of fresh leaves, at variable concentrations, was active[AV021].

Protein kinase inhibition. Polysaccharide fraction of fresh leaves was active[AV057].

Protein synthesis inhibition. Chromatographic fraction of fresh leaf gel, in broth culture, was active on *Bacillus subtilis*[AV134]. Dried leaves, at a concentration of 1.0 mg, were active. Incorporation of leucine into protein was inhibited, as well as elongation factors EF-1 and EF-2[AV074].

Skin pigmentation effect. Water extract of undiluted leaf gel, applied externally to human adults, was active. A preparation containing extract was patch-tested on skin exposed to UVA radiation for 30–180 seconds. Areas treated with preparation showed pigmentation for more than 1 year after treatment[AV088].

Smooth muscle stimulant activity. Tincture of leaf juice was active on rabbit intestine, and produced weak activity on the bladder[AV004].

Teratogenic activity. Water extract of dried entire plant, administered intragastrically to pregnant rats at a dose of 125.0 mg/kg, was active[AV063]. Water extract of dried leaves, administered intragastrically to pregnant rats at a dose of 125.0 mg/kg, was active[AV035].

Toxic effect (general). Ethanol (95%) extract of the dried aerial parts, in the drinking water of mice at a dose of 100.0 mg/kg for 3 months, was active. Toxic signs included alopecia, degeneration, and putrefaction of the sex organs, sperm damage and decreased RBC levels. When the extract was administered intragastrically at a concentration of 3.0 gm/kg to mice, it was inactive[AV140]. Frozen leaf and stem, administered intragastrically to rats at a dose of 925.0 mg/kg, was inactive. Administration of test substance was temporally paired with introduction of sodium saccharin solution. Consumption of saccharin solution 2 days after test was used to estimate aversiveness of test substance, which is related to its toxicity[AV127].

Toxicity assessment (quantitative). Ethanol/water (1:1) extract of dried leaves, administered intraperitoneally to mice, produced $LD_{50} > 1.0$ gm/kg[AV011]. Ethanol/water (50%) extract of the entire plant, administered intraperitoneally to mice, produced LD_{50} 250.0 mg/kg. The maximum tolerated dose was 100.0 mg/kg[AV007].

Ultraviolet B protective activity. Gel, applied topically immediately after exposure of shaved abdominal skin of mice to 2.4 Kj/m² ultraviolet B, resulted in suppression of contact sensitization through the skin to 41.1%, compared to normal irradiated skin. The percentage of recovery of ultraviolet B–suppressed contact hypersensitivity response was 52.3, 77.3, and 86.6% when irradiated skin was treated once with 0.1, 0.5, and 2.5 mg/ml of gel-containing cream, respectively. The gel did not show nonspecific stimulatory activity on contact hyper-sensitivity response[AV215].

Uterine stimulant effect. Tincture of leaf juice was active on the non-pregnant uterus of rabbits. Stimulation of amplitude of contraction with tonic contraction and loss of rhythmic contraction was observed[AV004]. Water extract of leaves, at a concentration of 250.0 mg/liter, was active on guinea pig uterus[AV008].

Wound healing acceleration. Ethanol (95%) extract of fresh leaf gel, applied externally on guinea pigs at a concentration of 5.0%, was active. Partial thickness burn healing assessed. Similar effect was seen in the use of antithromboxane U38485, lipid peroxidation inhibitor U75412E, and xanthine oxidase inhibitor U4285E[AV032]. A concentration of 5.0% applied externally to human adults was active on intra-arterial drug use-induced injury, frostbite injuries, and partial thickness burns. When applied externally to rabbits, at a concentration of 5.0% the extract, was active alone and in combination with methimazole improved tissue survival in intra-arterial drug abuse in rabbit ear model. The extract was not as effective against frostbite injury as methylprednisolone or acetylsalicyclic acid. In rats, 5.0% concentration of the extract alone and in combination with methimazole, improved tissue survival in electrical injury model[AV032]. Ethanol/water (1:1) extract of fresh leaves, administered subcutaneously to mice at a dose of 150.0 mg/kg, was active[AV148]. Fresh leaf homogenates in cell culture was active on CA-ME-180 and human embryonic lung cells[AV135]. Fresh leaves, applied topically to human adults, were active. Eighteen dermabrasion patients with acne vulgaris were included in the study[AV143]. Fresh leaf juice, applied topically at a concentration of 25.0% and in the drinking water at a dose of 100.0 mg/kg, were active. Both groups were dosed daily for 2 months; the wound healing (6-mm

punch biopsy wounds) was significantly faster than the untreated control[AV146]. Fresh leaf juice, applied topically to human adults at a concentration of 40.0%, was active in several cases of Roentgen ray dermatitis[AV172]. Undiluted leaf juice was active in one case of radiation ulcers of the tongue, floor of the mouth and mandible resulting from intraoral radium therapy and external deep X-ray therapy[AV170]. Fresh leaf gel, administered intragastrically to male rats at a dose of 2.0 ml/kg, was active[AV040]. Fresh leaf juice, applied to wounds induced with sterile sandpaper in tips of the fingers of human adults at a concentration of 50.0% in the form of an ointment using petroleum as a base, was active[AV168]. Juice, administered subcutaneously to mice at a dose of 300.0 mg/kg, was active. The juice blocked 100% of the wound healing suppression of hydrocortisone acetate[AV039]. When applied, undiluted from 1–4 weeks externally on cats, dogs and horses for a variety inflammatory condition, the juice was active[AV108]. A case of Roentgen ray dermatitis with ulceration in human adults was treated with undiluted fresh leaf juice with positive results. External application produced weak activity on surgically induced skin wounds[AV165]. It was active in rats vs dermatitis produced by 14,000 Rep of beta radiation and in rabbits on 28,000 Rep of beta radiation[AV171]. The juice, when applied for 14 days, was equivocal in rat vs third degree Roentgen radiation[AV166]. Leaf pulp, applied externally on human adults at a concentration of 20.0%, was active. Epidermal cell proliferation was 168% of untreated skin[AV173]. Ophthalmic application of undiluted fresh leaf juice was active in rabbits. Traumatic corneal ulcers were produced in 30 animals, and the juice was used as eye drops 3 times daily[AV097]. The juice increased the rate of wound healing in patients with chronic leg ulcers and improved skin conditions in human patients with acne vulgaris, seborrheic alopecia and alopecia areata[AV173]. Water extract of fresh leaves, applied externally to human adults of both sexes, was active[AV105]. Fresh leaf pulp, applied externally to patients with chronic and acute injuries 3 times per week for 3 weeks, was active[AV066]. Leaf gel cream was applied to frostbitten rabbit ears. Recovery of tissue was enhanced. The effect was increased by co-administration of pentoxyphylline[AV050]. Undiluted leaf juice, applied externally on female human adults, was active. In one patient with roentgen dermatitis, treatment with fresh leaf juice subsided itching and burning in 24 hours. After 5 weeks, there was complete regeneration of skin, new hair growth, complete restoration of sensation, and lack of scar tissue[AV153]. After treatment of Roentgen ray ulcers in a 40-year-old man by daily application of fresh leaf juice, healing began 4–6 weeks after initiation of treatment, with no pain relief for 2–3 weeks after start of treatment. In the treatment of Roentgen ray dermatitis in a 46-year-old man, pain subsided 48 hours following initiation of treatment. Epithelization started in 48–72 hours after start of treatment[AV155]. Leaf juice, applied externally on rabbits at a concentration of 30%, was active. When ointment was applied twice daily on experimentally induced thermal burns on the back of rabbits, the lesions healed in 2 weeks without gross evidence of scarring[AV154]. Undiluted leaf juice was active on human adults[AV130]. Water extract of fresh leaf gel (undiluted), applied externally, was active. The treatment was found to promote fibroblast generation, fibrocytic activity and collagen proliferation in patients who have undergone nasal surgery[AV149]. The leaf gel, administered subcutaneously to mice at a dose of 300.0 mg/kg, was active[AV033]. Water extract of fresh leaf juice, administered subcutaneously to mice at a dose of 1.0 mg/kg, was active. The decolorized extract was used. A 6-mm circular piece of skin was removed from both sides of bodies of normal and diabetic rats. Test groups were dosed daily for 7 days. Treated diabetic animals showed a wound reduction of 47% after 7 days, relative to a 35% reduction in untreated normal controls and 28% for untreated diabetic controls vs carrageenin-induced pedal edema[AV062]. Water extract, administered subcutaneously to mice at a dose of 10.0 mg/kg, was active. Wound healing was more rapid when decolorized aloe (e.g. with anthraquinone removed) was used. When administered subcutaneously to rats, aloe powder (anthraquinone fraction present) was more effective than aloe powder combined with RNA and vitamin C[AV058]. Water extract of fresh leaves, applied topically to human adults at a concentration of 0.5%, was active. The biological activity reported has been patented[AV087]. Undiluted water extract of leaves, applied externally to human adults following dental surgery, was active[AV024]. When applied externally on guinea pig, the extract was active vs burn injury[AV043]. On human adults, the juice improved laparotomy wounds healing by secondary intention[AV043]. Lyophilized gel, applied to induced second degree wounds in rats, was effective. A total of 48 male rats were equally divided into sham controls, untreated burn wound, those treated with once-daily application of normal saline, and those treated with once-daily application of the gel. The animals in each group were equally subdivided into 2 subgroups for the study of cutaneous microcirculation and wound healing on day 7 and 14 after burn. Dorsal skin fold chamber preparation and intravital fluorescence microscopic technique were performed to examine dermal microvascular changes, including arteriolar diameter, postcapillary venular permeability and leukocyte adhesion on postcapillary venules. On day 7, the vasodilation and increased postcapillary venular permeability was encountered in the untreated burn were found to be reduced significantly ($P < 0.05$) in both the normal saline and gel treated groups, but to a greater extent in the latter. Leukocyte adhesion was not different among the untreated, saline and gel treated groups. On day 14, vasoconstriction occurred after the wound had been left untreated. Only in the gel treated groups was arteriolar diameter increased up to normal condition and postcapillary venular permeability was not different from the sham controls. The amount of leukocyte adhesion was also less observed compared to the untreated and saline treated groups. The healing area of the gel treated wound was better than that of the untreated and saline treated groups at 7 and 14 days after burn. It was evident that the gel exhibits the actions of both wound healing and anti-inflammatory activity when applied on a second-degree burn wound[AV210].

REFERENCES

AV001 Suwal, P. N. Medicinal Plants of Nepal. Ministry of Forests, Department of Medicinal Plants, Thapathali, Kathmandu, Nepal 1970.

AV002 Quisumbing, E. Medicinal plants of the Philippines. **Tech Bull 16**, Rep Philippines, Dept Agr Nat Resources, Manila 1951; 1.

AV003 Schifferli, E. Abortion and attempted abortion with plant substances. **Ditsch Z Ges Gerichtl Med** 1939; 31: 239.

AV004 Boyd, L. J. The pharmacology of the homeopathic drugs. I. **J Amer Inst Homeopathy** 1928; 21: 7.

AV005 Mukerji, B. The Indian Pharmaceutical Codex. Volume 1 – Indigenous Drugs. Council of Scientific and Industrial Research, New Delhi, India, 1953.

AV006 Bhaduri, B., C. R. Ghose, A. N. Bose, B. K. Moza and U. P. Basu. Antifertility activity of some medicinal plants. **Indian J Exp Biol** 1968; 6: 252–253.

AV007 Dhar, M. L., M. M. Dhar, B. N. Mehrotra and C. Ray. Screening of Indian plants for biological activity: Part I. **Indian J Exp Biol** 1968; 6: 232–247.

AV008 Saha, J. C., E. C. Savini and S. Kasinathan. Ecbolic properties of Indian medicinal plants. Part I. **Indian J Med Res** 1961; 49: 130–151.

AV009 Garg, S. K., S. K. Saksena and R. R. Chaudhury. Antifertility screening of plants. Part VI. Effect of five indigenous plants on early pregnancy in albino rats. **Indian J Med Res** 1970; 58: 1285–1289.

AV010 Baquar, S. R. and M. Tasnif. Medicinal plants of Southern West Pakistan. **Pak PCSIR Bull Monogr 3** 1967.

AV011 Bhakuni, D. S., M. L. Dhar, M. M. Dhar, B. N. Dhawan, B. Gupta and R. C. Srimali. Screening of Indian plants for biological activity. Part III. **Indian J Exp Biol** 1971; 9: 91.

AV012 Perrot, E. and P. Hurrier. Matiere Medicale et Pharmacopee Sino-Annamites. Vigot Freres, Edit., Paris, 1907; 292pp.

AV013 Wren, R. C. Potter's New Cyclopedia of Botanical Drugs and Preparations. Sir Isaac Pitman & Sons, Inc., London, 1956.

AV014 Morton, J. F. Folk-remedy plants and esophageal cancer in Coro, Venezuela. **Morris Arboretum Bull** 1974; 25: 24–34.

AV015 Manfred, L. Siete Mil Recetas Botanicas a Base de Mil Trescientas Plantas. Edit Kier, Buenos Aires, 1956.

AV016 Anon. The Lilly Hand Book, 7th Rev, Eli Lilly Co. Indianapolis, Indiana, 1917.

AV017 Burkhill, I. H. Dictionary of the Economic Products of the Malay Peninsula. Ministry of Agriculture and Cooperatives, Kuala Lumpur, Malaysia, Vol. 1, 1966.

AV018 Doff, W. In vitro tuberculostatic action of aloe and its important components. **Arzniemittel-Forsch** 1953; 3: 627–630.

AV019 Gottshall, R. Y., J. C. Jennings, L. E. Weller, C. T. Redemann, E. H. Lucas and H. M. Sell. Antibacterial substances in seed plants active against tubercle bacilli. **Amer Rev Tuberculosis** 1950; 62: 475–480.

AV020 Gottshall, R. Y., E. H. Lucas, A. Lickfeldt and J. M. Roberts. The occurrence of antibacterial substances active against *Mycobacterium tuberculosis* in seed plants. **J Clin Invest** 1949; 28: 920–923.

AV021 Hart, L. A., P. H. Van Enckevort, H. Van Dijk, R. Zaat, K. T. D. De Silva and R. P. Labadie. Two functionally and chemically distinct immunomodulatory compounds in the gel of *Aloe vera*. **J Ethnopharmacol** 1988; 23(1): 61–71.

AV022 Maret, R. H. and H. R. Cobble. Extracts of *Aloe vera*. **Patent-US** 3,878,197: 1975.

AV023 Galal, E. E., A. Kandila, R. Hegazy, M. El-Ghoroury and W. Gobran. Aloe vera and gastrogenic ulceration. **J Drug Res (Egypt)** 1975; 7(2): 73.

AV024 Cobble, H. H. Stabilized *Aloe vera* gel. **Patent US**-3,892,853: 1975.

AV025 Morton, J. F. Current folk remedies of Northern Venezuela. **Q J Crude Drug Res** 1975; 13: 97–121.

AV026 Wong, W. Some folk medicinal plants from Trinidad. **Econ Bot** 1976; 30: 103–142.

AV027 Keys, J. D. Chinese Herbs, Botany, Chemistry and Pharmacodynamics. Charles E. Tuttle Co., Rutland, Vermont, USA, 1976.

AV028 Nieto Burgos, C. Hair regenerator based on aloe extract. **Patent-Spain**-2,019,828: 1991.

AV029 Mahmoud, I., A. Alkofahi and A. Abdelaziz. Mutagenic and toxic activities of several spices and some Jordanian medicinal plants. **Int J Pharmacog** 1992; 30(2): 81–85.

AV030 Yaron, A., E. Cohen and S. Arad. Stabilization of *Aloe vera* gel by interaction with sulfated polysaccharides from red microalgae and with xanthan gum. **J Agr Food Chem** 1992; 40(8): 1316–1320.

AV031 Roman-Ramos, R., J. L. Flores-Saenz, G. Partida-Hernandez, A. Lara-Lemus, F. Alarcon-Aguilar. Experimental study of hypoglycemic activity of some antidiabetic plants. **Arch Invest Med (Mex)** 1991; 22(1): 87–93.

AV032 Heggers, J. P., R. P. Pelley and M. C. Robson. Beneficial effects of aloe in wound healing. **Phytother Res** 1993; 7: 848–852.

AV033 Davis, R. H., J. J. Donato, G. M. Hartman and R. C. Haas. Anti-inflammatory and wound healing activity of a growth substance in *Aloe vera*. **J Amer Pod Med Assoc** 1994; 84(2): 77–81.

AV034 Kavoussi, H. and H. P. Kavoussi. Saturated solution of purified sodium chloride in purified *Aloe vera* for inducing and stimulating hair growth and for decreasing hair loss. **Patent US**-5,215,760: 1993.

AV035 Nath, D., N. Sethi, R. K. Singh and A. K. Jain. Commonly used Indian abortifacient plants with special reference to their teratologic effects in rats. **J Ethnopharmacol** 1992; 36(2): 147–154.

AV036 Zamora-Martinez, M. C. and C. N. P. Pola. Medicinal plants used in some rural populations of Oaxaca, Puebla and Veracruz, Mexico. **J Ethnopharmacol** 1992; 35(3) 229–257.

AV037 Yamaguchi, I., N. Mega and H. Sanada. Components of the gel of Aloe vera (L.) Burm. F. **Biosci Biotech Biochem** 1993; 57(8): 1350–1352.

AV038 Jeong, H. Y., J. H. Kim, S. J. Hwang and D. K. Rhee. Anticancer effects of aloe on Sarcoma 180 in ICR mouse and on human cancer cell lines. **Yakhak Hoeji** 1994; 38(3): 311–321.

AV039 Davis, R. H., J. J. Di Donato, R. W. Johnson and C. B. Stewart. *Aloe vera*, hydrocortisone and sterol influence on wound tensile strength and anti-inflammation. **J Amer Pod Med Assoc** 1994; 84(12): 612–621.

AV040 Upupa, S. L., A. L. Udupa and D. R. Kulkarni. Anti-inflammatory and wound healing properties of *Aloe vera*. **Fitoterapia** 1994; 65(2): 141–145.

AV041 Yamamoto, M., K. Sugiyama, M. Yokoto, Y. Maeda, K. Nakagomi and H. Nakazawa. Inhibitory effects of aloe extracts on antigen- and compound 48/80-induced histamine release from rat peritoneal mast cells. **Jap J Toxicol Environ Health** 1993; 39(5): 395–400.

AV042 Garnick, J., P. J. Hanes, J. Hardin and W. Thompson. Changes in root sensitivity with toothpastes containing *Aloe vera* and allantoin. **Arch Oral Biol** 1994; 39-S: 1325.

AV043   Hormann, H. P. and H. C. Korting. Evidence for the efficacy and safety of topical herbal drugs in dermatology. Part I. Anti-inflammatory agents. **Phytomedicine** 1994; 1(2): 161–171.

AV044   Koo, M. W. L. *Aloe vera.* Antiulcer and antidiabetic effects. **Phytother Res** 1994; 8(8): 461–464.

AV045   Holdsworth, D. K. Traditional medicinal plants of Rarotonga, Cook Islands. Part I. **Int J Crude Drug Res** 1990; 28(3): 209–218.

AV046   Bouthet, C. F., V. R. Schirf and W. D. Winters. Stimulation of neuron-like cell growth by aloe substances. **Phytother Res** 1995; 9(3): 185–188.

AV047   Winters, D. Immunoreactive lectins in leaf gel from *Aloe barbadensis* Miller. **Phytother Res** 1993; 7: S23–S25.

AV048   Singh, K. K. and J. K. Maheshwari. Traditional phytotherapy of some medicinal plants used by the Tharus of the Nainital District, Uttar Pradesh, India. **Int J Pharmacog** 1994; 32(1): 51–58.

AV049   Bhattarai, N. K. Folk herbal remedies for gynaecological complaints in Central Nepal. **Int J Pharmacog** 1994; 32(1): 13–26.

AV050   Miller, M. B. and P. J. Koltai. Treatment of experimental frostbite with pentoxifylline and *Aloe vera* cream. **Arch Otolaryngol Head Neck Surg** 1995; 121(6): 678–680.

AV051   Leung, A. Y. *Aloe vera* in cosmetics. **Drug Cosmet Ind** 1977; 120: 34.

AV052   Tewari, P. V., H. C. Mapa and C. Chaturvedi. Experimental study on estrogenic activity of certain indigenous drugs. **J Res Indian Med Yoga Homeopathy** 1976; 11: 7–12.

AV053   Heinerman, J. Medical Doctor's Guide to Herbs. Biworld Publishers, Provo, Utah (ISBN-0-89557-016-5), 1977.

AV054   Hikino, H. and T. Hayashi. Hypoglycemic polysaccharides extraction from Aloe species. **Patent-Japan Kokai Tokkyo Koho**-60,214,741: 1985.

AV055   Hikino, H., M Takahashi, M. Murakami, C. Konno, Y. Mirin, M. Karikura and T. Hayashi. Isolation and hypoglycemic activity of arborans A and B, glycans of *Aloe arborescens* var. *natalensis* leaves. **Int J Crude Drug Res** 1986; 24(4): 183–186.

AV056   Hart, L. A., P. H. Van Enckevort and R. F. Labadie. Analysis of two functionally and chemically different immunomodulators from *Aloe vera* gel. **Pharm Weekbl (Sci Ed)** 1987; 9(2): 157.

AV057   Hart, L. A., P. H. Van Enckevort and R. F. Labadie. Analysis of two functionally different immunomodulators from *Aloe vera* gel. **Pharm Weekbl (Sci Ed)** 1987; 9(4): 219.

AV058   Davis, R. H., J. M. Kabbani and N. P. Maro. *Aloe vera* and wound healing. **J Amer Podiatr Med Assoc** 1987; 77(4): 165–169.

AV059   Kaufman, T., N. Kalderon, Y. Ullmann and J. Berger. *Aloe vera* gel hindered wound healing of experimental second-degree burns: A quantitative controlled study. **J Burn Car Rehab** 1988; 9(2): 156–159.

AV060   Rodriquez-Bigas, M., N. I. Cruz and A. Suarez. Comparative evaluation of *Aloe vera* in the management of burn wounds in guinea pigs. **Plastic & Reconstructive Surgery** 1988; 81(3): 386–389.

AV061   Davis, R. H., M. G. Leitner and J. M. Russo. Topical anti-inflammatory activity of *Aloe vera* as measured by ear swelling. **J Amer Podiatr Med Assoc** 1987; 77(11): 610–612.

AV062   Davis, R. H., M. G. Leitner and J. M. Russo. *Aloe vera.* A natural approach for treating wounds, edema, and pain in diabetes. **J Amer Podiatr Med Assoc** 1988; 78(2): 60–68.

AV063   Sethi, N., D. Nath and R. K. Singh. Teratological evaluation of some commonly used indigenous antifertility plants in rats. **Int J Crude Drug Res** 1989; 27(2): 118–120.

AV064   Audy-Rowland, J. Natural aloe gel: Cosmetic composition with anti-acne and moisturizing properties. **Patent-Fr Demande**-2,555,445: 1983.

AV065   Al-Awadi, F. and M. Shoukry. The lipid lowering effect of an anti-diabetic plant extract. **Acta Diabetol Lat** 1988; 25(1): 1–5.

AV066   Lerner, F. N. Investigation of effects of proteolytic enzymes, aloe gel, and iontophoresis on chronic and acute athletic injuries. **Chiropractic Sports Med** 1987; 1(3): 106–110.

AV067 Mohsin, A., A. H. Shah, M. A. Al-Yahya, M. Tariq, M. O. M. Tanira and A. M. Ageel. Analgesic antipyretic activity and phytochemical screening of some plants used in traditional Arab system of medicine. **Fitoterapia** 1989; 60(2): 174–177.

AV068 Hart, L. A., A. J. J. Van den Berg, L. Kuis, H. Van Dijk and R. P. Labadie. An anti-complementary polysaccharide with immunological adjuvant activity from the leaf parenchyma gel of *Aloe vera*. **Planta Med** 1989; 55(6): 509–512.

AV069 Ghannam, N., M. Kingston, I. A. Al-Meshaal, M. Tariq, N. S. Parman and N. Woodhouse. The antidiabetic activity of aloes: Preliminary clinical and experimental observations. **Horm Res** 1986; 24: 288–294.

AV070 Chen, C. P., C. C. Lin and T. Namba. Screening of Taiwanese crude drugs for antibacterial activity against *Streptococcus mutans*. **J Ethnopharmacol** 1989; 27(3): 285–295.

AV071 Mossa, J. S. A study on the crude antidiabetic drugs used in Arabian folk medicine. **Int J Crude Drug Res** 1985; 23(3): 137–145.

AV072 Ajabnoor, M. A. Effect of aloes on blood glucose levels in normal and alloxan diabetic mice. **J Ethnopharmacol** 1990; 28(2): 215–220.

AV073 Davis, R. H., K. Y. Rosenthal, L. R. Cesario and G. A. Rouw. Processed *Aloe vera* administered topically inhibits inflammation. **J Amer Podiatr Med Assoc** 1989; 79(8): 395–397.

AV074 Paszkiewicz-Gadek, A., J. Chlabicz and W. Galasinski. The influence of selected potential oncostatics of plant origin on the protein biosynthesis in vitro. **Polish J Pharmacol Pharm** 1989; 40(2): 183–190.

AV075 Davis, R. H., M. G. Leitner, J. M. Russo and M. E. Byrne. Anti-inflammatory activity of *Aloe vera* against a spectrum of irritants. **J Amer Podiatr Med Assoc** 1989; 79(6): 263–276.

AV076 Davis, R. H. and N. P. Maro. *Aloe vera* and gibberellin anti-inflammatory activity in diabetes. **J Amer Podiatr Med Assoc** 1989; 79(1): 24–26.

AV077 Jain, S. P. Tribal remedies from Saranda Forest, Bihar, India. I. **Int J Crude Drug Res** 1989; 27(1): 29–32.

AV078 Kaufman, T., A. R. Newman and M. R. Wexler. *Aloe vera* and burn wound healing. **Plastic and Reconstructive Surgery** 1990; 83(6): 1075–1076.

AV079 Davis, R. H., W. L. Parker and D. P. Murdoch. *Aloe vera* as a biologically active vehicle for hydrocortisone acetate. **J Amer Podiatr Med Assoc** 1991; 81(1): 1–9.

AV080 Crowell, J., S. Hilsenbeck and N. Penneys. *Aloe vera* does not affect cutaneous erythema and blood flow following ultraviolet B exposure. **Photodermatology** 1989; 6(5): 237–239.

AV081 Nagaraju, N. and K. N. Rao. A survey of plant crude drugs of Rayalaseema, Andhra Pradesh, India. **J Ethnopharmacol** 1990; 29(2): 137–158.

AV082 Davis, R. H., W. L. Parker, R. T. Samson and D. P. Murdoch. The isolation of an active inhibitory system from an extract of *Aloe vera*. **J Amer Podiatr Med Assoc** 1991; 81(5): 258–261.

AV083 Joshi, P. Herbal drugs used in Guinea worm disease by the tribals of Southern Rajasthan (India). **Int J Pharmacog** 1991; 29(1): 33–38.

AV084 Al-Awad, F. M. and K. A. Gumaa. Studies on the activity of individual plants of an antidiabetic plant mixture. **Acta Diabetol Lat** 1987; 24(1): 37–41.

AV085 Lin, C. C. and W. S. Kan. Medicinal plants used for the treatment of hepatitis in Taiwan. **Am J Chin Med** 1990; 18(1/2): 35–43.

AV086 Carbajal, D., A. Casaco, L. Arruzazabala, R. Gonzalez and V. Fuentes. Pharmacological screening of plant decoctions commonly used in Cuban folk medicine. **J Ethno-pharmacol** 1991; 33(1/2): 21–24.

AV087 Egawa, M., K. Ishida, M. Maekawa and Y. Sato. Anti-inflammatory and wound-healing topical skin preparations containing aloe extract and ellagic acids. **Patent-Japan Kokai Tokkyo Koho** – 02 231,408: 1990.

AV088 Dominguez-Soto, L. Photodermatitis to *Aloe vera*. **Int J Dermatol** 1992; 31(5): 372.

AV089 Chauhan, J. S., N. K. Singh and S. V. Singh. Screening of higher plants for specific herbicidal principles active against dodder, *Cuscuta reflexa* Roxb. **Indian J Exp Biol** 1989; 27(10): 877–884.

AV090   Davis, R. H., G. J. Stewart and P. J. Bregman. *Aloe vera* and the inflamed synovial pouch model. **J Amer Pod Med Assoc** 1992; 82(3): 140–148.

AV091   Caceres, A., E. Jauregu, D. Herrera and H. Logemann. Plants used in Guatemala for the treatment of dermatomucosal infections. I. Screening of 38 plant extracts for anticandidal activity. **J Ethnopharmacol** 1991; 33(3): 277–283.

AV092   Estevez, A., R. Magdan and G. Marquina. Chemical study and antitumor activity on Cuban plants. **First Latin American & Caribbean Symposium on Pharmacologically Active Natural Products, Havana, Cuba, UNESCO** 1982.

AV093   Apisariyakul, A. Investigation of fractions isolated from Thai medicinal plants affecting on isolated rat ileum. **Abstr 10th Conference of Science and Technology, Thailand** 1984; 450–451.

AV094   Goswami, C. S. and M. M. Bokadia. The effect of extracts of *Aloe barbadensis* leaves on the fertility of female rats. **Indian Drugs** 1979; 16: 124–125.

AV095   Halberstein, R. A. and A. B. Saunders. Traditional medical practices and medicinal plant usage on a Bahamian Island. **Cul Med Psychiat** 1978; 2: 177–203.

AV096   Ayensu, E. S. Medicinal plants of the West Indies. **Unpublished Manuscript** 1978.

AV097   Hegazy, M. A., A. Mortada, M. R. Hegazy and M. Helal. The use of *Aloe vera* extract in the treatment of experimental corneal ulcers in rabbits. **J Drug Res (Egypt)** 1978; 10: 199–209.

AV098   Gupta, M. P., T. D. Arias, M. Correa and S. S. Lamba. Ethnopharmacognostic observations on Panamanian medicinal plants. Part 1. **Q J Crude Drug Res** 1979; 17(3/4): 115–130.

AV099   Coutts, B. C. Stabilized *Aloe vera* gel. **Patent Japan Kokai Tokkyo Koho**-79 119,018 1979: 6pp.

AV100   Abraham, Z. and P. N. Prasad. Occurrence of triploidy in *Aloe vera* Tourn Ex Linn. **Curr Sci** 1979; 48: 1001–1002.

AV101   Heggers, J. P., G. R. Pineless and M. C. Robson. Dermaide Aloe/*Aloe vera* gel: Comparison of the antimicrobial effects. **J Amer Med Technol** 1979; 41: 293–294.

AV102   Singh, M. P., S. B. Malla, S. B. Rajbhandari and A. Manandhar. Medicinal plants of Nepal-Retrospects and prospects. **Econ Bot** 1979; 33(2): 185–198.

AV103   Crewe, J. E. Aloes in the treatment of burns and scalds. **Minnesota Med** 1939; 22: 538–539.

AV104   Kandil, A. and W. Gobran. Protection of gastric mucosa by *Aloe vera*. **J Drug Res (Egypt)** 1979; 11: 191–196.

AV105   Sayed, M. D. Traditional medicine in health care. **J Ethnopharmacol** 1980; 2(1): 19–22.

AV106   Medina, F. R. and R. Woodbury. Terrestrial plants molluscicidal to Lymnaeid hosts of *Fasciliasis hepatica* in Puerto Rico. **J Agr Univ Puerto Rico** 1979; 63: 366–376.

AV107   Weninger, B., M. Haag-Berrurier and R. Anton. Plants of Haiti used as antifertility agents. **J Ethnopharmacol** 1982; 6(1): 67–84.

AV108   Northway, R. B. Experimental use of *Aloe vera* extract in clinical practice. **Vet Med Small Animal Clinic** 1975; 70: 89.

AV109   Prakash, A. O., R. B. Gupta and R. Mathur. Effect of oral administration of forty-two indigenous plant extracts on early and late pregnancy in albino rats. **Probe** 1978; 17(4): 315–323.

AV110   Ship, A. G. Is tropical *Aloe vera* plant mucus helpful in burn treatment? **J Amer Med Assn** 1977; 238: 1770.

AV111   Gupta, R. A., B. N. Singh and R. N. Singh. Preliminary study on certain Vedanasthapana (analgesic) drugs. **J Sci Res Pl Med** 1981; 2: 110–112.

AV112   Hafez, E. S. E. Abortifacients in primitive societies and in experimental animal models. **Contraceptive Delivery Systems** MTP Press, Ltd., Lancaster, England. (ISSN: 0143-6112). 1982; 3(3): 452.

AV113   Kandel, A. and W. Gobran. Protection of gastric mucosa by *Aloe vera*. **Bull Islamic Med** 1982; 2: 508–511.

AV114   Mazumder, R. C. and S. R. Dasgupta. Studies on the pharmacological properties of "Ghritakumar" (*Aloe perfoliata*) on gross behaviour on conscious animals. **Indian Med J** 1982; 76(7): 84–87.

AV115 Guillot, J. P., J. Y. Giauffret, M. C. Martini, J. F. Gonnet and G. Soule. Safety evaluation of cosmetic raw materials: Results obtained with 160 samples from various origins. **IFREB Lancaster CEO** 1980.

AV116 Bastien, J. W. Pharmacopeia of Qollahuaya Andeans. **Journal of Ethnopharmacol** 1983; 8(1): 97–111.

AV117 Gupta, R. A., B. N. Singh and R. N. Singh. Screening of Ayurvedic drugs for analgesic activity. **J Sci Res Pl Med** 1982; 3: 115–117.

AV118 Elvin-Lewis, M. and W. H. Lewis. The dental use of plants in Amazonia. **Odontostomatol Trop** 1983; 6(4): 179–186.

AV119 Boukef, K., H. R. Souissi and G. Balansard. Contribution to the study on plants used in traditional medicine in Tunisia. **Plant Med Phytother**1982; 16(4): 260–279.

AV120 Suga, T. and T. Hirata. The efficacy of the aloe plants chemical constituents and biological activities. **Cosmet Toiletries** 1983; 98(6): 105–108.

AV121 Sebastian, M. K. and M. M. Bhandari. Medico-ethno botany of Mount Abu, Rajasthan, Indian. **J Ethnopharmacol** 1984; 12(2): 223–230.

AV122 Woo, W. S., E. B. Lee, K. H. Shin, S. S. Kang and H. J. Chi. A review of research on plants for fertility regulation in Korea. **Korean J Pharmacog** 1981; 12(3): 153–170.

AV123 Mossa, J. S. A study on the crude antidiabetic drugs used in Arabian folk medicine. **Int J Crude Drug Res** 1985; 23(3): 137–145.

AV124 Darias, V., L. Bravo, E. Barquin, D. M. Herrera and C. Fraile. Contribution to the ethnopharmacological study of the Canary Islands. **J Ethnopharmacol** 1986; 15(2): 169–193.

AV125 Anderson, E. F. Ethnobotany of Hill Tribes of Northern Thailand. 1. Medicinal plants of Akha. **Econ Bot** 1986; 40(1): 38–53.

AV126 Parmar, N. S., M. Tariq, M. A. Alyahya, A. M. Ageel and M. S. Al

Said. Evaluation of *Aloe vera* leaf exudate and gel for gastric and duodenal antiulcer activity. **Fitoterapia** 1986; 57(5): 380–383.

AV127 Winters, W. D., R. Benavides and W. J. Clouse. Effects of aloe extracts on human normal and tumor cells in vitro. I. **Econ Bot** 1981; 35(1): 89–95.

AV128 Sydiskia, R. J. and D. G. Owen. Aloe emodin and other anthraquinones and anthraquinone-like compounds from plants virucidal against herpes simplex viruses. **Patent US-4,670,265**: 1987.

AV129 Weniger, B., M. Rouzier, R. Daguilh, D. Henrys, J. H. Henrys and R. Anton. Popular medicine of the Central Plateau of Haiti. 2. Ethnopharmacological inventory. **J Ethnopharmacol** 1986; 17(1): 13–30.

AV130 Bernhard, J. D. *Aloe vera* and Vitamin E as dermatologic remedies. **J Amer Med Assn** 1988; 259(1): 101.

AV131 Kamboj, V. P. A review of Indian medicinal plants with interceptive activity. **Indian J Med Res** 1988; 4: 336–355.

AV132 Yokel, R. A. and C. D. Ogzewalla. Effects of plant ingestion in rats determined by the conditioned taste aversion procedure. **Toxicon** 1981; 19(2): 223–232.

AV133 Hart, L. A., P. H. Van Enckevort and R. P. Labadie. Anionic polymers with anti-complementary activity from *Aloe vera* gel. **Pharm Weekbl (Sci Ed)** 1987; 9(4): 223.

AV134 Levin, H., R. Hazenfratz, J. Friedman, D. Palevitch and M. Perl. Partial purification and some properties of an antibacterial compound from *Aloe vera*. **Phytother Res** 1988; 2(2): 67–69.

AV135 Winters, W. D., R. Benavides and W. J. Clouse. Effects of aloe extracts on human normal and tumor cells in vitro. **Econ Bot** 1981; 35(1): 89–95.

AV136 Ramirez, V. R., L. J. Mostacero, A. E. Garcia, C. F. Mejia, P. F. Pelaez, C. D. Medina and C. H. Miranda. Vegetales Empleados en Medicina Tradicional Norperuana. **Banco Agrario Del Peru & NACL Univ Trujillo, Trujillo, Peru**, June 1988.

AV137 Caceres, A., L. M. Giron, S. R. Alvarado, and M. F. Torres. Screening of antimicrobial activity of plants popularly used in Guatemala for the treatment of dermatomucosal diseases. **J Ethnopharmacol** 1987; 20(3): 223–237.

AV138   Yagi, A., T. Shida and H. Nishimura. Effect of amino acids in aloe extract on phagocytosis by peripheral neutrophil in adult bronchial asthma. **Jap J Allergol** 1987; 36(12): 1094–1101.

AV139   Singh, V. P., S. K. Sharma, and V. S. Khare. Medicinal plants from Ujjain District Madhya Pradesh. Part II. **Indian Drugs Pharm Ind** 1980; 5: 7–12.

AV140   Shah, A. H., S. Qureshi, M. Tariqu and A. M. Ageel. Toxicity studies on six plants used in the traditional Arab system of medicine. **Phytother Res** 1989; 3(1): 25–29.

AV141   Darias, V., L. Brando, R. Rabanal, C. Sanchez Mateo, R. M. Gonzalez Luis and A. M. Hernandez Perez. New contribution to the ethnopharmacological study of the Canary Islands. **J Ethnopharmacol** 1989; 25(1): 77–92.

AV142   Hirschmann, G. S. and A. Rojas de Arias. A survey of medicinal plants of Minas Gerais, Brazil. **J Ethnopharmacol** 1990; 29(2): 159–172.

AV143   Fulton Jr, J. E. The stimulation of postdermabrasion wound healing with stabilized *Aloe vera* gel - polyethlene oxide dressing. **J Dermatol Surg Oncol** 1990; 16(5): 460–467.

AV144   Kivett, W. F. *Aloe vera* for burns. **Plastic & Reconstructive Surgery** 1989; 83(1): 195.

AV145   Hart, L. A., P. H. Nibbering, M. T. Van Den Barselaar, H. Van Dijk, A. J. J. Van Den Berg and R. P. Labadie. Effects of low molecular constituents from *Aloe vera* gel on oxidative metabolism and cytotoxic and bactericidal activities of human neutrophils. **Int J Immunopharmacol** 1990; 12(4): 427–434.

AV146   Davis, R. H., M. G. Leitner, J. M. Russo and M. E. Byrne. Wound healing oral and topical activity of *Aloe vera*. **J Amer Podiatr Med Assn** 1989; 79(11): 559–562.

AV147   Verma, S. B. S., H. J. Schulze and G. K. Steigleder. The effect of externally applied remedies containing *Aloe vera*

gel on the proliferation of the epidermis. **Parfumerie Und Kometik** 1989; 70(8): 452–459.

AV148   Davis, R. H., W. L. Parker, R. T. Samson and D. P. Murdoch. Isolation of a stimulatory system in an aloe extract. **J Amer Pod Med Assn** 1991; 81(9): 473–478.

AV149   Thompson, J. E. Topical use of *Aloe vera* derived allantoin gel in otolaryngology. **Ear Nose Throat** 1991; 70(2): 119.

AV150   Schmidt, J. M. and J. S. Greenspoon. *Aloe vera* dermal wound gel is associated with a delay in wound healing. **Obstet Gynecol** 1991; 78(1): 115–117.

AV151   Strickland, F. M., R. P. Pelley and M. L. Kripke. Prevention of ultraviolet radiation–induced suppression of contact and delayed hypersensitivity by *Aloe barbadensis* gel extract. **J Invest Dermatol** 1994; 102(2): 197–204.

AV152   Khurana, S. M. P. and K. S. Bhargava. Effect of plant extracts on the activity of three papaya viruses. **J Gen Appl Microbiol** 1970; 16: 225–230.

AV153   Collins, C. E. and Collins, C. Roentgen dermatitis treated with fresh whole leaf of *Aloe vera*. **Amer J Roentgen** 1935; 33: 396.

AV154   Rovatii, B. and R. J. Brennan. Experimental thermal burns. **Induct Med Surg** 1959; 28: 364.

AV155   Loveman, A. B. Leaf of *Aloe vera* in treatment of roentgen ray ulcers: Report on two additional cases. **Arch Dermatol Syphilol** 1937; 36: 838.

AV156   Lorenzetti, L. J., R. Salisbury, J. L. Beal and J. N. Baldwin. Bacteriostatic property of *Aloe vera*. **J Pharm Sci** 1964; 53: 1287.

AV157   Mausert, O. Herbs For Health, Clavering Press, San Francisco, California, 1932; 1–204.

AV158   Prakash, A. O. and R. Mathur. Screening of Indian plants for antifertility activity. **Indian J Exp Biol** 1976; 14: 623–626.

AV159   Gupta, M. L., T. K. Gupta and K. P. Bhargava. A study of antifertility effects of some indigenous drugs. **J Res Indian Med** 1971; 6: 112–116.

AV160   Rowe, T. D., B. K. Lovell and L. M. Parks. Further observations on the use of *Aloe vera* leaf in the treatment of third degree x-ray reactions. **J Amer Pharm Assn Sci Ed** 1941; 30: 266–269.

AV161 Collins, C. E. and Collins, C. Roentgen dermatitis treated with fresh whole leaf of *Aloe vera*. **Amer J Roentgen** 1937; 33: 396–397.

AV162 Wright, C. S. *Aloe vera* in the treatment of Roentgen ulcers and telangiectasis. **J Amer Med Assn** 1936; 106: 1363–1364.

AV163 El-Dean Mahmoud, A. A. G. Study of indigenous (folk ways) birth control methods in Alexandria. **Thesis-MS-University of Alexandria-Higher-Inst of Nursing** 1972.

AV164 Roig Y Mesa, J. T. Plantas Medicinales, Aromaticas o Venenosas de Cuba. Ministerio De Agricultura, Republica De Cuba, Havana 1945.

AV165 Goff, S. and I. Levenstein. Measuring the effects of tropical preparations upon the healing of skin wounds. **J Soc Cosmet Chem** 1964; 15: 509–518.

AV166 Rowe, T. D. Effect of fresh *Aloe vera* jell in the treatment of third degree Roentgen reactions on white rats, a preliminary report. **J Amer Pharm Assn Sci Ed** 1940; 29: 348–350.

AV167 Gjerstad, G. and T. D. Riner. Current status of aloe as a cure-all. **Amer J Pharm** 1968; 140: 58–64.

AV168 Barnes, T. C. The healing action of extracts of *Aloe vera* leaf in abrasions of human skin. **Amer J Bot** 1947; 34: 597A.

AV169 Rattner, H. Roentgen ray dermatitis with ulcers. **Arch Dermatol Syphilol** 1936; 33: 593–594.

AV170 Mandeville, F. B. *Aloe vera* in the treatment of radiation ulcers of mucous membranes. **Radiology** 1939; 32: 598–599.

AV171 Lushbaugh, C. C. and D. B. Hale. Experimental acute radiodermatitis following beta irradiation. V. Histopathological study of the mode of action of therapy with *Aloe vera*. **Cancer** 1953; 6: 690–698.

AV172 Kesten, B. and R. Mc Laughlin. Roentgen ray dermatitis treated with ointment containing viosterol. **Arch Dermatol Syphilol** 1936; 34: 901–903.

AV173 El Zawahry, M., M. R. Hegazy and M. Helal. Use of aloe in treating leg ulcers and dermatoses. **Int J Dermatol** 1973; 12: 68–73.

AV174 Anon. More Secret Remedies. What They Cost and What They Contain. British Medical Association, London, 1912.

AV175 Noskov, A. D. Treatment of parodontosis by injections of aloe extract and their effect on phosphorus-calcium metabolism. **Stomatologiya** 1966; 45(4): 13–15.

AV176 Chopra, R. N. Indigenous Drugs of India. Their Medical and Economic Aspects. The Art Press, Calcutta, India, 1933; 550 pp.

AV177 Belkin, M. and D. B. Fitzgerald. Tumor-damaging capacity of plant materials. I. Plants used as cathartics. **J Nat Cancer Inst** 1952; 13: 139–155.

AV178 Wasuwat, S. A list of Thai medicinal plants, ASRCT, Bangkok, Report No. 1 on Res. Project. 17. **A.S.R.C.T. Bangkok Thailand** 1967; 17: 22 pp.

AV179 Rowe, T. D. and L. M. Parks. A phytochemical study of *Aloe vera* leaf. **J Amer Pharm Ass Sci Ed** 1941; 30: 262–266.

AV180 Rienniyom, S. and S. Wongsangaroonsri. The extractive and preparation of *Aloe vera*. **Undergraduate Special Project Report** 1981; 33 pp.

AV181 Kringstad, R. and A. Nordal. Lactone-forming acids in succulent plants. **Phytochemistry** 1975; 14: 1868–1870.

AV182 Manna, S. and B. H. McAnalley. Determination of the position of the o-acetyl group in a beta-(1-4)-mannan (acemannan) from *Aloe barbardensis* Miller. **Carbohydr Res** 1993; 241(1): 317–319.

AV183 Winter, W. D. and C. Bouthet. Polypeptides of *Aloe barbadensis* Miller. **Phytother Res** 1995; 9(6): 395–400.

AV184 Zwaving, J. H. and E. T. Elema. A comparative investigation of two methods for the determination of 1,8-dihydroxyanthracene derivatives in vegetable drugs. **Pharm Weekbl** 1976; 111: 1315.

AV185 Rauwald, H. W. New hydroxyaloins: The 'periodate-positive' substance from Cape aloes and cinnamoyl esters from Curacao aloes. **Pharm Weekbl (Sci Ed)** 1987; 9(4): 215.

AV186   Sydiskis, R. J., D. G. Owen, J. L. Lohr, K. H. A. Rosler and R. N. Blowster. Inactivation of enveloped viruses by anthraquinones extracted from plants. **Antimicrob Agents Chemother** 1991; 35(12): 2463–2466.

AV187   Waller, G. R., S. Mangiafico and C. R. Ritchey. A chemical investigation of *Aloe barbadensis*. **Proc Okla Acad Sci** 1978; 58: 69.

AV188   Gowda, D. C., B. Nellisiddaiah and Y. V. Anjaneyalu. Structural studies of polysaccharides from *Aloe vera*. **Carbohydr Res** 1979; 72: 201–205.

AV189   Haq, Q. N. and A. Hannan. Studies on glucogalactomannam from the leaves of *Aloe vera*. **Bangladesh J Sci Ind Res** 1981; 16: 68–72.

AV190   Mandal, G., R. Ghosh and A. Das. Characterisation of polysaccharides of *Aloe barbadensis* Miller: Part III. Structure of an acidic oligosaccharide. **Indian J Chem Ser B 22** 1984; 890–893.

AV191   Haq, Q. N. and A. Hannan. Studies on glucogalactomannan from the leaves of *Aloe vera* Tourn. (Ex. Linn). **Bangladesh J Sci Ind Res** 1981; 16 (1/4): 68–72.

AV192   Mandal, G. and A. Das. Characterization of the polysaccharides of *Aloe barbadensis*, Part l. Structure of the D-galactan isolated from the *Aloe barbadensis* Miller. **Carbohyhydr Res** 1980; 86: 247–257.

AV193   Mandal, G. and A. Das. Characterization of the polysaccharides of *Aloe barbadensis*, Part ll. Structure of the glucomannan isolated from the leaves of *Aloe barbadensis* Miller. **Carbohyhydr Res** 1980; 87: 249–256.

AV194   Womble, D. and J. H. Helderman. Enhancement of allo-responsiveness of human lymphocytes by acemannan (carrisyn TM). **Int J Immunopharmacol** 1988; 10(8): 967–974.

AV195   Madis, V. H., M. M. Omar and V. Madis. Aloefoeron isolation manufacture, and pilliciations. **Patent-US-4,861,761** 1984; 8 pp.

AV196   Afzal, M., M. Ali, R. A. H. Hassan, N. Sweedan and M. S. I. Dhami. Iden-

tification of some prostanoids in *Aloe vera* extracts. **Planta Med** 1991; 57(1): 38–40.

AV197   Mary, N. Y., B. V. Christensen and J. L. Beal. A paper chromatographic study of aloe, aloin and *Cascara sagrada*. **J Amer Pharm Ass Sci Ed** 1956; 45: 229–232.

AV198   Segal, A., J. A. Taylor and J. C. Eoff III. A re-investigation of the polysaccharide material from *Aloe vera* mucilage. **Lloydia** 1968; 31: 423E.

AV199   Lee, J. K., M. K. Lee, Y. P. Yun, Y. Kim, J. S. Kim, Y. S. Kim, K. Kim, S. S. Han and C. K. Lee. Acemannan purified from *Aloe vera* induces phenotypic and functional maturation of immature dendritic cells. **Int Immunopharmacol** 2001; 1(7): 1275–1284.

AV200   Olsen, D. L., W. Raub Jr, C. Bradley, M. Johnson, J. L. Macias, V. Love and A. Markoe. The effect of aloe vera gel/mild soap verus mild soap alone in preventing skin reactions in patients undergoing radiation therapy. **Oncol Nurs Forum** 2001; 28(3): 543–547.

AV201   Okyar, A., A. Can, N. Akev, G. Baktir and N. Sutlupinar. Effects of Aloe vera leaves on blood glucose level in type I and type II diabetic rats. **Phytother Res** 2001; 15(2): 157–161.

AV202   Pugh, N., S. A. Ross, M. A. El Sohly and D. S. Pasco. Characterization of Aloeride, a new high-molecular-weight polysaccharide from *Aloe vera* with potent immunostimulatory activity. **J Agric Food Chem** 2001; 49(2): 1030–1034.

AV203   Estaban, A., J. M. Zapata, L. Casano, M. Martin and B. Sabater. Peroxidase activity in *Aloe barbadensis* commercial gel: probable role in skin protection. **Planta Med** 2000; 66(8): 724–727.

AV204   Singh, R. P., S. Dhanalakshmi and A. R. Rao. Chemomodulatory action of *Aloe vera* on the profiles of enzymes associated with carcinogen metabolism and antioxidant status regulation in mice. **Phytomedicine** 2000; 7(3): 209–219.

AV205   Lee, K. H., H. S. Hong, C. H. Lee and C. H. Kim. Induction of apoptosis in human leukemic cell lines K562, HL60, and U937 by diethylhexylphthalate isolated from *Aloe vera* Linn. **J Pharm Pharmacol** 2000; 52(8): 1037–1041.

AV206 Lee, K. H., J. H. Kim, D. S. Lim and C. H. Kim. Antileukemic and anti-mutagenic effects of di(2-ethylhexyl)-phthalate isolated from *Aloe vera* Linn. **J Pharm Pharmacol** 2000; 52(5): 593–598.

AV207 Gauntt, C. J., H. J. Wood, H. R. McDaniel and B. H. McAnalley. Aloe polymannose enhances anti-coxsackie virus antibody titres in mice. **Phytother Res** 2000; 14(4): 261–266.

AV208 Pecere, T., M. V. Gazzola, C. Mucignat, C. Parolin, F. D. Vecchia, A. Cavaggioni, G. Basso, A. Diaspro, B. Salvato, M. Carli and G. Palu. Aloe-emodin is a new type of anticancer agent with selective activity against neuroectodermal tumors. **Cancer Res** 2000; 60(11): 2800–2804.

AV209 Andriani, E., T. Bugli, M. Aalders, S. Castelli, G. De Luigi, N. Lazzari and G. P. Rolli. The effectiveness and acceptance of a medical device for the treatment of aphthous stomatitis. Clinical observation in pediatric age. **Minerva Pediatr** 2000; 52(1–2): 15–20.

AV210 Somboonwong, J., S. Thanamittramanee, A. Jariyapongskul and S. Patumraj. Therapeutic effects of *Aloe vera* on cutaneous microcirculation and wound healing in second degree burn model rats. **J Med Assoc Thai** 2000; 83(4): 417–425.

AV211 Friedman, R. N. and K. Si. Initial characterization of the effects of *Aloe vera*

at a crayfish neuromuscular junction. **Phytother Res** 1999; 13(7): 580–583.

AV212 Akev, N. and A. Can. Separation and some properties of *Aloe vera* L. leaf pulp lectins. **Phytother Res** 1999; 13(6): 489–493.

AV213 Kim, H. S., S. Kacew and B. M. Lee. In vitro chemopreventive effects of plant polysaccharides (*Aloe barbadensis* Miller, *Lentinus edodesm*, *Ganoderma lucidum*, and *Coriolus versicolor*). **Carcinogenesis** 1999; 20(8): 1637–1640.

AV214 Yagi, A., J. Nakamori, T. Yamada, H. Iwase, T. Tanaka, Y. Kaneo, J. Qiu and S. Orndorff. In vivo metabolism of aloemannan. **Planta Med** 1999; 65(5): 417–420.

AV215 Lee, C. K., S. S. Han, Y. K. Shin, M. H. Chung, Y. I. Park, S. K. Lee and Y. S. Kim. Prevention of ultraviolet radiation-induced suppression of contact hypersensitivity by *Aloe vera* gel components. **Int J Immunopharmacol** 1999; 21(5): 303–310.

AV216 Izzo, A. A., L. Sautebin, F. Borrelli, R. Longo and F. Capasso. The role of nitric oxide in aloe-induced diarrhoea in the rat. **Eur J Pharmacol** 1999; 368(1): 43–48.

AV217 Strickland, F. M., A. Darvill, P. Albersheim, S. Eberhard, M. Pauly and R. P. Pelley. Inhibition of UV-induced immune suppression and interleukin-10 production by plant oligosaccharides and polysaccharides. **Photochem Photobiol** 1999; 69(2): 141–147.

5 | Annona muricata
L.

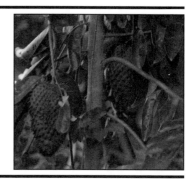

Common Names

Anyigli	Togo	Quanabana	Nicaragua
Apele	Togo	Saput	Nicaragua
Apple leaf	West Indies	Sarifa	Nicaragua
Beleda	Borneo	Seremaia	Nicaragua
Corosol	West Indies	Sorsaca	Curacao
Corossol	Dominica	Soursop leaf	West Indies
Corossol	Rodrigues Islands	Soursop tree	USA
Custard apple	Rodrigues Islands	Soursop	Barbados
Dian	Borneo	Soursop	Dominica
Guanabana	Barbados	Soursop	Dominican Republic
Guanabana	Cuba	Soursop	Guam
Guanabana	Dominican Republic	Soursop	Guyana
Guanabana	Panama	Soursop	Jamaica
Guanabana	Puerto Rico	Soursop	Jamaica
Katara ara tara	Cook Islands	Soursop	Nicaragua
Korosol	Haiti	Soursop	Puerto Rico
Kowosol	West Indies	Soursop	Virgin Islands
Laguana	Guam	Soursop	West Indies
Pumo	Nicaragua	Sowasap	Nicaragua
Puntar waithia	Nicaragua	Ualapana	Dominica

BOTANICAL DESCRIPTION

This small tree of the ANNONACEAE family is 5 to 7 meters in height. The leaves are oblong-obovate to oblong, 2 to 15 cm long, pointed at both ends, smooth, shiny, usually with petioles 5 cm long. Flowers are large and solitary, yellowish or greenish-yellow in color. Three outer petals are broadly ovate with heart-shaped base, inner 3 also large, elliptical and rounded. The fruit ovoid, 18 cm long or more, is covered with scattered spine-like structures. The pulp is soft white, and rather fibrous and fleshy, with an agreeable sour flavor.

ORIGIN AND DISTRIBUTION

Native of tropical America, it is now commonly cultivated worldwide.

From: *Medicinal Plants of the World, vol. 1: Chemical Constituents, Traditional and Modern Medicinal Uses, 2nd ed.*
By: Ivan A. Ross © Humana Press Inc., Totowa, NJ

TRADITIONAL MEDICINAL USES

Barbados. Hot water extract of dried leaves is taken orally as a sedative[AM001].

Brazil. Hot water extract of fresh leaves is taken orally as an analgesic[AM038].

Cook Islands. Decoction of dried leaves is used externally to treat rashes, skin diseases and skin infections. Patient is bathed in the cool green solution obtained by boiling the leaves in water. The decoction is taken orally to treat indigestion. Crushed leaves produce a scent that is inhaled for dizziness and fainting spells[AM034].

Curacao. Hot water extract of leaves is taken orally for gall bladder trouble. The extract is taken orally with *Citrus aurantium* every morning to relieve nervousness. The extract is also taken orally for easy childbirth[AM012].

Dominica. Fruit, when eaten by women, is believed to induce lactation. Women in labor take hot water extract of leaves as a tea[AM060].

Guam. Hot water extract of leaves is used as a tea for asthma sufferers[AM002].

Guatemala. Hot water extract of dried leaves is used in a poultice for ringworm[AM042].

Haiti. Decoction of dried leaves is taken orally for grippe, coughs, and asthenia. Fresh fruit juice is taken orally for asthenia[AM056].

India. Hot water extract of dried leaves is taken orally as an antiphlogistic[AM013].

Jamaica. Hot water extract of dried parts is used as bush tea[AM063]. Infusion of hot water extract of leaves is used as an antispasmodic; beverage is prepared as a lactagogue. The heart of the fruit is given to children orally, as a remedy for worms. Fruit is taken on an empty stomach as a cure for intermittent fevers, and as a diuretic[AM061].

Mexico. Decoction of dried bark is taken orally to treat diarrhea[AM033]. Fruit is used as a food[AM057].

Nigeria. Fresh fruit juice is taken orally as an antipyretic; applied externally it is an astringent[AM053]. Hot water extract of dried stem is taken orally to treat arthritis[AM052].

Panama. Decoction of the plant is used as an anthelmintic. Piscicidal activity is reported. Hot water extract of the bark is taken orally to treat diarrhea. Pulp is taken orally to treat stomach ulcers[AM046].

Togo. Decoction of dried leaves is taken orally for malaria[AM040].

Trinidad. Hot water extract of dried leaves is taken orally to lower high blood pressure and as a galactagogue[AM001].

Virgin Islands. Water extract of leaves is used externally as a cooling agent; taken orally, excess of 3 leaves will make one drowsy[AM059].

West Indies. Decoction of hot water extract of leaves is taken orally to ease delivery. Tea is used for hypertension; tea with castor oil for worms; tea with *Stachytarpheta jamaicensis* and *Chenopodium ambrosioides* is used for worms and the extract is taken orally for diarrhea and as a lactagogue. Fruit is eaten or applied externally as a poultice on the breast to induce lactation[AM045].

CHEMICAL CONSTITUENTS
(ppm unless otherwise indicated)

Acetaldehyde: Fr[AM055]
Amylcaproate: Pl[AM015]
Amyloid: Pl[AM015]
Annomonicin: Sd 56.5[AM019]
Annomontacin: Sd 60.3[AM019]
Annomuricin-D-one, cis: Lf[AM066]
Annomuricin-D-one, trans: Lf[AM066]
Annomuricine A: Lf 4[AM026]
Annomuricine B: Lf 3.5[AM026]
Annomuricine C: Lf 4[AM027]
Annonacin A: Lf [AM028]
Annonacin, cis: Sd[AM065]
Annonacin, iso, 2-4 trans: Lf[AM028]
Annonacin, iso: Sd 27.7[AM030]
Annonacin: Pl[AM079]
Annonacin: Sd 1.0%[AM035], Lf [AM026]
Annonacin-10-one, cis: Sd[AM065]
Annonacin-10-one, iso, neo: Sd[AM024]
Annonacin-10-one, iso: Sd 11.3[AM030]
Annonacin-10-one, neo: Sd[AM024]
Annonacin-10-one: Sd 13.6[AM030]
Annonacinone: Sd 0.007–1.07%[AM018,AM035]

Annonain: Pl[AM011]
Annonaine: Fr, Lf[AM067]
Annopentocin A: Lf[AM066]
Annopentocin B: Lf[AM066]
Annopentocin C: Lf[AM066]
Anomuricine: Rt[AM048], Bk, Lf[AM049]
Anomurine: Rt[AM048], Bk, Lf[AM049]
Anoniine: Pl[AM011]
Anonol: Lf[AM005,AM062]
Arginine: Pu[AM010]
Arianacin: Sd[AM065]
Ascorbic acid: Fr 0.019–0.154%[AM007]
Asimilobine: Fr, Lf[AM067]
Atherospermine: St Bk[AM004]
Atherosperminine: Rt[AM048], Bk, Lf[AM049]
Beta carotene: Fr 0.6[AM003]
Beta sitosterol: Lf[AM005,AM062], Sd oil[AM047]
Caffeic acid: Pl[AM015]
Campesterol: Sd oil[AM047]
Caproic acid methyl ester: Fr[AM055]
Caprylic acid methyl ester: Fr[AM055]
Carbohydrate: Fr 8.9–14.9%[AM003]
Cellobiose: Pl[AM015]
Cholesterol: Pl[AM015]
Citric acid: Pl[AM015]
Citrulline: Pu[AM010]
Coclaurine, (+): Rt[AM048], Bk, Lf[AM049]
Cohibins C: Sd[AM075]
Cohibins D: Sd[AM075]
Corepoxylone: Sd 6.2[AM020]
Coreximine, (–): Bk, Lf[AM048]
Coreximine, (+): Rt[AM048]
Coronin: Rt[AM078]
Corossolin: Sd 0.0029–1.01%[AM018,AM035]
Corossolone: Sd 0.0004–1.02[AM023,AM035]
Deacetyl uvaricin: Sd[AM036]
Dextrose: Pl[AM015]
D-Sucrose: Fr[AM006]
Epomuricenin A: Sd 27.8[AM023]
Epomuricenin B: Sd 27.8[AM023]
Epoxy murin A: St Bk[AM021]
Epoxy murin B: St Bk[AM021]
Ethanol: Fr[AM055]
Fiber: Fr 0.6–6.5%[AM003]
Fixed oil: Sd 23.86%[AM009]
Folic acid: Pl[AM015]
Fructose: Pl[AM015]
Galactomannan: Pl[AM015]
Gamma amino butyric acid: Pu[AM010]
Gentisic acid: Lf [AM014]
Geranyl caproate: Pl[AM015]
Gigantetrocin A: Sd 18.1[AM022]

Gigantetrocin B: Sd 13.6[AM022]
Gigantetrocin: Sd 22.1[AM030]
Gigantetronenin: Lf [AM027]
Glucose: Lf[AM062]
Goniothalamicin, cis: Sd[AM065]
Goniothalamicin: Lf[AM026], Sd 5.9–166[AM030,AM019]
HCN: Pl[AM004]
Hex-trans-2-en-1-ol: Fr[AM055]
Howiicin A: Sd[AM025]
Howiicin B, 4-deoxy: Sd[AM025]
Howiicin B: Sd[AM025]
Howiicin F: Sd[AM036]
Howiicin G: Sd[AM036]
Iron: Fr 5–33[AM003]
Isocitric acid: Pl[AM015]
Javoricin: Sd[AM065]
Lignoceric acid: Lf[AM005,AM062]
Linoleic acid: Sd oil[AM009], Lf[AM062]
Longifolicin: Sd[AM077]
Malic acid: Pl[AM015]
Mericyl alcohol: Pl[AM015]
Methanol: Fr[AM055]
Methyl-hexanoate: Pl[AM015]
Montanacin: Sd 249[AM019]
Montecristin: Rt[AM080]
Muricanin, diepoxy: St Bk[AM021]
Muricapentocin: Lf[AM068]
Muricatacin: Sd[AM016]
Muricatalicin: Pl[AM079]
Muricatalin: Pl[AM079]
Muricatetrocin A: Sd[AM022], Lf[AM026]
Muricatetrocin B: Sd 6.8[AM022], Lf[AM026]
Muricatocin A: Lf 4.5[AM028]
Muricatocin B: Lf 4[AM028]
Muricatocin C: Lf[AM027]
Muricin A: Sd[AM077]
Muricin B: Sd[AM077]
Muricin C: Sd[AM077]
Muricin D: Sd[AM077]
Muricin E: Sd[AM077]
Muricin F: Sd[AM077]
Muricin G: Sd[AM077]
Muricine: Bk[AM008,AM011]
Muricinine: Bk[AM008,AM011]
Muricoreacin: Lf[AM071]
Murihexocin C: Lf[AM071]
Murihexol: Sd[AM081]
Murisolin: Sd 6–93[AM023,AM018]
Myricyl alcohol: Lf[AM062]
Myristic acid: Sd oil[AM009]
Nornuciferine: Fr, Lf[AM067]

Oleic acid: Sd oil[AM009], Lf[AM062]
Ornithine: Pu[AM010]
Palmitic acid: Sd oil[AM009]
Panatellin, cis: Rt[AM069]
Paraffin: Pl[AM015]
P-Coumaric acid: Pl[AM015]
Potassium chloride: Lf[AM005,AM062]
Procyanidin: Pl[AM015]
Resin: Pl[AM015]
Reticulatacin, cis: Rt[AM069]
Reticulatacin-10-one: Rt[AM069]
Reticuline, (+): Rt[AM048], Bk, Lf[AM049]
Reticuline: St Bk[AM004]
Rolliniastatin 1: Sd[AM035]
Rolliniastatin 2: Sd[AM035]
Scyllitol: Pl[AM015]
Solamin, cis: Rt[AM069]
Solamin: Rt[AM069], Sd 3.6–11.6[AM023,AM017],
    St Bk[AM021]
Stearic acid: Lf[AM005], Sd oil[AM009]
Stepharine: Pl[AM015]
Stigmasterol: Sd oil[AM047]
Tannin: Lf[AM005]
Uvariamicin I, cis: Rt[AM069]
Uvariamicin IV, cis: Rt[AM069]
Xylosyl cellulose: Pl[AM015]

PHARMACOLOGICAL ACTIVITIES AND CLINICAL TRIALS

Analgesic activity. Ethanol/water (1:1) extract of fresh leaves, administered intragastrically to mice at a dose of 1.0 gm/kg, was inactive vs writhing and tail flick tests[AM038].

Anti-amoebic activity. Ethanol (95%) extract of dried bark was active on *Entamoeba histolytica*, MIC 63.0 mcg/ml[AM033].

Antibacterial activity. Acetone extract of dried leaves, on agar plate, was active on *Escherichia coli, Pseudomonas aeruginosa, Salmonella B, Salmonella newport, Salmonella typhosa, Serratia marcescens, Shigella flexneri, Staphylococcus albus* and *Staphylococcus aureus*, and inactive on *Sarcina lutea*. The ethanol (95%) extract was inactive on *E. coli, P. aeruginosa, Salmonella B, S. newport, S. typhosa, S. lutea, S. marcescens, S. flexneri, S. flexneri 3A, S. albus* and *S. aureus*. The water extract was active on *E. coli, P. aeruginosa* and *S. flexneri*, and inac-

tive on *Salmonella B, S. newport, S. typhosa, Sarcina lutea, Serratia marcescens, S. flexneri, S. albus*, and *S. aureus*[AM029]. Ethanol (95%) extract of dried bark, at a concentration of 10.0 mcg/disk on agar plate, was active on *Escherichia coli* and *Micrococcus luteus*. At a concentration of 5.0 mcg/disk, the extract was active on *Bacillus subtilis*[AM033]. Acetone extract of dried stem, on agar plate, was active on *Escherichia coli, Salmonella B, Salmonella newport, Salmonella typhosa, Shigella flexneri* and *Shigella flexneri 3A* and inactive on *Pseudomonas aeruginosa, Sarcina lutea, Serratia marcescens, Staphylococcus albus*, and *Staphylococcus aureus*. Ethanol (95%) extract was inactive on *Pseudomonas aeruginosa, Salmonella B, Salmonella newport, Salmonella typhosa, Sarcina lutea, Serratia marcescens, Shigella flexneri, Shigella flexneri 3A, Staphylococcus albus*, and *Staphylococcus aureus*. Water extract was active on *Escherichia coli, Pseudomonas aeruginosa, Salmonella newport, Salmonella typhosa* and *Shigella flexneri*, and inactive on *Salmonella B, Sarcina lutea, Serratia marcescens, Shigella flexneri 3A, Staphylococcus albus* and *Staphylococcus aureus*[AM029]. Ethanol (95%) extract of dried root bark, at a concentration of 2–3 mcg/plate on agar plate, was active on *Bacillus subtilis* and *Staphylococcus albus*, and inactive on *Klebsiella pneumoniae* and *Pseudomonas aeruginosa*. Ethanol (95%) extract of dried seeds, at a concentration of 2–3 mcg/liter on agar plate, was active on *Bacillus subtilis* and *Staphylococcus albus*, and inactive on *Klebsiella pneumoniae* and *Pseudomonas aeruginosa*. Ethanol (95%) extract of dried stem bark, on agar plate at a concentration of 2–3 mg/plate, was active on *Bacillus subtilis* and *Staphylococcus albus*, and inactive on *Klebsiella pneumoniae* and *Pseudomonas aeruginosa*[AM031].

Anticonvulsant activity. Ethanol (95%) extract of fresh fruit, at variable dosages administered intraperitoneally to mice of both sexes, was inactive vs strychnine and metrazole-induced convulsions[AM053].

Anticrustacean activity. Ethanol (95%) extract of dried leaves was active on *Artemia salina* larvae, LC_{50} 0.17 mg/ml[AM026]. Hexane extract of dried seeds was active on *Artemia salina*, LD_{50} 30.0 ppm and LC_{50} 0.8 ppm[AM016]. Methanol extract was also active on adults, LD_{50} 5.0[AM023] and 40.0 mg/liter as active on larvae[AM043]. Methanol/water (1:1) extract produced strong activity, LD_{50} 0.8 ppm[AM022].

Antidepressant activity. The fruit has been shown to produce anti-depressive effects, possibly induced by annonaince, nornuciferine and asimilobine[AM067].

Antifungal activity. Acetone, ethanol (95%) and water extracts of dried leaves, at a concentration of 50.0% on agar plate, was inactive on *Neurospora crassa*[AM054]. Ethanol (95%) extract of bark, at a concentration of 5.0 mcg/disc on agar plate, was active on *Penicillum oxalicum* and on *Cladosporium cucumerinum* at a concentration of 7.0 mcg/disk[AM033]. Hot water extract of dried leaves, at a concentration of 1.0 ml in broth culture, was inactive on *Epidermophyton floccosum, Microsporum canis, Microsporum gypseum, Trichophyton mentagrophytes* vars. algodonosa and granulare, and *Trichophyton rubrum*[AM042]. Acetone, water and ethanol (95%) extracts of dried stem, at concentrations of 50% on agar plate, were inactive on *Neurospora crassa*[AM054]. Aqueous, alcoholic, and ketonic extracts of the leaf were active on *Neurospora crassa*[AM083].

Antihepatotoxic activity. Decoction of dried leaves, at a concentration of 1.0 mg/plate in cell culture, produced weak activity on hepatocytes when measured by leakage of LDH and ASAT. It reduced the leakage of ASAT[AM037].

Antileishmanial activity. Hexane, ethyl acetate, and methanol extracts of the pericarp was active on *Leishmania braziliensis* and *Leishmania panamensis promastigotes*. The ethyl acetate extract was more active

than the other extracts and even of Glucantime, used as a reference substance[AM074].

Antimalarial activity. Chloroform extract of wood, administered subcutaneously to chicken at a dose of 118.0 mg/kg, and water extract, administered orally at a dose of 3.675 gm/kg, were inactive on *Plasmodium gallinaceum*[AM001]. Ethanol (95%) extract of dried leaves produced weak activity on *Plasmodium falciparum* W-2, IC_{50} 20.0 mcg/ml, and inactive on *Plasmodium falciparum* D-6[AM032].

Antiparasitic activity. Methanol extract of dried seeds, in broth culture, was active on *Nippostrongylus brasiliense* LD_{50} 20.0 mg/liter, *Molinema dessetae*, LD_{50} 6.0 mg/liter, *Trichomonas vaginalis*, MIC 30.0 mg/liter, inactive on *Entamoeba histolytica*, MIC > 100 mg/liter[AM043]. Methanol extract of the seed was active on the infective larvae of *Molinema desetae*[AM082].

Antitumor activity. Methanol extract of the leaves showed some antiherpetic activity with acceptable therapeutic indexes[AM072].

Antiviral activity. Ethanol extract of the fruit inhibited the cytopathic effect of Herpes simplex virus –1 on vero cells as indicative of anti-Herpes simplex virus-1 potential, MIC 1 mg/ml[AM070].

Cardiac depressant activity. Water extract of bark was active on the heart of rabbits[AM008].

Cytotoxic activity. Ethanol (95%) extract of leaves, in cell culture, was active on CA-9KB, ED_{50} < 20.0 mcg/ml. Ethanol (95%) extract of stem, in cell culture, was active on CA-9KB, ED_{50} < 20.0 mcg/ml[AM064]. Annopentocin, isolated from leaves, was selectively cytotoxic to pancreatic carcinoma cells (PACA-2). Annopentocins B and C were selectively cytotoxic to lung carcinoma cells (A-549). The mixture of cis- and trans-annomuricin-D-ones was selectively cytotoxic to lung (A-549), colon (HT-29), and pancreatic (PACA-2) cell lines with potencies equal to or exceeding those of Adriamycin[AM066]. Compounds annomuricine and muricapentocin has showed significant cytotoxicities against six types of human tumors, with selectivities to the pancreatic carcinome (PACA-2) and colon adenocarcinoma (HT-29) cell lines[AM068]. Muricoreacin and murihexocin C showed significant cytotoxicities among six human tumor cell lines with selectivities to the prostate adenocarcinoma (PC-3) and pancreatic carcinoma (PACA-2) cell lines[AM071]. Muricins A-G, muricatetrocins A-B, Longifolicin, corossolin, and corossolone showed significantly selective in vitro cytotoxicities toward the human hepatoma cell lines Hep G(2) and 2,2,15[AM077].

Hypertensive activity. Ethanol (95%) and water extracts of leaves and stem, administered intravenously to dogs at doses of 0.1 ml/kg, were active[AM003].

Hypotensive activity. Hot water extract of dried leaves, at a dose of 1.0 ml/animal administered intravenously to rats, was active. Blood pressure was lowered by more than 30%[AM044].

Inotropic effect positive. Hot water extract of dried leaves, at a concentration of 320.0 microliters, was inactive on the guinea pig atria[AM044].

Insecticidal activity. Ethanol (95%) extract of leaves, at a concentration of 5.0%, produced weak activity on *Macrosiphoniella sanborni*. Ethanol (95%) extract of dried seeds, at a concentration of 5.0%, was inactive on *Macrosiphoniella sanborni*. Ethanol (95%) extract of root, at a concentration of 5.0%, produced weak activity on *Macrosiphoniella sanborni*. Ethanol (95%) extract of seeds, at a concentration of 5.0%, was active on *Callosobruchus chinensisi*[AM041] and strongly active on *Macrosiphoniella sanbornii*[AM058].

Larvicidal activity. Water extract of dried leaves and stem, at a concentration of 0.03 gm of fresh plant material per ml of water, was inactive on *Culex quinquefasciatus*[AM039].

Lipid peroxidation formation inhibition. Decoction of dried leaves, at a concentration of 1.0 mg/plate in cell culture, was inactive on hepatocytes. It was monitored by production of malonaldehyde[AM037].

Molluscicidal activity. Aqueous slurry (homogenate) of fresh entire plant (fruits, leaves and roots) was inactive on *Lymnaea columella* and *Lymnaea cubensis*, $LD_{100} > 1M$ ppm[AM050]. Leaf homogenate produced significant activity against *Biomphalaria glabrata* with LD_{50} values of 11.86 ppm for adult and 49.62 ppm for eggs[AM073]. Ethanol extract of the leaf was active on *Biomphalaria glabrata*, LD_{90} 8.75 ppm[AM076].

Radical scavenging effect. Decoction of dried leaves, at a concentration of 250.0 mg/liter, was inactive. Measured by decoloration of diphenylpicryl hydroxyl radical solution; 16% decoloration[AM037].

Smooth muscle relaxant activity. Ethanol (95%) and water extracts of leaves and stem, at concentrations of 3.3 ml/liter, were active on rabbit duodenum[AM003].

Spasmogenic activity. Ethanol (95%) and water extracts of leaves and stem, at a concentration of 0.033 ml/liter, were active on the guinea pig ileum[AM003].

Toxicity assessment (quantitative). Water extract of leaves and stem, administered intraperitoneally to mice, produced a minimum toxic dose of 1.0 ml/animal[AM003].

Uterine stimulant effect. Ethanol (95%) and water extracts of leaves and stem, at a concentration of 0.033 ml/liter, were active on the rat uterus[AM003].

Vasodilator activity. Ethanol (95%) extract of leaves and stem, at a concentration of 0.033 ml/liter, was active on the isolated hindquarter of rats[AM003].

REFERENCES

AM001   Spencer, C. F., F. R. Koniuszy, E. F. Rogers, et al. Survey of plants for antimalarial activity. **Lloydia** 1947; 10: 145–174.

AM002 Haddock, R. L. Some Medicinal Plants of Guam Including English and Guamanian Common Names. Report Regional Tech Mtg Med Plants, Papeete, Tahiti, Nov, 1973, South Pacific Commissioner, Noumea, New Claedonia 1974; 79.

AM003 Feng, P. C., L. J. Haynes, K. E. Magnus, J. R. Plimmer and H. S. A. Sherrat. Pharmacological screening of some West Indian medicinal plants. **J Pharm Pharmacol** 1962; 14: 556–561.

AM004 Santos, G. A., J. R. Librea, A. C. Santos. The alkaloids of *Annona muricata*. **Philippine J Sci** 1967; 96: 399.

AM005 Callan, T. and F. Tutin. Chemical examination of the leaves of *Annona muricata*. **Pharm J** 1914; 87: 743.

AM006 Cutolo, A. The composition of the fruit *Annona cherimolia*. **Staz Sper Agr ital** 1915; 48: 889.

AM007 Hermano, A. J. and G. Sepulveda Jr. The vitamin content of Philippine foods. II. Vitamin C in various fruits and vegetables. **Philippine J Sci** 1934; 53: 379.

AM008 Meyer, T. M. The alkaloids of *Annona muricata*. **Ing Ned Indie** 1941; 8(6): 64.

AM009 Asenjo, C. F. and J .A. Goyco. Puerto Rican fatty oils. II. The characteristics and composition of guanabana seed oil. **J Amer Chem Soc** 1943; 65: 208.

AM010 Ventura, M. M. and I. H. Lima. Ornithine cycle amino acids and other free amino acids in fruits of *Annona squamosa* and *A. muricata*. **Phyton (Buenos Aires)** 1961; 17: 39.

AM011 Willaman, J. J. and B. G. Schubert. Alkaloid bearing plants and their contained alkaloids. **ARS, USDA, Tech Bull 1234, Supt Documents, Govt Print Off, Washington DC** 1961.

AM012 Morton, J. F. A survey of medicinal plants of Curacao. **Econ Bot** 1968; 22: 87.

AM013 Watt, J. M. and M. G. Breyer-Brandwijk. The Medicinal and Poisonous Plants of Southern and Eastern Africa. 2nd Ed, E. S. Livingstone, Ltd., London, 1962.

AM014 Griffiths, L. A. On the distribution of gentisic acid in green plants. **J Exp Biol** 1959; 10: 437.

AM015 Ur-Rahman, A., H. M. Said and V. U. Ahmad. Pakistan Encyclopaedia Planta Medica, Vol. I. Hamdard Foundation Press, Karachi, Pakistan 1986; 373pp.

AM016 Reiser, M. J., J. F. Kozlowski, K. V. Wood and J. L. Mc Laughlin. Muricatacin: A simple biologically active acetogenin derivative from the seeds of *Annona muricata* (Annonaceae). **Tetrahedron Lett** 1991; 32(9): 1137–1140.

AM017 Myint, S. H., D. Cortes, A. Laurens, R. Hocquemiller, M. Lebceuf, A. Cave, J. Cotte and A. M. Quero. Solamin, a cytotoxic mono-tetrahydrofuranic gamma-lactone acetogenin from *Annona muricata* seeds. **Phytochemistry** 1991; 30 (10): 3335–3338.

AM018 Cortes, D., S. H. Myint, A. Laurens, R. Hocquemiller, M. Leboeuf and A. Cave. Corossolone and corossoline, two new monotetrahydrofuran gamma lactones. **Can J Chem** 1991; 69(1): 8–11.

AM019 Jossang, A., B. Dubaele, A. Cave, M. H. Bartoli and H. Beriel. Cytotoxic gamma lactone monotetrahydrofuran annomontacin: A new acetogen from *Annona muricata*. **J Nat Prod** 1991; 54(4): 967–971.

AM020 Gromek, D., B. Figadere, R. Hoc0quemiller and A. Cave. Corepoxylone, a possible precursor of mono-tetrahydrofuran gamma-lactone acetogenins: Biometric synthesis of corossolone. **Tetrahedron** 1993; 49 (24): 5247–5252.

AM021 Hisham, A., U. Sreekala, L. Pieters, T. De Bruyne, H. Vanden Heuvel and M. Claeys. **Tetrahedron** 1993; 49(31): 6913–6920.

AM022 Rieser, M. J., X. P. Fang, J. E. Anderson, L. R. Miesbauer, D. L. Smith and J. L. Mc Laughlin. Muricatetrocins A and B and gigantetrocin B: Three new citotoxic monotetrahydrofuran-ring acetogenins from *Annona muricata* I. **Helv Chim Acta** 1993; 76(7): 2433–2444.

AM023 Roblot, F., T. Laugel, M. Lebqueue, A. Cave and O. Laprevote. Two acetogenins from *Annona muricata* seeds. **Phytochemistry** 1993; 34(1): 281–285.

AM024 Yang, R. Z., S. J. Wu, R. S. Su and G. W. Qin. Annonaceous acetogenins from *Annona muricata*. **Yun-Nan Chih Wu Yen Chiu** 1994; 16(2): 187–190.

AM025 Yang, R. Z., S. J. Wu, R. S. Su, D. J. Fan and G. W. Qin. Annonaceous acetogenins from *Annona muricata*. **Chih Wu Hsueh Pao** 1994; 36(10); 805–808.

AM026 Wu, F. E., Z. M. Gu, L. Zeng, G. X. Zhao, Y. Zhang and J. L. Mc Laughlin. Two new cytotoxic monotetra-hydrofuran annonaceous acetogenins, annomuricins A and B, from the leaves of *Annona muricata*. **J Nat Prod** 1995; 58(6): 830–836.

AM027 Wu, F. E., L. Zeng, Z. M. Gu, G. X. Zhao, Y, Zhang, J. T. Schwedler, J. L. Mc Laughlin and S. Sastrodihardjo. New bioactive monotetrahydrofuran annonaceous acetogenins, anno-muricin C and muricatocin C, from the leaves of *Annona muricata*. **J Nat Prod** 1995; 58(6): 909–915.

AM028 Wu, F. E., L. Zeng, Z. M. Gu, G. X. Zhao, Y, Zhang, J. T. Schwedler, J. L. Mc Laughlin and S. Sastrodihardjo. Muricatocins A and B, two new bioactive monotetrahydrofuran anno-naceous acetogenins from the leaves of *Annona muricata*. **J Nat Prod** 1995; 58(6): 902–908.

AM029 Misas, C. A. J., N. M. R. Hernandez and A. M. L. Abraham. Contribution to the biological evaluation of Cuban plants. 1V. **Rev Cub Med Trop** 1979; 31(1): 29–35.

AM030 Rieser, M. J., X. P. Fang, J. K. Rupprecht, Y. H. Hui, D. L. Smith and J. L. Mc Laughlin. Bioactive single-ring acetogenins from seeds extracts of *Annona muricata*. **Planta Med** 1993; 59(1): 91–92.

AM031 Sundarrao, K., I. Burrows, M. Kuduk, Y. D. Yi, M. H. Chung, N. J. Suh, I. M. Chang. Preliminary screening of anti-bacterial and antitumor activities of Papua, New Guinean native medicinal plants. **Int J Pharmacog** 1993; 31(1): 3–6.

AM032 Antoun, M. D., L. Gerena and W. K. Milhous. Screening of the flora of Puerto Rico for potential antimalarial bioactives. **Int J Pharmacog** 1993; 31(4): 255–258.

AM033 Heinrich, M., M. Kuhnt, C. W. Wright, H. Rimpler, J. D. Phillipson, A. Schandelmaier and D. C. Warhurst. Parasitological and microbiological evaluation of Mixe Indian medicinal plants (Mexico). **J Ethnopharmacol** 1992; 36(1): 81–85.

AM034 Holdsworth, D. K. Traditional medici-nal plants of Rarotonga, Cook Islands, Part 1. **Int J Crude Drug Res** 1990; 28(3): 209–218.

AM035 Gromek, D., R. Hocquemiller and A. Cave. Qualitative and quantitative evaluation of annonaceous aceto-genins by high performance liquid chromatography. **Phytochem Anal** 1994: 5(3): 133–140.

AM036 Yang, R. Z. and S. J. Wu. Annonaceous acetogenins from *Annona muricata* (lll). **Yunnan Zhiwu Yanjiu** 1994; 16(3): 309–310.

AM037 Joyeux, M., F. Mortier and J. Fleurentin. Screening of antiradical, antilipoperoxidant and hepatoprotec-tive effects of nine plant extracts used in Caribbean folk medicine. **Phytother Res** 1995; 9(3): 228–230.

AM038 Di Stasi, L. C., M. Costa, L. J. Mendacolli, M. Kirizawa, C. Gomes and G. Trolin. Screening in mice of some medicinal plants used for analge-sic purposes in the state of Sao Paulo. **J Ethnopharmacol** 1988; 24 (2/3): 205–211.

AM039 Evans, D. A. and R. K. Raj. Extracts of Indian plants as mosquito larvicides. **Indian J Med Res** 1988; 88(1): 38–41.

AM040 Greassor, M., A. Y. Kedjagni, K. Koumaglo, C. DeSouza, K. Agbo, K. Aklikokou and K. A. Amegbo. In vitro antimalarial activity of six medicinal plants. **Phytother Res** 1990; 4(3): 115–117.

AM041 Ohsawa, K., S. Kato, H. Honda and I. Yamamoto. Pesticidal substances in tropical plants. Insecticidal substances from annonaceae seeds. **Nogaku Shuho (Tokyo Nagyo Daigaku)** 1990; 34(4): 253–258.

AM042 Caceres, A., B. R. Lopez, M. A. Giron and H. Logemann. Plants used in Gua-temala for the treatment of dermatophytic infections. I. Screening for anti-mycotic activity of 44 plant extracts. **J Ethnopharmacol** 1991; 31(3): 263–276.

AM043 Bories, C., P. Loiseau, S. H. Myint, R. Hocquemiller, P. Gayral, A. Cave and A. Laurens. Antiparasitic activity of *Annona muricata* and *Annona cherimoiai* seeds. **Planta Med** 1991; 57(5): 434–436.

AM044 Carbajal, D., A. Casaco, L. Arruzazabala, R. Gonzalez and V. Fuentes. Pharmacological screening of plant decoctions commonly used in Cuban folk medicine. **J Ethnopharmacol** 1991; 33(1/2): 21–24.

AM045 Ayensu, E. S. Medicinal plants of the West Indies. **Unpublished Manuscript** 1978; 110 pp.

AM046 Gupta, M. P., T. D. Arias, M. Correa and S. S. Lamba. Ethnopharmacognostic observations on Panamanian medicinal plants. Part 1. **Q J Crude Drug Res** 1979; 17(3/4): 115–130.

AM047 Izzo, R. Composition of *Annona muricata* seed oil. **Riv Soc Ital Sci Aliment** 1979; 8: 241–244.

AM048 Leboeuf, M., C. Leguet, A. Cave, J. F. Desconclois and P. Forgascs. Anomurine and anomuricine, two new isoquinoline alkaloids from *Annona muricata*. (Abstract). **Planta Med** 1980; 39: 204–205.

AM049 Leboeul, M., C. Legueut, A. Cave, J. F. Desconclois, P. Forgacs and H. Jacquemin. Alkaloids of annonaceae. XXXIX. Alkaloids of *Annona muricata*. **Planta Med** 1981; 42: 37–44.

AM050 Medina, F. R. and R. Woodbury. Terrestrial plants molluscicidal to Lymnaeid hosts of *Fasciliasis hepatica* in Puerto Rico. **J Agr Univ Puerto Rico** 1979; 63: 366–376.

AM051 Morton, J. F. Caribbean and Latin American folk medicine and its influence in the United States. **Q J Crude Drug Res** 1980; 18(2): 57–75.

AM052 Iwu, M. M. and B. N. Anyanwu. Phytotherapeutic profile of Nigerian herbs. 1. Anti-inflammatory and anti-arthritic agents. **J Ethnopharmacol** 1982; 6(3): 263–274.

AM053 Adesina, S. K. Studies on some plants used as anticonvulsants in Amerindian and African traditional medicine. **Fitoterapia** 1982; 53: 147–162.

AM054 Lopez Abraham, A. N., N. M. Rojas Hernandez and C. A. Jimenez Misas. Potential antineoplastic activity of Cuban plants. IV. **Rev Cubana Farm** 1981; 15(1): 71–77.

AM055 Escarraman Mata, S., M. Del Refugio, F. Juarez and A. Gonzalez Perez. Determination of seven flavor components of custard apple by gas chromatography. **Tecnol Aliment (Mexico City)** 1982; 17(6): 3,4,6,7.

AM056 Weniger, B., M. Rouzier, R. Daguilh, D. Henrys, J. H. Henrys and R. Anthon. Popular medicine of the Central Plateau of Haiti. 2. Ethnopharmacological inventory. **J Ethnopharmacol** 1986; 17(1): 13–30.

AM057 Vietmeyer, N. D. Lesser-known plants of potential use in agriculture and forestry. **Science** 1986; 232(4756): 1379–1384.

AM058 Tattersfield, F. and C. Potter. The insecticidal properties of certain species of annona and an Indian strain of *Mundulea sericea* (Suppl). **Ann Appl Biol** 1940; 27: 262–273.

AM059 Oakes, A. J. and M. P. Morris. The West Indian weedwoman of the United States Virgin Islands. **Bull Hist Med** 1958; 32: 164.

AM060 Hodge, W. H. and D. Taylor. The ethnobotany of the island Caribes of Dominica. **WEBBIA** 1956; 12: 513–644.

AM061 Asprey, G. F. and P. Thornton. Medicinal plants of Jamaica. III. **West Indian Med** 1955; J4: 69–82.

AM062 Callan, T. and F. Tutin. Chemical examination of the leaves of *Annona muricata*. **Pharm J** 1912; 87: 743–745.

AM063 Jelliffe, D. B., G. Bras and K. L. Stuart. The clinical picture of veno-occlusive disease of the liver in Jamaican children. **Ann Trop Med Parasitol** 1954; 48: 386–396.

AM064 ANON. Unpublished data, National Cancer Institute. **National Cancer Inst. Central Files** 1976.

AM065 Rieser, M. J., M. Z. Gu, X. P. Fang, L. Zeng, K. V. Wood and J. L. McLaughlin. Five novel mono-tetrahydrofuran ring acetogenins from the seeds of *Annona muricata*. **J Nat Prod** 1996; 59(2): 100–108.

AM066 Zeng, L., F. E. Wu, N. H. Oberlies, J. H. McLaughlin and S. Sastrodihadjo. Five new monotetrahydrofuran ring acetogenins from the leaves of *Annona muricata*. **J Nat Prod** 1996; 59(11): 1035–1042.

AM067 Hasrat, J. A., T. De Bruyne, J. P. De Backer, G. Vauquelin and A. J. Vlietinck. Isoquinoline derivatives isolated from the fruit of *Annona muricata* as 5-Htergic 5-HT1A receptor agonist in rats: unexploited antidepressive (lead) products. **J Pharm Pharmacol** 1997; 49(11): 1145–1149.

AM068 Kim, G. S., L. Zeng, F. Alali, L. L. Rogers, F. E. Wu, J. L. McLaughlin and S. Sastrodihardjo. Two new mono-tetrahydrofuran ring acetogenins, annomuricin E and muricapentocin, from the leaves of *Annona muricata*. **J Nat Prod** 1998; 61(4): 432–436.

AM069 Gleye, C., P. Duret, A. Laurens, R. Hocquemiller and A. Cave. Cis monotetrahydrofuran acetogenins from the roots of *Annona muricata* I. **J Nat Prod** 1998; 61(5): 576–579.

AM070 Padma, P., N. P. Pramod, S. P. Thyagarajan and R. L. Khosa. Effect of the extract of *Annona muricata* and *Petunia nyctaginiflora* on Herpes simplex virus. **J Ethnopharmacol** 1998; 61(1): 81–83.

AM071 Kim, G. S., L. Zeng, F. Alali, L. L. Rogers, F. E. Wu, S. Sastrodihardjo and J. L. McLaughlin. Muricoreacin and murihexocin C, monotetrahydrofuran acetogenins, from the leaves of *Annona muricata*. **Phytochemistry** 1998; 49(2): 565–571.

AM072 Betancur-Galvis, L., J. Saez, H. Granados, A. Salazar and J. Ossa. Antitumor and antiviral activity of Colombian medicinal plant extracts. **Mem Inst Oswaldo Cruz** 1999; 94(4): 531–535.

AM073 Dos Santos, A. F. and A. E. Sant' Ana. The molluscicidal activity of plants used in Brazilian fold medicine. **Phytomedicine** 2000; 6(6): 431–438.

AM074 Jarmaillo, M. C., G. J. Arango, M. C. Gonzlalez, S. M. Robeldo and I. D. Velez. Cytotoxicity and antileishmanial activity of *Annona muricata* pericarp. **Fitoterapia** 2000; 71(2): 183–186.

AM075 Gleye, C., S. Raynaud, C. Fourneau, A. Laurens, O, Laprevote, L. Serani, A. Fournet and R. Hocquemiller. Cohibins C and D, two important metabolites in the biogenesis of acetogenins from *Annona muricata* and *Anona nutans*. **J Nat Prod** 2000; 63(9): 1192–1196.

AM076 Dos Santos, A. F. and A. E. Sant'Ana. Molluscicidal properties of some species of *Annona*. **Phytomedicine** 2001; 8(2): 115–120.

AM077 Chang, F. R. and Y. C. Wu. Novel cytotoxic annonaceous acetogenins from *Annona muricata*. **J Nat Prod** 2001; 64(7): 925–931.

AM078 Gleye, C., B. Akendengue, A. Laurens and R. Hocquemiller. Coronin from roots of *Annona muricata*, a putative intermediate in acetogenin biosynthesis (I). **Planta Med** 2001; 67(6): 570–572.

AM079 Yu, J. G., H. Q. Gui, X. Z. Luo, L. Sun, P. Zhu and Z. L. Yu. Studies on the chemical constituents of *Annona muricata*. **Yao Xue Bao** 1997; 32(6): 431–437.

AM080 Gleye, C., A. Lauren, R. Hocquemiller, A. Cave, O. Laprevote and L. Serani. Isolation of monte-cristin, a key metabolite in biogenesis of acetogenins from *Annona muricata* and its structure elucidation by using tandem Mass Spectrometry. **J Org Chem** 1997; 62(3): 510–513.

AM081 Yu, J. G., H. Q. Gui, X. Z. Luo and L. Sun. Murihexol, a linear acetogenin from *Annona muricata*. **Phytochemistry** 1998; 49(6): 1689–1692.

AM082 Bories, C., P. Loiseau, D. Cortes, S. H. Myint, R. Hocquemiller, P. Gayral, A. Cave and A. Laurens. Antiparasitic activity of *Annona muricata* and *Annona cherimolia* seeds. **Planta Med** 1991; 57(5): 434–436.

AM083 Lopez Abraham, A. M., N. M. Rojas Hernandez and C. A. Jimenez Misas. Plant extracts with cytostatic properties growing in Cuba. I. **Rev Cubana Med Trop** 1979; 31(2): 97–104.

6 | Carica papaya
L.

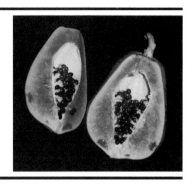

Common Names

Aanabahe-hindi	India	Jhad-chibhadi	India
Ababau	Nicaragua	Karumusa	India
Amita	India	Karutha kapalam	India
Badie	Ivory Coast	Kath	India
Bake	Ivory Coast	Kunam-paran popo	Admiralty Islands
Bedon-al-babo	Guinea-Bissau	Lesi	Admiralty Islands
Bepaia	Guinea-Bissau	Lesi tangata	Tonga
Boppai	India	Lo hong phle	Vietnam
Boppaya	India	Mak hung	Vietnam
Buah betek	Malaysia	Malako	Thailand
Buah ketela	Malaysia	Mama	Angola
Buah papaya	Malaysia	Mamioko	Bougainville
Budibaga	Senegal	Mamoeiro	Paraguay
Bumpapa	Senegal	Mande	Ghana
Bupapay	Senegal	Mande	Senegal
Chibda	India	Manjan	Borneo
Chichihualxochitl	Mexico	Melon tree	India
Chirbhita	India	Melon tree	Nigeria
Common papaw	India	Mewa	Nepal
Du du	Vietnam	Mikana	Hawaii
Ebabayo	Tanzania	Mokka	Japan
Ehi	Tanzania	Mupapawe	Venda
Eranda-kakadi	India	Nita	Cook Islands
Esi	India	O rabana	Senegal
Fafy	Oman	Ojo-mgbimgbi	Nigeria
Fakai	Sierra Leone	Olesi	Nigeria
Fakai laa	Sierra Leone	Omita	India
Fruta bomba	Cuba	Ommal	India
Fruto bomba	Cuba	Pace	Guinea-Bissau
Goppe	India	Papae	Guinea-Bissau
Gwanda	Nigeria	Papai	India
I'ita	Nigeria	Papai	West Indies
Ibepe	Nigeria	Papaia	Guinea-Bissau
Ipi	Papua-New Guinea	Papapa	Fiji

From: *Medicinal Plants of the World, vol. 1: Chemical Constituents, Traditional and Modern Medicinal Uses, 2nd ed.*
By: Ivan A. Ross © Humana Press Inc., Totowa, NJ

Papaw	Guyana	Papeya	India
Papaw	Jamaica	Papia	Senegal
Papaw	Malaysia	Papita	Fiji
Papaw	USA	Papita	India
Papaw	West Indies	Papitha	India
Papay	Haiti	Papoia	Guinea-Bissau
Papay	India	Parimi	India
Papaya	India	Parindakaya	India
Papaya	Brazil	Paupau	India
Papaya	Fiji	Paw paw	Nigeria
Papaya	Gold Coast	Pawpaw	East Africa
Papaya	Guatemala	Pawpaw	England
Papaya	India	Pawpaw	Fiji
Papaya	Indonesia	Pawpaw	India
Papaya	Japan	Pawpaw	Malaysia
Papaya	Malaysia	Pawpaw	Oman
Papaya	Nepal	Pawpaw	Papua-New Guinea
Papaya	Papua-New Guinea	Pawpaw	Philippines
Papaya	Peru	Poi poi	Kenya
Papaya	Tanzania	Popai	India
Papaya	USA	Poyam	Admiralty Islands
Papaya tree	India	Puppai	India
Papaye	Guadeloupe	Tree melon	India
Papaye	Rodrigues Islands	Tuunuk	Nicaragua
Papayer	Ivory Coast	Twas	Nicaragua
Papayer	Vietnam	Ulmak	Nicaragua
Papayer	Zaire	Vatakumba	India
Papayi	Guadeloupe	Vatre	Ivory Coast
Papayo	Mexico	Vi nita	Ivory Coast
Papayu	India	Wayoye	Papua
Papeeta	Pakistan	Weleti	Papua
Papeta	India	Wi	Papua

BOTANICAL DESCRIPTION

This is a perennial, herbaceous plant of the CARICACEAE family, with copious milky latex reaching to as high as 10 meters. The stem is about 25 cm thick, simple or branched above the middle and roughened with leaf scars. Leaves, clustered around the apex of the stem and branches, have nearly cylindrical stalks, 25 to 100 cm long; the leaf blade has 7 to 11 main lobes and some secondary irregular pointed lobes and prominent veins; leaf surface is yellow-green to dark-green above and paler beneath. Usually male and female flowers are borne on separate plants, but hermaphrodite flowers often occur, and a male plant may convert to a female after being beheaded. Flowers emerge singly or in clusters from the main stem among the lower leaves, the female short-stalked, the male with drooping peduncles 25 to 100 cm long. Corolla is 1.25 to 2.5 cm long, with 5 oblong recurved white petals. Fruit is extremely variable in form and size; it may be nearly round, pear-shaped, oval, or oblong; that of the wild plants may be as small as an egg, whereas in cultivation, the fruit ranges from 10 cm to 60 cm in length and up to 20 cm thick. Its skin is smooth, relatively thin, and deep yellow to orange when the fruit is ripe. Flesh is succulent, yellow to orange or salmon-red, sweet and more or less musky.

The central cavity is lined with a dryish pulpy membrane to which adhere numerous black rough peppery seeds, each with a glistening transparent gelatinous coating.

ORIGIN AND DISTRIBUTION

It is believed that papaya originated in Southern Mexico and Central America, though it was cultivated as far south as Lima, Peru, in pre-Spanish times. Today, papaya is grown in all tropical and subtropical countries as a commercial crop.

TRADITIONAL MEDICINAL USES

Admiralty Islands. Fresh leaf sap is applied to skin with Siponia eruptions twice daily. The treatment is repeated in 5 days, if needed. Fresh soft bark is scraped onto a leaf and heated over a fire. The soft material is rubbed onto a new cut to promote healing[CP124].

Bougainville. Fresh leaves are squeezed to a pulp and plastered onto cuts or wounds to promote healing[CP115].

Brazil. Latex is taken orally as an anthelmintic[CP039]. Unripe fruit is applied to the skin for ringworm and dermatitis. Ripe fruit is eaten for constipation[CP101].

Cook Islands. Fresh seeds are eaten whole as a treatment for intestinal worms[CP137]. Fresh unripe fruit is used externally to treat cuts and sores, skin infections[CP072]. For boils and carbuncles, the unripe fruit is grated, mixed with coconut oil, and rubbed in affected part[CP137].

Cuba. Unripe fruit is eaten for hypertension[CP033].

East Africa. Hot water extract of leaves is taken orally as an anthelmintic[CP106]. Hot water extract of dried roots is taken orally for syphilis and as an anthelmintic[CP037]. Hot water extract of latex is taken orally as an anthelmintic. Hot water extract of roots is taken orally as an anthelmintic. Hot water extract of seeds is taken orally as an anthelmintic[CP106]. Unripe fruit juice is taken orally as an abortifacient[CP010].

Ecuador. Hot water extract of fresh fruit is taken orally as a contraceptive[CP151].

Fiji. Fresh sap is used externally for ringworm. Ground dried leaf is taken with salt for coughs. Fresh ripe fruit pulp is taken orally for indigestion, as an appetizer, and for diarrhea and dysentery[CP141].

Ghana. Hot water extract of seeds is taken orally as an abortifacient. Latex is used as an abortifacient[CP106]. Root blended with salt and triturated with water is used as a douche to induce abortion[CP003]. Hot water extract of root is taken orally as an abortifacient[CP106].

Gold Coast. Hot water extract of root is taken orally as an abortifacient[CP001].

Guadeloupe. Seeds are eaten as a vermifuge[CP127].

Guinea-Bissau. Decoction of hot water extract is taken orally as an abortive. Unripe fruits are crushed and part of the pulp is used to massage the breasts as an emmenagogue; the remaining part is mixed with water and boiled with vapors, being placed on the woman's breasts. After cooling, the decoction is administered orally in divided doses throughout the day[CP002].

Guinea. Decoction of hot water extract of leaves is taken orally to provoke abortion. Decoction of hot water extract of unripe fruit is taken orally to provoke milk secretion. Latex of unripe fruits is massaged over the breasts to provoke milk secretion. Seeds are eaten to induce abortion[CP003].

Haiti. Fresh fruit juice is taken orally for hypertension. Fresh latex is taken orally for toothache. Water extract of dried root is taken orally for urethritis[CP143].

Hawaii. Unripe fruit is claimed to be beneficial in producing lactation. The fruit is washed, cut into cubes, and boiled as for soup. The broth is taken by new mothers. Within a few days, stinging sensations in the breasts begin, and the breasts then fill up with milk[CP159]. Water extract of unripe fruit is taken orally for asthma[CP071].

India. A mixture of *Carica papaya* root and *Ferula marthex* resin is used to induce abortion. The root of *Carica papaya* with girth able to penetrate the vagina and about 8- to 10-in long is obtained. At one end, an incision a half an inch deep in the shape of a cross is made in such a way that the root does not break into separate portions. In these cuts, the *Ferula marthex* resin is put, better if somewhat crushed and refined. The vagina is penetrated with the portion containing the *Ferula marthex* to go deep inside and most probably to touch the os uteri. Penetration and maintaining the root in this way daily for 7–8 hours in the vagina is said to result in abortion, even in a fetus 3–4 months old[CP122]. Decoction of inner stem-bark is taken orally twice daily for dental caries[CP096]. Dried seed eaten by pregnant women will produce abortion and is a powerful emmenagogue[CP037]. Powdered seed is taken orally as an anthelmintic[CP090]. Hot water extract of seeds is taken orally as an anti-inflammatory and analgesic[CP152]. Fresh fruit is eaten as an abortifacient. Tender fruits are used in different forms. To expel intestinal worms, ripe fruits are eaten[CP129]. Fruit is taken orally as an emmenagogue[CP008] and abortifacient[CP016]. Pregnant women are strictly prohibited from eating papaya during pregnancy for fear of inducing labor. Some tribal people believe that papaya has a powerful antifertility property[CP104]. Hot water extract of flowers is taken orally as a heart tonic. Hot water extract of leaves is taken orally as a febrifuge and heart tonic[CP106]. Hot water extract of ripe-dried fruit is taken orally as an emmenagogue[CP147]. Hot water extract of ripe fresh fruit is said to be astringent to the bowels, an aphrodisiac, and is used for biliousness[CP152]. Unripe fresh fruit is taken orally for abortion. Ripe fruits are taken orally, as a diuretic and treatment of flatulence[CP063]. Latex is taken orally for indigestion, abdominal colic, hemorrhoids, worms, and for liver and spleen enlargement[CP152]. To treat worms, leaf extract and latex of raw fruit are taken orally[CP059]. Hot water extract of root is taken orally, as an abortifacient and for the treatment of yaws[CP106]. Latex is applied to the os uteri for inducing abortion[CP001]. Latex is taken orally as an anthelmintic[CP109]. Plant juice taken orally is said to be a powerful anthelmintic, and when applied to the os uteri it produces abortion[CP154]. Seeds are taken orally as a powerful emmenagogue, an abortifacient when mixed with *Zingiber officinale* and honey[CP001]. Unripe fruit is eaten for gastric disorders. Young fruit is eaten together with the young seeds to cause abortion[CP125]. Unripe fruit juice, taken orally is claimed to a powerful galactagogue, emmenagogue, and abortifacient. Application to the os uteri is believed to interrupt pregnancy[CP100]. Young fresh leaves are made into a fine paste and taken orally for a week at doses of 5–6 gm, for severe jaundice[CP099].

Indonesia. Seed and flesh of fruit are eaten to promote abortion[CP056].

Ivory Coast. Decoction of hot water extract of leaves is taken orally in case of difficult delivery; if the decoction is drunk, it can cause abortion; externally it is used as a galactagogue[CP019]. Fresh leaves are used externally as a hemostatic[CP150].

Jamaica. Fresh latex is used externally in the treatment of ringworm[CP162].

Kenya. Decoction of dried root is taken orally for venereal diseases. *Carica papaya* and *Carissa edulis* and other species are combined[CP095].

Malawi. Water extract of dried root is taken orally to cure yellow fever[CP093].

Malaysia. Fresh unripe fruit juice is taken orally as an emmenagogue. Hot water extract of flowers is taken orally as an emmenagogue[CP106]. Hot water extract of roots is taken orally as an abortifacient[CP106]. Latex is applied to the os uteri to induce abortion[CP001]. The latex is taken orally as an abortifacient[CP007,CP015]. Seeds are taken orally to induce abortion in early pregnancy[CP007]. Hot water extract of seeds is taken orally as an abortifacient and emmenagogue[CP106]. Unripe fruit is considered dangerous to be eaten by women during pregnancy[CP015].

Mexico. Fresh latex is taken orally to treat constipation. The exudation is taken as a purgative[CP065]. Fresh unripe fruit juice is taken orally as an emmenagogue[CP106]. Hot water extract of latex is applied externally to skin rash. Orally, it is taken for ulcers and as a digestive[CP051]. Hot water extract of seeds is taken orally as an emmenagogue[CP106]. Water[CP001] and hot water[CP106] extracts of flowers are taken orally as emmenagogue.

Mozambique. Hot water extract of leaves is taken orally as a febrifuge[CP019].

Myanmar. Unripe fruit is eaten as an abortifacient[CP009].

Nigeria. Dried leaves cooked with *Musa sapientum* in equal proportions is taken orally or as a bath to treat body infections. The leaf extract is taken with salt, orally, to treat yellow fever, and the infusion prepared from leaves is taken orally to treat stomachache. Fresh fruit is eaten as a treatment for beri-beri[CP059]. Hot water extract of fresh leaves is taken orally as a purgative, antipyretic, analgesic, and anthelmintic. Hot water extract of fresh root is taken orally as an anthelmintic, antipyretic, and analgesic. Fruit is eaten for nausea, as a carminative, for yaws, as an antipyretic, purgative, and for dysentery[CP120].

Panama. Fruit juice is taken orally for diarrhea and dysentery. Toasted and powdered seeds mixed with honey are taken orally, 1 teaspoon, followed by a laxative (castor oil) as an anthelmintic[CP105].

Papua-New Guinea. Dried seeds of a ripe fruit are chewed for cough and stomachache[CP069]. Fresh sap from any part of the plant mixed with lime is rubbed into *Tinea imbricaton* and other skin eruptions[CP068,CP135].

Paraguay. Dried seeds are eaten as a vermifuge[CP070].

Peru. Hot water extract of dried fruit is taken orally for gall bladder and liver conditions and for disorders of fat digestion and dyspepsia. Hot water extract of dried leaves is taken orally for gallbladder and liver conditions, and for disorders of fat digestion and dyspepsia[CP149].

Senegal. Decoction of dried fruit and citrus species is taken orally for venereal diseases[CP094]. Decoction of young leaves is taken orally as an abortifacient, for blennorrhagia, and for yellow fever. Hot water extract of dried root is taken orally for gonorrhea and venereal disease, yellow fever, toothache, and dysentery. Hot water extract of dried seeds is taken orally for fungal infections of the skin. Hot water extract of fresh latex is used externally for sores. Hot water extract of unripe fruit is taken orally for coughs, and externally for sores[CP089]. Seeds are taken orally as an abortifacient and emmenagogue[CP011].

Sierra Leone. Old yellowish leaves are rubbed in a calabash, with water added the liquid is taken orally to stimulate labor[CP134]. Decoction of dried leaves is taken orally for yellow fever[CP138].

Tanzania. Hot water extract of dried root is taken orally as an anthelmintic[CP112]. Hot water extract of fresh leaves is taken orally for gonorrhea[CP140].

Thailand. Hot water extract of dried root is used as a diuretic[CP168].

Tonga. Dried stem scrapings are used to prepare an infusion that is taken orally to remedy failure of lactation[CP132].

Vanuatu. Unripe fruit is taken to induce abortion. Four small unripe fruits are eaten together with 4 tablets of nivaquine and the juice of 2 limes[CP067].

Venda. Decoction of dried root of *Carica papaya*, *Terminalia sericea*, *Parinari curatellifolia*, and *Citrus limon* is used. One tablespoonful of the decoction is taken orally[CP133].

Vietnam. Unripe fruit is eaten as an abortive[CP018].

West Africa. Hot water extract of dried root is taken orally as an abortifacient[CP037].

West Indies. Hot water extract of flowers is taken orally as an emmenagogue. Hot water extract of fresh unripe fruit is taken orally as an emmenagogue. Hot water extract of seeds is taken orally as an emmenagogue[CP106]. Latex of milk from incisions in stem is taken orally as a diuretic. It is said that "it burns but it makes the urine flow"[CP073]. Unripe fruit juice and hot water extracts are taken orally for hypertension[CP103].

CHEMICAL CONSTITUENTS

(ppm unless otherwise indicated)

(E)-beta-ocimene: Fr[CP049]
(Z)- beta-ocimene: Fr[CP049]
2-6-Dimethyl-3-7-diene-2-6-diol: Fr EO[CP085]
2-6-Dimethyl-oct-7-ene-2-3-6-triol: Fr EO[CP085]
2-6-Dimethyl-octa-1-7-diene-3-6-diol: Fr EO[CP085]
2-6-Dimethyl-octa-cis-2-7-diene-1-6-diol: Fr EO[CP085]
2-6-Dimethyl-octa-trans-2-7-diene-1-6-diol: Fr EO[CP085]
Butan-1-al, 2-methyl: Fr 6.0 mcg/kg[CP079]
3-Methyl-butyl benzoate: Fr[CP049]
4-Hydroxy-4-methyl-pentan-2-one: Fr[CP049]
4-Terpineol: Fr[CP049]
Avenasterol, 5-dehydro: Sd oil[CP075]
6-7-epoxy linalool: Fr EO[CP085]
6-Methylkept-5-en-2-one: Fr[CP049]
Avenasterol, 7-dehydro: Sd oil[CP075]
Cycloartenol, 24-methylene: Sd oil[CP075]
5,6-Monoepoxi-beta carotene: Fr[CP048]
Alanine: Fr 140–1253[CP050]
Alpha linolenic acid: Fr 250–2238[CP050]
Alpha terpinene: Fr[CP049]
Alpha tocopherol: Lf[CP171]
Alpha-phellandrene: Fr[CP049]
Beta-phellandrene: Fr[CP049]
Amyl iso-acetate: Fr[CP040]
Amyl-acetate: Fr[CP040]
Arachidic acid: Sd oil 0.5–1.0%[CP161]
Arginine: Fr 100–895[CP050]
Ascorbic acid: Fr 0.015–0.050%[CP041]
Ash: Fr 0.58–5.73%[CP050], Sd 8.8%[CP047]
Aspartic acid: Fr 490–4387[CP050]
Behenic acid: Sd oil 1.6%[CP023]

Benzaldehyde: Fr 0.3 mcg/mg[CP079]
Benzyl alcohol: Fr 0.2 mcg/kg[CP079]
Benzyl glucosinolate: Fr[CP165]
Benzyl-iso-thiocyanate: Fr[CP049], Sd 0.2–0.5%[CP028]
Sitosterol, beta: Lf; Sd, Fl, Fr[CP136]
Carotene, beta: Fr[CP172], Fr peel[CP029], Sd oil[CP075]
Carotene, beta-beta: Lf[CP061]
Carotene-3-diol, beta-beta: Lf[CP061]
Carotene, beta-epsilon: Lf[CP061]
Beta-phellandrene: Fr[CP049]
Carotene, beta-pseudo: Lf[CP061]
Boron: Fr 5–15[CP045]
But-2-enoic acid benzyl ester: Fr 0.1 mcg/kg[CP079]
But-2-enoic acid methyl ester: Fr 0.3 mcg/kg[CP079]
Butanedione: Fr[CP079]
Butanoic acid methyl ester: Fr 46.7 mcg/kg[CP079]
Butanoic acid, Fr pulp 1.2[CP082]
Butyl-acetate, Fr[CP040]
Butyl-alcohol: Fr[CP048]
Butyl-benzoate: Fr[CP049]
Butyl-hexanoate: Fr[CP049]
Caffeic acid: Lf[CP087]
Calcium: Fr 100–2729[CP046,CP050,CP047]
Callose: Lx[CP048]
Campesterol: Sd oil[CP075]
Caoutchouc: Lx 4.5%[CP047]
Caproic acid: Fr[CP079]
Carbohydrates: Fr 9.5–99.1%[CP046,CP047], Sd 15.5%[CP047]
Carica papaya amylase: Fr[CP041]
Carica papaya anticoagulant: Fr Lx[CP021]
Carica papaya polysaccharide P-1: Lx[CP076]
Carica papaya polysaccharide PP-11: Lx[CP076]
Carica papaya polysaccharide: Lx[CP116]
Caricacin: Fr[CP035]
Caricin: Sd[CP047]
Carpaine: Lf 0.015–0.400%[CP106], Sd[CP013], Fr 0.02%[CP033]
Carpasamine: Sd 0.35%[CP024]
Carpasemine: Sd 0.35%[CP027]
Carposide: Lf[CP047]
Caryophyllene: Fr[CP049]
Cholesterol: Sd oil[CP075]
Choline: Lf 0.02%[CP025]
Chrysanthemexanthin: Fr[CP048]
Chymopapain A: Lx[CP081]

Chymopapain: Lx[CP074]
Chymopapain B: Lx[CP048]
Cis-beta ocimene: Fr 0.4 mcg/kg[CP079]
Citric acid: Fr[CP047]
Copper: Fr 0.1–5[CP050,CP045]
Cotinine: Lf 27.8[CP034]
Cryptoxanthin monoepoxide: Fr peel[CP029]
Cryptoxanthin: Fr peel[CP029]
Cycloartanol: Sd oil[CP075]
Cycloartenol: Sd oil[CP075]
Cyclobranol: Sd oil[CP075]
D-galactose: Fr[CP048]
D-galacturonic acid: Fr[CP048]
Decanal: Fr[CP049]
Dehydrocarpaine 1: Lf[CP106]
Dehydrocarpaine 11: Lf[CP106]
Dehydrocarpamines: Pl[CP044]
Octalactone, delta: Fr 0.1 mcg/kg[CP079]
Delta-5-stigmasterol: Sd oil[CP075]
Essential oil: Sd 900[CP047]
Carotene, epsilon: Fr peel[CP029]
Ethanol: Fr[CP040]
Ethyl acetate: Fr[CP040]
Ethyl alcohol: Fr[CP048]
Ethyl benzoate: Fr[CP049]
Ethyl butyrate: Fr[CP049]
Ethyl octanoate: Fr[CP049]
Fat: Fr 0.098–2.2%[CP046,CP047], Lx 2.4%,
    Sd 25.3%[CP047]
Fatty acids: Sd oil[CP130]
Fiber: Fr 0.696–7.554%[CP050], Sd 17%[CP047]
Fixed oil (Carica papaya): Sd 25.0%[CP161]
Flavonols: Lf 0–2000[CP043]
Fructose: Fr[CP173], Lf[CP087], Tr Bk[CP110]
Galactose: Tr Bk[CP110]
Gamma carotene: Fr[CP048]
Gamma terpinene: Fr[CP049]
Gamma octalactone: Fr[CP049]
Gentisic acid: Lf[CP038]
Geranyl acetone: Fr[CP049]
Germacrene-D: Fr[CP049]
Glucotropaeolin: Pl[CP048]
Glutamic acid: Fr[CP050]
Glycine: Fr 180–1611[CP050]
Heptan-2-one: Fr[CP040]
Heptanal: Fr[CP049]
Hex-2-enoic acid methyl ester:
    Fr 0.1 mcg/kg[CP079]
Hexadecenoic acid: Sd oil 0.8%[CP023]
Hexanal: Fr[CP049]
Hexanoic acid methyl ester:
    0.1 mcg/kg[CP079]

Hexyl acetate: Fr[CP040]
Hexyl alcohol: Fr[CP040]
Histidine: Fr 50–448[CP050]
Iron: Fr 0.8–38[CP046,CP047,CP050]
Iso-butyl acetate: Fr[CP040]
Iso-propyl alcohol: Fr[CP040]
Iso-butyl alcohol: Fr[CP040]
Isoamyl acetate: Fr[CP048]
Isoleucine: Fr 80–716[CP050]
Kilocalories: Fr 390–3491[CP050]
Kryptoflavin: Fr[CP048]
Kryptoxanthin: Fr[CP047]
Lauric acid: Lf, Fl, Fr[CP136], Sd oil 0.40%[CP023]
Leucine: Fr 160–1432[CP050]
Lignoceric acid: Sd oil[CP075]
Linalool oxide-A: Fr[CP049]
Linalool oxide-B: Fr[CP049]
Linalool oxide, cis: Fr 7.1 mcg/kg[CP079]
Linalool: Fr 0.3 mcg/kg[CP079]
Linoleic acid: Fr, Fl, Lf [CP136],
    Sd oil 0.40%[CP023]
Linolenic acid: Sd oil[CP170]
Lycopene: Fr Peel[CP029]
Lysine: Fr 250–2238[CP050]
Lysozyme: Lx[CP074]
Magnesium: Fr 82–1058[CP050]
Malic acid: Lx 4400, Fr[CP047]
Manganese: Fr 0.1–1.1[CP050]
Methanol: Fr[CP040]
Methionine: Fr 20–179[CP050]
Methyl acetate: Fr [CP040]
Methyl cyclohexane: Fr 4.5 mcg/kg[CP079]
Methyl hexanoate: Fr[CP049]
Methyl nicotinate: Fr 0.5 mcg/kg[CP079]
Methyl octanoate: Fr[CP049]
Methyl salicyclate: Fr[CP049]
Methyl thiocyanate: Fr[CP049]
Methylgeranate: Fr[CP049]
MUFA: Fr 380–3,402[CP050]
Mutatochrom: Fr[CP050]
Myosmine: Lf 1.4[CP034]
Myrcene: Fr[CP049]
Myristic acid: Fr, Sd, Lf, Fl[CP136]
Myristoleic acid: Fl, Fr[CP136]
Myrosin: Sd[CP047]
Butanol, N: Fr[CP040]
Docosane, N: Sd oil[CP075]
Dodecane, N: Sd oil[CP075]
Dotriacontane, N: Sd oil[CP075]
Eicosane, N: Sd oil[CP075]
Heneicosane, N: Sd oil[CP075]
Hentriacontane, N: Sd oil[CP075]

Heptadecane, N: Sd oil[CP075]
Hexacosane, N: Sd oil[CP075]
Hexadecane, N: Sd oil[CP075]
Formamide, N-N-dimethyl: Fr 0.1%[CP079]
Nonacosane, N: Sd oil[CP075]
Nonadecane, N: Sd oil[CP075]
Octacosane, N: Sd oil[CP075]
Octadecane, N: Sd oil[CP075]
Pentacosane, N: Sd oil[CP075]
Pentadecane, N: Sd oil[CP075]
Tetracosane, N: Sd oil[CP075]
Tetradecane, N: Sd oil[CP075]
Triacontane, N: Sd oil[CP075]
Tricosane, N: Sd oil[CP075]
Tridecane, N: Sd oil[CP075]
Tritriacontane, N: Sd oil[CP075]
Neoxanthin: Fr[CP048]
Niacin: Fr 3–33[CP050]
Nicotine: Lf 0.01028%[CP034]
Nonanal: Fr[CP049]
Octadecadienoic acid: Sd oil[CP075]
Octadecenoic acid: Sd oil[CP075]
Octan-3-ol: Fr[CP079]
Octanal: Fr[CP049]
Octanoic acid methyl ester:
    Fr 0.2 mcg/kg[CP079]
Octanoic acid: Fr[CP079]
Oleic acid: Sd oil 75.0%[CP161], Lf, Fl[CP136]
Ortho-xylene: Fr[CP079]
Palmitic acid: Sd oil 16.2–19.0%[CP023,CP161],
    Fr, Lf, Fl[CP136]
Palmitoleic acid: Fr, Fl[CP136]
Pantothenic acid: Fr 2–19[CP050]
Papain: Fr[CP171], Fr Lx 5.1–8.4%[CP077],
    St Lx 13.5%[CP042]
Papaya peptidase A: Lx[CP121,CP107]
Papaya peptidase B: Lx[CP107]
Papaya polysaccharide II: Fr[CP084]
Papaya proteinase omega: Lx[CP081]
Pectin (Carica papaya): Fr (unripe)[CP032]
Pentan-2,4-Dione: Fr[CP049]
Phenyl acetonitrile: Fr 17.1 mcg/kg[CP079]
Phenylalanine: Fr 90–806[CP050]
Phosphatidyl glycerol: Lf[CP083]
Phosphorus: Fr 45–1,260[CP050]
Phytoene: Fr[CP050]
Phytofluene: Fr[CP050]
Potassium: Fr 0.2294–2.5469%[CP050]
Proline: Fr 100–895[CP050]
Prop-2-yl-butyrate: Fr[CP049]
Propyl acetate: Fr[CP040]
Propyl alcohol: Fr[CP048]

Protease: Call Tiss[CP102,CP005]
Protein: Sd 40.0%[CP170], Lf 20.90%[CP158]
Proteinase: Lx[CP074]
Prunasin: Lf[CP080]
Carpaine, pseudo: Lf 0.01%[CP031]
Carotene, pseudo-pseudo: Lf[CP061]
PUFA: Fr 310–2,775[CP050]
Pyridine: Fr[CP079]
Resin: Lx 2.8%[CP047]
Riboflavin: Fr 0.3–3[CP050]
Serine: Fr 150–1,343[CP050]
SFA: Fr 430–3,850[CP050]
Sodium: Fr 26–554[CP046]
Squalene: Sd oil[CP075]
Stearic acid: Lf, Fr, Fl[CP136],
    Sd oil 5.0%[CP161,CP023]
Stigmasterol: Sd oil[CP075]
Styrene: Fr 0.1%[CP079]
Sucrose: Fr[CP047], Trunk Bk[CP110], Lf[CP087]
Sulfoquinovosyl-diacyl glycerol:
    Fr, Lf, Fr peel[CP083]
Sulfur: Fr 300–900[CP045]
Tartaric acid: Fr[CP047]
Terpinolene: Fr[CP049]
Tetraphyllin B: Lf[CP080]
Thiamin: Fr 0.2–2.6[CP050]
Threonine: Fr 110–985[CP050]
Toluene: Fr 4.6 mcg/kg[CP079]
Trans-linalool oxide: Fr 0.7 mcg/kg[CP079]
Triacetin: Fr[CP049]
Tricosanoic acid: Sd oil[CP075]
Tryptophan: Fr 80–716[CP050]
Tyrosine: Fr 50–448[CP050]
Valine: Fr 100–895[CP050]
Violaxanthin: Fr[CP047]
Vitamin B6: Fr 0.2–1.7[CP050]
Water: Fr 86.5–91.8%[CP047,CP046],
    Lx 75.0%[CP047]
Xylitol: Trunk Bk[CP110]
Zeaxanthin: Fr[CP047]
Zinc: Fr 1.8–5.4[CP045]

PHARMACOLOGICAL ACTIVITIES AND CLINICAL TRIALS

Abortifacient effect. Extract of ripe dried fruit was active. Percentage effectiveness in studies reviewed was 100%[CP147]. Fruit, in the ration of pregnant rats at a dose of 300.0 gm/kg, was equivocal. Saponifiable fraction of unripe fruit, in the ration of pregnant rats at a dose of 300.0 gm/kg, was active. Seeds, in the ration of pregnant rats at a dose of 300.0 gm/kg, were inactive[CP100].

Allergenic activity. Water extract of pollen, administered intradermally to human adults of both sexes at a concentration of 1:50, was active[CP164].

Analgesic activity. Ethanol (100%) extract of dried leaves, administered intraperitoneally to rats at a dose of 20.0 mg/kg, was active[CP153]. Ethanol (95%) extract of dried seeds was inactive[CP126]. Ethanol/water (1:1) extract of the aerial parts, administered intraperitoneally to mice at a dose of 500.0 mg/kg, was inactive vs tail pressure method[CP157].

Anthelmintic activity. Ethanol (95%) extract of dried seeds, administered to chicken, was active on *Ascaridia galli*[CP126]. Ethanol (95%) extract of fruit juice, at a concentration of 0.11 ml, produced weak activity on *Ascaridia galli*[CP055]. Ethanol (95%) extract of latex from the stem, at a concentration of 7.5 mg/ml, produced weak activity on *Ascaridia galli*[CP091]. Ethanol (95%) extract of seeds, at a concentration of 25.0 mg/ml, was active on *Ascaridia galli*[CP055].

Antiandrogenic effect. Dried seeds, administered by gastric intubation to rats at a dose of 20.0 mg/animal, were inactive[CP108].

Antiascariasis activity. Water extract of leaves, at a concentration of 10.0 mg/ml, was active on earthworms. Water extract of seeds, at a concentration of 10.0 mg/ml, produced strong activity on earthworms[CP036].

Antibacterial activity. Acetone extract of dried leaves, on agar plate, was active on *Pseudomonas aeruginosa, Salmonella newport, Sarcina lutea, Serratia marcescens,* and *Shigella flexneri* 3A; inactive on *Escherichia coli, Propionibacterium acnes, Salmonella typhosa, Shigella flexneri, Staphylococcus albus,* and *Staphylococcus aureus.* The ethanol (95%) extract was active on *Escherichia coli, Propionibacterium acnes, Pseudomonas aeruginosa,* and *Salmonella newport*; inactive on *Salmonella typhosa, Sarcina lutea, Serratia*

marcescens, Shigella flexneri, Shigella flexneri 3A, *Staphylococcus albus,* and *Staphylococcus aureus.* Water extract was active on *Escherichia coli, Propionibacterium acnes, Pseudomonas aeruginosa, Salmonella newport, Sarcina lutea, Serratia marcescens, Shigella flexneri,* and *Staphylococcus aureus*; inactive on *Salmonella typhosa, Shigella flexneri* 3A, and *Staphylococcus albus*[CP060]. Ethanol (95%) extract of undiluted dried fruit, on agar plate, was active on *Escherichia coli* and *Staphylococcus aureus.* Ethanol (95%) extract of undiluted dried leaves, on agar plate, was inactive on *Escherichia coli* and *Staphylococcus aureus.* Ethanol (95%) extract of undiluted dried root, on agar plate, was active on *Escherichia coli* and *Staphylococcus aureus*[CP166]. Methanol extract of dried root, at a concentration of 1.0% on agar plate, was equivocal on *Escherichia coli* and inactive on *Staphylococcus aureus*[CP112]. Ethanol (95%) extract of undiluted dried seeds, on agar plate, was active on *Escherichia coli* and *Staphylococcus aureus*[CP166]. Ethanol (95%) extract of undiluted latex, on agar plate, was inactive on *Escherichia coli* and *Staphylococcus aureus*[CP166]. Ethanol/water (1:1) extract of aerial parts, on agar plate at a concentration of 25.0 mg/ml, was inactive on *Bacillus subtilis, Escherichia coli, Salmonella typhosa, Staphylococcus aureus,* and *Agrobacterium tumefaciens*[CP157]. Juice of unripe dried fruit, on agar plate, was active on *Bacillus subtilis*, MIC 500.0 mcg/ml and zone of thinning 15.0; *Enterobacter cloacae*, MIC 500.0 mcg/ml, zone of thinning 13.0; *Escherichia coli*, MIC 500.0 mcg/ml, zone of thinning 13.5; *Klebsiella pneumoniae*, MIC 500.0 mcg/ml, zone of thinning 10.5; *Proteus vulgaris*, MIC 500.0 mcg/ml, zone of thinning 5.0; *Pseudomonas aeruginosa*, MIC 500.0 mcg/ml, zone of thinning 9.5; *Salmonella typhi*, MIC 500.0 mg/ml, zone of thinning 8.0 and *Staphylococcus aureus*, MIC 500.0 mg/ml, zone of thinning 10.5[CP064]. Protein fraction of fresh leaves, on agar plate at a concentration of 2.0 mg/ml, was active on

Bacillus cereus, Escherichia coli, Pseudomonas aeruginosa, Shigella flexneri, and *Staphylococcus aureus;* inactive on *Streptococcus faecalis,* and produced weak activity on *Proteus vulgaris* and *Salmonella typhimurium*[CP118]. Protein fraction of fresh, ripe seeds, on agar plate at a concentration of 2.0 mg/ml, was active on *Bacillus cereus, Escherichia coli, Pseudomonas aeruginosa,* and *Shigella flexneri;* inactive on *Streptococcus faecalis,* and produced weak activity on *Proteus vulgaris* and *Salmonella typhimurium*[CP118]. Acetone extract of dried stem, on agar plate, was active on *Escherichia coli, Propionibacterium acnes, Pseudomonas aeruginosa, Salmonella typhosa, Sarcina lutea, Serratia marcescens, Shigella flexneri, Shigella flexneri 3A,* and *Staphylococcus aureus* and inactive on *Salmonella newport* and *Staphylococcus albus.* Ethanol (95%) extract was active on *Escherichia coli, Propionibacterium acnes, Pseudomonas aeruginosa, Salmonella newport, Shigella flexneri, Shigella flexneri 3A,* and *Staphylococcus albus;* inactive on *Salmonella typhosa, Sarcina lutea, Serratia marcescens,* and *Staphylococcus aureus.* Water extract was active on *Escherichia coli, Propionibacterium acnes, Pseudomonas aeruginosa, Salmonella newport, Sarcina lutea, Serratia marcescens, Shigella flexneri, Shigella flexneri 3A,* and *Staphylococcus albus;* inactive on *Salmonella typhosa* and *Staphylococcus aureus*[CP060]. Protein fraction of ripe endocarp tissue on agar plate, at a concentration of 2.0 mg/ml, was active on *Bacillus cereus, Escherichia coli, Pseudomonas aeruginosa, Shigella flexneri,* and *Staphylococcus aureus;* inactive on *Streptococcus faecalis;* and produced weak activity on *Proteus vulgaris* and *Salmonella typhimurium*[CP118]. Protein fraction of ripe-fresh epicarp, on agar plate at a concentration of 2.0 mg/ml, was active on *Bacillus cereus, Escherichia coli, Pseudomonas aeruginosa, Shigella flexneri,* and *Staphylococcus aureus;* inactive on *Streptococcus faecalis;* and produced weak activity on *Proteus vulgaris* and *Salmonella typhimurium*[CP118].

Water extract of fresh bark, at a concentration of 1.0% on agar plate, was inactive on *Neisseria gonorrhea*[CP140]. Water extract of fresh latex, on agar plate at a concentration of 335.0 units/ml, was active on *Micrococcus leisodeikticus*[CP163]. Water extract of fresh root, on agar plate at a concentration of 1.0%, was inactive on *Neisseria gonorrhea*[CP140].

Anticlastogenic activity. Fruit and seed juice, administered intraperitoneally to mice at a dose of 50.0 ml/kg, was active on marrow cells vs tetracycline-, mitomycin-, and dimethylnitrosamine-induced micronuclei[CP066].

Anticoagulant activity. Fresh leaf, at a concentration of 50%, was active on human whole blood[CP150].

Anticonvulsant activity. Ethanol (100%) extract of dried leaves, administered intraperitoneally to rats at a dose of 100.0 mg/kg, was active vs maximal electroshock-induced convulsions. A dose of 20.0 mg/kg was active vs pentylenetetrazole-induced seizures[CP153]. Ethanol (70%) extract of fresh root, administered intraperitoneally to mice of both sexes at a dose of 100.0 mg/kg, was equivocal vs strychnine-induced convulsions, 20% protection was observed. Weak activity was observed vs metrazole-induced convulsions, 30% protection[CP120]. Ethanol/water (1:1) extract of aerial parts, administered intraperitoneally to mice at a dose of 500.0 mg/kg, was inactive vs electroshock-induced convulsions[CP157].

Antiedema activity. Methanol extract of fruit, applied onto the ear of mice at a dose of 2.0 mg/ear, was active vs 12-0-tetradecanoylphorbol-13-acetate(TPA)-induced ear inflammation. Inhibition ratio (IR) was 5[CP062].

Antiestrogenic effect. Seeds, administered orally to mice at a dose of 1.5 gm/kg, were active[CP012].

Antifertility effect. Dried seeds, administered by gastric intubation to male rats at a dose of 20.0 mg/animal, were active[CP108].

Acetone and water extracts of dried leaves, on agar plate at a concentration of 50%, was inactive on *Neurospora crassa*[CP131]. Acetone/water (50:50) extract of fresh latex, on agar plate, was inactive on *Microsporum gypseum* and *Trichophyton mentagrophytes*[CP088]. Ethanol (100%) extract of fresh leaves, at a concentration of 10.0%, ethanol/acetone (50%) extract at a concentration of 50.0%, ethanol/water (1:1) at a concentration of 1.0%, and water extract at a concentration of 1.0%, on agar plate, were active on *Neurospora crassa*[CP128]. Ethanol/water (1:1) extract of aerial parts, on agar plate at a concentration of 25.0 mcg/ml, was inactive on *Microsporum canis*, *Trichophyton mentagrophytes*, and *Aspergillus niger*[CP157]. Methanol extract of unripe fruit, on agar plate at a concentration of 0.03%, was inactive on *Trichophyton mentagrophytes*[CP117].

Antihepatotoxic activity. Water extract of trunkbark, administered orally to male rats at a dose of 500.0 mg/kg, was active vs jaundice induced by intraperitoneal injection of *Brenania brieyi* fruit saponin fraction[CP078].

Anti-implantation effect. Ethanol (95%) extract of unripe fruit, administered orally to rats at a dose of 500.0 mg/kg, produced weak activity[CP014]. Ethanol (95%), petroleum ether, and water extracts of seeds, administered orally to pregnant rats, were inactive[CP052]. Petroleum ether extract of seeds, administered orally to rats at a dose of 500.0 mg/kg, was active. Pregnancy was prevented in 60% of the rats. No activity was observed at lower doses[CP054]. Unripe, dried fruit pulp, administered intraperitoneally to rats, was active[CP147]. Ethanol/water (1:1) extract of aerial parts, administered orally to male rats at a dose of 500.0 mg/kg, was inactive vs carrageenin-induced pedal edema. Animals were dosed one hour before carrageenin injections[CP157].

Antimalarial activity. Chloroform and water extracts of flowers, administered orally to chicken at doses of 166.0 mg/kg

and 3.72 gm/kg, respectively, were inactive on *Plasmodium gallinaceum*[CP004].

Antimycobacterial activity. Water extract of fresh leaves, (one part of fresh leaves to three parts of water) on agar plate, produced weak activity on *Mycobacterium tuberculosis*[CP160].

Antioxidant activity. Juice of unripe dried fruit, at concentrations of 25.0 and 58.0 mg/ml, was active. Superoxide radicals were generated using the hypoxanthine oxidase system[CP064].

Antisickling activity. Water extract of unripe fresh fruit was active on RBC[CP144].

Antispasmodic activity. Ethanol/water (1:1) extract of aerial parts was inactive on the ileum of guinea pigs vs ACh- and histamine-induced spasms[CP157].

Antispermatogenic effect. Dried seed, administered by gastric intubation to male rats at a dose of 20.0 mg/animal daily for eight weeks, was inactive. Animals were mated with adult females of proven fertility at estrus following treatment[CP108].

Antitumor activity. Ethanol (95%) extract of dried leaves, administered intraperitoneally to mice at a dose of 100.0 mg/kg, was inactive on Sarcoma 180(ASC)[CP092].

Antiulcer activity. Fresh fruit latex, administered by gastric intubation to rats at a dose of 0.75 gm/kg twice daily for six days, was inactive vs aspirin-, prednisolone-, and stress-induced ulcers (water immersion). Fresh latex, administered by gastric intubation to rats at a dose of 0.75 gm/kg twice daily for six days, was active vs stress- (water-immersion) and prednisolone-induced ulcers. The treatment was inactive vs aspirin-induced ulcers. Fresh seeds, administered by gastric intubation to rats at a dose of 0.75 gm/kg twice daily for six days, was inactive vs aspirin, prednisolone-, and stress-induced (water immersion) ulcers. Fresh unripe fruit, administered by gastric intubation to rats at a dose of 0.75 gm/kg twice daily for six days, was active vs stress-induced ulcers (water-immersion), and inactive vs aspirin- and prednisolone-induced ulcers[CP123].

Antiviral activity. Ethanol (80%) extract of freeze-dried leaves, in cell culture at variable concentrations, was equivocal on Coxsackie B2 virus vs Plaque-inhibition; inactive on Adenovirus, Herpes virus type 1, measles virus, poliovirus, and Semlicki-forest virus vs plaque inhibition[CP119]. Ethanol (95%) extract of leaves, in cell culture, was active on distortion ringspot virus, mild mosaic virus, and ringspot virus[CP156]. Latex, in cell culture, was active on tobacco mosaic virus[CP017].

Antiyeast activity. Ethanol/water (1:1) extract of aerial parts, at a concentration of 25.0 mcg/ml, was inactive on *Candida albicans* and *Cryptococcus neoformans*[CP157]. Fresh latex, on agar plate, was active on *Candida albicans*, LC$_{100}$ 138.0 mcg/ml[CP057]. Fresh latex, at a concentration of 10.0% on agar plate, was active on *Candida albicans*, *Candida guilliermondii*, and *Candida tropicalis*[CP113]. Methanol extract of unripe fruit, on agar plate at a concentration of 0.03%, was inactive on *Candida albicans*[CP117]. Water extract of dried root, on agar plate, was active on *Candida albicans* using hole-plate diffusion method and produced weak activity in broth culture using test-tube dilution method. Chloroform and methanol extracts were inactive on agar plate using hole-plate diffusion method, and in broth culture using test-tube dilution method. Petroleum ether extract was active on agar plate using hole-plate diffusion method, and in broth culture using test-tube dilution method[CP142].

Ascaricidal activity. Fruit latex, administered orally to dogs at a dose of 1.50 ml/kg, was active on *Ascaris lumbricoides*[CP020].

Cardiac depressant activity. Hot water extract of fruit, taken orally by human adults at a dose of 0.02 gm/person, was active[CP033].

Chronotropic effect positive. Ethanol (100%) extract of dried leaves, administered

intraperitoneally to rats at a dose of 200.0 mg/kg, was active[CP153].

Detoxifying effect (non-immunologic). Methanol extract of dried leaves, at a concentration of 100.0 ppm, was inactive on *Bulinus globosus*[CP114].

Diuretic activity. Ethanol/water (1:1) extract of aerial parts, administered intraperitoneally to male rats at a dose of 250.0 mg/kg, was inactive on saline-loaded animals. Urine was collected for four hours post-treatment[CP157].

Embryotoxic effect. Fruit, in the ration of pregnant rats at a dose of 300.0 gm/kg, was equivocal[CP100]. Water and petroleum ether extracts of seeds, administered orally to pregnant rats, were active[CP052]. Seeds, in the ration of pregnant rats at a dose of 300.0 gm/kg, were inactive[CP100].

Fish poison. Water extract of fresh bark was inactive[CP146].

Gastric antisecretory activity. Fresh latex, administered by gastric intubation to rats at a dose of 0.75 gm/kg twice daily for six days, was active vs histamine-induced ulcer[CP123].

Gastric secretory stimulation. Fruit juice, taken orally by human adults, was inactive[CP026].

Hemagglutinin activity. Water extract of dried seeds was active on human RBC. No specificity for any particular blood group was observed[CP167].

Hypoglycemic activity. Ethanol/water (1:1) extract of aerial parts, administered orally to rats at a dose of 250.0 mg/kg, was inactive. Less than 30% drop in blood sugar level was observed[CP157]. Fruit, administered orally to rabbits, was inactive[CP030].

Hypotensive activity. Ethanol (95%) extract of seeds, administered intravenously to dogs, was active. Respiration was also depressed[CP022].

Hypothermic activity. Ethanol/water (1:1) extract of aerial parts, administered intraperitoneally to mice at a dose of 500.0 mg/kg, was inactive[CP157].

Inflammation induction. Fresh latex, injected into rats at a dose of 0.25%, was active vs aspirin, prednisolone, levamisole, and boswellic acid anti-inflammatory treatment. The dose was inactive vs piroxicam, ibuprofen, and chloroquine phosphate anti-inflammatory treatment[CP058].

Insecticide activity. Ethanol (95%) extract of dried seeds, at a concentration of 50.0 mg, was inactive on *Rhodnius neglectus*[CP070]. Fruit juice was active on *Leptinotarsa decemlineata*[CP053].

Larvicidal activity. Water extract of dried latex was active on *Culex quinquefasciatus*, LC_{100} 0.004 ml/ml. Concentration given in gm of fresh plant material per ml of water needed for 100% mortality in six hours. The extract was tested in 100 ml of water[CP086].

Molluscicidal activity. Water extract of oven-dried fruit was inactive on *Biophalaria pfeifferi*[CP145].

Ovulation inhibition effect. Ethanol (95%), water, and petroleum ether extracts, administered orally to rabbits at a dose of 100.0 mg/kg, were inactive[CP006].

Plant germination inhibition. Chloroform extract of dried leaves was active vs *Amaranthus spinosus*, 49.5% inhibition. Chlorform extract of dried seeds was active vs *Amaranthus spinosus*, 58% inhibition[CP111].

Radical scavenging effect. Fresh fruit juice, at a concentration of 20.0 microliters, was active[CP091]. Juice of unripe dried fruit was active, IC_{50} 25.0 mg/ml when scavenging of 1,1-diphenyl-1-2-picrylhydrazyl radicals was assayed and IC_{50} 67.1 mg/ml when scavenging of hydroxyl radicals was assayed[CP064].

Semen coagulation. Ethanol/water (1:1) extract of aerial parts, at a concentration of 2.0%, was inactive on the semen of rats[CP157].

Skeletal muscle relaxant effect (central). Ethanol (100%) extract of dried leaves, administered intraperitoneally to rats at a dose of 50.0 mg/kg, was active[CP153].

Smooth muscle stimulant activity. Ethanol (95%) extract of dried seeds was active on the ileum of guinea pigs vs ACh, and barium-induced contractions[CP126]. Ethanol (95%), and water extracts of seeds were active on the rat intestine. Atropine or antihistamine did not block the activity[CP118].

Spasmolytic activity. Butanol extract of dried leaves, at a concentration of 0.2 mg/ml, was active on the ileum of guinea pigs, 35.67% reduction in contraction was seen vs ACh-induced contractions and 53.37% reduction vs KCl-induced contractions. Chloroform extract was inactive vs ACh- and KCl-induced contractions. Isopentyl alcohol extract was active, 89.34% reduction vs ACh-induced contractions and 72.43% reduction vs KCl-induced contractions. Methanol extract was active, 20.17% reduction vs ACh-induced contractions and inactive vs KCl-induced contractions[CP098].

Spermicidal activity. Water extract of seeds was active in rodents. The effect was 100% reversible after three months[CP139].

Spermicidal effect. Dried seeds, administered by gastric intubation to male rats at a dose of 20.0 mg/animal, were inactive[CP108]. Ethanol/water (1:1) extract of aerial parts, at a concentration of 2.0%, was inactive on the spermatozoa of rats[CP157].

Superoxide radical scavenging activity. Juice of unripe dried fruit was active, IC_{50} 114.5 mg/ml when scavenging of superoxide was assayed[CP064].

Toxicity assessment (quantitative). Ethanol (95%) extract of dried seeds, administered intraperitoneally to rats, produced LD_{50} 208.0 mg/kg[CP126]. Ethanol/water (1:1) extract of aerial parts, administered intraperitoneally to mice, produce LD_{50} >1.0 gm/kg[CP157].

Tranquilizing effect. Ethanol (100%) extract of dried leaves, administered intraperitoneally to rats at a dose of 10.0 mg/kg, was active[CP153].

Tumor promotion inhibition. Methanol extract of fresh fruit, in cell culture at a concentration of 200.0 mg, was inactive on Epstein-Barr virus vs 12-0-hexadecanoyl-phorbol-13-acetate-induced Epstein-Barr virus activation[CP148].

Uterine relaxation effect. Ethanol (95%) and water extracts of seeds produced weak activity on the rat uterus[CP022]. Ethanol (95%) extract of seeds was active on the rat uterus vs oxytocin-induced contractions[CP126].

Uterine stimulant effect. Ethanol (95%) extract of seeds, administered intravenously to guinea pigs at a concentration of 2.0 mg/ml, was inactive on the non-pregnant uterus[CP169]. Latex, at a concentration of 0.22 ml/liters, was active on the uterus of guinea pigs[CP008].

WBC-macrophage stimulant. Water extract of freeze-dried fruit, at a concentration of 2.0 mg/ml, was inactive. Nitrite formation was used as an index of the macrophage stimulating activity to screen effective foods[CP097].

REFERENCES

CP001 Quisumbing, E. Medicinal plants of the Philippines. **Tech Bull 16, Rep Philippines, Dept Agr Nat Resources**, Manila 1951; 1.

CP002 Alvaro Viera, R. Subsidio para o Estudio da Flora Medicinal da Guinea Portuguesa. Agencia-General do Ultramar, Lisboa, 1959.

CP003 Vasileva, B. Plantes Medicinales de Guinee. Conarky, Republique, 1969.

CP004 Spencer, C. F., F. R. Koniuszy, E. F. Rogers et al. Survey of plants for antimalarial activity. **Lloydia** 1947; 10: 145–174.

CP005 Medora, R. S., J. M. Campbell and G. P. Mell. Proteolytic enzymes in papaya tissue cultures. **Lloydia** 1973; 36: 214.

CP006 Kapoor, M., S. K. Garg and V. S. Mathur. Antiovulatory activity of five indigenous plants in rabbits. **Indian J Med Res** 1974; 62: 1225–1227.

CP007 Gimlette, J. D. Malay Poisons and Charm Cures. J & A Churchill, London, 3rd Edition, 1929.

CP008 Hikino, H., K. Aota and T. Takemoto. Structure and absolute configuration of cyperotundone. **Chem Pharm Bull** 1966; 14: 890.

CP009 Milne, L. Shans at Home. John Murray, London, 1910; 181.

CP010 Maugham, R. C. F. Portuguese East Africa, the History, Scenery and Great Game of Manica and Sofala. John Murray, London, 1906; 271.

CP011 Berhault, J. Flore Illustree du Senegal II. Govt. Senegal, Min Rural Dev, Water and Forest Div. Dakar, 2. 1974.

CP012 Sareen, K. N., N. Misra, D. R. Varma, M. K. P. Amma and M. L. Gujral. Oral contraceptives. V. Anthelmintics as antifertility agents. **Indian J Physiol Pharmacol** 1961; 5: 125–135.

CP013 Burdick, E. M. Carpaine: An alkaloid of *Carica papaya*, its chemistry and pharmacology. **Econ Bot** 1971; 25: 363.

CP014 Garg, S. K. and G. P. Garg. Antifertility screening of plants. Part VII. Effect of five indigenous plants on early pregnancy in albino rats. **Indian J Med Res** 1970; 59: 302.

CP015 Gimlette, J. D. A Dictionary of Malayan Medicine, Oxford Univ. Press., New York, USA, 1939.

CP016 Murray, J. A. Plants and Drugs of Sind. Richardson and Co., London, 1881.

CP017 Khurana, S. M. P. Studies on *Calotropis procera* latex as an inhibitor of tobacco mosaic virus. **Phytopathol** 1972; Z 73: 341.

CP018 Petelot, A. Les Plantes Medicinales du Cambodge, du Laos et du Vietnam, Vol. 1–4. Archives des Recherches Agronomiques et Pastorales au Vietnam No. 23, 1954.

CP019 Kerharo, J. and A. Bouquet. Plantes Medicinales et Toxiques de La Cote-D'Ivoire - Haute-Volta. Vigot Freres, Paris, 1950; 297pp.

CP020 Nagaty, H. F., M. A. Rifatt and T. A. Morsy. Trials on the effect on dog ascaris In vivo produced by the latex of *Ficus carica* and *Papaya carica* growing in Cairo gardens. **Ann Trop Med Parasitol** 1959; 53: 215.

CP021 Pillai, N. C., C. S. Vaidyanathan and K. V. Giri. A blood anticoagulant factor from the latex of *Carica papaya*. 1. Purification and general properties. **Proc Indian Acad Sci Ser** B 1955; 42: 316.

CP022 Bose, B. C., A. Q. Saifi, R. Vijay-vargiya and A. W. Bhagwat. Pharma-cological study of Carica papaya seeds, with special reference to its anthelm-intic action: Preliminary report. **Indian J Med Sci** 1961; 15: 888.

CP023 Badami, R. C. and C. D. Daulatabad. The component acids of Carica papaya (Caricaceae) seed oil. **J Sci Food Agr** 1967; 18: 360.

CP024 Panse, T. B. and A. S. Paranjpe. Carpasemine isolated from Carica papaya seeds. **Proc Indian Acad Sci Ser A** 1943; 18: 140.

CP025 Ogan, A. U. West African medicinal plants. II. Basic constituents of the leaves of Carica papaya. **Phytochemistry** 1971; 10: 2544.

CP026 Brailski, K., K. Mao and K. Kuk. The action of certain tropical fruits on the gastric function. **VOPR Pitaniya** 1960; 19(4): 39.

CP027 Panse, T. B. and A. S. Paranipe. An alkaloid substance isolated from Carica papaya seeds. **Rasayanam** 1941; 1: 215.

CP028 Ettlinger, M. G. and J. E. Hodgkins. The mustard of papaya seeds. **J Org Chem** 1956; 21: 204.

CP029 Yamamoto, H. Y. Comparison of the carotenoids in yellow- and red-fleshed Carica papaya. **Nature (London)** 1964; 201: 1049.

CP030 Bischoff, F., M. L. Long and M. Sahyun. Investigations of the hypogly-cemic properties of reglykol pancrea-tine and papaw. **J Pharmacol Exp Ther** 1929; 36: 311.

CP031 Govindachari, T. R., B. R. Pai and N. S. Narasimhan. Pseudocarpaine, a new alkaloid from Carica papaya. **J Chem Soc** 1954; 1954: 1847.

CP032 Biswas, A. B. and C. V. N. Rao. Struc-tural investigation of the galactan component of the pectic substance from Carica papaya. **Aust J Chem** 1969; 22: 2001.

CP033 Noble, I. G. Fruta bomba (Carica pa-paya) in hypertension. **An Acad Cienc Med Fis Nat Habana** 1947; 85: 198.

CP034 Smalberger, T. M., G. J. H. Rall and H. L. Waal. Carica papaya alkaloids. **Tydskr Natuurwetr** 1968; 8: 156.

CP035 Cairns, T. M. Isolation and indenti-fication of caricacin, a plant growth inhibitor in the methanolic extract of Carica papaya. **Diss Abstr Int B** 1969; 29: 2689.

CP036 Krishnakumari, M. K. and S. K. Majumder. Bioassay of piperazine & some plant products with earthworms. **J Sci Ind Res** 1960; C 19: 202.

CP037 Watt, J. M. and M. G. Breyer-Brandwijk. The Medicinal and Poison-ous Plants of Southern and Eastern Africa. 2nd Ed, E. S. Livingstone, Ltd., London, 1962.

CP038 Griffiths, L. A. On the distribution of gentisic acid in green plants. **J Exp Biol** 1959; 10: 437.

CP039 Peckolt, G. Brazilian anthelmintic plants. **Rev Flora Med** 1942; 9(7): 333.

CP040 Katague, D. B. and E. R. Kirch. Chro-matographic analysis of the volatile components of papaya fruit. **J Pharm Sci** 1965; 54: 891.

CP041 Ritthibut, A. and R. Charoenphol. Enzymes and vitamins in raw and ripe papaya fruit. Undergraduate Special Project Report 1971; 19pp.

CP042 Sornsuchaat, T. Isolation of papain from papaya latex. Undergraduate Special Project Report, Chulalong-korn University, Bangkok, Thailand 1951; 10pp.

CP043 Economic Botany. 1991; Volume 45.

CP044 Glasby, J. H. **Dictionary of Plants Con-taining Secondary Metabolites**. Taylor and Francis. New York. 1991; 488pp.

CP045 **Journal of Food Science** 1961; Vol. 14.

CP046 Pederson, M. Nutritional Herbology. Pederson Publishing. Bountiful, UT, 1987; 377pp.

CP047 The Wealth of India. Council of Sci-entific and Industrial Research. New Delhi, 1948–1976.

CP048 List, P. H. and L. Horhammer. Hager's Handbuch der Pharmazeutischen Praxis. Springer-Verlag, Berlin. 1969–1079.

CP049 **Journal of Agriculture and Food Chemistry** 1992; Volume 40.

CP050 USDA Agricultural Handbook No. 8 and sequels; strictly nutritional data.

CP051 Ortiz De Montellano, B. Empirical Aztec medicine. **Science** 1975; 188: 215–220.

CP052 Bodhankar, S. L., S. K. Garg and V. S. Mathur. Antifertility screening of plants. Part IX. Effect of five indigenous plants on early pregnancy in female albino rats. **Indian J Med Res** 1974; 62: 831–837.

CP053   Yagashi, R. Papain for the control of termites. **Patent-Japan Kokai**-74 125,520: 1974.

CP054   Garg, S. K. Antifertility effect of oil from few indigenous plants on female albino rats. **Planta Med** 1974; 26: 391–393.

CP055   Lal, J., S. Chandra, V. Raviprakash and M. Sabir. In vitro anthelmintic action of some indigenous medicinal plants on *Ascardia galli* worms. **Indian J Physiol Pharmacol** 1976; 20: 64.

CP056   Devereux, G. A Study of Abortion in Primitive Societies. The Julian Press, Inc, New York, 1976.

CP057   Giordani, R., M. Siepaio, J. Moulin-Traffort and P. Regli. Antifungal action of *Carica papaya* latex. Isolation of fungal cell wall hydrolysing enzymes. **Mycoses** 1991; 34(11/12): 469–477.

CP058   Gupta, O. P., N. Sharma and D. Chad. A sensitive and relevant model for evaluating anti-inflammatory activity, papaya latex-induced rat paw inflammation. **J Pharmacol Toxicol Meth** 1992; 28(1): 15–19.

CP059   Bhat, R. B., E. O. Eterjere and V. T. Oladipo. Ethnobotanical studies from Central Nigeria. **Econ Bot** 1990; 44(3): 382–390.

CP060   Misas, C. A. J., N. M. R. Hernandez and A. M. L. Abraham. The biological assessment of Cuban plants. III. **Rev Cub Med Trop** 1979; 31(1): 21–27.

CP061   Topuriya, L. I. Pigments of the plastids and flavonoids of the leaves of *Carica papaya*. **Chem Nat Comp** 1990; 26(1): 98–99.

CP062   Yasukawa, K., A. Yamaguchi, J. Arita, S. Sakurai, A. Ikeda and M. Takido. Inhibitory effect of edible plant extracts on 12-0-Tetradecanoyl-phorbol-13-Acetate-induced ear oedema in mice. **Phytother Res** 1993; 7(2): 185–189.

CP063   Reddy, M. B., K. R. Reddy and M. N. Reddy. A survey of plant crude drugs of Anantapur District, Andhra Pradesh, India. **Int J Crude Drug Res** 1989; 27(3): 145–155.

CP064   Osato, J. A., L. A. Santiago, G. M. Reno, M. S. Cuadra and A. Mori. Antimicrobial and antioxidant activities of unripe papaya. **Life Sci** 1993; 53(17): 1383–1389.

CP065   Zamora-Martinez, M. C. and C. N. P. Pola. Medicinal plants used in some rural populations of Oaxaca, Puebla and Veracruz, Mexico. **J Ethnopharmacol** 1992; 35(3) 229–257.

CP066   Lim-Sylianco, C. Y., J. A. Concha, A. P. Jocano and C. M. Lim. Antimutagenic effects of expressions from twelve medicinal plants. **Philippine J Sci** 1986; 115(1): 23–30.

CP067   Bourdy, G. and A. Walter. Maternity and medicinal plants in Vanuatu I. The cycle of reproduction. **J Ethnopharmacol** 1992; 37(3): 179–196.

CP068   Holdsworth, D. Medicinal plants of the Gazelle peninsula, New Britain Island, Papau, New Guinea. Part 1. **Int J Pharmacog** 1992; 30(3): 185–190.

CP069   Holdsworth, D and L. Balun. Medicinal plants of the East and West Sepik Provinces, Papau, New Guinea. **Int J Pharmacog** 1992; 30(3): 218–222.

CP070   Schmeda-Hirschmann, G. and A. Rojas de Arias. A screening method for natural products on Triatomine bugs. **Phytother Res** 1992; 6(2): 68–73.

CP071   Hope, B. E., D. G. Massey and G. Fournier-Massey. Hawaiian materia medica for asthma. **Hawaii Med J** 1993; 52(6): 160–166.

CP072   Holdsworth, D. K. Traditional medicinal plants of Rarotonga, Cook Islands Part 1. **Int J Crude Drug Res** 1990; 28(3): 209–218.

CP073   Morton, J. F. Medicinal and other plants used by people on North Caicos (Turks and Caicos Islands, West Indies). **J Crude Drug Res** 1977; 15: 1–24.

CP074   Anon. Pure proteolytic active enzymes from the latex of *Carica papaya*. **Patent-Belg**-838,750: 1976.

CP075   Strocchi, A., G. Lercker, G. Bonaga, and A. Maye. Composition of papaya seed oil. **Riv Ital Sistanze Grasse** 1977; 54: 429.

CP076   Chandrasekaran, E. V., J. N. Bemiller and S. C. D. Lee. Isolation, partial characterization, and biological properties of polysaccharides from crude papain. **Carbohydr Res** 1978; 60: 105.

CP077 Marrero, M., J. Garcia, M. Bonera and F. Alonso. Industrial process for obtaining purified papain from the latex of the *Carica papaya* fruit. **Rev Cubana Farm** 1977; 11(1): 35.

CP078 Boum, R., J. L. Pousset, F. Lemonnier and M. Hadchouel. Action of extracts of *Carica papaya* on experimental jaundice induced in the rat by saponins extracted from *Brenani brieyi*. **Toxicol Appl Pharmacol** 1978; 46: 353.

CP079 MacLeod, A. J., and N. M. Pieris. Volatile components of papaya (*Carica papaya* L.) with particular reference to glucosinolate products. **J Agr Food Chem** 1983; 31(5): 1005–1008.

CP080 Spencer, K. C. and D. S. Seigler. Cyanogenic glycosides of *Carica papaya* and its phylogenetic position with respect to the volatiles and capparales. **Amer J Bot** 1984; 71(10): 1444–1447.

CP081 Brocklehurst, K., E. Salih, R. Mc Kee and H. Smith. Fresh non-fruit latex of *Carica papaya* contains papain, multiforms of chymopapain A and papaya proteinase omega. **Biochem J** 1985; 228(2): 525–527.

CP082 Idstein, H., C. Bauer and P. Schreier. Volatile acids from tropical fruits: Cherimoya (*Annona cherimolia*, Mill.) guava, (*Psidium guajava*, L.) mango (*Mangifera indica*, L., var. Alphonso) and papaya (*Carica papaya*, L). **Z Lebensm-Unters Forsch** 1985; 180(5): 394–397.

CP083 Kenrick, J. R. and D. G. Bishop. Phosphatidylglycerol and sulphoquinovosyldiacylglycerol in leaves and fruits of chilling-sensitive plants. **Phytochemistry** 1986; 25(6): 1293–1295.

CP084 Bemiller, J. N. and S. B. Dikko. Structural analysis of papaya polysaccharide ll. **Carbohydr Res** 1986; 158: 173–181.

CP085 Schreier, P. and P. Winterhalter. Precursors of papaya (*Carica papaya*, L.) fruit volatiles. **ACS Symp Ser** 1986; 317: 85–98.

CP086 Evans, D. A. and R. K. Raj. Extracts of Indian plants as mosquito larvicides. **Indian J Med Res** 1988; 88(1): 38–41.

CP087 Saleh, N. A. M., A. E. A. El Sherbeiny and H. I. El Sissi. Local plants as potential sources of tannins in Egypt. Part IV. (Aceraceae to Flacourtiaceae). **Qual Plant Mater Veg** 1969; 17(4): 384–394.

CP088 Asthana, A., H. V. Mall, K. Dixit and S. Gupta. Fungitoxic properties of latex of plants with special reference to that of croton *Bonplandianus baill*. **Int J Crude Drugs Res** 1989; 27(1): 25–58.

CP089 Le Grand, A. Anti-infectious phytotherapy of the tree-savannah, Senegal (Western Africa) III: A review of the phytochemical substances and antimicrobial activity of 43 species. **J Ethnopharmacol** 1989; 25(3): 315–338.

CP090 Shah, G. L. and G. V. Gopal. Ethnomedical notes from the tribal inhabitants of the North Gujarat (India). **J Econ Taxon Botany** 1985; 6(1): 193–201.

CP091 Webman, E. J., G. Edling and H. F. Mower. Free radical scavenging activity of papaya juice. **Int J Rad Biol** 1989; 55(3): 347–351.

CP092 Itokawa, H., F. Hirayama, S. Tsuruoka, K. Mizuno, K. Takeya and A. Nitta. Screening test for antitumor activity of crude drugs (III). Studies on antitumor activity of Indonesian medicinal plants. **Shoyakugaku Zasshi** 1990; 44(1): 58–62.

CP093 Msonthi, J. D. and D. Magombo. Medicinal herbs in Malawi and their uses. **Hamdard** 1983; 26(2): 94–100.

CP094 Le Grand, A. and P. A. Wondergem. Antiinfective phytotherapy of the savannah forests of Senegal (West Africa). I. An inventory. **J Ethnopharmacol** 1987; 21(2): 109–125.

CP095 Johns, T., J. O. Kokwaro and E. K. Kimanani. Herbal remedies of the Luo of Siaya District, Kenya. Establishing quantitative criteria for consensus. **Econ Bot** 1990; 44(3): 369–381.

CP096 Nagaraju, N. and K. N. Rao. A survey of plant crude drugs of Rayalaseema, Andhra Pradesh, India. **J Ethnopharmacol** 1990; 29(2): 137–158.

CP097 Miwa, M., Z. L. Kong, K. Shinohara and M. Watanabee. Macrophage stimulating activity of foods. **Agr Biol Chem** 1990; 54(7): 1863–1866.

CP098 Kambu, K., L. Tona, S. Kaba, K. Cimanga and N. Mukala. Antispasmodic activity of extracts proceeding of plant antidiarrheic traditional preparations used in Kinshasa, Zaire. **Ann Pharm Fr** 1990; 48(4): 200–208.

CP099 Raja Reddy, K. Folk medicine from Chittoor District, Andhra Pradesh, India, used in the treatment of jaundice. **Int J Crude Res** 1988; 26(3): 127–140.

CP100 Gopalakrishnan, M. and M. R. Rajasekharasetty. Effect of papaya (*Carica papaya*) on pregnancy and estrous cycle in albino rats of wistar strain. **Indian J Physiol Pharmacol** 1978; 22: 66–70.

CP101 Halberstein, R. A. and A. B. Saunders. Traditional medical practices and medicinal plant usage on a Bahamian Island. **Cul Med Psychiat** 1978; 2: 177–203.

CP102 Mell, G. P., R. S. Medora and D. E. Bilderback. Substrate specificity of enzymes from papaya callus cultures. **Z Pflanzenphysiol** 1979; 91: 279–282.

CP103 Ayensu, E. S. Medicinal Plants of the West Indies. **Unpublished Manuscript** 1978; 110pp.

CP104 Devi, S. and S. Singh. Changes in placenta of rat fetuses induced by maternal administration of papain. **Indian J Exp Biol** 1978; 16: 1256–1260.

CP105 Gupta, M. P., T. D. Arias, M. Correa and S. S. Lamba. Ethnopharmacognostic observations on Panamanian medicinal plants. Part 1. **Q J Crude Drug Res** 1979; 17(3/4): 115–130.

CP106 Tang, C. S. Macrocyclic piperidine and piperideine alkaloids in *Carica papaya*. **Trop Foods Chem Nutr** 1979; 1: 55–68.

CP107 Lynn, K. R. A purification and some properties of two proteases from papaya latex. **Biochim Biophys Acta** 1979; 569: 193–201.

CP108 Das, R. P. Effect of papaya seed on the genital organs and fertility of male rats. **Indian J Exp Biol** 1980; 18: 408–409.

CP109 Chan Jr, H. T. and C. S. Tang. The chemistry and biochemistry of papaya. **Trop Foods: Chem Nutr (Proc Int Conf)** 1979; 1979: 33–53.

CP110 Pousset, J., B. Boum and A. Cave. Antihemolytic activity of xylitol isolated from the bark of *Carica papaya*. **Planta Med** 1981; 41: 40-47.

CP111 Rizvi, S. J. H., D. Mukerji and S. N. Mathur. A new report of some possible source of natural herbicide. **Indian J Exp Biol** 1980; 18: 777–781.

CP112 Khan, M. R., G. Ndaalio, M. H. Nkunya, H. Wevers and A. N. Sawhney. Studies on African medicinal plants. Part l. Preliminary screening of medicinal plants for antibacterial activity. **Planta Med** (Suppl) 1980; 40: 91–97.

CP113 Tezuka, H. and K. Kitabatake. Growth-inhibitory activity in papaya latex against Candida species. **Bull Brew Sci** 1980; 26: 47–49.

CP114 Sofowora, E. A. and C. O. Adewunmi. Preliminary screening of some plant extracts for molluscicidal activity. **Planta Med** 1980; 39: 57–65.

CP115 Holdsworth, D. K. Traditional medicinal plants of the North Solomons Province Papau, New Guinea. **Q J Crude Drug Res** 1980; 18: 33–44.

CP116 Dikko, S. B. and J. N. Be Miller. Structural elucidation of a polysaccharide isolated from crude papain. **Diss Abstr Int** 1982; B(43): 1483.

CP117 Sawhney, A. N., M. R. Khan, G. Ndaalio, M. H. H. Nkunya and H. Wevers. Studies on the rationale of African traditional medicine. Part III. Preliminary screening for antifungal activity. **Pak J Sci Ind Res** 1978; 21: 193–196.

CP118 Emeruwa, A. C. Antibacterial substance from *Carica papaya* fruit extract. **J Nat Prod** 1982; 45: 123–127.

CP119 Van Den Berghe, D. A., M. Ieven, F. Mertens, A. J. Vlietinck and E. Lammens. Screening of higher plants for biological activities. II. Antiviral activity. **J Nat Prod** 1978; 41: 463–467.

CP120 Adesina, S. K. Studies on some plants used as anticonvulsants in Amerindian and African traditional medicine. **Fitoterapia** 1982; 53: 147–162.

CP121 Baines, B. S. and K. Brocklehurst. Characterization of papaya peptidase A as a cysteine proteinase of *Carica papaya* L. with active-center properties that differ from those of papain by using 2,2'-dipyridyl disulfide and 4-chloro-7-nitrobenzofuran as reactivity probes. **Biochem J** 1982; 205: 205–211.

CP122 Tiwari, K. C., R. Majumder and S. Bhattacharjee. Folklore information from Assam for family planning and birth control. **Int J Crude Drug Res** 1982; 20: 133–137.

CP123 Chen, C. F., S. M. Chen, S. Y. Chow and P. W. Han. Protective effects of *Carica papaya* Linn. on the exogenous gastric ulcers in rats. **Amer J Chin Med** 1981; 9: 205–212.

CP124 Holdsworth, D. and B. Wamoi. Medicinal plants of the Admiralty Islands, Papau, New Guinea. Part I. **Int J Crude Drug Res** 1982; 20(4): 169–181.

CP125 Rao, R. R. and N. S. Jamir. Ethnobotanical studies in Nagaland. I. Medicinal plants. **Econ Bot** 1982; 36: 176–181.

CP126 Rao, V. S. Pharmacological screening and comparative efficacy of some indigenous anthelmintics. **Abstr 4th Asian Symp Med Plants Spices** Bangkok, Thailand 1980; 1980: 145.

CP127 Vitalyos, D. Phytotherapy in domestic traditional medicine in Matouba-Papaye (Guadeloupe). **Dissertation** - Ph.D.- Univ Paris 1979; 110pp.

CP128 Rojas Hernandez, N. M., C. A. Jimienez Misas, A. M. Lopez Abraham and C. Hernandez Suarez. Study of the inhibitory activity of plant extracts on microbial growth. Part V. **Rev Cubana Farm** 1981; 15: 139–145.

CP129 John, D. One hundred useful raw drugs of the Kani Tribes of Trivandrum Forest Division, Kerala, India. **Int J Crude Drug Res** 1984; 22(1): 17–39.

CP130 Miralles, J. Research on new sources of vegetable oils. **Oleagineux** 1983; 38(12): 665-667.

CP131 Lopez Abraham, A. N., N. M. Rojas Hernandez and C. A. Jimenez Misas. Potential antineoplastic activity of Cuban plants. IV. **Rev Cubana Farm** 1981; 15(1): 71–77.

CP132 Singh, Y. N., T. Ikahihifo, M. Panuve and C. Slatter. Folk medicine in Tonga. A study of the use of herbal medicines for obstetric and gynaecological conditions and disorders. **J Ethnopharmacol** 1984; 12(3): 305–329.

CP133 Arnold, H. J. and M. Gulumian. Pharmacopoeia of traditional medicine in Venda. **J Ethnopharmacol** 1984; 12(1): 35–74.

CP134 Kargbo, T. K. Traditional practices affecting the health of women and children in Africa. **Unpublished Manuscript** 1984.

CP135 Sircar, N. N. Pharmaco-therapeutics of Dasemani drugs. **Ancient Sci Life** 1984; 3(3): 132–135.

CP136 Hashem, F. M., M. Y. Haggag and A. M. S. Galal. A phytochemical study of *Carica papaya* L. growing in Egypt. **Egypt J Pharm Sci** 1980; 21(3/4): 199–214.

CP137 Whistler, W. A. Traditional and herbal medicine in Cook Islands. **J Ethnopharmacol** 1985; 13(3): 239–280.

CP138 Macfoy, C. A. and A. M. Sama. Medicinal plants in Pujehun District of Sierra Leone. **J Ethnopharmacol** 1983; 8(2): 215–223.

CP139 Chinoy, N. J., R. J. Verma, M. G. Sam and O. M. D'Souza. Reversible antifertility effects of papaya seed extract in male rodents. **J Androl** 1985; 6(2): Abstr-M10

CP140 Khan, M. R., G. Ndaalio, M. H. H. Nkunya, H. Wevers. Studies on the rationale of African traditional medicine. Part II. Preliminary screening of medicinal plants for anti-gonoccoci activity. **Pak J Sci Ind Res** 1978; 27(5/6): 189–192.

CP141 Singh, Y. N. Traditional medicine in Fiji. Some herbal folk cures used by Fiji Indians. **J Ethnopharmacol** 1986; 15(1): 57–88.

CP142 Gundidza, M. Screening of extracts from Zimbabwean higher plants II: Antifungal properties. **Fitoterapia** 1986; 57(2): 111–113.

CP143 Weniger, B., M. Rouzier, R. Daguilh, D. Henrys, J. H. Henrys and R. Anthon. Popular medicine of the Central Plateau of Haiti. 2. Ethnopharmacological inventory. **J Ethnopharmacol** 1986; 17(1): 13–30.

CP144 Thomas, K. D. and B. Ajani. Antisickling agent in an extract of unripe pawpaw fruit (*Carica papaya*). **Trans Roy Soc Trop Med Hyg** 1987; 81(3): 510-511.

CP145 Kloss, H., F. W. Thiongo, J. H. Ouma and A. E. Butterworth. Preliminary evaluation of some wild and cultivated plants from snail control in Machakos

District, Kenya. **J Trop Med Hyg** 1987; 90(4): 197–204.

CP146   Kulakkattolickal, A. Piscicidal plants of Nepal. Preliminary toxicity screening using grass carp (Ctenopharyngodon idella) fingerlings. **J Ethnopharmacol** 1987; 21(1): 1–9.

CP147   Kamboj, V. P. A review of Indian medicinal plants with interceptive activity. **Indian J Med Res** 1988; 4: 336–355.

CP148   Koshimizu, K., H. Ohigashi, H. Tokuda, A. Kondo and K. Yamaguchi. Screening of edible plants against possible anti-tumor promoting activity. **Cancer Lett** 1988; 39(3): 247–257.

CP149   Ramirez, V. R., L. J. Mostacero, A. E. Garcia, C. F. Mejia, P. F. Pelaez, C. D. Medina and C. H. Miranda. Vegetales Empleados en Medicina Tradicional Norperuana. Banco Agrario Del Peru & NACL Univ Trujillo, Trujillo, Peru, June 1988; 54pp.

CP150   Kone-Bamba, D., Y. Pelissier, Z. F. Ozoukou and D. Kouao. Hemostatic activity of 216 plants used in traditional medicine in the Ivory Coast. **Plant Med Phytother** 1987; 21(2): 122–130.

CP151   Gonzalez, F and M. Silva. A survey of plants with antifertility properties described in the South American folk medicine. **Abstr Princess Congress I** Thailand, Dec. 1987; 20pp.

CP152   Singh, V. P., S. K. Sharma, and V. S. Khare. Medicinal plants from Ujjain District Madhya Pradesh. Part II. **Indian Drugs Pharm Ind** 1980; 5: 7–12.

CP153   Gupta, A., C. O. Wambebe and D. L. Parsons. Central and cardiovascular effects of the alcoholic extract of the leaves of *Carica papaya*. **Int J Crude Drug Res** 1990; 28(4): 257–266.

CP154   Chopra, R. N., R. L. Badhwar and S. Ghosh. Poisonous Plants of India. Manager of Publications, Government of India Press, Calcutta. Volume 1, 1949.

CP155   Garg, S. K. and G. P. Garg. A preliminary report on the smooth muscle stimulating property of some indigenous plants on isolated rat uterus. **Bull P. G. I.** 1970; 4: 162.

CP156   Khurana, S. M. P. and K. S. Bhargava. Effect of plant extracts on the activity

CP157   of three papaya viruses. **J Gen Appl Microbiol** 1970; 16: 225–230.

CP157   Dhawan, B. N., G. K. Patnaik, R. P. Rastogi, K. K. Singh and J. S. Tandon. Screening of Indian plants for biological activity. VI. **Indian J Exp Biol** 1977; 15: 208–219.

CP158   Malik, M. Y., A. A. Sheikh and W. H. Shah. Chemical composition of indigenous fodder tree leaves. **Pak J Sci** 1967; 19: 171.

CP159   Kobayashi, J. Early Hawaiian uses of medicinal plants in pregnancy and childbirth. **J Trop Pediatr Environ Child Health** 1976; 22: 260.

CP160   Frisbey, A., J. M. Roberts, J. C. Jennings, R. Y. Gottshall and E. H. Lucas. The occurrence of antifungal substances in seed plants with special reference to Mycobacterium tuberculosis (Third report). **Mich State Univ Agr Appl Sci Quart Bull** 1953; 35: 392–404.

CP161   Kafuku, K. and C. Hata. Mokka seed oil. **J Chem Soc Japan** 1932; 53: 439-441.

CP162   Asprey, G. F. and P. Thornton. Medicinal plants of Jamaica. III. **West Indian Med** 1955; J4: 69–82.

CP163   Shukla, O. P. and C. R. Krishna Murti. Bacteriolytic activity of plants latices. **J Sci Ind Res** 1961; C 20: 225–226.

CP164   Shivpuri, D. N. and K. L. Dua. Allergy to papaya tree (*Carica papaya*). **Ann Allergy** 1963; 21: 139–144.

CP165   Tang, C. S. Localization of benzyl glucosinolate and thioglucosidase in *Carica papaya* fruit. **Phytochemistry** 1973; 12: 769-773.

CP166   George, M. and K. M. Pandalai. Investigations on plant antibiotics. Part IV. Further search for antibiotic substances in Indian medicinal plants. **Indian J Med Res** 1949; 37: 169–181.

CP167   Osman, H. G. and E. W. Jwanny. Serological and chemical investigation on the agglutinins of Phaseolus montcalm. **J Chem U A R** 1963; 6(2): 191–204.

CP168   Wasuwat, S. A list of Thai medicinal plants, ASRCT, Bangkok, Report No. 1 on Res. Project. 17. A.S.R.C.T. Bangkok Thailand 1967; 17: 22pp.

CP169   Jamwal, K. S. and K. K. Anand. Preliminary screening of some reputed abortifacient indigenous plants. **Indian J Pharm** 1962; 24: 218–220.

CP170 Chan Jr, H. T., R. A. Heu, C. S. Tang, E. N. Okazaki and S. M. Ishizaki. Composition of papaya seeds. **J Food Sci** 1978; 43: 255.

CP171 Der Marderosian, A. H. Pharmacognosy: Medicinal teas – Boon or bane? **Drug Therapy** 1977; 7: 178–186.

CP172 Giri, J., V. Bhuvaneswari and R. Tamilarasu. Evaluation of the nutritive content of five varieties of papaya in different stages of ripening. **Indian J Nutr Diet** 1980; 17: 319–325.

CP173 Ratwijit, P. and Y. Tanphaibuun. Reducing sugars in fresh raw papaya. Undergraduate Special Project Report 1971: 18pp.

CP174 Pathak, N., P. K. Mishra, B. Manivannan and N. K. Lohiya. Sterility due to inhiobition of sperm motility by oral administration of benzene chromatographic fraction of the chloroform extract of the seeds of *Carica papaya* in rats. **Phytomedicine** 2000; 7(4): 325–333.

CP175 Bhat, G. P. and N. Surolia. In vitro antimalarial activity of extracts of three plants used in the traditional medicine of India. **Am J Trop Med Hyg** 2001; 65(4): 304–308.

CP176 Vieira , R. H., D. Rodrigues, F. A. Goncalves, F. G. Menezes, J. S. Aragao and O. V. Sousa. Microbicidal effect of medicinal plant extracts (*Psidium guajava* Linn. and *Carica papaya* Linn.) upon bacteria isolated from fish muscle and known to induce diarrhea in children. **Rev Inst Med Trop Sao Paulo** 2001; 43(3): 145–148.

CP177 Verma, R. J. and N. J. Chinoy. Effect of papaya seed extract on microenvironment of cauda epididymis. **Asian J Androl** 2001; 3(2): 143–146.

CP178 Kermanshai, R., B. E. McCarry, J. Rosenfeld, P. S. Summers, E. A. Weretilnyk and G. J. Sorger. Benzyl isothiocyanate is the chief or sole anthelmintic in papaya seed extracts. **Phytochemistry** 2001; 57(3): 427–435.

CP179 Sripanidkulchai, B., V. Wongpanich, P. Laupattarakasem, J. Suwansaksri and D. Jirakulsomchok. Diuretic effects of selected Thai indigenous medicinal plants in rats. **J Ethnopharmacol** 2001; 75(2-3): 185–190.

CP180 Lohiya, N. K., L. K. Kothari, B. Manivannan, P. K. Mishra and N. Pathak. Human sperm immobilization effect of *Carica papaya* seed extracts: an in vitro study. **Asian J Androl** 2000; 2(2): 103–109.

CP181 Gandhi, N. N. and K. D. Mukherjee. Papaya (*Carica papaya*) lipase with some distinct acyl and alkyl specificities as compared with microbial lipases. **Biochem Soc Trans** 2000; 28(6): 977–978.

CP182 Udoh, P. and A. Kehinde. Studies on antifertility effect of pawpaw seeds (*Carica papaya*) on the gonads of male albino rats. **Phytother Res** 1999; 13(3): 226–228.

CP183 Sarma, H. N. and H. C. Mahanta. Modulation of morphological changes of endometrial surface epithelium by administration of composite root extract in albino rat. **Contraception** 2000; 62(1): 51–54.

CP184 Lohiya, N. K., P. K. Mishra, N. Pathak, B. Manivannan and S. C. Jain. Reversible azoospermia by oral administration of the benzene chromatographic fraction of the chloroform extract of the seeds of *Carica papaya* in rabbits. **Adv Contracept** 1999; 15(2): 141–161.

CP185 Eno, A. E., O. I. Owo, E. H. Itam and R. S. Konya. Blood pressure depression by the fruit juice of *Carica papaya* (L.) in renal and DOCA-induced hypertension in the rat. **Phytother Res** 2000; 1494): 235–239.

CP186 Cherian, T. Effect of papaya latex extract on gravid and non-gravid rat uterine preparations in vitro. **J Ethnopharmacol** 2000; 70(3): 205–212.

CP187 Hewitt, H., S. Whittle, S. Lopez, E. Bailey and S. Weaver. Topical use of papaya in chronic skin ulcer therapy in Jamaica. **West Indian Med J** 2000; 49(1): 32–33.

CP188 Lans, C., T. Harper, K. George and E. Bridgewater. Medicinal plants used for dogs in Trinidad and Tobago. **Prev Vet Med** 2000; 45(3-4): 201–220.

CP189 Lohiya, N. K., N. Pathak, P. K. Mishra and B. Manivannan. Contraceptive evaluation and toxicological study of aqueous extract of the seeds of *Carica papaya* in male rabbits. **J Ethnopharmacol** 2000; 70 (1): 17–27.

CP190 Starley, I. F., P. Mohammed, G. Schneider and S. W. Bickler. The treatment of pediatric burns using topical papaya. **Burns** 1999; 25(7): 636–639.

CP191 Lohiya, N. K., N. Pathak, P. K. Mishra and B. Manivannan. Reversible contraception with chloroform extract of *Carica papaya* Linn. Seeds in male rabbits. **Reprod Toxicol** 1999; 13(1): 59–66.

7 | Cassia alata

L.

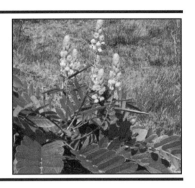

Common Names

Aaku pero	Buka Island	La'au fai lafa	Nicaragua
Akapulko	Philippines	Maliof	Papua-New Guinea
Akapulko	West Africa	Mata pasto	Brazil
Akoria	West Africa	Mhingu	Tanzania
Awunwon	West Africa	Mongrang-jangtong	India
Ayengogo	Guinea	Mula mula	India
Bai nicagi	Guinea	Mulu mulu	Papua
Bakua	Guinea	Njepaa	Sierra Leone
Balilang	Malaysia	Okpo Ndichi	Sierra Leone
Barajo	Guatemala	Palotsina	Philippines
Candelabra bush	Thailand	Pui-chi	Bangladesh
Candle tree	Malaysia	Qanabisi	Nicaragua
Christmas blossom	Nicaragua	Ringworm bush	Fiji
Chum het thet	Thailand	Ringworm bush	Guyana
Chumhet yai	Thailand	Ringworm bush	West Indies
Cortalinde	Guinea-Bissau	Ringworm cassia	Malaysia
Dadmardan	India	Ringworm shrub	Australia
Dadmurdan	Fiji	Roman candle tree	Fiji
Dadrughna	India	Sengseng	India
Galinggang hutan	Indonesia	Serocontil	Nicaragua
Gelenggang	Malaysia	Sindjo-el	Guinea-Bissau
Gelenngang	Indonesia	Sus saika	Nicaragua
Grili	Papua-New Guinea	Sus tara saika	Nicaragua
Kabaiura	Papua-New Guinea	Sus waha tara	Nicaragua
Ketapeng	Indonesia	Tarantan	West Indies
Ketepeng	Indonesia	Te'elango	West Indies
King of the forest	Jamaica	Totoncaxihuitl	Mexico
Kinkeliba	Gabon	Wasemu	Papau
Kislin	Nicaragua	Wild senna	West Indies

BOTANICAL DESCRIPTION

This shrub of the LEGUMINOSAE family may grow up to about 3 meters tall. Leaves are pinnately compound, 30 to 40 cm long, with 6–12 pairs of broad oblong leaflets, blunt at the tip, unequal at the base, the ter-

From: *Medicinal Plants of the World, vol. 1: Chemical Constituents, Traditional and Modern Medicinal Uses, 2nd ed.*
By: Ivan A. Ross © Humana Press Inc., Totowa, NJ

minal pair much larger, about 15 cm long and 8 cm wide. Flowers are roundish in compact axillary racemes, golden-yellow and very showy, about 20 to 30 cm long and 3–4 cm wide. The bracts are 2–3 by 1–2 cm. There are 5 unequal, oblong, 10–20 by 6–7 mm green sepals. The petals are bright yellow, ovate-orbicular to spathulate, short-clawed, 2 by 1–1.5 cm. There are 9–10 stamens; 2 large, 4 small, and 3–4 reduced. The anthers open via apical pores. There is only 1 pistil and glabrous ovary. Fruit are 4-winged pods, 10–15 cm long, dark brown when ripe. There are about 50 seeds, more or less quadrangular, arranged transversely in the pod.

ORIGIN AND DISTRIBUTION

A native of tropical America, it is now widespread in warm countries. The plant grows in waste places, often along streams, banks, and in swamps.

TRADITIONAL MEDICINAL USES

Australia. Hot water extract of dried leaves is taken orally as a cathartic[CA067].

Bangladesh. Fresh leaves are squeezed and rubbed into ringworm[CA016].

Brazil. Decoction of dried leaves is taken orally as an emmenagogue and abortifacient[CA063]. Decoction of dried root is taken orally for malaria. Data were obtained by interviews with more than 8000 natives of various parts of Brazil[CA013].

Buka Island. Fresh leaves are squeezed until soft and rubbed regularly onto the affected part of the body to treat ringworm[CA046].

Fiji. Hot water extract of dried leaves and stem is used externally for ringworm and skin diseases[CA055]. The juice of the leaves and stem is squeezed out and rubbed on the affected area for ringworm and skin infections[CA015]. Infusion of dried leaves is taken orally as a blood purifier for worms and diarrhea[CA055].

Guatemala. Hot water extract of dried bark, leaves, and root is used externally for ringworm[CA034].

Guinea-Bissau. Hot water extract of root is taken orally as an emmenagogue[CA002].

Guinea. A strong decoction of hot water extract of leaves is taken orally to promote abortion, and to treat leprosy[CA034].

India. Fresh leaf juice is used for eczema. Juice from leaves is applied to affected area 3 times daily until cured[CA054]. Fresh leaves are crushed and used for skin diseases, especially ringworm, eczema and scabies[CA051,CA050]. Leaf juice is used externally to treat leukoderma; a poultice of tender leaves is applied for over a month[CA051].

Ivory Coast. Decoction of dried leaves is used externally to treat infections caused by dermatophytes, and orally[CA019] and externally to treat yeast infections caused by *Candida albicans*, as well as orally to treat bacterial infections caused by *Escherichia coli*[CA018].

Jamaica. Hot water extract of dried leaves is taken orally for diabetes[CA049].

Malaysia. Decoction of root is taken orally to ease stomachache[CA028]. Hot water extract of dried leaves is taken orally as a laxative; leaves are used externally against ringworm and scabies; the sap is used externally against external ulcers[CA026].

Mexico. Hot water extract of the plant is used externally as an astringent and against inflammation of rashes, orally as a purgative, anthelmintic and to relieve fever[CA010].

Nicaragua. Fresh leaves are used externally for ringworm and athlete's foot; decoction of the fresh leaves is taken orally for stomachache. It should not be given medicinally to pregnant women; it will induce abortion[CA030].

Nigeria. Dried leaf, powdered with equal amounts of *Piper guineense*, is divided into small portions and taken orally with hot "Pap" to treat indigestion. Decoction of the dried leaves is taken orally to hasten delivery during labor; a strong decoction is taken orally to produce abortion[CA015]. Decoction of dried leaves is used externally for ringworm, eczema and pustular skin infections[CA038]. Infusion of dried leaves is taken orally as a purgative[CA021]. Fresh leaf juice is used externally to treat skin infections[CA047]. Leaf mixed with fruit pulp of *Cucurbita pepo* and *Termitomyces microcarpus* (mushroom) is taken orally to treat gonorrhea[CA029]. The ground inflorescence is mixed with "Pap" and taken orally to treat constipation[CA015].

Papau-New Guinea. Dried leaves are used externally for skin eruptions such as *Tinea imbricata*. Crushed leaves are rubbed on the skin[CA056]. Fresh leaves are used to treat grille, a skin fungus. Crushed leaves are rubbed into the skin affected by grille[CA024,CA025]. Leaf juice is used externally for skin eruptions such as *Tinea imbricata* and ringworm[CA052].

Philippines. Fresh leaves are used to treat fungal infection of the skin. The leaves are crushed and rubbed vigorously on the infected area of the skin[CA037].

Sierra Leone. Decoction of dried leaves is taken orally as a laxative[CA053].

Suriname. Fresh leaves are used externally for ringworm and skin diseases[CA056].

Tanzania. Decoction of leaves is taken orally as a purgative[CA060].

Thailand. Decoction of dried leaves is taken orally for asthma[CA062]; the hot water extract is taken orally as an antipyretic[CA066]. Hot water extract of dried entire plant is taken orally as a cathartic[CA068]. Pulverized flower is taken orally for asthma[CA062]. Hot water extract of dried seeds is taken orally as an anthelmintic[CA068].

Trinidad. Seeds and leaves are used as anthelmntics[CA077].

West Africa. Hot water extract of dried leaves is taken orally as an ecbolic and emmenagogue[CA044]. Hot water extract of fresh leaf juice is used for parasitic skin diseases[CA031]. Strong decoction of hot water extract of leaves is taken orally as an abortifacient[CA001]. Water extract of the leaf is used to treat bacterial infections caused by *Escherichia coli* and fungal infections caused by *Candida albicans* and dermatophytes[CA074].

West Indies. Hot water extract of flowers is used externally as an antibacterial[CA043]. Leaf teas are used for intestinal worms[CA043]. Seeds are taken orally as a vermifuge[CA043].

CHEMICAL CONSTITUENTS

(ppm unless otherwise indicated)

Alatonal: St[CA009]
Aloe emodin: Pl[CA012]
Alquinone: Rt 10[CA008]
Anthraquinone,1-5-dihydroxy-2-methyl: St[CA027]
Anthraquinone,5-hydroxy-2-methyl 1-0-rutinoside: St[CA027]
Benzoquinone, 2-6-dimethoxy: St[CA007]
Beta sitosterol: Rt[CA027]
Chrysarobin: Lf [CA005]
Chrysophanol: Pl[CA004]
Chrysophanol glycoside: Lf[CA005]
Chrysophanic acid: Lf[CA012]
Chrysoeriol-7-0(2-0-beta-D-mannopyranosyl)-beta D-allopyranoside: Sd[CA006]
Dalbergin: St[CA007]
Daucosterol: St[CA007]
Deoxycoeluatin: Lf[CA011]
Emodin: St 3.3[CA020,CA007]
Kaempferol: Lf[CA017]
Luteolin: St[CA007]
Phytosterol: Lf, St Bk[CA017]
Rhamnetin-3-O-(2-O-beta-D-mannopyranosyl)-beta-D-allopyranoside: Sd[CA072]
Rhein: Pl[CA004]
Rhein glycoside: Lf[CA003]
Santal: St[CA007]
Tannin: Lf[CA005]

PHARMACOLOGICAL ACTIVITIES AND CLINICAL TRIALS

Abortifacient effect. Ethanol/water (50%) extract of dried leaves, administered by gastric intubation to rats at a dose of 125.0 mg/kg, was inactive[CA063].

Analgesic activity. Ethanol (85%) extract of dried leaves, administered intraperitoneally to mice at a dose of 100.0 mcg/kg, was active[CA058]. Ethanol/water (1:1) extract of aerial parts, administered intraperitoneally to mice at a dose of 500.0 mg/kg, was inactive vs tail pressure method[CA064]. Leaf extract, administered intraperitoneally to mice and rats, was active using tail clip, tail flick, tail immersion, and acetic acid-induced writhing methods. Maximum analgesic activity was apparent 2 hours after injection of the extract. Fifty mg of kaempferol 3-0-sophoroside appeared equivalent to 100 mg of the extract[CA073].

Antibacterial activity. Chloroform extract of dried leaves, at a concentration of 5.0 mcg/ml on agar plate, was active on *Pseudomonas aeruginosa, Bacillus subtilis, Escherichia coli, Micrococcus luteus,* and *Staphylococcus aureus*[CA038]. The chromatographic fraction, undiluted on agar plate, was active on several Gram positive and Gram negative organisms[CA047]. The acetic acid extract of dried leaves, at a concentration of 5.0 mg/ml, was active on *Bacillus subtilis, Escherichia coli, Micrococcus luteus, Pseudomonas aeruginosa,* and *Staphylococcus aureus*[CA038]. Chloroform extract of dried stem bark, at a concentration of 1.0 mg/disk on agar plate, was active on *Bacillus cereus, Bacillus subtilis, Pseudomonas aeruginosa, Salmonella paratyphi* B, *Salmonella typhi, Shigella dysenteriae, Shigella flexneri, Shigella sonnei* and *Staphylococcus aureus*. It was inactive on *Aeromonas hydrophilia, Escherichia coli, Salmonella paratyphi* A, *Vibrio cholera, Vibrio mimicus* and *Vibrio parahemolyticus*. The methanol extract was active on *Bacillus cereus, Bacillus subtilis, Escherichia coli, Salmonella paratyphi* B, *Salmonella typhi, Shigella flexneri, Shigella sonnei* and *Vibrio cholera,* and inactive on *Aeromonas hydrophilia, Pseudomonas aeruginosa, Salmonella paratyphi* A, *Vibrio mimicus* and *Vibrio parahemolyticus*. The petroleum ether extract was active on

Salmonella paratyphi B and *Shigella flexneri,* and inactive on *Aeromonas hydrophilia, Bacillus cereus, Bacillus subtilis, Escherichia coli, Salmonella paratyphi* A, *Salmonella typhi, Vibrio cholera, Vibrio mimicus,* and *Vibrio parahemolyticus;* active on *Shigella sonnei* at a concentration of 1.4 mg/disk, and *Shigella dysenteriae* and *Staphylococcus aureus,* MIC 0.8 mg/disk[CA017]. Ethanol (85%) extract of dried leaves, at a concentration of 10.0% on agar plate, was active on *Escherichia coli, Proteus vulgaris, Pseudomonas aeruginosa,* and *Staphylococcus aureus*[CA035]. Methanol extract of the dried leaves, at a concentration of 1.0 mg/disk on agar plate, was active on *Bacillus subtilis, Escherichia coli, Salmonella paratyphi* B, *Shigella flexneri, Shigella sonnei,* and *Vibrio cholera,* and inactive on *Aeromonas hydrophilia, Bacillus cereus, Pseudomonas aeruginosa, Salmonella paratyphi* A, *Salmonella typhi, Vibrio mimicus,* and *Vibrio parahemolyticus*. The methanol extract of dried leaves, on agar plate, showed MIC 0.2 mg/disk for *Shigella dysenteriae* and 0.4 mg/disk for *Staphylococcus aureus*. Petroleum ether extract of dried leaves, at a concentration of 1.0 mg/disk on agar plate, was active on *Salmonella paratyphi* B, *Shigella flexneri,* and *Shigella sonnei,* and inactive on *Aeromonas hydrophilia, Bacillus cereus, Bacillus subtilis, Escherichia coli, Pseudomonas aeruginosa, Salmonella paratyphi* A, *Salmonella typhi, Staphylococcus aureus, Vibrio cholera, Vibrio mimicus, Vibrio parahemolyticus,* and *Shigella dysenteriae*[CA017]. Ethanol (95%) extract of dried leaves, at a concentration of 100.0 mg/disk (expressed as dry weight of plant) on agar plate, was active on *Bacillus subtilis,* and inactive on *Escherichia coli, Salmonella typhosa, Shigella dysenteriae,* and *Staphylococcus aureus*. Water extract, at a concentration of 20.0 mg/disk, was inactive on *Bacillus subtilis, Escherichia coli, Salmonella typhosa, Shigella dysenteriae,* and *Staphylococcus aureus*[CA040]. Ethanol (95%) extract of dried leaves, at a concentration of 500.0 mg/

ml on agar plate, was inactive on *Escherichia coli*, *Proteus mirabilis*, *Proteus vulgaris*, and *Staphylococcus epidermidis*. A concentration of 500.0 micromols/ml was inactive on *Staphylococcus aureus*[CA026]. A concentration of 5.0 mg/ml was active on *Bacillus subtilis*, *Escherichia coli*, *Micrococcus luteus*, *Pseudomonas aeruginosa* and *Staphylococcus aureus*[CA038]. Ethanol (95%) extract of leaves, on agar plate, was active on *Bacillus subtilis*, *Escherichia coli*, *Klebsiella pneumonia*, *Serratia marcescens*, and *Staphylococcus aureus*[CA045]. Ethanol/water (1:1) extract of aerial parts, at a concentration of 25.0 mcg/ml on agar plate, was inactive on *Bacillus subtilis*, *Escherichia coli*, *Salmonella typhosa*, *Staphylococcus aureus* and *Agrobacterium tumefaciens*[CA064]. Water extract of dried leaves, at variable concentrations, was active on *Pseudomonas aeruginosa* and *Staphylococcus aureus*[CA014]. The water extract of dried leaves, on agar plate, was active on *Escherichia coli*, LC_{50} 1.0 mg/unit and MIC 1.6 mg/ml[CA019,CA018]. The methanol extract of leaves, flowers, stem, and root bark produced a broad spectrum of antibacterial activity. The activity was increased on fractionation with petrol, dichloromethane and ethyl acetate. The dichloromethane fraction of the flower extract being the most effective[CA076]. Methanol extract of leaves, flowers, stem, and root barks produced a broad spectrum activity. The activity was increased on fractionation with petrol, dichloromethane, ethyl acetate. The dichloromethane fraction of the flower extract was the most effective[CA078].

Anticlastogenic activity. Juice of leaves, administered by gastric intubation to mice at a dose of 25.0 ml/kg, was active on bone marrow cells vs mitomycin C-, dimethylnitrosamine-, and tetracycline-induced micronuclei[CA022].

Anticonvulsant activity. Ethanol/water (1:1) extract of aerial parts, administered intraperitoneally to mice at a dose of 500.0 mg/kg, was inactive vs electroshock-induced convulsions[CA064].

Antifungal activity. Chloroform, acetic acid and ethanol (95%) extracts of dried leaves, at concentrations of 5.0 mg/ml on agar plate, showed weak activity on *Aspergillus fumigatus*, *Lasiodiplodia theobromae*, *Penicillium italicum* and *Trichophyton mentagrophytes*[CA038]. Dried leaf, at a concentration of 20.0% on agar plate, was inactive on *Aspergillus flavus*, *Aspergillus fumigatus*, *Mucor* species, *Penicillium* species, and *Rhizopus* species. Water extract of dried leaves, at concentrations of 80.0%, 90.0%, and 100.0% applied externally on human adults, was active on *Malassezia furfur*. The extract was applied to the neck, hands, and trunk. Pityriasis versicolor was treated[CA069]. Methanol (85%) extract of dried leaves, at a concentration of 2.5% on agar plate, was active on *Microsporum gypseum*, *Trichophyton mentagrophytes*, and *Trichophyton rubrum*[CA059]. Ethanol (95%) extract of dried leaves, at a concentration of 500 mg/ml on agar plate, was active on *Microsporum canis*, *Microsporum gypseum*, *Trichophyton mentagrophytes*, and *Trichophyton rubrum*, and weakly active on *Aspergillus niger*, *Cladosporium werneckii*, *Fusarium solani*, and Penicillium species, and inactive on *Candida albicans*, *Rhodotorula rubra*, and *Saccharomyces cerevisiae*[CA026]. Ethanol/water (1:1) extract of aerial parts, at a concentration of 25.0 mcg/ml, was inactive on *Microsporum canis*, *Trichophyton mentagrophytes*, and *Aspergillus niger*[CA064]. Hot water extract of dried bark, leaf and root, at a concentration of 1.0 ml in broth culture, was inactive on *Epidermophyton floccosum*, *Microsporum canis*, *Microsporum gypseum*, *Trichophyton mentagrophytes* vars. Algodonosa and Granulare, and *Trichophyton rubrum*[CA034]. Juice of the dried entire plant, on agar plate, was inactive on *Epidermophyton floccosum*, *Microsporum gypseum* and *Trichophyton rubrum*[CA041]. Hot water extract of dried leaves, at a concentration of 5.0% on agar plate, was active on *Trichophyton mentagrophytes*[CA048].

Antihistamine activity. Ethanol/water (1:1) extract of dried leaves, at variable concentrations, was active on guinea pig ileum[CA066].

Antihyperglycemic activity. Petroleum ether extract of shade-dried leaves, administered by gastric intubation at a dose of 100.0 mg/kg to rats, was active vs streptozotocin-induced hyperglycemia[CA057].

Anti-inflammatory activity. Ethanol (85%) extract of dried leaves, administered intraperitoneally to mice at a dose of 100.0 mg/kg, was active vs carrageenin-induced pedal edema and cotton pellet granuloma[CA039]. Ethanol/water (1:1) extract of aerial parts, administered orally to rats at a dose of 500.0 mg/kg, was active vs carrageenin-induced pedal edema. Animals were dosed 1 hour before carrageenin injections[CA064]. Shade-dried leaves, administered by gastric intubation to rats at dose of 150.0 mg/kg, were active[CA033].

Antimutagenic activity. Methanol-insoluble fraction of dried flowers was active vs methylnitrosamine, methyl methane sul-fonate, or tetracycline-induced genotoxicity [CA023].

Antipyretic activity. Ethanol/water (1:1) extract of dried leaves, administered by gastric intubation at variable concentrations to rabbit, was inactive vs yeast-induced pyrexia[CA066].

Antispasmodic activity. Ethanol/ water (1:1) extract of dried leaves, at variable concentrations, was active on guinea pig ileum[CA066]. Ethanol/water (1:1) extract of aerial parts was inactive on guinea pig ileum vs ACh- and histamine-induced spasms[CA064].

Antitumor activity. Acid/water, ethanol (95%) and water extracts of dried leaves, administered subcutaneously to mice of both sexes at doses of 0.02 gm/kg, showed weak activity on Sarcoma 37[CA067].

Antiyeast activity. Chloroform, acetic acid, and ethanol (95%) extracts of dried leaves,

at concentrations of 5.0 mg/ml on agar plate, showed weak activity on *Candida albicans*[CA038]. Dried leaf, at a concentration of 20.0% on agar plate, was inactive on *Candida albicans*[CA059]. Ethanol (95%) extract of dried leaves, at concentrations of 20.0 and 100.0 mg/disk on agar plate, were inactive on *Candida albicans*[CA040]. Ethanol/water (1:1) extract of aerial parts, at a concentration of 25.0 mcg/ml on agar plate, was inactive on *Candida albicans* and *Cryptococcus neoformans*[CA064]. Juice of the dried entire plant, on agar plate, was inactive on *Candida albicans*, *Cryptococcus neoformans*, and *Saccharomyces cerevisiae*[CA041]. Water extract of dried leaves, on agar plate, showed IC_{50} 28.0 mg/ml and MIC 0.39 mg/ml on *Candida albicans*[CA019,CA018].

Barbiturate potentiation. Ethanol/ water (1:1) extract of aerial parts, administered intraperitoneally to mice at a dose of 500.0 mg/kg, was inactive[CA064].

Choleretic effect. Leaf extract, administered orally to rats at doses of 15, 30, and 60 mg/kg, was active. Choleretic activity at the 15 mg/kg dose level was better that a group treated with 15 mg/kg of hydroxycyclohexenyl butyrate, a synthetic choleretic. At elevated doses, the extract tends to inhibit bile secretion[CA074].

Diuretic activity. Ethanol/water (1:1) extract of aerial parts, administered intraperitoneally to male rats at a dose of 250.0 mg/kg, was active. Urine was collected for 4 hours post-treatment from saline-loaded animals[CA064].

Embryotoxic effect. Ethanol/water (50%) extract of dried leaves, administered by gastric intubation to rats at a dose of 125.0 mg/kg, was inactive[CA063].

Estrous cycle disruption effect. Ethanol/water (50%) extract of dried leaves, administered by gastric intubation to rats at a dose of 125.0 mg/kg, was equivocal[CA063].

Hypoglycemic activity. Ethanol/ water (1:1) extract of aerial parts, administered orally to rats at a dose of 250.0 mg/kg, was inactive. Less than 30% drop in blood sugar level was observed[CA064]. Hot water extract of dried leaves, administered by gastric intubation to dogs at a dose of 200.0 ml/animal, produced weak activity[CA049]. Petroleum ether extract of shade-dried leaves, administered by gastric intubation to rats at a dose of 400.0 mg/kg, was inactive[CA057]. Leaf extract, administered orally to streptozotocin-induced hyperglycemic rats, reduced the blood sugar value in streptozotocin-induced hyperglycemic rats. The extract had no effect on glucose levels in normoglycemic animals[CA071].

Hypotensive activity. Ethanol/water (1:1) extract of dried leaves, administered intravenously to dogs at variable dosages, was inactive[CA066].

Hypothermic activity. Ethanol/water (1:1) extract of aerial parts, administered intraperitoneally to mice at a dose of 500.0 mg/kg, was inactive[CA064].

Laxative effect. Ethanol/water (1:1) extract of dried leaves, administered orally at variable dosages to human adults, was active. Patients with at least 72 hours of constipation were treated with either placebo or Cassia. Out of 24 patients treated with Cassia, 83% passed stools in 24 hours. The success rate in the placebo group was only 18%[CA032]. Hot water extract of dried leaves, administered by gastric intubation at a dose of 500.0 mg/kg to rats, was active. The extract had 70% of the activity of senna, *Cassia acutifolia*[CA036]. The infusion, at a dose of 800.0 mg/kg, was also active[CA021]. Leaves, administered orally to male albino rats, were active. The leaves of *Cassia acutifolia* Del. was used as reference standard[CA070].

Molluscicidal activity. Ethanol (95%) and water extracts of dried trunk bark, at concentrations of 10,000 ppm, were inactive on *Biomphalaria glabrata* and *Biomphalaria straminea*[CA065].

Pityriasis versicolor effect. Leaf extract has been effective in a 10-year human study with no side effect[CA075].

Semen coagulation effect. Ethanol/water (1:1) extract of aerial parts, at a concentration of 2.0%, was inactive on rat semen[CA064].

Spermicidal effect. Ethanol/water (1:1) extract of aerial parts, at a concentration of 2.0%, was inactive on rat sperm[CA064].

Toxic effect (general). Ethanol (85%) extract of dried leaves, administered intraperitoneally to mice at a dose of 2.0 gm/kg, was inactive[CA058,CA039]. Ethanol/water (1:1) extract of dried leaves, administered by gastric intubation and subcutaneously at doses of 10.0 gm/kg to mice, was inactive[CA042].

Toxicity assessment (quantitative). Ethanol/water (1:1) extract of aerial parts, administered intraperitoneally to mice, showed LD_{50} 1.0 gm/kg[CA064].

Wound healing acceleration. Petrol (gasoline) extract of dried leaves, applied externally to rabbits at a dose of 10.0%, was active. The extract, in the form of a polyethylene glycol ointment, was applied daily to a skin wound that had been inoculated with *Staphylococcus aureus* or *Pseudomonas aeruginosa*. By 21 days, area of wound was 87.6% healed over vs 56.2% on controls[CA061].

REFERENCES

CA001 Quisumbing, E. Medicinal plants of the Philippines. **Tech Bull 16, Rep Philippines, Dept Agr Nat Resources,** Manila 1951; 1.

CA002 Alvaro Viera, R. Subsidio para o Estudio da Flora Medicinal da Guinea Portuguesa. Agencia-Geral do Ultramar, Lisboa, 1959.

CA003 List, P. H. and L. Horhammer. Hager's Handbuck der Pharmazeutischen Praxis. Vols. 2–6. Springer-Verlag. Berlin, 1969–1979.

CA004 Glasby, J. H. Dictionary of Plants Containing Secondary Metabolites. Taylor and Francis. New York. 1991, 488pp.

CA005 Morton, J. F. Major Medicinal Plants, C. C. Thoman , Springfield, IL. 1977. 431pp.

CA006 Gupta, D. and J. Singh. Flavonoid glycosides from *Cassia alata*. **Phytochemistry** 1991; 30(8): 2761–2763.

CA007 Kalidhar, H. S. B. Alatinone, an anthraquinone from *Cassia alata*. **Phytochemistry** 1993; 32(6): 1616–1617.

CA008 Yadav, S. K. and S. B. Kalidhar. Alquinone, an anthraquinone from *Cassia alata*. **Planta Med** 1994; 60(6): 601.

CA009 Kalidhar, S. B. Altonal, an anthraquinone from *Cassia alata*. **Indian J Chem Ser B** 1994; 33(1): 92–93.

CA010 Ortiz de Montellano, B. Empirical Aztec medicine. **Science** 1975; 188: 215–220.

CA011 Mulchandani, N. B. and S. A. Hassarajani. Isolation of 1,3,8-trihydroxy-2-methylanthraquinone from *Cassia alata* leaves. **Phytochemistry** 1975; 14: 2728B.

CA012 Harrison, J. and C. V. Garro. Study on anthraquinone derivatives from *Cassia alata* L. (Leguminosae). **Rev Peru Bioquim** 1977; 1(1): 31–32.

CA013 Brandao, M. G. L., T. S. M. Grandi, E. M. M. Rocha and D.R. Sawyer. Survey of medicinal plants used as antimalarials in the Amazon. **J Ethnopharmacol** 1992; 36(2): 175–182.

CA014 Setiodihardjo, S. H. Tests of antibacterial effect of ointment containing *Cassia alata* L. leaves. **Thesis-MS-Dept Pharm Fac Math & Sci Univ Padjadjaran, Indonesia** 1986.

CA015 Bhat, R. B., E. O. Eterjere and V. T. Oladipo. Ethnobotanical studies from Central Nigeria. **Econ Bot** 1990; 44(3): 382–390.

CA016 Alam, M. K. Medicinal ethnobotany of the Marma Tribe of Bangladesh. **Econ Bot** 1992; 46(3): 330–335.

CA017 Hasan, C. M., S. N. Islam, K. Begum, M. Ilias and A. Hussain. Antibacterial activities of the leaves and stem bark of *Cassia alata* L. **Bangdladesh J Bot** 1988; 17(2): 135–139.

CA018 Crockett, C. O., F. Guede-Guina, D. Pugh, M. Vangah-Manda, T. J. Robinson, J. O. Qlubadewo and R. F. Ochillo. *Cassia alata* and the preclinical search for therapeutic agents for the treatment of opportunistic infections in AIDS patients. **Cell Mol Biol** 1992; 38(5): 505–511.

CA019 Crockett, C. O., F. Guede-Guina, D. Pugh, M. Vangah-Manda, T. J. Robinson, J. O. Qlubadewo and R. F. Ochillo. *Cassia alata* and the preclinical search for therapeutic agents for the treatment of opportunistic infections in AIDS patients. **Cell Mol Biol** 1992; 38(7): 799–902.

CA020 Elisabethsky, E. and Z. C. Castilhos. Plants used as analgesics by Amazonian Caboclos as a basis for selecting plants for investigation. **Int J Crude Drug Res.** 1990; 28(4): 309–320.

CA021 Vu, V. D. and T. T. Mai. Study on analgesic effect of *Cyperus stoloniferus* Retz. **Tap Chi Duoc Hoc** 1994; 1: 16–17.

CA022 Lim-Sylianco, C. Y., J. A. Concha, A. P. Jocano and C. M. Lim. Antimutagenic effects of eighteen Philippine plants. **Philippine J Sci** 1986; 115(4): 293–296.

CA023 Balboa, J. G. and C. Y. Lim-Sylianco. Antigenotoxic effects of drug preparations Akapulko and Ampalaya. **Philipp J Sci** 1992; 121(4): 399–411.

CA024 Holdsworth, D. Medicinal plants of the Gazelle peninsula, New Britain Island, Papau, New Guinea. Part 1. **Int J Pharmacog** 1992; 30(3): 185–190.

CA025 Holdsworth, D and L. Balun. Medicinal plants of the East and West Sepik Provinces, Papau, New Guinea. **Int J Pharmacog** 1992; 30(3): 218–222.

CA026 Ibrahim D. and H. Osman. Antimicrobial activity of *Cassia alata* from Malaysia. **J Ethnopharmacol** 1995; 45(3): 151–156.

CA027 Rai, K. N. and S. N. Prashad. Chemical examination of the stem of *Cassia alata*, Linn. **J Indian Chem Soc** 1994; 71(10): 653–654.

CA028 Ahmad, F. B. and D. K. Holdsworth. Traditional medicinal plants of Sabah, Malaysia, Part III. The Rungus people of Kudat. **Int J Pharmacog** 1995; 33(3): 262.

CA029 Oso, B. A. Mushrooms in Yoruba and medicinal practices. **Econ Bot** 1977; 31: 367.

CA030 Dennis, P. A. Herbal medicine among the Miskito of Eastern Nicaragua. **Econ Bot** 1988; 42(1): 16–28.

CA031 Comley, J. C. W. New macrofilaricidal leads from plants. **Trop Med Parasitol** 1990; 41(1): 1–9.

CA032 Thamlikitkul, V., T. Dechatiwongse et al. Randomized controlled trial of *Cassia alata* Linn. for constipation. **J Med Assoc Thailand** 1990; 73(4): 217–221.

CA033 Abatan, M. O. A note of the anti-inflammatory action of plants of some Cassia species. **Fitoterapia** 1990; 61(4): 336–338.

CA034 Caceres, A., B. R. Lopez, M. A. Giron and H. Logemann. Plants used in Guatemala for the treatment of dermatophytic infections. I. Screening for antimycotic activity of 44 plant extracts. **J Ethnopharmacol** 1991; 31(3): 263–276.

CA035 Palacinchamy, S., E. Amal Bhaskar and S. Nagarajan. Antibacterial activity of *Cassia alata*. **Fitoterapia** 1991; 62(3): 249–252.

CA036 Elujoba, A. A., O. O. Ajulo and G. O. Iweibo. Chemical and biological analyses of Nigerian Cassia species for laxative activity. **J Pharm Biomed Anal** 1989; 7(12): 1453–1457.

CA037 Madulid, D. A., F. J. M. Gaerlan, E. M. Romero and E. M. G. Agoo. Ethnopharmacological study of the Ati tribe in Nagpana, Barotac Viejo, Iloilo. **Acta Manilana** 1989; 38(1): 25–40.

CA038 Ogunti, E. O., A. J. Aladesanmi and S. A. Adesanya. Antimicrobial activity of *Cassia alata*. **Fitoterapia** 1991; 62(2): 537–539.

CA039 Palanichamy, S. and S. Nagarajan. Antiinflammatory activity of *Cassia alata* leaf extract and kaempferol 3-0-sophoroside. **Fitoterapia** 1990; 61(1): 44–47.

CA040 Avirutnant, W. and A. Pongpan. The antimicrobial activity of some Thai flowers and plants. **Mahidol Univ J Pharm Sci** 1983; 10(3): 81–86.

CA041 Achararit, C., W. Panyayong and E. Ruchatakomut. Inhibitory action of some Thai herbs to fungi. **Undergraduate Special Project Report** 1983.

CA042 Mokkhasmit, M., K. Swasdimongkol and P. Satrawaha. Study on toxicity of Thai medicinal plants. **Bull Dept Med Sci** 1971; 12(2/4): 36–65.

CA043 Ayensu, E. S. Medicinal plants of the West Indies. **Unpublished Manuscript** 1978; 110pp.

CA044 Anton, R. and M. Haag-Berrurier. Therapeutic use of natural anthraquinone for other than laxative actions. **Pharmacology Suppl** 1980; 20: 104–112.

CA045 Benjamin, T. V. Analysis of the volatile constituents of local plants used for skin disease. **J Afr Med Pl.** 1980; 3: 135–139.

CA046 Holdsworth, D. K. Traditional medicinal plants of the North Solomons Province Papau, New Guinea. **Q J Crude Drug Res** 1980; 18: 33–44.

CA047 Benjamin, T. V. and A. Lamikanra. Investigations of *Cassia alata*, a plant used on Nigeria in the treatment of skin diseases. **Q J Crude Drug Res** 1981; 19: 93–96.

CA048 Fuzellier, M. C., F. Mortier and P. Lectard. Antifungic activity of *Cassia alata* L. **Ann Pharm Fr** 1982; 40: 357–363.

CA049 Morrison, E. Y. S. A. and M. West. A preliminary study of the effects of some West Indian medicinal plants on blood sugar levels in the dog. **West Indian Med J** 1982; 31: 194–197.

CA050 Rao, R. R. and N. S. Jamir. Ethnobotanical studies in Nagaland. I. Medicinal plants. **Econ Bot** 1982; 36: 176–181.

CA051 Pushpangadan, P. and C. K. Atal. Ethnomedico-botanical investigations on Kerala. I. Some primitive tribals of Western Ghats and their herbal medicine. **J Ethnopharmacol** 1984; 11(1): 59–77.

CA052 Sircar, N. N. Pharmaco-therapeutics of Dasemani drugs. **Ancient Sci Life** 1984; 3(3): 132–135.

CA053 Macfoy, C. A. and A. M. Sama. Medicinal plants in Pujehun District of Sierra Leone. **J Ethnopharmacol** 1983; 8(2): 215–223.

CA054 Tiwari, K. C., R. Majumder and S. Bhattacharjee. Folklore medicines from Assam and Arunachal Pradesh (District Tirap). **Int J Crude Res** 1979; 17(2): 61–67.

CA055 Singh, Y. N. Traditional medicine in Fiji. Some herbal folk cures used by Fiji Indians. **J Ethnopharmacol** 1986; 15(1): 57–88.

CA056 Holdsworth, D., B. Pilokos and P. Lambes. Traditional medicinal plants of New Ireland, Papau New Guinea. **Int J Crude Drug Res** 1983; 21(4): 161–168.

CA057   Palinichamy, S., S. Nagarajan and
        M. Devasagayam. Effect of *Cassia
        alata* leaf extract on hyperglycemic
        rats. **J Ethnopharmacol** 1988; 22(1):
        81–90.

CA058   Palanichamy, S. and S. Nagarajan.
        Analgesic activity of *Cassia alata* leaf
        extract and kaempferol 3-0-sophoro-
        side. **J Ethnopharmacol** 1990; 29(1):
        73–78.

CA059   Palanichamy, S. and S. Nagarajan.
        Antifungal activity of *Cassia alata* leaf
        extract. **J Ethnopharmacol** 1990;
        29(3): 337–340.

CA060   Chabra, S. C., R. L. A. Mahunnah and
        E. N. Mshiu. Plants used in traditional
        medicine in Eastern Tanzania. I. Pteri-
        dophytes and angiosperms (Acan-
        thaceae to Canellaceae). **J Ethno-
        pharmacol** 1987; 21(3): 253–277.

CA061   Palanichamy, S., E. Amala Bhaskar, R.
        Bakthavathsalam and S. Nagarajan.
        Wound healing activity of *Cassia alata*.
        Fitoterapia 1991; 62(2): 153–156.

CA062   Panthong, A., D. Kanjanapothi and
        W. C. Taylor. Ethnobotanical review
        of medicinal plants from Thai tradi-
        tional books, Part 1. Plants with anti-
        inflammatory, anti-asthmatic and
        antihypertensive properties. **J Ethno-
        pharmacol** 1986; 18(3): 213–228.

CA063   Rao, V. S. N., A. M. S. Menezes and
        M. G. T. Gadelha. Antifertility screen-
        ing of some indigenous plants of Bra-
        zil. **Fitoterapia** 1988; 59(1): 17–20.

CA064   Dhawan, B. N., G. K. Patnaik, R. P.
        Rastogi, K. K. Singh and J. S. Tandon.
        Screening of Indian plants for biologi-
        cal activity. VI. **Indian J Exp Biol**
        1977; 15: 208–219.

CA065   Pinheiro de Sousa, M. and M. Z.
        Rouquayrol. Molluscicidal activity of
        plants from Northeast Brazil. **Rev
        Bras Fpesq Med Biol** 1974; 7(4):
        389–394.

CA066   Mokkhasmit, M., K. Swasdimongkol,
        W. Ngarmwathana and U. Permphi-
        phat. Study on toxicity of Thai medici-
        nal plants. (Continued). **J Med Assoc
        Thailand** 1971; 54(7): 490–504.

CA067   Belkin, M. and D. B. Fitzgerald. Tumor-
        damaging capacity of plant materials. 1.
        Plants used as cathartics. **J Nat Cancer
        Inst** 1952; 13: 139–155.

CA068   Wasuwat, S. A list of Thai medicinal
        plants, ASRCT, Bangkok, Report No.
        1 on Res. Project. 17. **A.S.R.C.T.
        Bangkok Thailand** 1967; 17: 22pp.

CA069   Damodaran, S. and S. Venkataraman.
        A study of the therapeutic efficacy of
        Cassia alata Linn. Leaf extract against
        pityriasis versicolor. **J Ethnophar-
        macol** 1994; 42(1): 19–23.

CA070   Elujoba, A. A., O. O. Ajulo and G. O.
        Iweibo. Chemical and biological
        analyses of Nigerian Cassia species for
        laxative activity. **J Pharm Biomed
        Anal** 1989; 7(12): 1453–1457.

CA071   Palanichamy, S., S. Nagarajan and M.
        Devasagayam. Effect of *Cassia alata* leaf
        extract on hyperglycemic rats. **J
        Ethnopharmacol** 1988; 22(1): 81–90.

CA072   Gupta, D. and J. Singh. Flavonoid gly-
        cosides from *Cassia alata*. **Phytochem-
        istry** 1991; 30(8): 2761–2763.

CA073   Palanichamy, S. and S. Nagarajan. An-
        algesic activity of *Cassia alata* leaf ex-
        tract and kaempferol 3-O-sophoroside.
        J Ethnopharmacol 1990; 29(1): 73–78.

CA074   Assane, M., M. Traore, E. Bassene and
        A. Sere. Choleretic effects of *Cassia
        alata* Linn. in the rat. **Dakar Med**
        1993; 38(1): 73–77.

CA075   Damodaran, S. and S. Venkataraman.
        A study on the therapeutic efficacy of
        Cassia alata, Linn. leaf extract against
        Pityriasis versicolor. **J Ethnophar-
        macol** 1994; 42(1): 19–23.

CA076   Khan, M. R., M. Kihara and A. D.
        Omolso. Antimicrobial activity of
        Cassia alata. **Fitoterapia** 2001; 72(5):
        561–564.

CA077   Lans, C., T. Harper, K. George and E.
        Bridgewater. Medicinal plants used
        for dogs in Trinidad and Tobago. **Prev
        Vet Med** 2000; 45(3-4): 2012–2020.

CA078   Khan, M. R., M. Kihara and A. D.
        Omoloso. Antimicrobial activity of
        Cassia alata. **Fitoterapia** 2001; 72(5):
        561–564.

8 | Catharanthus roseus

G. Don.

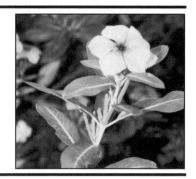

Common Names

Ainskati	India	Patti-poo	Sri Lanka
Atay-biya	Philippines	Periwinkle	Guyana
Billaganneru	India	Periwinkle	India
Boa-noite	Brazil	Periwinkle	Jamaica
Brown man's fancy	West Indies	Periwinkle	Philippines
Caca poule	Dominica	Periwinkle	USA
Chatilla	Guatemala	Periwinkle	West Indies
Chavelita	Peru	Pervenchede	French Guiana
Chichirica	Philippines	Phaeng phoi farang	Thailand
Congorca	Brazil	Phang-puai-fa-rang	Thailand
Consumption bush	West Indies	Pink flower	West Indies
Dua can	Vietnam	Ram goat rose	West Indies
Kantotan	Philippines	Rattanjot	India
Liluvha	Venda	Red rose	West Indies
Madagascan periwinkle	Madagascar	Sada bahar	India
Maua	Kenya	Sada-bahar	Pakistan
Mini-mal	Sri Lanka	Sadaphul	India
Nayantara	Bangladesh	Sailor's flower	West Indies
Nayantara	India	Saponaire	Rodrigues Islands
Nichinich-so	Japan	Tiare-tupapaku-kimo	Cook Islands
Nichinichi-so	Japan	Tsitsirika	Philippines
Ninfa	Mexico	Ushamanjairi	India
Nityakalyani	India	White tulip	West Indies
Old maid	West Indies		

BOTANICAL DESCRIPTION

An erect, bushy perennial herb of the APOCYNACEAE family which grows to 75 cm high, becoming subwoody at the base and profusely branched, the stems containing some milky latex; leaves are opposite in pairs, smooth, oblong-oval, blunt, or rounded at the apex, 2.5 to 9 cm long and 1.5 to 4 cm wide, short-petioled. Flowers borne all year in upper leaf axils, are tubular, 1.5 to 4 cm long, 5-lobed, flaring to a width of 5 cm; color may be white with a yellow eye, white with a crimson eye, or lavender-pink with a crimson eye.

From: *Medicinal Plants of the World, vol. 1: Chemical Constituents, Traditional and Modern Medicinal Uses, 2nd ed.*
By: Ivan A. Ross © Humana Press Inc., Totowa, NJ

ORIGIN AND DISTRIBUTION

The periwinkle is believed to be native of the West Indies but was originally described from Madagascar. It is cultivated as an ornamental plant almost throughout the tropical and subtropical world. It is abundantly naturalized in many regions, particularly in arid coastal locations.

TRADITIONAL MEDICINAL USES

Australia. Hot water extract of dried leaves is taken orally for menorrhagia[CR222]. Hot water extract of leaves is taken orally by human adults for diabetes[CR029]. Hot water extract of root bark is taken orally as a febrifuge[CR029].

Brazil. Decoction of dried root is taken orally for fevers and malaria[CR064]. Hot water extract of dried leaves is taken orally for diabetes[CR109].

China. Hot water extract of the aerial parts is taken orally as a menstrual regulator[CR023,CR127].

Cook Islands. Decoction of dried leaves is taken orally to treat diabetes, hypertension, and cancer; eighteen leaves are boiled in a kettle of water and the cool solution is taken orally as necessary[CR083].

Dominica. Hot water extract of the leaf is taken orally by pregnant women to combat primary inertia in childbirth; the tea is used to treat diabetes[CR215].

England. Hot water extract of dried entire plant is taken orally by human adults for diabetes[CR194].

Europe. Decoction of dried leaf is taken orally for diabetes mellitus[CR112].

France. Hot water extract of entire plant is taken orally as an antigalactagogue[CR023]. Hot water extract of the leaf is taken orally by human adults as an antigalactagogue[CR127].

French Guiana. Hot water extract of entire plant is taken orally as a cholagogue[CR056].

India. Hot water extract of dried entire plant is taken orally by human adults for cancer[CR040]. Hot water extract of the dried leaf is taken orally for Hodgkin's disease[CR134],

menorrhagia, and diabetes[CR222]. Hot water extract of entire plant is taken orally to treat a confirmed (by needle biopsy) case of Hodgkin's disease[CR120]. Hot water extract of leaf[CR207], root[CR127], and twig[CR024] are taken orally for menorrhagia. Pulp of nodes mixed with cow dung is used externally for cuts and wounds[CR085].

Jamaica. Hot water extract of dried leaves is taken orally for diabetes[CR174].

Kenya. Decoction of dried root is taken orally for stomach problems[CR111].

Mexico. Infusion of whole plant is taken orally for cancer[CR078].

Mozambique. Hot water extract of leaves is taken orally for diabetes and rheumatism. Hot water extract of root is taken orally as a hypotensive and febrifuge[CR090].

North Vietnam. Hot water extract of the aerial parts is taken orally as a menstrual regulator[CR023,CR127].

Pakistan. Hot water extract of dried ovules is taken orally for diabetes[CR062].

Peru. Hot water extract of dried entire plant is taken orally by human adults for cancer, heart disease and leishmaniasis[CR200].

Philippines. Hot water extract of dried root is taken orally as an emmenagogue[CR138]. Hot water extract of leaves is taken orally for diabetes mellitus, amenorrhea and menorrhagia[CR002]. Hot water extract of root is taken orally by pregnant women to produce abortion, as an effective emmenagogue, and for dysmenorrhea with scanty flow[CR127,CR001,CR002,CR023,CR022,CR025].

South Africa. Hot water extract of dried leaves is taken orally for menorrhagia and diabetes[CR222]. Hot water extract of leaves is taken orally for menorrhagia[CR127].

South Vietnam. Hot water extract of entire plant is taken orally by human adults as an antigalactagogue[CR127,CR023].

Taiwan. Decoction of dried entire plant is taken orally by human adults to treat diabetes mellitus[CR063] and liver disease[CR199]. Decoction of dried entire plant is taken orally to treat diabetes mellitus[CR063]. Decoction of dried root and stem is taken orally to treat diabetes mellitus[CR073].

Thailand. Hot water extract of dried entire plant is taken orally for diabetes[CR218.]

USA. Hot water extract of leaves is taken orally, and dried leaves are smoked as a euphoriant[CR060.]

Venda. Water extract of dried root is taken orally for venereal disease. *Catharanthus roseus* and *Ximenia caffra* are macerated and soaked in cold water for several hours to 2 days[CR185].

Vietnam. Hot water extract of dried aerial parts is taken orally as a drug in Vietnamese traditional medicine listed in Vietnamese pharmacopoeia (1974 Edition)[CR154.]

West Indies. Hot water extract of leafy stems is taken orally for diabetes. Hot water extract of the entire plant is taken orally for diabetes; the extract of the white variety is used for high blood pressure. Root, infused with whiskey, is taken orally for diabetes. Tea of white flowers and leaves is taken orally by human adults for diabetes[CR125]. Tea prepared from leaf and stem is taken orally as a remedy for diabetes[CR089.]

CHEMICAL CONSTITUENTS

(ppm unless otherwise indicated)

(-)Tabersonine: Pl[CR155]
10-Geraniol hydroxylase: Pl[CR099]
10-Hydroxy deacetyl akuammiline: Call Tiss[CR165]
11-Methoxy tabersonine: Fl 0.10[CR183]
16-Epi vindolinine-N(B)-oxide: Pl 10[CR151]
16-Epi-19-(s) vindoline-N-oxide: Lf[CR175]
16-Epi-trans iso-sitsirikine: Lf 0.20[CR170]
16-Epi-Z-iso-sitsirikine: Lf[CR232]
16-Hydroxy tabersonine: Call Tiss 1.6[CR074], Rt, Co[CR077]
16-Methoxy tabersonine: Cot, Hyp[CR077]
17-Deacetoxy leurosine: Pl[CR187]
17-Deactoxy vincaleukoblastine: Pl[CR187]
19(s) 16-Epi-vindolinine: Lf 39[CR164]
19(s)-Vindolinine: Lf[CR096]
19-20-Cis 16(R) iso-sitsirikine: Pl[CR186]
19-20-Trans 16(R) iso-sitsirikine: Pl[CR186]

19-Acetoxy-11-hydroxy tabersonine: Pl[CR137]
19-Epi, 3-iso ajmalicine: Pl 0.01%[CR169]
19-Epi-ajmalicine: Pl[CR091]
19-Epi-vindolinine: Pl[CR137]
19-Hydroxy-11-methoxy tabersonine: Pl[CR137]
20-Epi-vindolinine: Pl 20.0[CR151]
20-Hydroxy tabersonine: Pl[CR167]
21-Hydroxy cyclochnerine: Pl[CR186]
21'-Oxo leurosine: Lf[CR131]
24-Methylene cholesterol: Pl[CR068]
2-Hydroxy-6-methoxy benzoic acid: Lf[CR105]
3'-4'-Anhydro-vincaleukoblastine: Lf[CR118]
3-Epi-ajmalicine: Call Tiss[CR165]
3-Hydroxy voafrine A: Pl[CR044]
3-Hydroxy voafrine B: Pl[CR044]
3-Iso-ajmalicine: Pl 8[CR151]
4-Deacetoxy vincaleukoblastine: Lf[CR057]
4-Deacetoxy-3'-hydroxy vincaleukoblastine: Lf[CR059]
5' Phosphodiesterase: Call Tiss[CR217]
7-Hydroxy-indolenine ajmalicine: Call Tiss[CR165]
Adenine phosphoribosyltransferase: Pl[CR176]
Adenoside diphosphate: Pl[CR161]
Adenoside triphosphate: Pl[CR161]
Adenosine: Lf[CR048]
Ajmalicine synthetase: Pl[CR088]
Ajmalicine: Call Tiss 100[CR075], Fl 0.3[CR183], Lf 0.2[CR146], St[CR092], Rt 250[CR115]
Ajmaline: Res[CR084]
Akuamicine: Pl[CR168]
Akuammicine: Rt 4[CR017], Lf 0.06[CR146]
Akuammigine: Pl[CR167]
Akuammiline: Pl 5[CR151]
Akuammine: Pl[CR036]
Alpha amyrin acetate: St[CR150]
Alpha-3, 4-anhydrovinblastine synthase: Lf[CR226]
Alstonine: Rt Bk 100[CR212], Rt[CR214]
Ammocalline: Rt 50[CR017]
Ammorosine: Rt 30[CR017]
Amotin: Pl[CR234]
Anthranilate synthetase: Pl[CR140]
Antirhine: Pl 200[CR169]
Aparicine: Lf, Fl[CR197]
Arginine: Pl[CR066]
ATP sulfurylase: Pl[CR124]
Bannucine: Lf 0.1[CR042]
Beta sitosterol: Pl 0.9[CR034]
Calmodulin: Pl[CR204]
Campesterol: Pl[CR068]

Cantharanthine: Pl[CR159]
Carosidine: Lf, Rt[CR219]
Carosine: Lf, Fl[CR036]
Cathalanceine: Pl[CR008]
Catharanhine: Pl[CR004]
Catharanthamine: Lf[CR145]
Catharanthine: Pl 27.8[CR034], Call Tiss 230[CR075]
Catharanthus roseus alkaloid (Mp 300+):
    Lf[CR055]
Catharanthus roseus alkaloid (MW 336):
    Pl[CR119]
Catharanthus roseus alkaloid B: Pl[CR119]
Catharanthus roseus alkaloid C: Pl[CR119]
Catharanthus roseus alkaloid D: Pl[CR119]
Catharanthus roseus iridoid glucoside
    (Mp 194-5): Pl 4[CR015]
Catharicine: Lf[CR219], Fl[CR036]
Catharine: Aer[CR036]
Catharosine: Aer[CR028]
Cathasterone: Pl[CR046]
Cathenamine: Pl[CR086]
Cathindine: Rt 0.7[CR017], Lf[CR016]
Cathovaline: Lf 2.0[CR103]
Cavincidine: Rt 0.2[CR017], Lf[CR016]
Cavincine: Lf, Rt[CR036]
Cholesterol: Pl[CR068]
Choline: Pl[CR066]
Cinnamate 4-hydroxylase: Pl[CR236]
Coronaridine: Pl[CR191]
Deacetoxy vincaleukoblastine: Lf[CR047]
Deacetoxy vindoline: Lf[CR201], Cot, Hyp[CR077]
Deacetyl aduammiline: Lf 0.3[CR184]
Deacetyl akuammiline: Call Tiss[CR165]
Deacetyl vincaleukoblastine: Lf[CR079]
Deacetyl vindoline acetyl transferase:
    Lf[CR094]
Deacetyl vindoline: Lf[CR014], Cot, Hyp[CR077]
Dehydro loganin: Lf, St[CR048]
De-n-methyl vincaleukoblastine: Lf[CR052]
Deoxy loganin: Pl 0.30[CR015]
Deoxy vincaleukoblastine: Lf[CR021]
Diacylglycerol pyrophosphate: Pl[CR045]
Dihydro sitsirikine: Lf, Rt[CR036]
Dihydro vindoline: Pl[CR005]
Dimethyl tryptamine: Pl[CR070]
Diol pseudo vincaleukoblastine: Lf[CR054]
Epi-vindolinine: Lf[CR201]
Extensin: Pl[CR190], Fixed oil, Sd[CR097]
Fluorocarpamine: Lf[CR175]
Fluorocarpamine-N-oxide: Lf[CR175]
Fructose-2-6-bis-phosphate: Pl[CR106]
Geissoschizine dehydrogenase: Pl[CR130]

Geissoschizine: Pl, Call Tiss[CR051]
Geraniol: Pl[CR093]
Glucose: Pl[CR066]
Glutamine: Pl[CR066]
Glycoprotein: Pl[CR132]
Gomaline: Lf 0.1[CR102]
Hemicellulose: Pl[CR172]
Hirsutidin: Call Tiss[CR058], Fl[CR157]
Horhammericine: Lf[CR201]
Indole-3-acetic acid: Fl[CR095]
Iso-fucosterol: Pl[CR068]
Iso-leurosine: Lf[CR011]
Iso-pent-2-enyl adenine riboside:
    Cr Gall 3.92 nMol/gm[CR182]
Iso-pent-2-enyl adenine riboside-5'-mono-
    phosphate: Cr Gall 10.98 nMol/gm[CR182]
Iso-pent-2-enyl adenine:
    Cr Gall 1.55 nMol/gm[CR182]
Isositsirikine: Lf, Rt[CR036]
Isositsirikine: Pl[CR169]
Isovallesiachotamine: Pl[CR069]
Isovincoside: Pl[CR178]
Kaempferol: Lf[CR105]
L-(+)-bornesitol: Rt[CR038]
Lanceine: Pl[CR008]
Leurocolombine: Pl[CR119]
Leurocristine: Pl[CR209]
Leurosidine: Pl[CR209]
Leurosidine-N'-B-oxide: Lf[CR149]
Leurosine: Pl[CR020]
Leurosine-N-oxide: Lf[CR135]
Leurosinone: Lf 1.5[CR043]
Leurosivine: Rt 1[CR017], Lf[CR036]
Linoleic acid: Pl[CR116]
Lirioresinol B, D-glucoside: Pl[CR039]
Lochnerallol: Lf[CR222]
Lochnericine: Pl 25.60[CR034]
Lochneridine: Lf[CR021]
Lochnerine: Pl 64.60[CR034]
Lochnerinine: Pl[CR211]
Lochnerivine: Rt 1[CR017], Lf[CR018]
Lochnerol: Lf[CR222]
Lochrovicine: Lf[CR219]
Lochrovidine: Lf[CR219]
Lochrovine: Lf[CR219]
Loganic acid: Pl, Sd[CR049]
Loganin: Lf[CR048]
Maandrosine: Rt 0.05[CR017]
Malic acid: Pl[CR101]
Malvidin: Call Tiss[CR058], Fl[CR157]
Mannoside: Pl[CR038]
Mevalonate kinase: Lf[CR227]

Minovincinine: Pl 2.0[CR151]
Mitraphylline: Fl 1.0[CR183]
Myricyl alcohol: Lf[CR037]
N-deformyl leurocristine: Lf[CR179]
N-demethyl vincaleukoblastine: Lf[CR012]
Neoleurocristine: Lf[CR219], Pl[CR036]
Neoleurosidine: Aer[CR036]
Nor harman: Lf[CR100]
Oleanolic acid: Pl[CR142]
Oleic acid: Sd oil 56.76%[CR097]
Para-coumaric acid: Lf[CR105]
Pericalline: Pl[CR171], Rt 0.20[CR017]
Pericyclivine: Lf 0.02[CR146]
Perimivine: Lf[CR018]
Perividine: Lf[CR011]
Perivine: Pl 9.30[CR034]
Perosine: Lf[CR016], Rt 0.05[CR017]
Petunidin: Fl[CR157], Call Tiss[CR058]
Phosphodiesterase: Call Tiss[CR210]
Phytochelatin A: Pl[CR041]
Pleiocarpamine: Pl 5.0[CR151]
Pleurosine: Aer[CR036]
Prolyl hydroxylase: Pl[CR152]
Protocatechuic acid: Lf[CR105]
Pseudo-vincaleukoblastinediol: Pl[CR038]
Putrescine: Pl[CR082]
Quercetin: Lf[CR105]
Quinone reductase: Pl[CR231]
Reserpine: Pl[CR167], Call Tiss[CR129]
Rhazimol: Lf 0.2[CR061]
Ricinoleic acid: Sd oil 3.27%[CR107]
Rosamine: Lf[CR181]
Roseadine: Lf[CR189]
Roseoside: Lf, St[CR048]
Rosicine: Lf[CR188]
Rovidine: Lf[CR219]
Seco loganic acid: Pl[CR013]
Seco loganin: Pl[CR049]
Seco loganoside: Pl[CR013]
Serpentine: Pl[CR098], Call Tiss[CR123]
Sitsirikine: Pl 2[CR169]
Stigmasterol: Pl[CR068]
Strictosideine glucosidase 1: Pl[CR139]
Strictosidine glucosidase 11: Pl[CR139]
Strictosidine lactam: Pl[CR168]
Strictosidine synthase: Pl[CR177]
Strictosidine synthetase: Pl[CR117]
Strictosidine: Pl[CR196]
Sulfotransferase: Pl[CR124]
Sweroside: Pl 10.0[CR015]
Syringic acid: Lf[CR105]
Tabersonine: Pl[CR203]

Tetrahydro alstonine: Rt 370[CR213], Fl[CR072], Pl[CR005]
Tetrahydroserpentine: Pl[CR211]
Tryptamine: Pl[CR080]
Tryptophan decarboxylase: Pl[CR113]
Tryptophan synthetase: Pl[CR140]
Tryptophan: Pl[CR140]
Tubotaiwine: Pl[CR104]
Uridine: Pl[CR162]
Ursolic acid: Lf[CR221]
Vallesiachotamine: Pl[CR144]
Vanillic acid: Lf[CR105]
Vinamidine: Lf[CR220]
Vinaphamine: Lf[CR016]
Vinaspine: Lf[CR219]
Vincadioline: Lf[CR050]
Vincaleukoblastine: Pl[CR147], Lf 45–70[CR143]
Vincaline 1: Rt Bk 40.0[CR003]
Vincaline 11: Rt Bk 20.0[CR003]
Vincamicine: Lf[CR021]
Vincarodine: Lf 0.06[CR146]
Vincathicine: Lf[CR016]
Vincolidine: Lf[CR018]
Vincoline: Lf[CR053]
Vincubine: Pl[CR087]
Vindolicine: Lf[CR219], Fl[CR036]
Vindolidine: Lf[CR219]
Vindoline: Lf[CR235], Pl[CR004], Call Tiss[CR129]
Vindolinine: Pl 0.2083%[CR136]
Vindolinine-N(B)oxide: Pl[CR151]
Vindolinine-N-oxide: Pl[CR136]
Vindorosine: Aer[CR027]
Vinosidine: Rt 3.0[CR017]
Vinsedicine: Sd[CR219]
Vinsedine: Sd[CR219]
Virosine: Pl 6.1[CR034], Rt 4.0[CR017]
Vivaspine: Lf[CR016]
Yohimbine: Pl 300[CR169]
Zeatin glucosyl: Rt, Lf, Fl[CR158]
Zeatin riboside-5'-monophosphate: Cr Gall[CR182]
Zeatin ribosyl: Rt, Fl, Lf[CR158]
Zeatin: Cr Gall, Rt, Lf, Fl[CR158]
Zeatin-9-riboside: Cr Gall[CR182]

PHARMACOLOGICAL ACTIVITIES AND CLINICAL TRIALS

Abortifacient effect. Ethanol/water (1:1) extract of seed pods, administered orally to rats at a dose of 100.0 mg/kg, was inactive[CR216].

Acid phosphatase inhibition. Ethanol (95%) extract of leaves, administered orally to male rats at a dose of 75.0 mg/kg daily for 24 days and autopsy on day 25, was active. The control group (10 animals) had an enzyme level of 102 mcg/100 mg in testes. Extract treated group was 162.5 mcg/100 mg. Control group enzyme level was 178.57 mcg/100 mg in prostate; extract treated group was 68.75 mcg/100 mg[CR126].

Acid phosphatase stimulation. Ethanol (95%) extract of leaves, administered orally to male rats at a dose of 300.0 mg/kg daily for 24 days and autopsy on day 25, was active. Control group (10 animals) enzyme level was 102 mcg/100 mg in testes; extract treated group was 400 mcg/100 mg. Control group enzyme level in prostate was 178.57 mcg/100 mg; extract treated group was 447.92 mg/100 mg. Ethanol (95%) extract of leaves, administered orally to male rats at a dose of 75.0 mg/kg daily for 24 days and autopsy on day 25, was active. Control group (10 animals) enzyme level was 132.14 mcg/100 mg in testes; extract treated group was 427.08 mcg/100 mg. Control group enzyme level in prostate was 720.83 mcg/100 mg; extract treated group was 1183.33 mcg/100 mg[CR126].

Alkaline phosphatase stimulation. Ethanol (95%) extract of leaves, administered orally to male rats at a dose of 300.0 mg/kg daily for 24 days and autopsy on day 25, was active. Control group (10 animals) enzyme level was 1132.14 mcg/100 mg in testes; extract treated group was 954.17 mcg/100 mg. Control group enzyme level in prostate was 720.83 mcg/100 mg; extract treated group was 1716.66 mcg/100 mg[CR126].

Alkylating activity reduction. Fresh root juice and hot water extract of dried leaves produced weak activity. There was reduction of alkylating activity of ethyl methane sulfonate toward 4-para-nitro-benzylpyridine[CR148].

Animal repellent activity. Dried leaf and stem, at variable concentrations, were active on Helix pomatia[CR180].

Antiascariasis activity. Alkaloid fraction of the entire plant produced weak activity on earthworm[CR031].

Antibacterial activity. Benzene extract of dried flowers, at a concentration of 5.0% on agar plate, was active on Proteus, Pseudomonas, Shigella and Staphylococcus species, and inactive on Salmonella species and Shigella paradysenteriae. Benzene extract of leaves, at a concentration of 5.0% on agar plate, was active on Proteus, Pseudomonas, Salmonella, Shigella and Staphylococcus species[CR197]. Ethanol (70%) extract of dried leaves, on agar plate, was active on Bacillus megaterium and Staphylococcus albus, and inactive on Bacillus cereus and Staphylococcus aureus[CR173]. Ethanol (95%) extract of fresh root, on agar plate, was active on Shigella flexneri, Streptococcus faecalis and Vibrio cholera, and produced weak activity on Corynebacterium diptheriae, Diplococcus pneumoniae, Salmonella paratyphi A, Shigella dysenteriae, and Staphylococcus aureus. Ethanol (95%) extract of fresh shoots, on agar plate, was active on Corynebacterium diphtheriae, Diplococcus pneumoniae and Staphylococcus aureus, and produced weak activity on Salmonella paratyphi B[CR224]. Total alkaloids of root, at a concentration of 500.0 mcg/ml in broth culture, were inactive on Escherichia coli, Salmonella typhosa, and Shigella dysenteriae. Weak activity was produced on Staphylococcus aureus, MIC 200.0 mcg/ml and Vibrio cholera, MIC 300.0 mcg/ml[CR026]. Water extract of entire plant, on agar plate at a concentration of 1:4, was inactive on Salmonella paratyphi A, Salmonella typhosa and Shigella flexneri, and produced weak activity on Escherichia coli, Salmonella paratyphi B, Staphylococcus aureus and Vibrio cholera[CR031].

Antidiuretic activity. Alkaloid fraction of the entire plant, administered subcutaneously to male rats at a dose of 50.0 mg/kg, was active[CR031].

Antifertility effect. Methanol/water (1:1) extract of dried leaf and stem, administered orally to male rats, was active[CR141]. The leaf extract, administered orally to rats, produced widespread testicular necrosis, hyalinization of tubules and sertoli cell-only-syndrome. Biochemical studies revealing notable reduction in glycogen and fructose levels in reproductive tissues supported the histological observations[CR233].

Antifungal activity. Acetone and water extracts of dried aerial parts, at a concentration of 50% on agar plate, was inactive on *Neurospora crassa*; the ethanol (95%) extract was active[CR225]. Aqueous low speed supernatant of fresh leaves, at a concentration of 100.0 ml/liters in broth culture, produced weak activity on *Hendersonula toroidea*[CR192]. Dried flower extract was active on *Trichophyton rubrum*[CR163]. Hot water extract of dried leaves, in broth culture, was active on *Trichophyton mentagrophytes*[CR108]. Hot water extract of dried stem, in broth culture, was active on *Trichophyton mentagrophytes*, and weakly active on *Trichophyton rubrum*[CR163]. Leaves and roots, on agar plate, were active on *Pythium aphanidermatum*[CR076].

Antihypercholesterolemic activity. Hot water extract of dried leaves, administered orally to rabbits, was active[CR128].

Antihyperglycemic activity. Dried leaves, in the ration of male mice at a concentration of 6.25% of the diet for 28 days, were inactive vs streptozotocin-induced hyperglycemia[CR112]. Ethanol (95%) extract of dried leaves, administered intragastrically to rats at a dose of 100.0 mg/kg, was active. In streptozotocin-induced diabetic animals, treatment with extract decreased serum glucose by 20.67%[CR206]. Extract, at a dose of 75.0 mg/animal administered intraperitoneally, was active vs streptozotocin-induced hyperglycemia[CR198]. Hot water extract of dried aerial parts,

administered intragastrically to dogs at a dose of 50.0 gm/kg (dry weight of plant), was inactive; a dose of 10.0 gm/kg administered intragastrically to rabbits was active vs alloxan-induced hyperglycemia[CR035]. Water extract of dried entire plant, administered intravenously to rats at a dose of 10.0 mg/kg, was inactive vs streptozotocin-induced hyperglycemia[CR063]. Water extract of fresh cells, administered intragastrically to male rats, was active vs streptozotocin-induced hyperglycemia. A 60% decrease in blood sugar was observed[CR081]. Hot water extract of dried entire plant, administered by gastric intubation to rats at a dose of 3.0 gm/kg daily for 3 days, was inactive vs alloxan-induced hyperglycemia[CR153].

Antihypertensive activity. Total alkaloids of root, administered intravenously to dogs at a dose of 4.0 mg/kg, were active. There was a drop in blood pressure of 40 to 50% for 2 hours in hypertension produced by slow intravenous epinephrine infusion[CR026].

Anti-inflammatory activity. Ethanol (95%) extract of dried leaves, administered intraperitoneally to rats at a dose of 400.0 mg/kg, was active. Edema was inhibited 65%[CR067].

Antimalarial activity. Chloroform extract of root, at a dose of 400.0 mg/kg, and water extract, at a dose of 4.42 gm/kg administered orally to chicken, produced weak activity on *Plasmodium gallinaceum*[CR006].

Antimitotic activity. Ethanol (70%) extract of leaves, administered intraperitoneally to female mice, was active on CA-Ehrlich ascites vs induction of metaphase arrest in ascitic cells. Dosing was done 4 days after tumor cell inoculation. Ascitic samples removed 2, 4, 6, and 24 hours post-treatment[CR121].

Antimutagenic activity. Hot water extract of dried leaves was active on red blood cells. There was a reduction in number of micronucleated polychromatic red blood cells caused by various mutagens[CR160].

Antineoplastic activity. The alkaloid, 16-epi-Z-iso-sitsirikine from the leaves, was active in the KB test system in vitro and the P-388 test system in vivo[CR232].

Antispasmodic activity. Total alkaloids of root, at a concentration of 1:20, were active on rabbit duodenum vs ACh-induced spasms[CR026].

Antispermatogenic effect. Hot water extract of dried leaves, administered intraperitoneally to male mice at a dose of 0.2 ml/animal, produced weak activity. Dosing was equivalent to 10 mg of dried material daily for 15 days followed by sacrifice. There was a slight decrease in sperm concentration, from about 77 million/ml to about 52 million/ml. The levels achieved, taking all parameters together, might impair fertility, but did not necessarily achieve 100% antifertility effectiveness. There was a slight decrease in motility parameters (% motility and duration of motility) and a slight increase in percentage of abnormal and dead sperm[CR202]. At a dose of 10.0 mg/animal, regressive changes in seminiferous tubules and Leydig cells, increased cholesterol in testes and degeneration of all germinal elements other than were observed[CR205]. Total alkaloids, administered intraperitoneally to male rats, were active[CR009].

Antitumor activity. Ethanol (70%) extract of leaves, administered intraperitoneally to female mice, was active on CA-Ehrlich ascites[CR122]. Alkaloid fraction of dried leaves, used externally, was active. Nineteen patients with either flat, verruca vulgaris, plantar or genital warts were treated in this study. Six patients had all warts disappear, 7 had the majority of their warts disappear, 5 had 50% disappear, and 1 showed no response[CR110]. Alkaloid fraction of dried leaves, administered intraperitoneally to mice at doses of 2.5 and 20.0 mg/kg, was active on Leuk-P388, 116% and 150% ILS, respectively[CR145]. Chloroform extract of leaves was active on Leuk-P388[CR007]. Ethanol (95%) extract of entire plant, administered intraperitoneally to mice at a dose of 120.0 mg/kg, was active on Leuk-P1534. Total alkaloids of the entire plant, administered to mice intraperitoneally at a dose of 10.0 mg/kg and orally at a dose of 75.0 mg/kg, were active on Leuk-P1534[CR019]. Leaf extract, administered intravenously to human adults of both sexes at a dose of 6.0 mg/sq. meter body surface, was active on human cancer. Eighty percent mean reduction of leukocyte count was observed in all of the 16 patients treated. Five patients were in the terminal phase of positive chronic myelocytic leukemia, 1 patient had chronic myelomonocytic leukemia[CR114]. Alkaloid fraction of leaf, administered intraperitoneally to mice at a dose of 35.0 mg/kg, was active on CA-Ehrlich ascites, 70% ILS. A dose of 10.0 mg/kg, administered intraperitoneally to rats, was inactive on hepatoma, 12% TWD, and a dose of 35.0 mg/kg was active on sarcoma (Yoshida ASC), 40% ILS vs resistance of heat-induced hemolysis of rat RBC[CR208]. Ethanol extract of the leaf, at a dose of 25.0 microgram/disc using potato disk bioassay technique, significantly inhibited crown gall tumors caused by *Agrobacterium tumefaciens*[CR230]. Amotin, a structure that differs in terpenoid moiety structure of the indole part of the molecule from vinblastine, exhibited a high antileukemic activity which was more expressed than that of vinblastine. Tolerant doses produced moderate reversible morphological alterations in hematopoietic organs, gastrointestinal mucosa, liver, kidney, adrenals, testes, and ovaries[CR234].

Antiviral activity (plant pathogens). Water extract of callus tissue, in cell culture, was active on Tobacco Mosaic virus[CR133].

Cardiotonic activity. Ethanol (70%) extract of leaf and stem, administered intravenously to guinea pigs, was inactive[CR030].

CNS depressant activity. Total alkaloids of root, administered intraperitoneally to rats at a dose of 120.0 mg/kg, were active[CR026].

Cytotoxic activity. Alkaloid fraction of dried leaves, in cell culture, was active on CA-9KB, ED_{50} 0.045 mcg/ml[CR145]. Chloroform extract and culture filtrate of callus tissue, in cell culture at doses of 50.0 gm (dry weight of plant), were active on Leuk-L1210 culture. Chloroform extract of culture filtrate, at a dose of 0.75 mg/ml in cell culture, was active on Leuk-L1210[CR193]. Chloroform extract of leaves was active on CA-9KB[CR007]. Ethanol (95%) extract of leaves, in cell culture, was active on CA-9KB, ED_{50} < 20.0 mcg/ml[CR055]. Ethanol (70%) extract of leaves, in cell culture, was active on CA-Ehrlich ascites[CR122]. Water extract of dried root, in cell culture, was active on CA-9KB, ED_{50} 11.0 mcg/ml[CR071]. Water extract of dried stem, in cell culture, was active on CA-9KB, ED_{50} < 17.0 mcg/ml[CR071]. Water extract of leaves, in cell culture, was active on CA-9KB, ED_{50} < 2.5 mcg/ml[CR071]. Ethanol (95%) extract of seed pods, administered orally to rats at a dose of 100.0 mcg/kg, was inactive[CR216].

Glutamate pyruvate transaminase inhibition. Ethanol/water (1:1) extract of dried entire plant, at a concentration of 1.0 mg/ml in cell culture, was inactive on rat liver cell vs carbon tetrachloride-induced hepatotoxicity and PGE-1-induced pedal edema[CR199].

Hyperglycemic activity. Ethanol/water (1:1) extract of dried entire plant, administered orally to rabbits at a dose of 5.0 gm/kg, was active. There was a 51% increase in blood sugar. All animals died 6 days after dosing[CR218]. Water extract of dried entire plant, administered intravenously to rats at a dose of 5.0 mg/kg, was active vs streptozotocin-induced hyperglycemia[CR063].

Hypoglycemic activity. Dried leaf, in the ration of male mice at a concentration of 6.25% of the diet for 28 days, was inactive[CR112]. Ethanol (95%) extract of dried leaves, administered intragastrically to rats at a dose of 100.0 mg/kg, was active. Serum glucose concentration fell 26.22% in treated animals. Extract potentiated effect of exogenous insulin as well. Hot water extract, administered orally to rabbits, was also active[CR128]. Ethanol/water (1:1) extract of dried entire plant, administered orally to rabbits at a dose of 5.0 gm/kg, was inactive. All of the animals died within 6 days of dosing[CR218]. Hot water extract of dried entire plant, administered by gastric intubation to rats at a dose of 3.0 gm/kg daily for 3 days, was inactive[CR153]. Hot water extract of dried leaves (20 gm of air-dried leaves), administered by gastric intubation to dogs at a dose of 200.0 ml/animal, was active[CR174]. Hot water extract of the dried aerial parts, administered intragastrically to dogs and rabbits at doses of 50.0 and 20.0 gm/kg (dry weight of plant), respectively, was inactive[CR035]. Dichloromethane/methanol (1:1) extract of leaves and twigs, administered orally to rats at a dose of 500 mg/kg for 7 and 15 days, showed 48.6 and 57.6% hypoglycemic activity, respectively. Prior treatment, at the same dose for 30 days, provided complete protection against streptozotocin challenged rats. Enzymatic activities of glycogen synthase, glucose 6-phosphate-dehydrogenase, succinate dehydrogenase, and malate dehydrogenase were decreased in the liver of diabetic rats in comparison to normal and were significantly improved after treatment with the extract for 7 days[CR229]. Leaf extract, administered orally to rats, was active vs streptozotocin-induced diabetes. Blood sugar lowering activity of the extract and tolbutamide was calculated by ED_{50} values, results significant at $P < 0.05$ level[CR238].

Hypotensive activity. Total alkaloids of root, administered intravenously to rabbits at a dose of 0.10 gm/kg, were active[CR032]. Total alkaloids of root, administered intravenously to dogs at a dose of 5.0 mg/kg, were active. There was a 50 to 60% drop in blood pressure over 2 hours[CR026]. Alkaloid fraction of the entire plant, administered intravenously to dogs at a dose of 5.0 mg/kg, produced weak activity[CR031].

Inotropic effect (negative). Total alkaloids of root, at a dose of 5.0 mg, were active on rabbit heart[CR026].

Insect feeding deterrent. Alkaloid fraction of fresh leaves at a concentration of 0.06%, water extract at a concentration of 0.60% and methanol extract at a concentration of 0.25% of the diet, were active on *Spodoptera littoralis*[CR156].

Insect sterility induction. Total alkaloids of dried leaves, at a concentration of 0.5%, were inactive on *Dysdercus cingulatus*. Total alkaloids of dried root, at a concentration of 0.5%, were active on *Dysdercus cingulatus*[CR166].

Insecticidal activity. Water extract of dried branch and leaf, at variable concentrations, was inactive on *Blatella germanica*. Intravenous dose of 40.0 ml/kg, administered to *Periplaneta americana*, was also inactive[CR223].

Insulin activity. Ethanol (95%) extract of dried leaves, at a concentration of 25.0 mg/ml, was inactive. Extract did not stimulate glucose uptake or glycogen deposition but inhibited insulin's activities[CR065].

Larvicidal activity. Petroleum ether extract of dried flower, leaf, seed, and stem, at a concentration of 100.0 ppm, was active on *Anopheles stephensi* larvae; a concentration of 50.0 ppm was active on *Aedes aegypti* and a concentration of 80.0 ppm was active on *Culex quinquefasciatus*[CR195].

Leukopenic activity. Alkaloid fraction of leaves, administered intravenously to dogs at a dose of 2.5 mg/kg, 10 daily injections, was active[CR208]. Water extract of leaves, administered intraperitoneally to rats, was active[CR010].

Peroxidase activity. Cell suspension cultured in the phytohormone, auxin 2,4-D, reduced the peroxidase activity in the medium and cellular compartments, and ionically cell wall bound peroxidase. Qualitative analysis showed that 2,4-D, but not cytokinins, regulated the synthesis of a basic isoform. The presence of the basic peroxidase is correlated with the capacity of cells to produce indole alkaloids. The isolated peroxidase is a haem protein with a M(r) of 33,000 and a pH close to 9. The effect of pH on peroxidase activity was studied using guaiacol as substrate and the optimum pH determined to be 6.0[CR237].

Phospholipase C activity. Roots, treated with aluminum (0.1 mM) for 0-4 hours, inhibited phospolipase activity. A concentration of 1 mM diminished root growth in approximately 50% when added on the first day of the culture cycle conditions in phospholipase activity was also affected. The activity was inhibited in a concentration and time-dependent fashion. The effect was similar for both soluble and membrane-associated activities. NAD+-GDH, NADH-GDH, NADH-GOGAT and HMGR were not affected when roots were treated with 0.1 mM aluminum for 1 hour[CR228].

Smooth muscle relaxant activity. Total alkaloids of root, administered intravenously to dogs at a dose of 2.0 mg/kg, were active[CR026].

Spasmogenic activity. Total alkaloids of root produced weak activity on rat intestine[CR032].

Toxic effect (general). Ethanol (95%) extract of leaves, administered orally to male rats at a dose of 75.0 mg/kg daily for 24 days and autopsy on day 25, was active. Marked reduction in weights of testes and prostate in extract-treated animals was observed[CR126]. Water extract of root, administered subcutaneously to mice at a dose of 10.0 gm/kg, was inactive. Total alkaloids, at a dose of 0.05 gm/kg, were active; 20% of the animals died[CR032].

Toxicity assessment (quantitative). Alkaloid fraction of entire plant, administered intraperitoneally to mice, produced LD_{50} 4.0 ml/kg[CR033]. Total alkaloids of root, administered intraperitoneally to rats, produced LD_{50} 100.0 mg/kg and MLD 150.0 mg/kg[CR026]. **Uterine relaxation effect.** Alkaloid fraction of the entire plant was inactive on the pregnant uterus of rats[CR031].

Uterine stimulant effect. Alkaloid fraction of the entire plant was inactive on the pregnant uterus of rats. Hot water extract of root was inactive on nonpregnant uterus of cat. Total alkaloids of root were inactive in guinea pigs[CR026].

Weight loss. Ethanol (95%) extract of leaves, administered orally to male rats at doses of 75.0 and 300.0 mg/kg daily for 24 days and autopsy on day 25, was inactive[CR126].

REFERENCES

CR001   Quisumbing, E. Medicinal plants of the Philippines. Tech Bull 16, Rep Philippines, Dept Agr Nat Resources, Manilla 1951; 1.

CR002   Zaguirre, J. C. Guide notes of bed-size preparations of most common local (Philippines) medicinal plants, 1944.

CR003   Ramiah, N. Occurrence of liquid alkaloids in *Vinca rosea*. **J Indian Chem Soc** 1964; 41: 552.

CR004   Leete, E., A. Ahmad and I. Kompis. Biosynthesis of the Vinca alkaloids. I. Feeding experiments with tryptophan-2-C14 and acetate-1-C14. **J Amer Chem Soc** 1965; 87: 4168.

CR005   Roger, D. and K. Stolle. A new alkaloid from *Catharanthus roseus*. **Naturwissenschaften** 1964; 51: 637.

CR006   Spencer, C. F., F. R. Koniuszy, E. F. Rogers et al. Survey of plants for antimalarial activity. **Lloydia** 1947; 10: 145–174.

CR007   Cordell, G. A., S. G. Weiss and N. R. Farnsworth. Structure elucidation and chemistry of Catharanthus alkaloids. XXX. Isolation and structure of vincarodine. **J Org Chem** 1974; 39(4): 431–434.

CR008   Patterson, B. D. and D. P. Carew. Growth and alkaloid formation in *Catharanthus roseus* tissue cultures. **Lloydia** 1969; 32: 131.

CR009   Joshi, M. S. and R. Y. Ambaye. Effect of alkaloids from *Vinca rosea* on spermatogenesis in male rats. **Indian J Exp Biol** 1968; 6: 256,257.

CR010   Noble, R. L., C. T. Beer and J. H. Cutts. Role of chance observations in chemotherapy: *Vinca rosea*. **Ann NY Acad Sci** 1958; 76: 882.

CR011   Svoboda, G. H. Alkaloids of *Vinca rosea* (*Catharanthus roseus*). XX. Perividine. **Lloydia** 1963; 26: 243.

CR012   Jovanovics, K., K. Szasz, G. Pekete, E. Bittner E. Dezseri and J. Eles. Increasing the yield of vincristine when separating vincristine from *Vinca rosea* drug. **Patent-S Afr** 08,534 1973; 72.

CR013   Guarnaccia, R. and C. J. Coscia. Occurrence and biosynthesis of secologanic acid in *Vinca rosea*. **J Amer Chem Soc** 1971; 93: 6320.

CR014   Groger, D., K. Stolle and C. P. Falshaw. Isolation of desacetylvindoline from *Catharanthus roseus*. **Naturwissenschaften** 1965; 52: 132.

CR015   Bhakuni, D. S. and R. S. Kapil. Monoterpene glycosides from *Vinca rosea*. **Indian J Chem** 1972; 10: 454.

CR016   Svoboda, G. H. and A. J. Barnes, Jr. Alkaloids of *Vinca rosea* Linn. (*Catharanthus roseus* G. Don) XXXIV. Vinaspine, vincathicine, rovidine, desacetyl vlb and vinphamine. **J Pharm Sci** 1964; 53: 1227.

CR017   Svoboda, G. H., A. T. Oliver and D. R. Bedwell. Alkaloids of *Vinca rosea* (*Catharanthus roseus*). XIX. Extraction and characterization of root alkaloids. **Lloydia** 1963; 26: 141.

CR018   Svoboda, G. H., M. Gorman and R. H. Tust. Alkaloids of *Vinca rosea* (*Catharanthus roseus*). XXV. Lochrovine, perimivine, vincoline, lochrovidine, lochrovicine and vincolidine. **Lloydia** 1964; 27: 203.

CR019   Johnson, I. S., H. F. Wright, G. H. Svoboda and J. Vlantis. Antitumor principles derived from *Vinca rosea*. 1. Vincaleukoblastine and leurosine. **Cancer Res** 1960; 20: 1016.

CR020   Svoboda, G. H. A note on several new alkaloids from *Vinca rosea*. I. Leurosine, virosine, perivine. **J Amer Pharm Ass Sci Ed** 1958; 47: 834.

CR021   Svoboda, G. H., M. Gorman, N. Neuss and A. J. Barnes, Jr. Alkaloids of *Vinca rosea* (*Catharanthus roseus*). VIII. Preparation and characterization of new minor alkaloids. **J Pharm Sci** 1961; 50: 409.

CR022   Steenis-Kruseman, M. J. Van. Select Indonesian medicinal plants. **Organiz Sci Res Indonesia Bull** 1953; 18: 1.

CR023   Farnsworth, N. R. The pharmacognosy of the periwinkles: Vinca and Catharanthus. **Lloydia** 1961; 24(3): 105–138.

CR024   Oliver-Bever, B. Selecting local drug plants in Nigeria. Botanical and Chemical relationship in three families. **Q J Crude Drug Res** 1968; 8(2): 1194.

CR025   ANON, Description of the Philippines. Part I., Bureau of Public Printing, Manila, 1903.

CR026   Chopra, I. C., K. S. Jamwal, C. L. Chopra, C. P. N. Nair and P. P. Pillay. Preliminary pharmacological investigations of total alkaloids of *Lochnera rosea* (Rattonjot). **Indian J Med Res** 1959; 47: 40.

CR027   Moza, B. K. and J. Trojanek. New alkaloids from *Catharanthus roseus*. **Chem Ind (London)** 1962; 1962: 1425.

CR028   Moza, B. K. and J. Trojanek. Catharosine, a new alkaloid from *Catharanthus roseus*. **Chem Ind (London)** 1965; 1965: 1260.

CR029   Webb, L. J. Guide to the medicinal and poisonous plants of Queensland. CSIR Bull 232, Melbourne, 1948.

CR030   Thorp, R. H. and T. R. Watson. A survey of the occurrence of cardio-active constituents in plants growing wild in Australia. 1. Families Apocynaceae and Asclepiadaceae. **Aust J Exp Biol** 1953; 31: 529.

CR031   Neogi, N. C. and M. C. Bhatia. Biological investigation of *Vinca rosea*. Indian J **Pharmacy** 1956; 18: 73.

CR032   Paris, R. R. and H. Moyse-Mignon. A sympatholytic Apocynaceae, *Vinca rosea*. **CR Acad Sci** 1953; 240: 1993.

CR033   Pernet, M., G. Meyer, J. M. Bosser and G. Ratsiandavana. The Catharanthus of Madagascar. **CR Acad Sci** 1956; 243: 1352.

CR034   Svoboda, G. H., N. Neuss and M. Gorman. Alkaloids of *Vinca rosea* Linn. (*Catharanthus roseus* G. Don). V. Preparation and characterization of alkaloids. **J Amer Pharm Ass Sci Ed** 1959; 48: 659–666.

CR035   Shorti, D. S., M. Kelkar, V. K. Deshmukh and R. Aiman. Investigation of the hyperglycemic properties of *Vinca rosea*, *Cassia auriculata* and *Eugenia jambolana*. **Indian J Med Res** 1963; 51(3): 464–467.

CR036   Willaman, J. J. and H. L. Li. Alkaloid-bearing plants and their contained alkaloids, 1957–1968. **Lloydia** 1970; 33S: 1–286.

CR037   Tangkongchitr, U. Extraction of organic compounds from *Vinca rosea* Linn. **Master Thesis** 1973; 43pp.

CR038   Rizk, A. F. M. The Phytochemistry of the Flora of Qatar, Scientific and Applied Research Centre, University of Qatar, Kingsprint, Richmond, UK 1986; 582pp.

CR039   Arfmann, H. A., W. Kohl and V. Wray. Effect of 5-azacytidine on the formation of secondary metabolites in *Catharanthus roseus* cell suspension cultures. **Z Naturforsch Ser C** 1985; 40: 21–25.

CR040   ANON. Ayurvedic drug to fight cancer. **Probe** 1985; 24(4): 234.

CR041   Grill, E., E. L. Winnacker and M. H. Zenk. Phytochelatins: The principal heavy-metal complexing peptides of higher plants. **Science** 1985; 230(4726): 674–676.

CR042   Atta-ur-Rahman, I. Ali and M. I. Chaudhary. Bannucine–A new dihydroindole alkaloid from *Catharanthus roseus* (L) G. Don. **J Chem Soc Perkin Trans I** 1986(6); 923-926.

CR043   Atta-ur-Rahman, M. Alam, I. Ali, Habib-ur-Rehman and I. Hag. Leurosine: A new binary indole alkaloid from *Catharanthus roseus*. **J Chem Soc Perkin Trans I** 1988(8); 2175–2178.

CR044   Fahn, W., V. Kaiser, H. Schubel, J. Stockigt and B. Daniel. *Catharanthus roseus* enzyme mediated synthesis of 3-hydroxyvoafrine A and B – A simple route to the voafrines. **Phytochemistry** 1990; 29(1): 127–133.

CR045   Wissing, J. B. and H. Behrbohm. Diacylglycerol pyrophosphate, a novel phospholipid compound. **Febs Lett** 1993; 315(1): 95–99.

CR046 Fujioka, S., T. Inoue, S. Takatsuto, T. Yanagisawa, T. Yokota and A. Sakurai. Identification of a new brassinosteroid, cathasterone, in cultured cells of *Catharanthus roseus* as a biosynthetic precursor of teasterone. **Biosci Biotech Biochem** 1995; 59(8): 1543–1547.

CR047 Neuss, N., A. J. Barnes and L. L. Huckstep. Vinca alkaloids. XXXV. Desacetoxyvinblastine: A new minor alkaloid from *Vinca rosea* (*Catharanthus roseus*). **Experientia** 1975; 31: 18.

CR048 Bhakuni, D. S., P. P. Joshi, H. Uprety and R. S. Kapil. Roseoside – A C-13 glycoside from *Vinca rosea*. **Phytochemistry** 1974; 13: 2541–2543.

CR049 Guarnaccia, R., L. Botta and C. J. Coscia. Biosynthesis of acdic iridoid monoterpene glucosides in *Vinca rosea*. **J Amer Chem Soc** 1974; 96: 7079.

CR050 Jones, W. E. and G. J. Cullinan. Vincadioline. **Patent-US-3,887,565** 1975; 4pp.

CR051 Scott, A. I and S. L. Lee. Biosynthesis of the indole alkaloids. A cell-free system from *Catharanthus roseus*. **J Amer Chem Soc** 1975; 97: 6906.

CR052 Jovanovics, K., K. Szasz, G. Fekete, E. Bittner, E. Dezseri and J. Eles. Isolation of vincristine and n-demethylvinblastine from *Vinca rosea*. **Patent-Ger Offen**-2,259,388 1974.

CR053 Aynilian, G. H., S. G. Weiss, G. A. Cordell, D. J. Abraham, F. A. Crane and N. R. Farnsworth. Catharanthus alkaloids. XXIX. Isolation and structure elucidation of vincoline. **J Pharm Sci** 1974; 63(4): 536–538.

CR054 Tafur, S. S., W. E. Jones, D. E. Dorman, E. E. Logsdon and G. H. Svoboda. Alkaloids of *Vinca rosea* (*Catharanthus roseus*). XXXVI. Isolation and characterization of new dimeric alkaloids. **J Pharm Sci** 1975; 64: 1953.

CR055 Weiss, S. G. Antitumor principles of *Linum album* and *Catharanthus roseus*. **Diss Abstr Int** 1974; 35: 2669.

CR056 Luu, C. Notes on the traditional pharmacopoeia of French Guyana. **Plant Med Phytother** 1975; 9: 125–135.

CR057 Neuss, N. and A. J. Barnes. 4-Deacetoxyvinblastine. **Patent-US**-3,954,773 1976.

CR058 Carew, D. P. and R. J. Krueger. Anthocyanidins of *Catharanthus roseus* callus cultures. **Phytochemistry** 1976; 15: 442A.

CR059 Tafur, S. S. 4-Desacetoxy-3-hydroxyvinblastine. **Patent-US**-3,944,554 1976.

CR060 Siegel, R. K. Herbal intoxication. Psychoactive effects from herbal cigarettes, tea, and capsules. **J Amer Med Assoc** 1976; 236(5): 473–476.

CR061 Atta-ur-Rahman, I. Ali and M. Bashir. Isolation of rhazimol from the leaves of *Catharanthus roseus*. **J Nat Prod** 1984; 47(2): 389–.

CR062 Atta-ur-Rahman. Some approaches to the study of indigenous medicinal plants. **Bull Islamic Med** 1982; 2: 562–568.

CR063 Hsu, F. L. and J T. Cheng. Investigation in rats of the antihyperglycaemic effect of plant extracts used in Taiwan for the treatment of diabetes mellitus. **Phytother Res** 1992; 6(2): 108–111.

CR064 Brandao, M., M. Botelho and E. Krettli. Antimalarial experimental chemotherapy using natural products. **Cienc Cult** 1985; 37(7): 1152–1163.

CR065 Chattopadhay, R. R., S. K. Sarkar, S. Ganguly, R. N. Banerjee and T. K. Basu. Effect of extract of leaves of *Vinca rosea* Linn. on glucose utilization and glycogen deposition by isolated rat hemidiaphragm. **Indian J Physiol Pharmacol** 1992; 36(2): 137–138.

CR066 Schripsema, J. and R. Verpoorte. Regulation of indole alkaloid biosynthesis in *Catharanthus roseus* cell suspension cultures, investigated with 1H-NMR. **Planta Med Suppl** 1992; 58(1): A608.

CR067 Chattopadhyay, R. R., R. N. Banerjee, S. K. Sarkar, S. Ganguly and T. K. Basu. Anti-inflammatory and acute toxicity studies with the leaves of *Vinca rosea* Linn. in experimental animals. **Indian J Physiol Pharmacol** 1992; 36(4): 291–292.

CR068 Duperon, P., J. P. Allais and A. Dupaix. Comparison of the sterol content of tonoplast and microsomal fractions from *Catharanthus roseus* suspension-cultured cells. **Plant Physiol Biochem (Paris)** 1992; 30(4): 495–498.

CR069   Petiard, V., D. Courtois, F. Gueritte, N. Langlois and B. Mompon. New alkaloids in plant tissue cultures. **Proc 5th Intl Cong Plant Tissue & Cell Culture** 1982; 309–310.

CR070   Kutney, J. P. Studies in plant tissue culture – potentially important sources of clinically important anti-cancer agents. **Proc F E C S Third Int Conference on Chemistry and Biotechnology of Biologically Active Natural Products**, Vol 1 PP168–179, VCH Publisher Inc NY, NY 1973; 1: 168–179.

CR071   Perdue Jr, R. E. Cell Culture. 1. Role in discovery of antitumor agents from higher plants. **J Nat Prod** 1982; 45(4): 418–426.

CR072   Ali, I. The alkaloids in flowers of *Catharanthus roseus* (L) G. Don. **Gomal Univ J Res** 1990; 10(1): 27–31.

CR073   Lin, C. C. Crude drugs used for the treatment of diabetes mellitus in Taiwan. **Amer J Chin Med** 1992; 20(3/4): 269–279.

CR074   Tabata, H. Manufacture of tabersonine derivatives by plant tissue culture. **Patent-Japan Kokai Tokkyo Koho**-05 1993; 219,975: 5pp.

CR075   Hars, Y. and F. Ito. Manufacture of indole alkaloids with plant tissue or organ culture. **Patent-Japan Kokai Tokkyo Koho**-04 1992; 91–785: 7pp.

CR076   Kulkarni, R. and N. Ravindra. Resistance to *Pythium aphanidermatum* in diploids and induced autotetraploids of *Catharanthus roseus*. **Planta Med** 1988; 54(4): 356–359.

CR077   De Luca, V., N. Brisson, J. Balsevich and W. G. W. Kurz. Regulation of vindoline biosynthesis in *Catharanthus roseus*: Molecular cloning of the first and last steps in biosynthesis. **Primary and Secondary Metabolism of Plant Cell Cultures II**. 1989; 154–161.

CR078   Zamora-Martinez, M. C. and C. N. P. Pola. Medicinal plants used in some rural populations of Oaxaca, Puebla and Veracruz, Mexico. **J Ethnopharmacol** 1992; 35(3) 229–257.

CR079   Nagy-Turak, A. and Z. Vegh. Extraction and in situ densitometric determination of alkaloids from *Catharanthus roseus* by means of overpressured layer chromatography on amino-bonded silica layers. I. Optimization and validation of the separation system. **J Chromatogr A** 1994; 668(2): 501–507.

CR080   Islas, I., V. M. Loyola-Vargas and M. De Lourdes Miranda-Ham. Tryptophan decarboxylase activity in transformed roots from *Catharanthus roseus* and its relationship to tryptamine, ajmalicine and catharanthine accumulation during the culture cycle. **In Vitro Cell Dev Biol** 1994; 30P: 81–83.

CR081   Benjamin, B. D., S. M. Kelkar, M. S. Pote, G. S. Kakli, A. T. Sipahimalani and M. R. Heble. *Catharanthus roseus* cell cultures: Growth, alkaloid synthesis and antidiabetic activity. **Phytother Res** 1994; 8(3): 185–186.

CR082   Zhou, X. H., R. Minocha and S. C. Minocha. Physiological response of suspension cultures of *Catharanthus roseus* to aluminum: Changes in polyamines and inorganic ions. **J Plant Physiol** 1995; 145(3): 277–284.

CR083   Holdsworth, D. K. Traditional medicinal plants of Rarotonga, Cook Islands Part 1. **Int J Crude Drug Res** 1990; 28(3): 209–218.

CR084   Kamata, H. Production of vinca-alkaloid. **Patent-Japan Kokai Tokkyo Koho**-61 1986; 274,694: 6pp.

CR085   Maikhuri, R. K. and A. K. Gangwar. Ethnobiological notes on the Khasi and Garo tribes of Meghalaya, Northeast India. **Econ Bot** 1993; 47(4): 345–357.

CR086   Stockigt, J., H. P. Husson, C. Kan-Fan and M. H. Zenk. Cathenamine, a central intermediate in the cell free biosynthesis of ajmalicine and related indole alkaloids. **Chem Commun** 1977; 164–166.

CR087   Cuellar, A. *Catharanthus roseus* alkaloids. The structure of vincubine. **Rev Cubana Farm** 1976; 10: 19.

CR088   Scott, A. I., S. L. Lee and W. Wan. Indole alkaloid biosynthesis: Partial purification of "ajmalicine synthetase" from *Catharanthus roseus* tissue cultures. **Heterocycles** 1977; 6: 1552.

CR089   Morton, J. F. Medicinal and other plants used by people on North Caicos (Turks and Caicos Islands, West Indies). **J Crude Drug Res** 1977; 15: 1–24.

CR090 Amico, A. Medicinal plants of Southern Zambesia. **Fitoterapia** 1977; 48: 101–139.

CR091 Treimer, J. F. and M. H. Zenk. Enzymic synthesis of corynanthe-type alkaloids in cell cultures of Catharanthus roseus: Quantation by radioimmunoassay. **Phytochemistry** 1978; 17: 227–231.

CR092 Sarin, J. P. S., R. C. Nandi, R. S. Kapil and N. M. Khanna. Estimation of ajmalicine in Catharanthus roseus. **Indian J Pharmacy** 1977; 39: 62.

CR093 Deus, B. Cell cultures of Catharanthus roseus. **Production of Natural Compounds by Cell Culture Methods. Proc Int Symp Plant Cell Cult**, Ges Strahlen Umweltforsch, Munich (Al Fermann, AW, Reinhard, EC, EDS) 1978; 118.

CR094 De Luca, V., J. Balsevich and M. G. W. Kurz. Purification and properties of deacetylvindoline acetyltransferase from Catharanthus roseus. **Abstr Internat Res Cong Nat Prod Coll Pharm Univ**, Chapel Hill NC July 7–12, 1985; Abstr-103.

CR095 Bandyopadhyay, M. N., B. B. Mukheruee and S. N. Ganguly. IAA from the pollen grains and style stigma segments of Catharanthus roseus (Linn.) G. Don. **Physiol Sex Reprod Flowering Plants Int Symp 1st 1976** 1978; 102–104.

CR096 Atta-ur-Rahman, S. Malik and K. Albert. Structural studies on vindolinine. **Z Naturforsch Ser B** 1986; 41(3): 386–392.

CR097 Dolya, V. S., N. V. Svinidze, Y. I. Kornievskii and T. R. Gokitidze. Fatty oils of four plants of the Subtropics. **Farm Zh (Kiev)** 1985(2); 76–77.

CR098 Kutney, J. P. Studies on plant tissue cultures. **Heterocycles** 1981; 15: 1405–1431.

CR099 Schiel, O. and J. Berlin. Geraniol-10-hydroxylase of Catharanthus roseus and its correlation with indole alkaloid biosynthesis. **Planta Med** 1986; 1986(1): 422A.

CR100 Atta-ur-Rahman, S. Hasan and M. R. Qulbi. Beta-carboline from Catharanthus roseus. **Planta Med** 1985; 1985(3): 287.

CR101 Marigo, G., H. Bouyssou and B. M. Mal. Vacuolar efflux of malate and its influence on nitrate accumulation in Catharanthus roseus cells. **Plant Sci** 1985; 39(2): 97–103.

CR102 Atta-ur-Rahman and I. Ali. 13-C NMR Spectroscopic studies on gomaline and rosamine. **Fitoterapia** 1986; 57(6): 438–440.

CR103 Atta-ur-Rahman, I. Ali and M. I. Chaudhry. Isolation and 13-C-NMR studies on cathovaline, an alkaloid from the leaves of Catharanthus roseus. **Planta Med** 1985; 1985(5): 447–448.

CR104 Schripsema, J., T. A. Van Beek, R. Verpoorte, C. Erkelens, P. Perera and C. Tibell. A reinvestigation of the stereochemistry of tubotaiwine using NMR spectroscopy. **J Nat Prod** 1987; 50(1): 89–101.

CR105 Daniel, M. and S. D. Sabnis. Chemotaxonomical studies on Apocynaceae. **Indian J Exp Biol** 1978; 16(4): 512–513.

CR106 Ashihara, H. changes in fructose-2,6-biphosphate level during the growth of suspension cultured cells of Catharanthus roseus. **Z Naturforsch Ser C** 1986; 41(5/6): 529–531.

CR107 Garg, S. P., M. R. K. Sherwani, A. Arora, R. Agarwal and M. Ahmad. Ricinoleic acid in Vinca rosea seed oil. **J Oil Technol Ass India (Bombay)** 1987; 19(3): 63–64.

CR108 Rai, M. K. and S. Upadhyay. Screening of medicinal plants of Chhindwara district against Trichophyton mentagrophytes: A casual organism of Tinea pedis. **Hindustan Antibiot Bull** 1988; 30(1/2): 33–36.

CR109 De Mello, J. F. Plants in traditional medicine in Brazil. **J Ethnopharmacol** 1980; 2(1): 49–55.

CR110 Chattopadhyay, S. P. and P. K. Das. Evaluation of Vinca rosea for the treatment of warts. **Indian J Dermatol Venereol Leprol** 1990; 56(2): 107–108.

CR111 Johns, T., J. O. Kokwaro and E. K. Kimanani. Herbal remedies of the Luo of Siaya District, Kenya. Establishing quantitative criteria for consensus. **Econ Bot** 1990; 44(3): 369–381.

CR112 Swanston-Flatt, S. K., C. Day, P. R. Flatt, B. J. Gould and C. J. Bailey. Glycaemia effects of traditional European plant treatments for diabetes studies in normal and streptozotocin diabetic mice. **Diabetes Res** 1989; 10(2): 69–73.

CR113   Pennings, E. J. M., R. Verpoorte, O. J. M. Goddijn and J. H. C. Hoge. Purification of trypophan decarboxylase from a *Catharanthus roseus* cell suspension culture. **J Chromatogr** 1989; 483(1): 311–318.

CR114   Gomez, G. A. and J. E. Sokal. Use of vinblastine in the terminal phase of chronic myelocytic leukemia. **Cancer Treat Rep** 1979; 63: 1385–1387.

CR115   Singh, J., K. L. Handa, P. R. Rao and C. K. Atal. Recovery of ajmalicine (raubasine) from *Vinca rosea*. **Res Ind** 1978; 23: 166–167.

CR116   Maccarthy, J. J. and P. K. Stumpf. Fatty acid composition and biosynthesis on cell suspension cultures of *Glycine max, Catharanthus roseus* and *Nicotiana tabacum*. **Planta (Berla)** 1980; 147: 384–388.

CR117   Mizukami, H., H. Norlov, S. L. Lee and A. I. Scott. Purification and properties of strictosidine synthetase (an enzyme condensing tryptamine and secologanin) from *Catharanthus roseus* cultured cells. **Biochemistry** 1979; 18: 3760–3763.

CR118   Anon. Isolating alkaloid compounds from *Vinca rosea*. **Patent-Belg**-867,670 1978.

CR119   Madati, P. J., H. A. Pazi and A. Ernest. Phytochemical investigation of *Catharanthus roseus* growing wildly in East Africa. **J Afr Med Pl** 1979; 2: 1.

CR120   Barrois, V. and N. R. Farnsworth. The value of plants indicated by traditional medicine in cancer therapy. **WHO, Geneva** Nov. 13–17, 1978.

CR121   El-Merzabani, M. M., A. A. El-Aaser, A. K. El-Duweini and A. M. El-Masry. A bioassay of antimitotic alkaloids of *Catharanthus roseus*. **Planta Med** 1979; 36: 87–90.

CR122   El-Merzabani, M. M., A. A. El-Aaser, M. A. Attia, A. K. El-Duweini and A. M. Ghazal. Screening system for Egyptian plants with potential anti-tumor activity. **Planta Med** 1979; 36: 150–155.

CR123   Wahl, J. Airlift fermenter for growing plant cell cultures. **Git Fachz Lab** 1979; 23: 169–171.

CR124   Schwenn, J. D., H. El-Shagi, A. Kemena and E. Petrak. On the role of s:sulfotransferases in assimilatory sulfate reduction by plant suspension cultures. **Planta** 1979; 144: 419–425.

CR125   Ayensu, E. S. Medicinal plants of the West Indies. **Unpublished Manuscript** 1978; 110pp.

CR126   Chauhan, S., S. Agrawal, R. Mathur and R. K. Gupta. Phosphatase activity in testis and prostate of rats treated with embelin and *Vinca rosea* extract. **Experientia** 1979; 35: 1183–1185.

CR127   Virmani, O. P., G. N. Srivastava and P. Singh. *Catharanthus roseus* - The tropical periwinkle. **Indian Drugs** 1978; 15: 231–252.

CR128   Asthana, R. B. and M. K. Misra. Orally effective hypoglycemic agent from *Vinca rosea*. **Indian J Biochem Biophys** 1979; 16: 30.

CR129   Erdelsky, K. and L. Holickova. Cultivation of plant tissue culture of *Vinca rosea* L. and its alkaloid contents. **Acta Fac Rerum Nat Univ Comenianae Physiol Plant** 1978(15); 1–10.

CR130   Rueffer, M., C. Kan-Fan, H. P. Husson, J. Stockigt and M. H. Zenk. 4,21-Dehydrogeissoschizine, an intermediate in heteroyohimbine alkaloid biosynthesis. **Chem Commun** 1979; 1016–1018.

CR131   El-Sayed, A., G. A. Handy and G. A. Cordell. Catharanthus alkaloids. XXXIII. 21'-Oxoleurosine from *Catharanthus roseus* (Apocynaceae). **J Nat Prod** 1980; 43: 157–161.

CR132   Tanaka, M. and T. Uchida. Heterogeneity of hydroxypyroline-containing glycoproteins in protoplasts from a *Vinca rosea* suspension culture. **Plant Cell Physiol** 1979; 20: 1295–1306.

CR133   Misawa, M. Production of natural substances by plant cell cultures described in Japanese patents. **Plant Tissue Culture ITS Bio-Technol Appl Int Cong 1976** 1977; 17–26.

CR134   Farnsworth, N. R. and C. J. Kaas. An approach utilizing information from traditional medicine to identify tumor-inhibiting plants. **J Ethnopharmacol** 1981; 3(1): 85–99.

CR135   El-Sayed, A., G. H. Handy and G. A. Cordell. Further dimeric indole alkaloids from *Catharanthus roseus* (L.) G.

Don (Apocynaceae). **J Nat Prod** 1979; 42: 687D.

CR136 Kohl, W., H. Vogelmann and G. Hofle. Alkaloids from *Catharanthus roseus* tissue cultures. **Planta Med** 1980; 39: 283–284.

CR137 Kurz, W. G. W., K. B. Chatson, F. Constabel, J.. P. Kutney, L. S. L. Choi, P. Kolodziejczyk, S. K. Sleigh and K. L. Stuart. The production of catharanthine and other indole alkaloids by cell suspension cultures of *Catharanthus roseus*. **Planta Med** 1980; 39: 284A.

CR138 Cantoria, M. Aromatic and medicinal herbs of the Philippines. **Q J Crude Drug Res** 1979; 14: 97–128.

CR139 Hemscheidt, T. and M. H. Zenk. Glucosidases involved in indole alkaloid biosynthesis of Catharanthus cell cultures. **Febs Lett** 1980; 110: 187–191.

CR140 Scott, A. I., H. Mizukami and S. L. Lee. Characterization of a 5-methyltryptophan resistant strain of *Catharanthus roseus* cultured cells. **Phytochemistry** 1979; 18: 795–798.

CR141 Anon. Antifertility studies on plants. **Annual Report of the Director General - Indian Council of Medical Research 1979–1980** 1979; 71–72.

CR142 Ali, M. E., N. Huq, A. K. M. M. Rahman, A. Moitra and A. Rahman. Chemical investigations on *Vinca rosea* Linn. (Nayantara). **Bangladesh J Sci Ind Res** 1979; 14: 354–358.

CR143 Pardasani, K. M., S. Singh and J. P. S. Sarin. Chromatographic estimation of vincaleukoblastine in *Catharanthus roseus* Linn. **Indian J Pharm Sci** 1979; 41: 207–213.

CR144 Kurz, W. G. W., K. B. Chatson, F. Constabel, J. P. Kutney, L. S. L. Choi, P. Kolodziejczyk, S. K. Sleigh, K. I. Stuart and B. R. Worth. Alkaloid production in *Catharanthus roseus* cell cultures: Initial studies on cell lines and their alkaloid content. **Phytochemistry** 1980; 19: 2583–2587.

CR145 El-Sayed, A. and G. A. Cordell. Catharanthus alkaloids. XXXIV. Catharanthamine, a new antitumor bisindole alkaloid from *Catharanthus roseus*. **J Nat Prod** 1981; 44: 289–293.

CR146 Mukhopadhyay, S. and G. A. Cordell. Catharanthus alkaloids. XXXVI. Isolation of vincaleukoblastine (VLB) and periformyline from *Catharanthus trichophyllus* and pericyclivine from *Catharanthus roseus*. **J Nat Prod** 1981; 44: 335–339.

CR147 Hutchinson, C. R. Biosynthetic studies of antitumor indole alkaloids. **Annu Proc Phytochem Soc Eur** 1980; 17: 143–158.

CR148 Meksongsee, L., Y. Jiamchaisri, P. Sinchaisri and L. Kasamsuksakan. Effects of some Thai medicinal plants and spices on the alkylating activity of ethyl methane sulfonate. **Abstr 4th Asian Sym Med Plants Spices Bangkok**, Thailand Sept. 15–19, 1980; 1980: 118.

CR149 Mukhopadhyay, S. and G. A. Cordell. Catharanthus alkaloids. XXXV. Isolation of leurosidine-n'-b-oxide from *Catharanthus roseus*. **J Nat Prod** 1981; 44: 611–613.

CR150 Khan, N. and D. P. Chakraborty. Alpha amyrin acetate from *Catharanthus roseus* Linn. **J Indian Chem Soc** 1981; 58: 628–629.

CR151 Kohl, W., B. Witte and G. Hofle. Alkaloids from *Catharanthus roseus* tissue cultures. II. **Z Naturforsch Ser B** 1981; 36: 1153–1162.

CR152 Tanaka, M., H. Shibata and T. Uchida. A new prolyl hydroxylase acting on poly-l-proline, from suspension cultured cells of *Vinca rosea*. **Biochim Biophys Acta** 1980; 616: 188–198.

CR153 Ghosh, R. K. and I. Gupta. Effect of *Vinca rosea* and *Ficus racemososus* on hyperglycaemia in rats. **Indian J Anim Health** 1980; 19: 145–148.

CR154 Nguyen, Van Dan. List of simple drugs and medicinal plants of value in Vietnam. **Proc Seminar of the Use of Medicinal Plants in Healthcare**, Tokyo 13–17 September 1977, WHO Regional Office Manila, 65–83.

CR155 Petiard, V., F. Gueritte, N. Langolis and P. Potier. Presence of (-) tabersonine in a tissue culture strain of *Catharanthus roseus* G. Don. **Physiol Veg** 1980; 18: 711–720.

CR156 Meisner, J., M. Weissenberg, D. Palevitch and N. Aharonson. Phagodeterrency induced by leaves and leaf extracts of *Catharanthus roseus* in the larva of *Spodoptera littoralis*. **J Econ Entomol** 1981; 74: 131–135.

CR157   Milo, J. Flower color inheritance and shoot and ajmalicine yield components in successive developmental stages of pure lines and F-1 hybrids in *Catharanthus roseus* (L.) G. Don. **Thesis-MS-Hebrew University** 1981; 1981: 74 pp.

CR158   Davey, J. E., J. Van Staden and G. T. N. De Leeuw. Endogenous cytokinin levels and development of flower virescence in *Catharanthus roseus* infected with mycoplasmas. **Physiol Plant Pathol** 1981; 19: 193–200.

CR159   Verzele, M., L. De Taeye, J. Van Dyck, G. De Decker and C. De Pauw. High-performance liquid chromatography of *Vinca rosea* alkaloids and the correlation of plate height and molecular weight. **J Chromatogr** 1981; 214: 95–99.

CR160   Lim-Sylianco, C. Y. and F. Blanco. Antimutagenic effects of some anticancer agents. **Bull Philipp Biochem Soc** 1981; 4(1): 1–7.

CR161   Shimazaki, A., F. Hirose and H. Ashihara. Changes in adenine nucleotide levels and adenine salvage during the growth of *Vinca rosea* cells suspension culture. **Z Pflanzenphysiol** 1982; 106: 191–198.

CR162   Kanamori-Fukuda, I., H. Ashihara and A. Komamine. Pyrimidine nucleotide biosynthesis in *Vinca rosea* cells: Changes in the activity of the de novo and salvage pathways during growth in a suspension culture. **J Exp Bot** 1981; 32(126): 69–78.

CR163   Chile, S. K., M. Saraf and A. K. Barde. Efficacy of *Vinca rosea* extract against human pathogenic strains of *Trichophyton rubrum* Sab. **Indian Drugs Pharm Ind** 1981; 16(1): 31–33.

CR164   Atta-Ur-Rahman, M. Bashir, S. Kaleem and T. Fatima. 16-Epi-19-s-vindolinine, an indoline alkaloid from *Catharanthus roseus*. **Phytochemistry** 1983; 22(4): 1021–1023.

CR165   Gueritte, F., N. Langlois and V. Petiard. Secondary metabolites isolated from a tissue culture of *Catharan-*

thus roseus. **J Nat Prod** 1983; 46(1): 144–148.

CR166   Sukumar, K. and Z. Osmani. Insect sterilants from *Catharanthus roseus*. **Curr Sci** 1981; 50: 552–553.

CR167   Kohl, W., B. Witte and G. Hofle. Quantitative and qualitative HPLC-analysis of indole alkaloids from *Catharanthus roseus* cell cultures. **Planta Med** 1983; 47(3): 177–182.

CR168   Constabel, F., S. Rambold, K. B. Chatson, W. G. M. Kurz and J. P. Kutney. Alkaloid production in *Catharanthus roseus* (L.) G. Don. VI. Variation in alkaloid spectra of cell lines derived from one single leaf. **Plant Cell Rep** 1981; 1(1): 3–5.

CR169   Kohl, W., B. Witte and G. Hofle. Alkaloids from *Catharanthus roseus* tissue cultures. 3. **Z Naturforsch Ser B** 1982; 37: 1346–1351.

CR170   Mukhopadhyay, S., A. El-Sayed, G. A. Handy and G. A. Cordell. Catharanthus alkaloids. XXXVII. 16-Epi-z-isositsirikine, a monomeric indole alkaloid with antineoplastic activity from *Catharanthus roseus* and *Rhazya stricta*. **J Nat Prod** 1983; 46(3): 409–413.

CR171   Rojas, N. M. and A. Cuellar. *Catharanthus roseus* G. Don. 1. Microbiological study of its alkaloids. **First Latin American & Caribbean Symposium on Pharmacologically Active Natural Products**, Cuba 1982 UNESCO 1982; 194.

CR172   Takeuchi, Y. and A. Komamine. Turnover of cell wall polysaccharides of a *Vinca rosea* suspension culture. I. Synthesis and degradation of cell wall components. **Physiol Plant** 1980; 48: 271–277.

CR173   Ross, S. A., S. E. Megalla, D. W. Bishay and A. H. Awad. Studies for determining antibiotic substances in some Egyptian plants. Part 1. Screening for antimicrobial activity. **Fitoterapia** 1980; 51: 303–308.

CR174   Morrison, E. Y. S. A. and M. West. A preliminary study of the effects of some West Indian medicinal plants on blood sugar levels in the dog. **West Indian Med J** 1982; 31: 194–197.

CR175   Rahman, A. U. and M. Bashir. Isolation of new alkaloids from *Catharan-*

thus roseus. **Planta Med** 1983; 49(2): 124–125.

CR176 Hirose, F. and H. Ashihara. Adenine phosphoribosyltransferase activity in mitochondria of *Catharanthus roseus* cells. **Z Naturforsch Ser** C 1982; 37(11/12): 1288–1289.

CR177 Treimer, J. F. and M. H. Zenk. Purification and properties of strictosidine synthase, the key enzyme in indole alkaloid formation. **Eur J Biochem** 1979; 101: 225–233.

CR178 Stoeckigt, J. and M. H. Zenk. Strictosidine (isovincoside): The key intermediate in the biosynthesis of monoterpenoid indole alkaloids. **Chem Commun** 1977; 1977(18): 646–648.

CR179 Simonds, R., A. De Bruyn, L. De Taeye, M. Verzele and C. De Pauw. N-deformyl vincristine: A bisalkaloid from *Catharanthus roseus*. **Planta Med** 1984; 1984(3): 274–276.

CR180 Wink, M. Chemical defense of lupins. Mollusc-repellent properties of quinolizidine alkaloids. **Z Naturforsch Ser C** 1984; 39(6): 553–558.

CR181 Atta-Ur-Rahman, I. Ali, M. Bashir and M. I. Choudhary. Isolation and structure of rosamine – A new pseudo-indoxyl alkaloid from *Catharanthus roseus*. **Z Naturforsch Ser B** 1984; 39(9): 1292–1293.

CR182 Scott, I. M., B. A. McGaw, R. Horgan and P. E. Williams. Biochemical studies on cytokinins in *Vinca rosea* crown gall tissue. **Plant Growth Subst Proc Int Conf 11th** 1982; 1982: 165–174.

CR183 Atta-Ur-Rahman, I. Ali and M. Bashir. Isolation and structural studies on the alkaloids in flowers of *Catharanthus roseus*. **J Nat Prod** 1984; 47(3): 554–555.

CR184 Rahman, A-U and S. Malik. Isolation of isovallesiachotamine from legumes of *Rhazya stricta*. **J Nat Prod** 1984; 47(2): 388–389.

CR185 Arnold, H. J. and M. Gulumian. Pharmacopoeia of traditional medicine in Venda. **J Ethnopharmacol** 1984; 12(1): 35–74.

CR186 Kohl, W., B. Witte, W. S. Sheldrick and G. Hofle. Indole alkaloids from *Catharanthus roseus* tissue cultures. IV. 16r-19,20-e-isositsirikin,16e-19,20-z-

isositsirikin and 21-hydroxycyclo-lochnerin. **Planta Med** 1984; 1984(3): 242–244.

CR187 De Bruyn, A., L. De Taeye, R. Simonds, M. Verzele and C. De Pauw. Alkaloids from *Catharanthus roseus*. Isolation and identification of 17 dessacetoxyvinblastine and 17-desacetoxyleurosine. **Bull Soc Chim Belg** 1982; 91(1): 75–85.

CR188 Atta-Ur-Rahman, J. Fatima and K. Albert. Isolation and structure of rosicine from *Catharanthus roseus*. **Tetrahedron Lett** 1984; 25(52): 6051–6054.

CR189 El-Sayed, A., G. A. Handy and G. A. Cordell. Catharanthus alkaloids. XXXVIII. Confirming structural evidence and antineoplastic activity of the bisindole alkaloids leurosine-n'(b)-oxide (pleurosine), roseadine and vindolicine from *Catharanthus roseus*. **J Nat Prod** 1983; 46(4): 517–527.

CR190 Tanaka, M., H. Shibata, K. Sato, S. Tanada and T. Uchida. Biosynthesis of extensin in suspension-cultured cells of *Vinca rosea*. **Plant Tissue Cult Proc Int Congr Plant Tissue Cell Cult 5th** 1982; 1982: 39–40.

CR191 De Taeye, L., A. De Bruyn, C. De Pauw and M. Verzele. Alkaloids of *Vinca rosea*: Isolation and identification of coronaridine. **Bull Soc Chim Belg** 1981; 90(1): 83–87.

CR192 Barde, A. K. and S. M. Singh. Activity of plant extracts against *Scytalidium anamorph* of Hendersonula toruloidea causing skin and nail diseases in man. **Indian Drugs** 1983; 20(9): 362–364.

CR193 Petiard, V. Antimitotic activities of *Catharanthus roseus* tissue cultures. **J Med** 1981; 447–469.

CR194 Thompson, W. A. R. Herbs that heal. **J Roy Coll Gen Pract** 1976; 26: 365–370.

CR195 Kalyanasundaram, M. and P. K. Das. Larvicidal and synergistic activity of plant extracts for mosquito control. **Indian J Med Res** 1985; 82(1): 19–23.

CR196 Chen, T. H. H., K. K. Kartha, N. L. Leung, W. G. W. Kurz, K. B. Chatson and F. Constabel. Cryopreservation of alkaloid-producing cell cultures of periwinkle (*Catharanthus roseus*). **Plant Physiol** 1985; 75: 726–731.

CR197 Rojas, M. C. N. and M. C. A. Cuellar. Comparative microbiological studies of the alkaloids of *Catharanthus roseus* and other related compounds. **Rev Cubana Farm** 1981; 15(2): 131–138.

CR198 Chakraborty, T. and G. Poddar. Herbal drugs in diabetes - Part 1: Hypoglycaemic activity of indigenous plants in streptozotocin (STZ) induced diabetic rats. **J Inst Chem (India)** 1984; 56(1): 20–22.

CR199 Yang, L. L., K. Y. Yen, Y. Kiso and H. Kikino. Antihepatotoxic actions of Formosan plant drugs. **J Ethnopharmacol** 1987; 19(1): 103–110.

CR200 Ramirez, V. R., L. J. Mostacero, A. E. Garcia, C. F. Mejia, P. F. Pelaez, C. D. Medina and C. H. Miranda. Vegetales empleados en medicina tradicional Norperuana. **Banco Agrario Del Peru & NACL Univ Trujillo**, Trujillo, Peru, June 1988; 54pp.

CR201 Balsevich, J., L. R. Hogge, A. J. Berry, D. E. Games and I. C. Mylchreest. Analysis of indole alkaloids from leaves of *Catharanthus roseus* by means of supercritical fluid chromatography/mass spectrometry. **J Nat Prod** 1988; 51(6): 1173–1177.

CR202 Murugavel, T., A. Ruknudin, S. Thangavelu and M. A. Akbarsha. Antifertility effect of *Vinca rosea* (Linn.) leaf extract on male albino mice-A sperm parametric study. **Curr Sci** 1989; 58(19): 1102–1103.

CR203 Auriola, S., T. Naaranlahti and S. P. Lapinjoki. Determination of *Catharanthus roseus* alkaloids by high-performance liquid chromatography isotope dilution thermospray-mass spectrometry. **J Chromatogr** 1991; 554(1/2): 227–231.

CR204 Radvany, L. G. and F. Di Cosmo. Purification and characterization of calmodulin from cultured cells of *Catharanthus roseus*. **Phytochem Anal** 1991; 2(6): 241–252.

CR205 Murugavel, T. and M. A. Akbarsha. Anti-spermatogenic effect of *Vinca rosea* Linn. **Indian J Exp Biol** 1991; 29(9): 810–812.

CR206 Chattopadhyay, R. R., S. K. Sankar, S. Ganguly, B. N. Banerjee and T. K. Basu. Hypoglycemic and antihyperglycemic effect of leaves of *Vinca rosea* Linn. **Indian J Physiol Pharmacol** 1991; 35(3): 145–151.

CR207 Chopra, R. N., R. L. Badhwar and S. Ghosh. Poisonous Plants of India. Manager of Publications, Government of India Press, Calcutta. Volume 1, 1949.

CR208 Chang, S. Y., D. Y. Mao and P. Hsu. The antitumor action and toxicity of the alkaloidal fraction AC-875 from *Vinca roseus*. **Yao Hsueh Hsueh Pao** 1965; 12: 772–777.

CR209 Svoboda, G. H., A. J. Barnes Jr. and R. J. Armstrong. Leurosidine and leurocristine and their production. **Patent-US**-3,205,220 1965.

CR210 Furuya, A., M. Ukita, Y. Kotani, M. Misawa and H. Tanaka. RNA hydrolysis to 5'-ribonucleotides by phosphodiesterase from plant callus. **Patent-Japan Kokai**-73 33,903 1973.

CR211 Moza, B. K. and J. Trojanek. On alkaloids. VII. New alkaloids from *Catharanthus roseus*. **Collect Czech Chem Commun** 1963; 28: 1419.

CR212 Pillay, P. P. and T. N. Santha Kumari. The occurrence of alstonine in *Lochnera rosea*. **J Sci Ind Res-B** 1961; 20: 458.

CR213 Shimuzu, M. and F. Uchimaru. The isolation of alkaloids from *Vinca (Lochnera) rosea*. **Chem Pharm Bull** 1959; 7: 713.

CR214 Shimuzu, M. and F. Uchimaru. Isolation of alkaloids from *Vinca (Lochnera) rosea*. **Chem Pharm Bull** 1958; 6: 324.

CR215 Hodge, W. H. and D. Taylor. The ethnobotany of the island Caribes of Dominica. **WEBBIA** 1956; 12: 513–644.

CR216 Prakash, A. O. and R. Mathur. Screening of Indian plants for antifertility activity. **Indian J Exp Biol** 1976; 14: 623–626.

CR217 Ukita, M., A. Furuya, H. Tanaka and M. Misawa. 5'Phosphodiesterase formation by cultured plant cells. **Agr Biol Chem** 1973; 37: 2849–2854.

CR218 Mueller-Oerlinghausen, B., W. Ngamwathana and P. Kanchanapee. Investigation into Thai medicinal plants said to cure diabetes. **J Med Assoc Thailand** 1971; 54: 105–111.

CR219   Svoboda, G. A. The alkaloids of Catharanthus roseus G. Donn (Vinca rosea L.). Current Topics in Plant Science. J. E. Gunckel (Ed.), Academic Press, New York 1969; 303–335.

CR220   Smith, S. L., W. E. Jones, D. E. Dorman, E. E. Logsdon and G. H. Svoboda. Alkaloids of Vinca rosea L. (Catharanthus roseus G. Don). XXXIII. Isolation and characterization of new dimeric alkaloids. (Abstract). **Lloydia** 1974; 37(4): 645D.

CR221   Tabgkongchitr, U. Extraction of organic compounds from leaves of Vinca rosea Linn. **Thesis-MS-Chulalongkorn Univ** 1973; 1973: 42pp.

CR222   Bhandari, P. R. and B. Mukerji. Lochnera rosea Linn Reichb. **Gauhati Ayurvedic Coll Mag** 1959; 8: 1–4.

CR223   Heal, R. E., E. F. Rogers, R. T. Wallace and O. Starnes. A survey of plants for insecticidal activity. **Lloydia** 1950; 13: 89–162.

CR224   Attia, M. S., S. Ahmad, S. A. H. Zaidi and Z. Ahmed. Studies on the bacteriostatic properties of wild medicinal plants of Karachi (Pakistan) Region 1. **Pak J Sci Ind Res** 1972; 15: 199–207.

CR225   Kubas, J. Investigations on known or potential antitumoral plants by means of microbiological tests. Part III. Biological activity of some cultivated plant species in Neurospora crassa test. **Acta Biol Cracov Ser Bot** 1972; 15: 87–100.

CR226   Sottomayor, M., M. Lopez Serrano, F. DiCosmo and A. RosBarcelo. Purification and characterization of alpha-3',4'-anhydrovinblastine synthase (peroxidase-like) from Catharanthus roseus (L.) G. Don. **FERBS lett** 1998; 428(3): 299–303.

CR227   Schulte, A. E., R. van der Heijden and R. Verporte. Purification and characterization of mevalonate kinase from suspension-cultured cells of Catharantus roseus (L.) G. Don. **Arch Biochem Biophys** 2000; 378(2): 287–98.

CR228   Pina-Chable, M. L. and S. M. Sotomayor. Phospholipase C activity from Catharanthus roseus transformed roots: aluminum effect. **Prostaglandins** 2001; 65(1): 45–56.

CR229   Singh, S. N., P. Vats, S. Suri, R. Shyam, M. M. Kumria, S. Rangana-than and K. Sridharan. Effect of an antidiabetic extract of Catharanthus roseus on enzymic activities on streptozotocin induced diabetic rats. **J Ethnopharmacol** 2001; 76(3): 269–277.

CR230   Haque, N., S. A. Chowdhury, M. T. Nutan, G. M. Rahaman, K. M. Rahaman and M. A. Rashid. Evaluation of antitumor activity of some medicinal plants of Bangladesh by potato disk bioassay. **Fitoterapia** 2000; 71(5): 547–552.

CR231   Spitsberg, V. L. and C. J. Coscia. Quinone reductases of higher plants. **Eur J Biochem** 1982; 127(1): 67–70.

CR232   Mukhopadhyay, S., A. El-Sayed, G. A. Handy and G. A. Cordell. Catharanthus alkaloids XXXVII. 16-Epi-Z-isositsirikine, a monomeric indole alkaloid with antineoplastic activity from Catharanthus roseus and Rhazya stricta. **J Nat Prod** 1983; 46(3): 409–413.

CR233   Mathur, R. and S. Chaudan. Antifertility efficacy of Catharanthus roseus Linn: a biochemical and histological study. **Acta Eur Fertil** 1985; 16(3): 203–205.

CR234   Sedakova, L. A., I. K. Bukharova, I. D. Treshchalin and A. B. Syrkin. Antitumor and toxic effects of amotin. **Eksp Onkol** 1987; 9(5): 76–77.

CR235   Song. K. M., S. W. Park, W. H. Hong, H. Lee, S. S. Kwak and J. R. Liu. Isolation of vindoline from Catharanthus roseus by supercritical fluid extraction. **Biotechnol Prog** 1992; 8(6): 583–586.

CR236   Hotze, M., G. Schroder and J. Schroder. Cinnamate 4-hydroxylase from Catharanthus roseus, and a strategy for the functional expression of plant cytochrome P450 proteins as translational fusions with P450 reductase in Escherichia coli. **FEBS Lett** 1995; 374(3): 345–350.

CR237   Limam, F., K. Chahed, N. Ouelhazi, R. Ghrir and L. Ouelhazi. Phytohormone regulation of isoperoxidases in Catharanthus roseus suspension cultures. **Phytochemistry** 1998; 49(5): 1219–1225.

CR238   Chattopadhyay, R. R. A comparative evaluation of some blood sugar lowering agents of plant origin. **J Ethnopharmacol** 1999; 67(3): 367–372.

9 | Cymbopogon citratus

(DC.) Stapf.

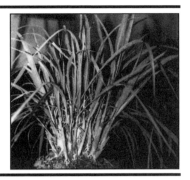

Common Names

Agin-ghas	Fiji	Lemon grass	Egypt
Agya-ghas	Fiji	Lemon grass	Guyana
Awaqa'pi l'ta	Argentina	Lemon grass	India
Bhoostrina	India	Lemon grass	Nicaragua
Black reed	USA	Lemon grass	Sierra Leone
Cana limon	Canary Islands	Lemon grass	Thailand
Capii cedron	Paraguay	Lemon grass	USA
Capim-cidrao	Brazil	Osang	Guinea
Capim-santo	Brazil	Paja de limon	Costa Rica
Chaywala ghas	Fiji	Sagadi abiruau	Nicaragua
Citronella	India	Sagadi	Nicaragua
Citronella	USA	Sakumau	Malaysia
Citronelle	Rodrigues Islands	Sitronel	Haiti
Erva cidreira capim	Brazil	Ta-khrai	Thailand
Erva-cidreira	Brazil	Tanglad	Indonesia
Fever grass	Belize	Tauj dub	USA
Fever grass	Guyana	Tauj qab	USA
Fever grass	Nicaragua	Te de limon	Guatemala
Gati-ma-nya	Ecuador	Tej-sar	Ethiopia
Ginger grass	Ecuador	Tiwahiwa	Nicaragua
Hierba de limon	Costa Rica	Vattu pulle	India
Hierba luisa	Ecuador	Yerba luisa	Easter Island
Hierba luisa	Peru	Zacate de limon	Nicaragua
Lemon grass	Argentina	Zacate limon	Belize
Lemon grass	Brazil	Zacate limon	Guatemala
Lemon grass	Ecuador	Zacate limon	Mexico

BOTANICAL DESCRIPTION

This densely tufted perennial of the GRAMINEAE family has leaf blades tapered to both ends up to 1 meter long and 5 to 10 mm wide. The flowering pannicles are rarely formed; inflorescence are 30 to 60 cm long and nodding; the partial inflorescence are paired racemes of spikelets subtended by spathes.

From: *Medicinal Plants of the World, vol. 1: Chemical Constituents, Traditional and Modern Medicinal Uses, 2nd ed.*
By: Ivan A. Ross © Humana Press Inc., Totowa, NJ

ORIGIN AND DISTRIBUTION

Probably originated in India, it is now widespread in the tropics and is frequently cultivated in gardens and along pathsides.

TRADITIONAL MEDICINAL USES

Argentina. Decoction of leaf is taken orally with "mate" tea for sore throat, empacho, and as an emetic[CC023].

Belize. Hot water extract of dried entire plant is taken orally for fever[CC048].

Canary Islands. Hot water extract of dried aerial parts is taken orally for high blood pressure and as a tranquilizer[CC067].

Colombia. Decoction of leaf is taken orally as a febrifuge[CC015].

Costa Rica. Hot water extract of leaves is taken orally as a carminative, with milk as a diaphoretic, depurative, expectorant, and for indigestion[CC047].

Cuba. Hot water extract of dried leaves is taken orally as a hypotensive, for catarrh and rheumatism[CC029].

Egypt. Hot water extract of dried leaves and stem is taken orally as a renal antispasmodic and diuretic[CC043].

Ethiopia. Hot water extract of aerial parts is taken orally to treat stomachaches[CC049].

Fiji. Decoction of dried leaves, in bath water, is used for colds, coughs, fever, flu, and pneumonia[CC056].

Guatemala. Hot water extract of dried leaves is used externally for wounds, ulcers, bruises, sores, infections of the skin and mucosa, skin eruptions and erysipelas. Orally the extract is used for urinary tract infections[CC064].

Haiti. Decoction of dried leaves is taken orally for stomachache[CC061].

India. Fresh entire plant is said to repel snakes[CC053]. Two to 3 drops of essential oil, in hot water, is taken orally for gastric troubles. For cholera, a few drops of oil with lemon juice is taken orally[CC055]. Hot water extract of dried leaves is used for bathing in cases of severe headache and fever. A fomentation of leaves is said to give immediate relief of colds[CC053].

Indonesia. Hot water extract of the entire plant is taken orally as an emmenagogue[CC001].

Malaysia. Hot water extract of entire plant is taken orally as an emmenagogue[CC003].

Mexico. An infusion prepared from the whole plant is taken orally to treat Varix and to promote the functions of the stomach[CC0017].

Paraguay. Hot water extract of dried leaves is used as an insecticide or vermifuge[CC020].

Peru. Hot water extract of dried entire plant is taken orally as an antispasmodic, stomachic and analgesic[CC063].

Thailand. Fresh entire plant is inhaled as a fragrance and eaten as a condiment[CC004]. Hot water extract of dried entire plant is taken orally as a stomachic[CC069]. Hot water extract of dried root is taken orally for diabetes[CC068].

USA. Hot water extract of entire plant is used externally by Laotian Hmong in Minnesota for healing wounds and bone fractures[CC066].

CHEMICAL CONSTITUENTS

(ppm unless otherwise indicated)

2'-0-Rhamnosyl orientin: Lf[CC037]
Alpha oxo-bisabolene: EO 12.1%[CC051]
Alpha pinene: Lf 1.3%[CC026]
Beta myrcene: EO[CC013]
Beta pinene: Lf EO 1.5%[CC026]
Beta sitosterol: Pl[CC027]
Beta-cadinene (+): EO[CC007]
Borneol: EO 5.0%[CC051]
Caffeic acid: Lf[CC037]
Camphene: EO 0.90%[CC026]
Camphor: EO 0.2%[CC051]
Car-3-ene: EO 0.1%[CC051]
Cineal: EO[CC006]
Citral: Lf EO 70.84–77.0%[CC050,CC044]
Citronellal: EO[CC006]
Citronellol acetate: Lf 1.3%[CC026]
Citronellol: EO[CC036]
Cymbopogenol: Lf[CC009]
Cymbopogone: Lf[CC005]

Cymbopogonol: Lf[CC042]
Cynaroside: Lf[CC037]
D-limonene: EO 5.0%[CC011]
Essential oil: Pl[CC004]
Farnesol: Lf EO 2.4%[CC026]
Fenchone: EO 0.3%[CC051]
Geranial: Lf EO 44.9%[CC044]
Geraniol acetate: Lf EO 9.9%[CC026]
Geraniol: EO[CC006]
Hept-5-en-2-one,6-methyl: Lf EO
    1.10%[CC026]
Heptan-2-one, 3-methyl: Lf EO[CC026]
Hexacosyl alcohol: Lf[CC027]
Humulene: EO 2.1%[CC007]
Iso-orientin: Lf[CC037]
Limonene: Lf EO[CC026]
Linalool oxide: Lf EO 1.0%[CC026]
Linalool: Lf, Pl[CC006]
Luteolin: Lf[CC037]
Luteolin-7-0-neohesperidoside: Lf[CC037]
Menthol: Lf EO 0.6%[CC026]
Menthone: EO 0.2%[CC051]
Methyl heptenol: EO[CC052]
Methyl heptenone: EO[CC052]
Myrcene: Lf EO[CC052]
Neral: EO 3.3–33.9%[CC051,CC044]
Nerol acetate: Lf EO 7.50%[CC026]
Nerol: EO[CC006]
Ocimene: EO 0.2%[CC051]
Para-coumaric acid: Lf[CC037]
Perilla alcohol: EO[CC045]
Terpineol: EO[CC052]
Terpinolene: Pl[CC051]
Triacontan 1-ol: Lf[CC027]

PHARMACOLOGICAL ACTIVITIES AND CLINICAL TRIALS

Aflatoxin-albumin adduct formation.
Leaf extract, administered to rats at a dose of 5 gm/kg daily for a week prior to the administration of 250 microgram/kg of aflatoxin B1 to rats, was effective. In control rats, maximum adduct levels were observed 12 hours after aflatoxin administration. No such effect was observed in animals treated with the extract. Daily treatment of rats with 250 microgram/kg of aflatoxin B1 for 3 weeks produced serum aflatoxin-albumin adduct levels to accumulate over a 10–14 day period and reached plateau levels 4.4-

fold higher that observed after a single dose. No significant alteration in the biomarker levels was seen in the rats treated with the extract[CC072].

Analgesic activity. Ethanol (95%) extract of fresh leaves, administered intragastrically to mice at a dose of 1.0 gm/kg, was inactive vs tail flick response to hot water and benzoyl peroxide-induced writhing [CC065]. Fresh leaf essential oil, administered intragastrically to mice, was active vs acetic acid- and Iloprost-induced writhing. A dose of 20% was active vs carrageenin- and PGE-2-induced pedal edema, and inactive vs dibutyl cyclic AMP-induced hyperalgesia in paw[CC036].

Antiamoebic activity. Essential oil, at a concentration of 0.25 microliters/ml in broth culture, was active on *Entamoeba histolytica*[CC022].

Antiascariasis activity. Ethanol (95%) extract of entire plant produced weak activity on earthworm. Paralysis was observed in 24 hours, no deaths[CC008].

Antibacterial activity. Chromatographic fraction of essential oil, at a concentration of 0.05% on agar plate, was active on *Bacillus subtilis*, *Escherichia coli* and *Staphylococcus aureus*. The essential oil was active on *Bacillus subtilis*, *Escherichia coli*, *Staphylococcus aureus*[CC025], *Salmonella paratyphi* A, IC_{100} 1600 ppm; *Shigella flexneri*, IC_{100} 1600 ppm; produced strong activity on *Staphylococcus aureus*, IC_{100} 400 ppm, and produced weak activity on *Escherichia coli*, IC_{90} 2400 ppm[CC024]. Essential oil, on agar plate at a concentration of 0.1 ml/disc, was active on *Bacillus mycoides*, *Bacillus subtilis* and *Escherichia coli*; and inactive on *Pseudomonas aeruginosa*[CC018]. Essential oil of fresh aerial parts, on agar plate, was active; a minimum toxic dose of 0.03% was observed for *Staphylococcus aureus*, 0.05% for *Bacillus subtilis*, 0.07% for *Escherichia coli* and 0.8% for *Pseudomonas aeruginosa*. The effects of pH, inoculum size and strength of nutrient broth were studied[CC058]. Essential oil, on agar plate, was active on *Escherichia coli* and *Staphylococcus aureus*. The extract was also active when the volatile oil extract was oxidized via the active oxygen method[CC012]. Essential oil, at a concentration of 20.0 mg/ml on agar plate, was active on *Bacillus subtilis* and *Staphylococcus aureus*, and produced weak activity on *Escherichia coli* and *Pseudomonas aeruginosa*[CC034]. Fresh stem, water and hot water extracts of fresh stem, at a concentration of 0.5 ml/disk on agar plate, were inactive on *Bacillus subtilis* H-17(Rec+) and M-45(Rec–)[CC054]. Tincture of dried leaves (extract of 10 gm plant material in 100 ml ethanol), at a concentration of 30.0 microliters/disk on agar plate, was inactive on *Escherichia coli*, *Pseudomonas aeruginosa* and *Staphylococcus aureus*[CC064]. Geranial and neral, extracted from the leaf, individually produced antibacterial action on Gram-negative and Gram-positive organisms. Myrcene did not show observable antibacterial activity on its own. However, myrcene provided enhanced activities when mixed with either geranial or neral [CC070]. Essential oil in the gaseous state produced weak activity on *Haemophilus influenza*, *Streptococcus pneumonia*, *Streptococcus pyogenes*, and *Staphylococcus aureus*[CC077].

Anticonvulsant activity. Hot water extract of leaves (10 gm powder/150 ml water), administered by gastric intubation to mice at a dose of 20–40 ml/kg, was inactive vs transcorneal electroshock and pentylenetetrazole-induced contractions[CC062].

Antifilarial activity. Fresh leaf was active on *Setaria digitata*, LC_{100} 75,000 ppm[CC035].

Antifungal activity. Distillate of leaf essential oil, on agar plate, was active on *Curvularia lunata*, *Rhizopus* species, *Ustilaginoidea virens* and *Ustilago maydis*[CC033]. The essential oil, at a concentration of 3000 ppm on agar plate, was active on *Aspergillus niger*[CC016]. Dried entire plant, at a concentration of 2.0% (expressed as dry weight of

plant) on agar plate, was active on *Absidia spinosa*, *Alternaria alternata*, *Ceratocystis paradoxa*, *Choanephora cucurbitarum*, *Colletotrichum denatium*, *Drechslera maydis*, *Fusarium solani*, *Geotrichum candidum*, *Melanconium fuligineum*, *Myrothecium roridum*, *Phytophthora* species, *Pleurotus ostreatus*, *Pythium aphanidermatum*, *Rhizopus microsporus*, *Sclerotium rolfsii*, *Sordaria fimicola*, *Thanatephorus cucumeris*, *Tri-choloma crassum*, *Ustilago maydis* and *Volvariella volvacea*[CC046]. Essential oil, at a concentration of 0.1 ml/disk on agar plate, was inactive on *Trichophyton rubrum*[CC018]. Concentration of 0.25% was active on *Aspergillus niger*. On agar plate, the essential oil was active on *Trichophyton mentagrophytes*, MIC 0.08% and *Aspergillus fumigatus*, MIC 0.1%[CC030]. A concentration of 20.0 mg/ml, on agar plate, was active on *Trichophyton mentagrophytes*, and produced weak activity on *Aspergillus flavus*[CC034]. On agar plate, the essential oil was active on several plant pathogenic fungi[CC002]. The inhibitory effect of the essential oil on the apical growth of hyphae of *Aspergillus fumigatus* was investigated using a bio cell tracer by vapor contact in a sealed vessel. The oil stopped the apical growth at a loading dose of 6.3 micrograms/ml air, and did not allow the regrowth after gaseous contact, indicative of fungicidal action. Suppression of the apical growth by vapor contact was ascribed to the direct deposition of the essential oil on fungal mycelia, together with an indirect effect via the agar medium absorbed[CC076].

Anti-inflammatory activity. Hot water extract of dried leaves, administered intragastrically to rats at a dose of 15.0 ml/kg, was active vs carrageenin-induced pedal edema[CC029].

Antimutagenic activity. Water extract of a commercial sample of the aerial parts, at a concentration of 50.0 mg (expressed as dry weight of plant), was active on *Salmonella typhimurium* TA98 vs TRP-P-2-induced mutation. Metabolic activation was required for activity[CC031]. Ethanol (80%) extract of freeze-dried aerial parts, at a concentration of 0.5 mg/plate on agar plate, was active on *Salmonella typhimurium* TA100 vs 2-amino-3-methylimidazo[4,5-F]quinoline-, n-methyl-n'-nitro-n-nitroso-guanidine (MNNG)- and furylfuramide(AF-2); and on TA98 vs aflatoxin B1-, 2-amino-6-methyl-dipyrido[1,2-A:3',2'-D]imidazole- and 2-aminodipyrido-1,2-A:3'2'-D-imidazole-induced mutagenesis. A concentration of 2.5 mg/plate was active on TA100 and TA98 vs Benzo(A)Pyrene- and 3-Amino-1-Methyl-5H-Pyrido[4,3-B]Indole-induced mutagenesis, respectively. A concentration of 5.0 mg/plate was active on TA98 vs 3-Amino-1,4-Dimethyl-5H-Pyrid[4,3-B]Indole (TRP-P-1) induced-mutagenesis and a concentration of 10.0 mg/plate was active on TA100 and TA98. Metabolic activation was not required of activity[CC019].

Antimycobacterial activity. Essential oil, at a concentration of 20.40 mg/ml on agar plate, was active on *Mycobacterium smegatis*[CC034].

Antinociceptive effect. The essential oil from leaves, administered orally to mice at a dose of 25 mg/kg and intraperitoneally at a dose of 25–100 mg/kg, increased the reaction time to thermal stimuli. Fifty to 200 mg/kg orally and intraperitoneally strongly inhibited acetic acid-induced writhing. In the formalin test, 50 and 200 mg/kg intraperitoneally, inhibited preferentially the second phase of the response, causing inhibitions of 100 and 48% at 200 mg/kg intraperitoneally and 100 mg/kg orally, respectively. The opoid antagonist, naloxone, blocked the central antinociceptive effect of the essential oil, suggesting the essential oil acts both at the peripheral and central levels[CC073].

Antioxidant activity. Leaf and stem, taken orally by human adults, was active. Biological activity reported has been patented[CC040]. Crude plant extract was evaluated for its influence on the survival of the *Escherichia coli* wild type (AB 1157) strain submitted to stannous chloride treatment. The results indicated that the extract produced a reduction of stannous chloride effect on the survival of the culture[CC074].

Antispasmodic activity. Unsaponifiable fraction of dried leaf and stem was active on rabbit ileum[CC043].

Antispermatogenic effect. Hot water extract of oven-dried leaves, administered by gastric intubation to female rats at a dose of 20–40 ml/kg, was inactive. Dose contained 2 mg powdered leaf/150 ml water. Dosing was for 70 days[CC060].

Antistress activity. Hot water extract of leaves (2 gm powdered leaf/150 ml water), administered by gastric intubation to mice at a dose of 40.0 ml/kg, was inactive[CC062].

Antiyeast activity. Dried entire plant, at a concentration of 2.0% (expressed as dry weight of plant) on agar plate, was active on *Saccharomyces cerevisiae*[CC046]. Essential oil, at a concentration of 20.0 mg/ml on agar plate, was active on *Cryptococcus neoformans* and *Saccharomyces cerevisiae*[CC034]. Essential oil, on agar plate, was active on *Candida albicans* and *Candida pseudotropicalis*, MIC 0.05%[CC030]. Tincture of dried leaves (extract of 10 gm dried leaves in 100 microliters ethanol), at a concentration of 30.0 ml/disk on agar plate, was inactive on *Candida albicans*[CC064].

Anxiolytic effect. Hot water extract of oven-dried leaves, taken orally by human adults at a dose of 2–10 gm/person, was inactive. Eighteen volunteers were exposed to an anxiety state using the Stroop color-word test. There were no differences in the pulse rates and error rates between the placebo and treated groups[CC059].

Ascaricidal activity. Fresh leaf essential oil, undiluted, was active. The oil concentration of 1:2 and 1:4 (oil/ethanol; v/v) showed high activity 5 days after dipping. The oil, at a concentration of 1:3 (oil/ethanol; v/v), was active when sprayed on the ticks on cattle[CC014].

Barbiturate potentiation. Hot water extract of leaves (10 gm powdered leaf/150 ml water), administered by gastric intubation to mice at a dose of 20.40 ml/kg, was inactive. Lyophilized extract (2 gm powder/150 ml water), administered intraperitoneally to mice, was inactive[CC062].

Barbiturate sleeping time decrease. Hot water extract of leaves (10 gm powdered leaf/150 ml water), administered by gastric intubation to mice at a dose of 20.40 ml/kg, was inactive. The lyophilized extract (2 gm powdered leaf/150 ml water), administered intraperitoneally to mice, was inactive[CC062].

Cataleptic effect. Hot water extract of leaves (2 gm powdered leaf/150 ml water), administered by gastric intubation to rats at a dose of 20.40 ml/kg, was inactive[CC062].

CNS depressant activity. Hot water extract of fresh leaves (10 leaves/150 ml water), administered by gastric intubation and intraperitoneally to mice at doses of 20.0 ml/kg, was inactive vs Rotarod test. Hot water extract of leaves (10 gm powder/150 ml water), administered intraperitoneally and by gastric intubation to mice at doses of 20.40 ml/kg, was inactive vs Rotarod test[CC062]. Hot water extract of oven-dried leaves, taken orally by human adults at a dose of 4.0 gm/day, was active. The extract did not significantly affect sleep parameters in 50 healthy volunteers[CC059].

Conditioned avoidance response decrease. Hot water extract of leaves (2 gm powder/150 ml water), administered by gastric intubation to rats at a dose of 40.0 ml/kg, was inactive[CC062].

Dermatitis producing effect. Essential oil, applied externally to male human adults, was active[CC021].

Diuretic activity. Hot water extract of dried leaves, administered intragastrically to rats at a dose of 25.0 ml/kg, produced weak activity[CC029].

Embryotoxic effect. Hot water extract of oven-dried leaves, administered by gastric intubation to pregnant rats at a dose of 20–40 ml/kg, was inactive[CC060].

Estrous cycle disruption effect. Hot water extract of oven-dried leaves (2 mg of powdered leaf/150 ml water), administered by gastric intubation to female rats at a dose of 40.0 ml/kg daily for 30 days, was inactive[CC060].

Glutamate oxaloacetate transaminase stimulation. Essential oil, in the ration of rats at a dose of 1500 ppm, was active[CC010].

Glutamate pyruvate transaminase stimulation. Essential oil, in the ration of rats at a dose of 1500 ppm, was active[CC010].

Glutathione-S-transferase induction. Essential oil, administered intragastrically to mice at a dose of 30.0 mg/animal, was active on the small intestine, and inactive on the liver and stomach. Dose was given every 2 days for a total of 3 doses[CC039].

Hyperglycemic activity. Hot water extract of oven-dried leaves (2 mg of powdered leaf/150 ml water), administered by gastric intubation to rats at a dose of 20–40 ml/kg daily for 8 weeks, was inactive[CC060].

Hyperthermic activity. Hot water extract of oven-dried leaves (2 mg of powdered leaf/150 ml water), administered by gastric intubation to rats at a dose of 20–40 ml/kg daily for 8 weeks, was inactive[CC060]. Hot water extract of leaves (2 gm powder/150 ml water), administered by gastric intubation to rats at a dose of 20.0 ml/kg, was inactive[CC062].

Hypnotic effect. Tea prepared from the dried leaves, taken orally by healthy volunteers daily for 2 weeks, produced no effect on sleep induction, sleep quality, dream recall, and rewakening[CC059].

Hypocholesterolemic activity. Essential oil, taken orally by human adults at a dose of 140.0 mg/day, was active. Twenty-two volunteers were given lemon grass oil capsules for 3 months. After 60 days, cholesterol level fell modestly, not significantly for a group of 8 responding subjects, but it was stable for 14 resistant subjects. A post-test showed no difference between responders and resistors after the oil was withdrawn[CC032].

Hypoglycemic activity. Hot water extract of dried root, administered orally to rabbits at a dose of 2.5 gm/kg, was inactive[CC068]. Hot water extract of oven-dried leaves (2 mg of powdered leaf/150 ml water), administered by gastric intubation to rats at a dose of 20–40 ml/kg daily for 8 weeks, was inactive[CC060].

Hypotensive activity. Hot water extract of dried leaves, administered intravenously to rats at doses of 1.0[CC038] and 3.0 ml/animal, was active. Blood pressure fell by more than 30%[CC029].

Hypothermic activity. Hot water extract of fresh leaves (2 leaves/150 ml water), administered intraperitoneally to rats at a dose of 40.0 ml/kg, was active. Results significant at $P < 0.05$ level. Hot water extract of leaves (2 gm powder/150 ml water), administered by gastric intubation at a dose of 20.0 ml/kg, was inactive; a dose of 40.0 ml/kg, administered intraperitoneally to rats, was active. Results significant at $P < 0.05$ level[CC062]. Hot water extract of oven-dried leaves (2 mg of powdered leaf/150 ml water), administered by gastric intubation to rats at a dose of 20–40 ml/kg daily for 8 weeks, was inactive[CC060].

Immunomodulator activity. Essential oil, in the ration of rats at a dose of 1500 ppm, was inactive. Polymorphocyte, eosinophil and monocyte counts were unaltered[CC010].

Inotropic effect positive. Hot water extract of dried leaves, at a concentration of 320.0 ml, was inactive on guinea pig atrium[CC038].

Insecticidal activity. Petroleum ether extract of dried leaves, at a concentration of 50.0 mcg, was inactive on *Rhodnius neglectus*[CC020]. Petroleum ether extract of dried leaves, at a concentration of 1.0 gm/liter, was inactive on *Lutzomyia longipalpis*[CC041].

Intestinal motility inhibition. Hot water extract of fresh leaves (10 leaves/150 ml water), administered by gastric intubation to rats at a dose of 20.40 ml/kg, was inactive vs charcoal meal intestinal transport assay. Hot water extract of leaves (10 gm powdered leaf/150 ml water), administered by gastric intubation to mice at a dose of 20.40 ml/kg, was inactive; intraperitoneally, at a dose of 40.0 ml/kg, the extract was active. Results significant at $P < 0.001$ level vs charcoal meal intestinal transport assay[CC062].

Intestinal motility stimulation. Hot water extract of fresh leaves (10 leaves/150 ml water), administered by gastric intubation to rats at a dose of 20.40 ml/kg, was inactive vs charcoal meal intestinal transport assay. Hot water extract of leaves (10 gm powdered leaf/150 ml water), administered by gastric intubation to mice at a dose of 20.40 ml/kg, was inactive vs charcoal meal intestinal transport assay[CC062].

Larvicidal activity. Fresh leaf essential oil, diluted with 95% ethanol and tested on larvae and engorged female cattle ticks, was active. It showed high activity at concentrations of 1:8, 1:12, and 1:16 (oil/ethanol, v/v)[CC014]. Water extract of dried leaves, at a concentration of 0.03 gm/ml (gm leaf per ml water), was inactive on *Culex quinquefasciatus*[CC028].

Mating inhibition. Hot water extract of oven-dried leaves (2 mg of powdered leaf/ 150 ml water), administered by gastric intubation to male rats at a dose of 20–40 ml/kg daily for 70 days, was inactive[CC060].

Mitogenic activity. Hot water extract of oven-dried leaves (2 mg of powdered leaf/ 150 ml water), administered by gastric intubation to pregnant rats at a dose of 40 ml/kg daily during the entire pregnancy, was inactive[CC060]. Fresh stem, water and hot water extracts of fresh stem, at concentrations of 0.5 ml/disk on agar plate, were inactive on *Bacillus subtilis* H-17(Rec+) and M-45(Rec-)[CC054].

Monooxygenases induction. Beta-myrcene, administered by gavage to Wistar rats at a dose of 1000 mg/kg for 1 to 3 consecutive days, produced 13 to 34-fold increases in the activities of pentoxy-resorufin-O-dealkylation and benzyloxy-resorufin-O-dealkylation, and only minor changes in ethoxycoumarin-O-deethylation, ethoxy-resorufin-O-dealkylation and methoxy-resorufin-O-dealkylation[CC071].

Mosquito repellant. Essential oil provides almost complete protection against *Anopheles culicifacies* and other anopheline species. Percent protection against *Culex quinquefasciatus* ranged from 95 to 96%[CC075].

Ovulation inhibition effect. Hot water extract of oven-dried leaves (2 mg of powdered leaf/150 ml water), administered by gastric intubation to female rats at a dose of 20–40 ml/kg daily for 51 days, was inactive[CC060].

Spontaneous activity reduction. Hot water extract of leaves (10 gm powdered leaf/150 ml water), administered by gastric intubation to mice at a dose of 20.40 ml/kg, was inactive[CC062].

Spontaneous activity stimulation. Hot water extract of leaves (10 gm powdered leaf/150 ml water), administered by gastric intubation to mice at a dose of 20.40 ml/kg, was inactive[CC062].

Spore germination inhibitor. Essential oil, at a concentration of 0.1%, was active on *Aspergillus fumigatus*[CC030].

Toxic effect. Hot water extract of oven-dried leaves (2 mg of powdered leaf/150 ml water), administered by gastric intubation to rats at a dose of 20–40 ml/kg daily for 8 weeks, was inactive[CC060]. The hot water extract, taken orally by human adults at a dose of 2–10 gm/day (dry weight of plant), was inactive. Serum levels of glucose, urea, creatinine, cholesterol, triglycerides, lipids, SGOT, SGPT, alkaline phosphatase, total protein, albumin, LDH, CPK, total bilirubin, and indirect bilirubin were unchanged after dosing for 2 weeks. A slight elevation of direct bilirubin and amylase was seen in some patients[CC060].

Weight loss. Hot water extract of oven-dried leaves (2 mg of powdered leaf/150 ml water), administered by gastric intubation to rats at a dose of 20–40 ml/kg daily for 8 weeks, was inactive[CC060].

REFERENCES

CC001   Quisumbing, E. Medicinal plants of the Philippines. **Tech Bull 16**, Rep Philippines, Dept Agr Nat Resources, Manilla 1951; 1.

CC002   Maruzzella, J. C. and J. Balter. The action of essential oils on phytopathogenic fungi. **Plant Disease Rept** 1959; 43: 1143–1147.

CC003   Burkill, I. H. Dictionary of the Economic Products of the Malay Peninsula. Ministry of Agriculture and Cooperatives, Kuala Lumpur, Malaysia. Vol. 1. 1966: 1.

CC004   Praditvarn, L. and C. Sambhandharaksa. A study of the volatile oil from Siam lemongrass. **J Pharm Assoc Siam** 1950; 3(2): 87–92.

CC005   Crawford, M., S. W. Hanson and M. E. S. Koker. The structure of cymbopogone, a novel triterpenoid from lemongrass. **Tetrahedron Lett** 1975; 1975: 3099.

CC006   Zaki, M. S. A., Y. H. Foda, M. M. Mostafa and M. A. Abd Allah. Identification of the volatile constituents of the Egyptian lemongrass oil. II. Thin-layer chromatography. **Nahrung** 1975: 19; 201.

CC007   Abd Allah, M. A., Y. H. Foda, M. Salem, M. S. A. Zaki and M. M. Mostafa. Identification of the volatile constituents of the Egyptian lemongrass oil. I. Gas-chromatographic analysis. **Nahrung** 1975; 19: 195.

CC008   Kaleysa Raj, R. Screening of indigenous plants for anthelmintic action against human *Ascaris lumbricoides*: Part 11. **Indian J Physiol Pharmacol** 1975; 19: 47–49.

CC009   Hanson, S. W., M. Crawford, E. S. Koker and F. A. Menezes. Cymbopogonol, a new triterpenoid from *Cymbopogon citratus*. **Phytochemistry** 1976; 15: 1074–1075.

CC010   Misbra, A. K., N. Kishore, N. K. Dubey and J. P. N. Chansouria. An evaluation of the toxicity of the oils of *Cymbopogon citratus* and *Citrus medica* in rats. **Phytother Res** 1992; 6(5): 279–281.

CC011 Zheng, G. Q., P. M. Kenney and L. K. T. Lam. Potential anticarcinogenic natural products isolated from lemongrass oil and galanga root oil. **J Agr Food Chem** 1993; 41(2): 153–156.

CC012 Orafidiva, L. O. The effect of autoxidation of lemon-grass oil on its antibacterial activity. **Phytother Res** 1993; 7(3): 269–271.

CC013 Zamith, H. P. S., M. N. P. Vidal, G. Speit and F. J. R. Paumgartten. Absence of genotoxic activity of beta-myrcene in the in vivo cytogenetic bone marrow assay. **Braz J Med Biol Res** 1993; 26(1): 93–98.

CC014 Chungsamarnvart, N. and S. Jiwajinda. Acaricidal activity of volatile oil from lemon and citronella grasses on tropical cattle ticks. **Kasetsart J Nat Sci** 1992; 26(5): 46–51.

CC015 Schultes, E. V. and R. F. Raffauf. De plantis Toxicariis e mundo novo tropicale commentationes XXXIX. Febrifuges of Northwest Amazonia. **Harvard Pap in Bot** 1994; 5: 50–68.

CC016 Mishra, A. and N. Dubey. Evaluation of some essential oils for their toxicity against fungi causing deterioration of stored food commodities. **Appl Environ Microbiol** 1994; 60(4): 1101–1105

CC017 Zamora-Martinez, M. C. and C. N. P. Pola. Medicinal plants used in some rural populations of Oaxaca, Puebla and Veracruz, Mexico. **J Ethnopharmacol** 1992; 35(3): 229–257.

CC018 Alam, K., T. Agua, H. Maven, R. Taie, K. S. Rao, I. Burrows, M. E. Huber and T. Rali. Preliminary screening of seaweeds, seagrass and lemongrass oil from Papua, New Guinea for antimicrobial and antifungal activity. **Int J Pharmacog** 1994; 32(4): 396–399.

CC019 Vinitketkummuen, U., R. Puatanachokchai, P. Kongtawelert, N. Lertprasetsuke and T. Matsushima. Antimutagenicity of lemon grass (*Cymbopogon citratus* Stapf) to various known mutagens in the Salmonella mutation assay. **Mutat Res** 1994; 341(1): 71–75.

CC020 Schmeda-Hirschmann, G. and A. Rojas De Arias. A screening method for natural products on Triatomine bugs. **Phytother Res** 1992; 6(2): 68–73.

CC021 Audicana, M. and G. Bernaola. Occupational contact dermatitis from citrus fruits: Lemon essential oils. **Contact Dermatitis** 1994; 31(3): 183–185.

CC022 De Blasi, V., S. Debrot, P. A. Menoud, L. Gendre and J. Schowing. Amoebicidal effect of essential oils in vitro. **J Toxicol Clin Exp** 1990; 10(6): 361–373.

CC023 Filipoy, A. Medicinal plants of the Pilaga of Central Chaco. **J Ethnopharmacol** 1994; 44(3): 181–193.

CC024 Syed, M., M. R. Khalid and F. M. Chaudhary. Essential oils of Gramineae family having antibacterial activity. Part 1. (*Cymbopogon citratus, C. martinii* and *C. jawarancusa* oils). **Pak J Sci Ind Res** 1990; 33(12): 529–531.

CC025 Onawunmi, G. O., W. A. Yisak and E. O. Ogunlana. Antibacterial constituents in the essential oil of *Cymbopogon citratus* (DC.) Stapf. **J Ethnopharmacol** 1984; 12(3): 279–286.

CC026 Ekundayo, O. Composition of the leaf volatile oil of *Cymbopogon citratus*. **Fitoterapia** 1985; 56(6): 334–342.

CC027 Olaniyi, A. A., E. A. Sofowora and B. O. Oguntimehin. Phytochemical investigation of some Nigerian plants used against fevers. II. *Cymbopogon citratus*. **Planta Med** 1975: 28; 186–189.

CC028 Evans, D. A. and R. K. Raj. Extracts of Indian plants as mosquito larvicides. **Indian J Med Res** 1988; 88(1): 38–41.

CC029 Carbajal, D., A. Casaco, L. Arruzazabala, R. Gonzalez and Z. Tolon. Pharmacological study of *Cymbopogon citratus* leaves. **J Ethnopharmacol** 1989; 25(1): 103–107.

CC030 Onawunmi, G. O. Evaluation of the antifungal activity of lemon grass oil. **Int J Crude Drug Res** 1989; 27(2): 121–126.

CC031 Natake, M., K. Kanazawa, M. Mizuno, N. Ueno, T. Kobayashi, G. I. Danno and S. Minamoto. Herb water-extracts markedly suppress the mutagenicity of TRP-P-2. **Agr Biol Chem** 1989; 53(5): 1423–1425.

CC032 Elson, C. E., G. L. Underbakke, P. Hanson, E. Shrago, R. H. Wainberg and A. A. Qureshi. Impact of lemongrass oil, an essential oil, on serum cholesterol. **Lipids** 1989; 24(8): 677–679.

CC033   Awuah, R. T. Fungitoxic effects of extracts from some West African plants. **Ann Appl Biol** 1989; 115(3): 451–453.

CC034   Lemos, T. L. G., F. J. A. Matos, J. W. Alencar, A. A. Craveiro, A. M. Clark and J. D. Mc Chesney. Antimicrobial activity of essential oils of Brazilian plants. **Phytother Res** 1990; 4(2): 82–84.

CC035   Suresh, M. and R. K. Rai. Cardol: The antifilarial principle from *Anacardium occidentale*. **Curr Sci** 1990; 59(9): 477–479.

CC036   Lorenzetti, B. B., G. E. P. Souza, S. J. Sarti, D. S. Filho and S. H. Ferreira. Myrcene mimics the peripheral analgesic activity of lemongrass tea. **J Ethnopharmacol** 1991; 34(1): 43–48.

CC037   De Matouschek, B. V. and E. Stahl-Biskup. Phytochemical investigation of nonvolatile constituents of *Cymbopogon citratus* (DC) Stapf. (Poaceae). **Pharm Acta Helv** 1991; 66(9/10): 242–245.

CC038   Carbajal, D., A. Casaco, L. Arruzazabala, R. Gonzalez and V. Fuentes. Pharmacological screening of plant decoctions commonly used in Cuban folk medicine. **J Ethnopharmacol** 1991; 33(1/2): 21–24.

CC039   Lam, L. K. T. and B. L. Zheng. Effects of essential oils on Glutathione S-Transferase activity in mice. **J Agr Food Chem** 1991; 39(4): 660–662.

CC040   Kobayashi, N. Pharmaceutical compositions containing lemongrass extracts and antioxidants. **Patent-Japan Kokai Tokkyo Koho**-01 221,320 : 2pp. 1989.

CC041   Arias, R. J., G. Schmeda-Hirschmann and A. Falcao. Feeding deterrency and insecticidal effects of plant extracts on *Lutzomyia longipalpis*. **Phytother Res** 1992; 6(2): 64–67.

CC042   Yokoyama, Y., T. Tsuyuki, N. Nakamura, T. Takahashi, S. W. Hanson and K. Matsushita. Revised structures of cymbopogone and cymbopogonol. **Tetrahedron Lett** 1980; 21: 3701–3702.

CC043   Locksley, H. D., M. B. E. Fayez, A. S. Radwan, V. M. Chari, G. A. Cordell and H. Wagner. Constituents of local plants. XXV. Constitution of the antispasmodic principle of *Cymbopogon proximus*. **Planta Med** 1982; 45: 20–22.

CC044   Tabata, M., N. Kiraoka and Y. Teranishi. Yield trial and tissue culture of Thai lemon grass. **Shoyakugaku Zasshi** 1981; 35: 128–133.

CC045   Semmler, F. W. and B. Zaar. Constituents of ethereal oils. (Identity of perilla alcohol with the alcohol, C10 H16 O, contained in ginger grass oil.) **Ber Dtsch Chem Ges** 1911; 44: 460–463.

CC046   Soytong, K., V. Rakvidhvasastra and T. Sommartya. Effect of some medicinal plants on growth of fungi and potential in plant disease control. **Abstr 11th Conference of Science and Technology**, Bangkok, Thailand October 24–26, 1985; 361.

CC047   Gupta, M. P., T. D. Arias, M. Correa and S. S. Lamba. Ethnopharmacognostic observations on Panamanian medicinal plants. Part 1. **Q J Crude Drug Res** 1979; 17(3/4): 115–130.

CC048   Arnason, T., F. Uck, J. Lambert and R. Hebda. Maya medicinal plants of San Jose Succotz, Belize. **J Ethnopharmacol** 1980; 2(4): 345–364.

CC049   Kloos, H. Preliminary studies of medicinal plants and plant products in markets of Central Ethiopia. **Ethnomedicine** 1977; 4(1): 63–104.

CC050   Sarer, E., J. J. C. Scheffer and A. Baerheim-Svendsen. Composition of the essential oil of *Cymbopogon citratus* (DC.) Stapf cultivated in Turkey. **Sci Pharm** 1983; 51(1): 58–63.

CC051   Abegaz, B., P. G. Yohannes and R. K. Dieter. Constituents of the essential oil of Ethiopian *Cymbopogon citratus*. **J Nat Prod** 1983; 46(3): 424–426.

CC052   Kasumov, F. Y. U. and R. I. Babaev. Components of the essential oil of lemongrass. **Chem Nat Comp** 1983; 19(1): 108.

CC053   Rao, R. R. and N. S. Jamir. Ethnobotanical studies in Nagaland. I. Medicinal plants. **Econ Bot** 1982; 36: 176–181.

CC054   Ungsurungsie, M., O. Suthienkul and C. Paovalo. Mutagenicity screening of popular Thai spices. **Food Chem Toxicol** 1982; 20: 527–530.

CC055 John, D. One hundred useful raw drugs of the Kani Tribes of Trivandrum Forest Division, Kerala, India. **Int J Crude Drug Res** 1984; 22(1): 17–39.

CC056 Singh, Y. N. Traditional medicine in Fiji: Some herbal folk cures used by Fiji Indians. **J Ethnopharmacol** 1986; 15(1): 57–88.

CC057 Chakraborty, D., P. K. Mahapatra and A. K. Nag Chaudhuri. A neurospsychopharmacological study of *Syzygium cumini*. **Planta Med** 1986; 2: 139–143.

CC058 Onawunmi, G. O. and E. O. Ogunlana. A study of the antibacterial activity of the essential oil of lemon grass (*Cymbopogon citratus* (DC.) Stapf). **Int J Crude Drug Res** 1986; 24(2): 64–68.

CC059 Leite, J. R., M. L. D. V. Seabra, E. Maluf, K. Assolant et al., Pharmacology of lemongrass (*Cymbopogon citratus* Stapf). III. Assessment of eventual toxic, hypnotic and anxiolytic effects on humans. **J Ethnopharmacol** 1986; 17(1): 75–83.

CC060 Souza Formigoni, M. L. O., H. M. Lodder, O. G. Filho, T. M. S. Ferriera and E. A. Carlini. Pharmacology of lemongrass (*Cymbopogon citratus* Stapf). II. Effects of daily two month administration in male and female rats and in offspring exposed "in utero". **J Ethnopharmacol** 1986; 17(1): 65–74.

CC061 Weniger, B., M. Rouzier, R. Daguilh, D. Henrys, J. H. Henrys and R. Anthon. Popular medicine of the Central Plateau of Haiti. 2. Ethnopharmacological inventory. **J Ethnopharmacol** 1986; 17(1): 13–30.

CC062 Carlini, E. A., J. D. D. P. Contar, A. R. Silva-Filho, N. G. Solveira-Filho, M. L. Frochtengarten and O. F. A. Bueno. Pharmacology of lemon grass (*Cymbopogon citratus* Stapf). Effects of teas prepared from the leaves on laboratory animals. **J Ethnopharmacol** 1986; 17(1): 37–64.

CC063 Ramirez, V. R., L. J. Mostacero, A. E. Garcia, C. F. Mejia, P. F. Pelaez, C. D. Medina and C. H. Miranda. Vegetales empleados en medicina tradicional Norperuana. **Banco Agrario Del Peru & NACL Univ Trujillo**, Trujillo, Peru, June 1988; 54pp.

CC064 Caceres, A., L. M. Giron, S. R. Alvarado, and M. F. Torres. Screening of antimicrobial activity of plants popularly used in Guatemala for the treatment of dermatomucosal diseases. **J Ethnopharmacol** 1987; 20(3): 223–237.

CC065 Costa, M., L. C. Di Stasi, M. Kirizawa, S. L. J. Mendacolli, C. Gomes and G. Trolin. Screening in mice of some medicinal plants used for analgesic purposes in the state of Sao Paulo. **J Ethnopharmacol** 1989; 27(1/2): 25–33.

CC066 Spring, M. A. Ethnopharmacological analysis of medicinal plants used by Laotian Hmong refugees in Minnesota. **J Ethnopharmacol** 1989; 26(1): 65–91.

CC067 Darias, V., L. Brando, R. Rabanal, C. Sanchez Mateo, R. M. Gonzalez Luis and A. M. Hernandez Perez. New contribution to the ethnopharmacological study of the Canary Islands. **J Ethnopharmacol** 1989; 25(1): 77–92.

CC068 Mueller-Oerlinghausen, B., W. Ngamwathana and P. Kanchanapee. Investigation into Thai medicinal plants said to cure diabetes. **J Med Assoc Thailand** 1971; 54: 105–111.

CC069 Wasuwat, S. A list of Thai medicinal plants, ASRCT, Bangkok, Report No. 1 on Res. Project. 17. A.S.R.C.T. Bangkok Thailand 1967; 17: 22pp.

CC070 Onawunmi, G. O., W. A. Yisak and E. O. Ogunlana. Antibacterial constituents in the essential oil of *Cymbopogon citratus* (DC.) Stapf. **J Ethnopharmacol**; 1984; 12(3): 279–283.

CC071 De-Oliveira, A. C., L. F. Ribeiro-Pinto, S. S. Otto, A. Gonsalves, F. J. Paumgartten. Induction of liver monooxygenases by beta-myrcene. **Toxicology** 1997; 124(2): 135–140.

CC072 Vinitketkumnuen, U., T. Chewonarin, P. Dhumtanom, N. Lertprasertsuk and C. P. Wild. Aflatoxin-albumin adduct formation after single and multiple doses of aflatoxin B(1) in rats treated with Thai medicinal plants. **Mutat Res** 1999; 428(1-2): 345–351.

CC073 Viana, G. S., T. G. Vale, R. S. Pinho and F. J. Matos. Antinociceptive effect of the essential oil from *Cymbopogon citratus* in mice. **J Ethnopharmacol** 2000; 70(3): 323–327.

CC074 Melo, S. F., S. F. Soares, R. F. da Costa, C. R. da Silva, M. B. de Oliviera, R. J. Bezerra, A. Caldeira-de-Araujo and M. Bernardo-Filho. Effect of the *Cymbopogon citrates*, Maytenus and *Baccharis genistelloides* extracts against the stannous chloride oxidative damage in *Escherichia coli*. **Mutat Res** 2001; 496(1-2): 33–38.

CC075 Ansari, M. A. and R. K. Razdan. Relative efficacy of various oils in repelling mosquitoes. **Indian J Malariol** 1995; 32(3): 104–111.

CC076 Inouye, S., T. Tsuruoka, M. Watanabe, K. Takeo, M. Akao, Y. Nishiyama nad H. Yamaguchi. Inhibitory effect of essential oils on apical growth of *Aspergillus fumigatus* by vapour contact. **Mycoses** 2000; 43(1–2): 17–23.

CC077 Inouye, S., T. Takizawa and H. Yamaguchi. Antibacterial activity of essential oils and their major constituents against respiratory tract pathogens by gaseous contact. **Antimicrob Chemother** 2001; 47(5): 565–573.

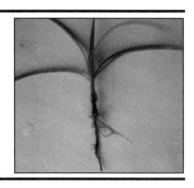

10 | *Cyperus rotundus*

L.

Common Names

Bhada	India	Motha sedge	India
Chido	India	Mothe	Nepal
Co cu	Malaysia	Musta	India
Coquinho	Madeira	Mustaka	India
Cu gau	Malaysia	Mustha	India
Cu gau	Vietnam	Mutha	India
Eldeis	Sudan	Muthanga	India
Galingale	Madeira	Nut grass	Brazil
Haeo muu	Thailand	Nut grass	Guyana
Haeo-mu	Thailand	Nut grass	Hawaii
Haew muu	Thailand	Nut grass	India
Hama-suge	Japan	Nut grass	Japan
Herbe a oignons	New Caledonia	Nut grass	Nepal
Hsiang fu	Vietnam	Nutsedge	Hawaii
Hsiang fu-tzu	China	Nutt grass	Iran
Hsiang-fu	China	Oniani tita	Cook Islands
Huai-mao ts'ao	China	Purple nutsedge	Hawaii
Hui-t'ou ch'ing	China	Purple nutsedge	Japan
Huong phu	Malaysia	Rhizoma cyperii	Taiwan
Hyang-boo-ja	Malaysia	S-s'ad	Morocco
Japanese nutgrass	Japan	Se'd	Qatar
Karimuthan	India	Sha-ts'ao	China
Kobushi	Japan	Siru	Nepal
Koraikizhangu	India	Souchet rond	Vietnam
Korchijhan	India	T'ien-t'ou ts'ao	China
Kraval chruk	Malaysia	Tamusayt	Morocco
Kravanh chruk	Malaysia	Tiao ma tsung	China
Mathe	India	Tungamuste	India
Moothoo	India	Tungamusti	India
Moth	India	Tungamuthalu	India
Motha	India	Xiangfu	China

From: *Medicinal Plants of the World, vol. 1: Chemical Constituents, Traditional and Modern Medicinal Uses, 2nd ed.*
By: Ivan A. Ross © Humana Press Inc., Totowa, NJ

BOTANICAL DESCRIPTION

Cyperus rotundus is a plant of the GRAMINEAE family, consisting of stems that are tuberous at the base, rising singly from a creeping, underground root-stock, about 10 to 25 cm tall. Leaves are linear, broadly grooved on the upper surface, and dark green in color. Flowers are in rather small inflorescence with 2–4 bracts. The longest bracts are usually longer than the inflorescence, but some are shorter. The inflorescence consists of a few slender branches, with the longest usually not more than about 7.5-cm spikes, consisting of about 2–10 spikelets. Each spikelet is narrow and flattened; glumes rather narrow, blunt, closely overlapping with 3 stamens, 3-branched. The nut is oblong-ovate, nearly half as long as the glume, strongly 3-angled, yellow, black when ripe.

ORIGIN AND DISTRIBUTION

Originated in India, it is now widely distributed in the tropics and subtropics. Because of its capacity to compete and adapt to diverse conditions, it has been recorded in more countries than any other weed in the world.

TRADITIONAL MEDICINAL USES

Cambodia. Hot water extract of dried tuber is taken orally for liver complaints with jaundice, and for malarial fevers[CR117].

China. Decoction of dried entire plant is taken orally for worms coming out of both the mouth and anus. *Cyperus rotundus, Berberis aristata, Embelia ribes, Piper longum,* and *Baliospermum* are used in the decoction. Mixed with honey and "Patola" (unidentified), the decoction is administered orally to bring unconscious patients to consciousness. For skin disease, decoction of *Tinospora cordifolia, Cyperus rotundus,* and *Zingiber officinale* is mixed with equal quantity of decoction of *Aconitum heterophyllum,* and taken orally[CR127]. For chronic bloody diarrhea

with abdominal pain, decoction of *Coleus vetiveroides, Aconitum heterophyllum, Cyperus rotundus* and *Holarrhea antidysenterica* is taken orally[CR127]. Dried tuber, mixed with *Rehmannia glutinosa* (root), *Scutellaria baicalensis* (root), *Phellodendron amurense* (bark), and *Ailanthus blandulosa* (bark) administered as a vaginal suppository, is used for leukorrhea with thirst, constipation, weak pulse, abdominal pain and backache in patients with vaginal cancer[CR135]. Hot water extract of dried rhizome is taken orally to restore menstrual regularity, to alleviate pain and for dysmenorrhea[CR096]. Hot water extract of tuber is used for dysmenorrhea[CR018], as a galactogogue, as an emmenagogue[CR025,CR043], to promote difficult labor[CR043], as an emmenagogue and for dysmenorrhea, in doses of 5–8 gm[CR045].

Cook Islands. Infusion of fresh bulb is taken orally as a treatment for sore throat. Twenty to 30 bulbs, a handful of *Pandanus tectoris* bark, and a handful of *Chrysopagon acriculatus* leaves are crushed into the water of 4 green coconuts. Half the mixture is drunk hot and the remainder cold. The treatment lasts for 3 days[CR054].

Europe. The rhizome is taken orally to induce menses[CR024].

India. Hot water extract of the tuber is taken orally to relieve thirst, decrease palpitations, reduce weight, strengthen memory and stimulate appetite; as an aphrodisiac, stomachic, carminative, astringent, tonic, diuretic and anthelmintic. The extract is used against alcoholism. One gram each of *Piper nigrum, Piper longum, Santalum album, Pterrocarpus santalinus, Nardostachys jatamansi, Symplocos racemosa, Andropogon muricatus, Elettaria cardamomum, Berris aristata, Plumbago zeylanica* and *Cyperus rotundus,* plus 5 gm *Woodfordia floribunda,* are soaked in 1 liter of water with sugar and raisins and fermented 30 days, strained and matured for 90 days, then taken orally[CR133]. Hot water extract of the tuber is taken orally as a diaphoretic, tonic, diuretic and demulcent. Externally, used as an astringent, and tuber paste is applied to the breast as a galactogogue[CR117]. Decoction of dried root is taken orally for diarrhea[CR049]. Decoction of *Melia azedarach* is mixed with bulbous root of *Cyperus rotundus* and taken orally as a treatment for dermatitis[CR077]. Extract of the root is taken as an emmenagogue[CR021]. Extract of the tuber is taken orally as an emmenagogue[CR021]. Hot water extract is taken orally as an anthelmintic and as an emmenagogue[CR138]. Hot water extract of dried entire plant is taken orally for fever. This is also used as an anti-inflammatory agent in Ayurveda[CR114]. Essential oil of the root is used externally as a treatment for dermatitis[CR077]. Hot water extract of dried leaves is taken orally for blood motions. Tuber and leaves are taken with bark, flowers and young fruit of *Plumbago zeylani*[CR071]. Hot water extract of dried rhizome is taken orally as a stimulant, anthelmintic, stomachic and carminative. Decoction, with the leaves of *Solanum nigrum*, is taken orally for recurring fever. The extract is also taken orally as an insect repellent, and for dysentery and stomach disorders[CR116]. Hot water extract of dried root is used as a diaphoretic and astringent[CR070]. Hot water extract of dried tuber is taken orally in Ayurvedic and Unani medicine as an emmenagogue[CR101]. Tuber is boiled in milk and given orally to improve digestion in infants[CR110]. A paste of the tuber is applied around the navel and throat to relieve pain, especially that caused by roundworms[CR110]. Hot water extract of rhizome is taken orally as an emmenagogue[CR002], and to regulate fat metabolism[CR030]. Rhizome, made into a paste, is applied to the breast as a galactagogue[CR002]. Tubers and rhizomes, crushed and boiled in goat's milk, are taken orally for colic, to treat diarrhea, vomiting in children and flatulence in children[CR106].

Indochina. Hot water extract of dried tuber is taken orally to aid childbirth and for indigestion in infants[CR117]. Hot water extract of tuber is administered orally to women in childbirth[CR031,CR032]. Rhizome is given to women in childbirth[CR002].

Indonesia. Hot water extract is taken orally to promote menses[CR003]. Hot water extract of dried tuber is taken orally for urinary disorders[CR117].

Japan. Extract of the tuber is taken orally in Chinese medicine for women's diseases[CR021]. Hot water extract of fresh tuber is used externally to promote hair growth[CR103]. Hot water extract of the rhizome is taken orally as an emmenagogue[CR026].

Malaysia. Extract of the rhizome is taken orally an emmenagogue[CR027]. Hot water extract of tuber is taken orally as an emmenagogue[CR032].

Nepal. Hot water extract of the tuber is administered orally as a diuretic, anthelmintic and emmenagogue[CR001].

New Caledonia. Hot water extract of rhizomes is taken orally as an emmenagogue[CR023].

Nigeria. Hot water extract of fresh root is used externally as an astringent, carminative, antimalarial and tonic[CR102].

Paraguay. Hot water extract is taken orally as a contraceptive[CR130].

Philippines. Hot water extract of dried tuber is taken orally for dysentery[CR117].

Puerto Rico. Hot water extract of dried entire plant is taken orally for kidney calculi[CR145].

South Korea. Hot water extract of rhizome is used for protection of the liver[CR086], and to induce menstruation and abortion[CR134]. Hot water extract of the dried rhizome is taken orally as an abortifacient and emmenagogue[CR118].

Sri Lanka. Hot water extract of dried tuber is taken orally as an astringent, stomachic, carminative, cholagogue and antiseptic, for anorexia, diarrhea and dysentery, liver congestion, laryngitis, bronchitis and pneumonia. For scorpion stings, ulcers and acne, a paste of tubers with lime juice is applied to the affected area[CR117].

Sudan. Hot water extract of dried entire plant is taken orally for indigestion, and as an antiemetic[CR122] and an astringent[CR107]. Hot water extract of dried root is taken orally as an antidiarrheal and antiemetic[CR122].

Taiwan. Hot water extract of dried rhizome is taken orally for liver disease[CR128].

Tanzania. Fresh tuber is used in traditional medicine[CR119]. Hot water extract of dried tuber is taken orally to aid in childbirth[CR092].

Thailand. Hot water extract of dried rhizome is taken orally for blood purification and as an antipyretic[CR144].

Vietnam. Hot water extract of dried tuber is taken orally as a diuretic, as an emmenagogue and for uterine hemorrhage[CR117]. Hot water extract of rhizome is taken orally for difficult delivery[CR027]. Hot water extract of the tuber is taken orally as an emmenagogue[CR031].

CHEMICAL CONSTITUENTS

(ppm unless otherwise indicated)

(–)-Isorotundene: Rh[CR151]
(–)-Cypera-2,4(15)-diene: Rh[CR151]
(–)-Norrotundene: Rh[CR151]
(+)-Nyperadione: Rh[CR151]
1,8-Cineole: Rt[CR037]
4,7-Dimethyl-tetral-1-one: Tu[CR038]
4-Alpha,5-alpha-oxo eudesm-11-en-3-alpha-ol: Rh[CR041]
2-Carboxy-arabinitol: Lf 34 nMol/g[CR146]
10,12-Peroxy-calamenene: Tu 0.45[CR038]
Alkaloids: Rt 0.21–0.24%[CR199]
Alpha copaene: Rh EO[CR066]
Alpha cyperone (+): Tu[CR043], EO[CR039]
Alpha cyperone: Tu[CR060], Rt EO[CR094], Rh 700[CR112]
Alpha humulene: Rh EO[CR066], Rt EO[CR094], Tu[CR100]
Alpha rotundol: Rh[CR013]
Alpha rotunol: Tu[CR137]
Alpha selinene: Tu[CR073]
Aristolone: Rh[CR154]
Arsenic: Rh 0.29[CR036]
Ascorbic acid: Rt 8.8 mg/%[CR015]
Aureusidin: Inf[CR033]

Beta caryophyllene: Rh EO[CR082]
Beta cyperone: Rh[CR035]
Beta elemene: Tu[CR100], Rh EO[CR066], Rt EO[CR094]
Beta guaiene: Rt EO[CR059]
Beta pinene: Rt[CR037]
Beta rotundol: Rh[CR013]
Beta rotunol: Tu[CR137]
Beta santalene: Rt EO[CR059]
Beta seliene: Rh EO[CR066]
Beta selinene: Rh[CR154], Rt EO[CR094], Tu[CR060]
Beta sitosterol: Tu[CR090], Rt[CR083]
Calamenene: Rh EO[CR066]
Calcium: Rh 0.318%[CR036]
Camphene: Rt[CR037]
Caryophylla-6-one: Tu 0.01%[CR055]
Caryophyllene: Tu 50.0[CR055], Rh EO[CR094]
Caryophyllene-6-7-oxide: Tu 33.3[CR055]
Caryophyllene-alpha-oxide: Tu 4.0[CR055]
Caryophyllenol: Tu EO[CR053]
Chlorophyll A: Lf[CR040]
Chlorophyll B: Lf[CR040]
Cineol: Tu[CR043]
Copadiene (+): EO[CR010]
Copaene: Rt[CR037]
Copper: Rh 10[CR036]
Cyperene II: Rh[CR141]
Cyperene: Rt EO[CR094], Tu[CR100], Rh EO[CR147]
Cyperenone: Tu[CR021], Rt EO[CR059], Rh 115[CR112]
Cyperol: Rh EO[CR066], Tu[CR011]
Cyperolone: Rh[CR009], EO[CR010]
Cyperotundone: Rh[CR143], Tu[CR052]
Cyperus rotudus germination inhibitor: Rh[CR006]
D-Copadiene: Rt[CR037]
Delta-cadinene: Rh EO[CR066], Tu[CR052], Rt EO[CR059]
D-Epoxyguaiene: Rt[CR037]
D-Fructose: Rt[CR037]
D-Glucose: Rt[CR037]
Epoxy-guaiene (+): EO[CR010]
Essential oil: Tu[CR028], Rh 0.6%[CR041]
Ferulic acid: Tu[CR100]
Flavonoids: Rt 1.25%[CR037]
Fluoride: Rh 3.7[CR131]
Fructose: Sh[CR029]
Gamma cymene: Rt[CR034]
Glucose: Sh[CR029]
Humulene: Rh EO[CR082], Tu[CR073]
Iron (inorganic): Sh[CR029]
Iso-cyperol: Rh 32.5[CR112], Rh EO[CR142], Tu[CR011]

Iso-kobusone: Rt EO[CR136]
Isocurcumenol: Rh[CR154]
Kobusone: Rt EO[CR136]
Limonene: EO[CR037]
Linoleic acid: Rh[CR035]
Linolenic acid: Rh[CR035]
Luteolin: Inf, Lf[CR104]
Magnesium: Rh 0.15%[CR036]
Manganese: Rh 28[CR036]
Mustakone: EO[CR012]
Myristic acid: Rh[CR035]
Nootkatone: Rh[CR154]
Oleanolic acid: Rh[CR154,CR090]
Oleanolic acid-3-0-neohesperidoside: Tu[CR090]
Oleic acid: Rh[CR035]
Para-coumaric acid: Tu[CR100]
Patchoulenol acetate: Tu[CR052]
Patchoulenone: Tu 30[CR038]
Patchouylenone: Rh EO[CR066]
P-cymol: Rt[CR037]
Pectin: Rt 3.72%[CR037]
Petchoulenyl acetate: Rh EO[CR066]
Phosphorus: Sh[CR029]
P-hydroxy-benzoic acid: Tu[CR100]
Pinene: Tu[CR043]
Polyphenols: Rt 1.62%[CR037]
Potassium: Rh 1.01%[CR036]
Protocatechuic acid: Tu[CR100]
Resin: Rt 4.21%[CR037]
Rhamnetin-3-0-rhamnosyl(1,4)rhamnoside: Tu[CR061]
Rotundene: Rt[CR034]
Rotundenol: Rt[CR058]
Rotundine A: Rh[CR152]
Rotundine B: Rh[CR152]
Rotundine C: Rh[CR152]
Rotundone (–): EO[CR010]
Selinatriene: Rt[CR034]
Sodium: Rh 254[CR036]
Starch: Rt 9.2%[CR037]
Stearic acid: Rh[CR036]
Sucrose: Sh[CR029]
Sugars: Rt 13.2–14.4%[CR037]
Sugenol: Rh[CR035]
Sugeonol acetate: Tu[CR052]
Sugeonol: Rh[CR014]
Sugeonyl acetate: Rh EO[CR066]
Sugetriol triacetate: Tu[CR052]
Sugetriol: Tu[CR148], Rh[CR017]
Vanillic acid: Tu[CR100]
Zinc: Rh 33[CR036]

PHARMACOLOGICAL ACTIVITIES AND CLINICAL TRIALS

Abortifacient effect. Ethanol/water (1:1) extract, at a dose of 100.0 mg/kg administered orally to pregnant rats, was inactive[CR091].

Adrenergic receptor blockade (A-2). Water extract of dried rhizome was inactive. The extract did not have any inhibitory effect on angiotensin II[CR064].

Aflatoxin inactivation. Water extract of dried leaf, at a concentration of 1.0 ml, was active on *Aspergillus flavus*[CR079].

Aldose reductase inhibition. Hot water extract, at a concentration of 0.1 mg/ml, produced strong activity. The effect was tested on bovine lens aldase reductase[CR047].

Analgesic activity. Ethanol (95%) extract of the entire plant (cultivated in Saudi Arabia), administered to mice at a dose of 500.0 mg/kg by gastric intubation, was inactive vs hot plate method[CR068]. Ethanol (95%) and hot water extracts of dried rhizome, at a dose of 12.7 gm/kg administered intraperitoneally to mice, were inactive vs hot plate method. Hot water extract, administered orally at a dose of 12.7 gm/kg, was also inactive vs acetic acid writhing inhibition test[CR088]. Alkaloid fraction, essential oil, and decoction of dried rhizome, administered to mice by gastric intubation, were active vs acetic acid-induced writhing[CR050].

Anthelmintic activity. Hot water extract of leaf, administered to mice, was inactive on *Nippostrongylus brasiliense, Trichostrongylus axei* and *Syphacia obvelata*[CR042]. Hot water extract of tuber, administered orally to mice, was inactive on *Nippostrongylus brasiliense, Syphacia obvelata*, and *Trichostrongylus axei*[CR042].

Antialcoholic activity. Fermented tuber, at a dose of 5.0 ml/animal in the ration of rats, was active. Dose given daily for 90 days reversed alcohol-induced changes on performance of neurologic tests, EEG and EKG, fat deposition in liver and signs of hemorrhage, demyelination and spongiosis in brain. Fermented extracts of the following plants, referred to as the SKV Indian herbal formula, were used: *Piper nigrum, Piper longum, Santalum album, Pterocarpus santalinus, Nardostachys jatamansi, Symplocos racemosa, Andropogon muricatus, Elettaria cardamomum,* and *Berber aristata.* Also included: *Plumbago zeylanica, Cyperus rotundus, Woodfordia floribunda* and raisins. Rats were given the herbal formula (SKV) for 3 months vs rats fed alcohol for 6 months[CR132,CR133].

Antibacterial activity. Chloroform and methanol extracts of dried entire plant, when tested on agar plate, were active, and the water extract was inactive on *Bacillus subtilis, Escherichia coli, Pseudomonas aeruginosa* and *Staphylococcus aureus*[CR122]. Decoction of dried entire plant, at MIC 125.0 mg/ml on agar plate, was inactive on *E. coli, Klebsiella pneumoniae* and *P. aeruginosa.* At MIC 15.63 mg/ml, the decoction had weak activity on *Staphylococcus aureus* and *Staphylococcus epidermidis.* At MIC 31.25 mg/ml, weak activity was shown on *Bacillus cereus, Bacillus subtilis, Bordetella bronchiseptica, Micrococcus flavus, Proteus vulgaris* and *Sarcina lutea.* At MIC 62.5 mg/ml, the decoction was inactive on *Salmonella typhi*[CR129]. Essential oil of dried rhizome, undiluted on agar plate, was active on *Staphylococcus aureus*[CR140]. Decoction of dried rhizome produced weak activity on *Streptococcus mutans* on agar plate, MIC 62.5 mg/ml[CR069]. Ethanol (95%) extract, at a concentration of 100.0 mg/disk, and water extract at 20.0 mg/disk on agar plate, were inactive on *Bacillus subtilis, E. coli, Salmonella typhosa, Shigella dysenteriae* and *Staphylococcus aureus.* Dose expressed as dry weight of plant[CR084]. Ethanol (95%) and petroleum ether extracts of shade-dried rhizomes, on agar plate, were inactive on *Enterobacter cloacae, Escherichia coli, Klebsiella pneumoniae, Proteus vulgaris, Pseudomonas aeruginosa, Serratia marcescens,* *Staphylococcus aureus* and *Streptococcus faecalis,* MIC >3.0 mg/ml[CR051]. Chloroform and methanol extracts of dried root, on agar plate, were active on *Bacillus subtilis, Escherichia coli, Pseudomonas aeruginosa* and *Staphylococcus aureus.* The water extract was inactive[CR122]. Decoction of dried stem, on agar plate, was active on *Pseudomonas aeruginosa, Salmonella paratyphi, Shigella sonnei, Staphylococcus aureus, Vibrio parahemolyticus* and *Yersinia enterolitica.* The decoction was inactive on *Bacillus subtilis, Escherichia coli, Klebsiella pneumonia* and *Proteus mirabilis*[CR067]. Chloroform and methanol extracts of dried stem, on agar plate, were active on *Bacillus subtilis, E. coli, Pseudomonas aeruginosa* and *Staphylococcus aureus.* The water extract was inactive[CR122]. Methanol extract of dried tuber, at a concentration of 1.0% on agar plate, was inactive on *Escherichia coli.* The extract produced weak activity on *Staphylococcus aureus*[CR092]. Water extract of fresh tuber, at a concentration of 1.0% on agar plate, was inactive on *Neisseria gonorrhea*[CR119].

Anticonvulsant activity. Ethanol (70%) extract of fresh roots, at variable dosage levels administered intraperitoneally to both sexes of mice, was active vs metrazole-induced and strychnine-induced convulsions[CR102].

Anticrustacean activity. Chloroform extract of dried root was active on *Artemia salina* larvae, LD_{50} 86.25 mg/ml. Water and methanol extracts were inactive, with LD_{50} of 1.0 mg/ml for each. Assay system is intended to predict for antitumor activity[CR075].

Antidiarrheal activity. Ethanol/water (1:1) extract of dried roots, at a concentration of 300.0 mg, was inactive on guinea pig and rabbit ileum vs coli-inte rotoxin-induced diarrhea[CR049].

Antiemetic activity. A commercial sample of roots, administered by gastric intubation to pigeons at a dose of 80.0 mg/kg, was active vs reserpine-induced emesis[CR062].

Antifungal activity. Rhizome, when tested on agar plate, was active on *Colletotrichum chardonianum*, *Phytophthora capsici* and *Sclerotinia sclerotiorum*[CR005]. Water extract of fresh shoots, undiluted on agar plate, was inactive on *Helminthosporium turcicum*[CR149].

Antihepatotoxic activity. Methanol extract of rhizome, at a dose of 670.0 mg/kg administered orally to mice, was active in CCl₄-treated mice[CR086]. Methanol extract of dried rhizome, at a dose of 670.0 mg/kg administered by gastric intubation to mice, showed strong activity vs CCl₄-induced hepatotoxicity[CR121]. Methanol extract of dried rhizome was active in rats. Activity was measured in terms of the elongation of hexobarbital sleeping time after CCl₄ treatment. Elongation of sleeping time indicated negative results vs CCl₄-induced hepatotoxicity[CR115]. Dried tuber, when administered to mice, was active. The duration of hexobarbital sleeping time was used as a measurement for this activity vs CCl₄-induced hepatotoxicity[CR124]. Ether extract of dried tuber, at a dose of 300.0 mg/kg administered to mice by gastric intubation, was inactive vs CCl₄-induced hepatotoxicity[CR113]. Water and methanol/water (1:1) extracts of dried rhizome, administered intraperitoneally to mice, were active vs CCl₄-induced hepatotoxicity[CR150,CR095].

Antihistamine activity. Ethanol/water (1:1) extract of dried rhizome, at a concentration of 0.001 gm/ml, was active on guinea pig ileum[CR144].

Antihypertensive activity. Dried root, at a dose of 2.0 gm/day taken by human adults, was active. Sixty-four patients were given this drug for 2 months. There was a significant reduction in weight. Blood pressure was lowered in hypertensive patients, but not in normotensive patients. Side effects were mild with some nausea initially, and appetite suppression in 12 subjects[CR123].

Anti-implantation effect. Ethanol/water (1:1) extract of dried rhizome, at a dose of 100.0 mg/kg administered orally to female rats, was inactive[CR091].

Anti-inflammatory activity. Chloroform extract of dried roots, at a dose of 10.0 mg/kg administered intraperitoneally to rats, and water extract, at a dose of 500.0 mg/kg administered by gastric intubation, were active vs carrageenin-induced pedal edema[CR111]. Water extract, at a dose of 2.0% administered ophthalmically to human adults, produced a decreased in redness and reduced pain and ocular discharge in patients with conjunctivitis[CR105]. Methanol extract, at doses of 10.0 mg/kg and 5.0 mg/kg administered intraperitoneally to rats, was active vs carrageenin-induced edema and formalin-induced pedal edema, respectively. Petroleum ether extract, at a dose of 10.0 mg/kg administered intraperitoneally to rats, was also active[CR016]. Water extract of rhizome was inactive in albumin stabilizing assay[CR004].

Antimalarial activity. Ethanol/water (50%) extract of dried aerial parts, at a concentration of 100 mcg/ml, was inactive on *Plasmodium berghei*. The extract was toxic at this dose. The extract, when administered by gastric intubation to mice at a dose of 1.0 gm/kg, was active on *Plasmodium berghei*. With daily dosing for 4 days, inhibition was 49%[CR080]. Chloroform extract of dried tuber was active on *Plasmodium falciparum*, IC₅₀ 10.0 mg/ml vs hypoxanthine uptake by plasmodia[CR074]. Both methanol and petroleum ether extracts were inactive. IC₅₀ 49.0 mg/ml was obtained for both extracts vs hypoxanthine uptake by plasmodia[CR074]. Hexane extract of dried tuber was active on *Plasmodium falciparum*, ED₅₀ 0.66 mcg/ml[CR038].

Antioxidant activity. Methanol extract of dried rhizome, at a dose of 1.6 gm/kg administered by gastric intubation to mice, was inactive vs ethanol-induced lipid peroxidation in mouse liver. Dose expressed as dry weight of plant[CR064].

Antipyretic activity. Ethanol (95%) extract of the entire plant (cultivated in Saudi Arabia), administered to mice at a dose of 500.0 mg/kg by gastric intubation, was active vs yeast-induced pyrexia[CR068]. Water extract of dried rhizome, at a dose of 0.5 gm/kg administered by gastric intubation to rats, was active. Effect was seen 4.5 hours after treatment vs yeast-induced pyrexia[CR081]. Methanol extract of dried root, at a dose of 5.0 mg/kg administered intraperitoneally to rats, was active vs pyrexia induced by yeast injection[CR016].

Antiradiation activity. Methanol extract of dried rhizome, at a dose of 1000 mg/kg administered intraperitoneally to mice, was inactive vs soft X-ray irradiation at lethal dose[CR126].

Antiscleroderma activity. Hot water extract of dried rhizome, taken by human adults of both sexes, was active. Thirty cases of generalized scleroderma were treated. The results claimed to be satisfactory in 28/30 cases. The preparation contained *Codonopsis pilosula* (root); *Astragalusi* (root); *Cinnamomum cassia* (bark); *ehmannia glutinosa* (root); *Paeonia rubra* (root); *Carthamus tinctorius* (flower); *Polygonum multiflorum*; *Millettia* species; *Salvia miltiorrhiza* (root); *Cyperus rotundus* (rhizome) and *Glycyrrhiza uralensis* (root)[CR089].

Antispasmodic activity. Ethanol (95%) extract of dried rhizome, at a concentration of 200.0 mcg/ml, was active on guinea pig ileum vs histamine-induced contractions and barium-induced contractions. Water extract was inactive vs barium-induced contractions, and showed weak activity vs histamine-induced contractions[CR109]. Ethanol/water (1:1) extract of dried rhizome, at a concentration of 0.001 gm/ml, was active on guinea pig ileum[CR144]. Methanol extract of rhizome, at a concentration of 1.0 mg/ml on rat ileum, was active vs ACh-induced contractions[CR044].

Antitumor activity. Water extract of the dried rhizome, at a concentration of 100.0 mg/ml, was active on Sarcoma 180(ASC) in mice[CR063]. Hot water extract of dried seeds, administered intravaginally to human adults, was active. Lacryma-Jobi uterine mycoma was treated. In 52.9% of cases, the symptoms completely disappeared, and in 27.2%, the tumors were reduced in size. A mixture was employed that contained *Angelica sinensis*, *Curcuma zedoaria*, *Prunus persica*, *Dipsacus asper*, *Cyperus rotundus*, *Prunella vulgaris*, *Achyranthes bidentata*, *Vaccaria segetalis*, *Sparganium stoloniferum*, *Laminaria japonica* and *coix*[CR098]. Ethanol (defatted with petroleum ether) extract of dried tuber, at a dose of 500.0 mg/kg administered to mice intraperitoneally, was active on CA-Erlich ascites, and inactive on LEUK-SN36 and Sarcoma 180(ASC)[CR099].

Antiviral activity. Decoction of dried entire plant, taken orally by human adults, was active. A patient with a typical chronic infectious hepatitis was treated with good results using a decoction of *Salvia miltiorrhiza*, *Isatis tinctoria*, *Taraxacum mongolicum*, *Paeonia lactiflora*, *Atractylodes macrocephala* and *Rehmannia glutinosa*[CR065]. Hot water extract of dried rhizome, at a concentration of 0.5 mg/ml in cell culture, was inactive on Herpes Simplex 1 virus, Measles virus and Poliovirus 1[CR048].

Antiyeast activity. Ethanol (95%) extract of dried rhizome, at a concentration of 100.0 mg/disk, and water extract, at a concentration of 20.0 mg/disk on agar plate, were inactive on *Candida albicans*. Dose expressed as dry weight of plant[CR084]. Ethanol (95%) extract of dried rhizome, on agar plate, was inactive on *Candida albicans*, MIC <3.0 mg/ml. The petroleum ether extract, however, was active, MIC 1.0 mg/ml[CR051].

Barbiturate potentiation. Methanol (75%) extract of rhizome, at a concentration of 500.0 mg/kg administered intraperitoneally to mice, was inactive[CR087]. Methanol extract of dried rhizome, at a dose of 500.0 mg/kg administered intraperitoneally to mice, was inactive. The extract did not affect barbiturate-sleeping time[CR120]. Methanol extract of rhizome, at a dose of 670.0 mg/kg administered orally to mice, decreases the barbiturate sleeping time in CCl_4-treated mice[CR086]. Methanol (75%) extract, at a dose of 500.0 mg/kg intraperitoneally, did not decrease the barbiturate sleeping time[CR087]. Ether extract of dried tuber, at a dose of 300.0 mg/kg administered by gastric intubation to mice, did not decrease the barbiturate sleeping time[CR113].

Bradycardia activity. Water extract of rhizome was active on the heart of frog. The extract was also active when administered intravenously to cats and rabbits[CR020].

Cardiac depressant activity. Water extract of rhizome, administered to frog subcutaneously, was active[CR020].

Coagulant activity. Hexane extract of dried leaves and stem was inactive[CR072].

Coronary vasodilator activity. Water extract of rhizome, administered intravenously to cats, rabbits and frogs, was active[CR020].

Cytotoxic activity. Hot water extract of dried aerial parts, at a dose of 500 mcg/ml in cell culture, showed weak activity on CA-JTC-26. The inhibition rate was 69%[CR078]. Chloroform, water, and methanol extracts, at concentrations of 100.0 mcg/ml in cell culture, were inactive on CA-A549[CR057]. Acetone extract of dried rhizome, at a concentration of 5.0% by cylinder plate method, was inactive on CA-Erlich ascites; 10 mm inhibition. The ether and water extracts, at concentrations of 5.0%, were both inactive; 15 mm inhibition. Methanol extract, at 5.0% concentration, was equivocal; 25 mm inhibition[CR057]. Water extract of dried roots, at a concentration of 500.0 mcg/ml in cell culture, was inactive on human embryonic cells HE-1. The extract produced weak activity on CA-Mammary-Microalveolar. Ethanol (defatted with petroleum ether) extract of dried tuber, in cell culture on HELA cells, produced ED_{50} 32.0 mcg/ml[CR099].

Diuretic activity. Ethanol (95%) extract of root, administered orally to dogs, increased urine output 12–60%. Chloride and urea concentrations were unchanged[CR015]. Water extract of rhizome, administered intraperitoneally to rats, was active[CR0198]. Ethanol/water (1:1) extract of dried rhizome, at a dose of 340.0 mg/kg administered orally to male rats, was active[CR091].

Estrogenic effect. Essential oil of the root, administered subcutaneously to female mice at variable dosage levels, was active[CR139].

Fibrinolytic activity. Hexane extract of dried leaves and stem was inactive[CR072].

Gamma-glutamyl transpeptidase inhibition. Fermented dried tuber, at a dose of 5.0 ml/day in the ration of rats, was active. Rats were given the SKV Indian herbal formula daily for 3–4 months vs rats fed alcohol for 6 months[CR133].

Glutamate pyruvate transaminase inhibition. Ethanol/water (1:1) extract, at a concentration of 1.0 mg/ml in cell culture on rat liver cells, was active vs PGE-1-induced pedal edema, but inactive vs CCl_4-induced hepatotoxicity[CR128].

Growth inhibitor activity. Water extract, at a dose of 0.5% in the drinking water of mice, was inactive. Strain SLN × C3H/HE F_1 obese mice, treated with extract in drinking water between ages 3 and 32 weeks, showed no lessening of obesity or decrease in glucose tolerance[CR046].

Hair stimulant effect. Ethanol (95%) extract of dried tuber, at a concentration of 0.4 gm/animal applied externally to male mice, was inactive. Dose expressed as dry weight of plant[CR103].

Hematopoietic activity. Powdered dried plant, administered to human adults at variable dosages, was active. Patients also received another preparation containing *Panax ginseng, Cervus elaphuus, Chinemys* *reevesii*, *Cervus* species and *Schisandra chinensis* concomitantly over 3 months[CR125].

Hypertensive activity. Water extract of dried fat, at a dose of 1.5 mg/kg administered intravenously to rats, was active. A vasopressor and then a vasodepressor response occur following administration of extract. Hypotensive response was blocked by administration of propanolol and atropine, but not by chlorisondamine, prazosin and cyproheptadine. Extract used was composed of roots of *Angelica koreana*, *Peucedanum japonicum*, *Angelica gigas*, *Lindera strychnifolia*, *Angelica dahurica*, *Glycyrrhiza glabra* and *Asiasarum* species. Also included were rhizomes of *Cnidium officinale*, *Pinellia ternata*, *Cyperus rotundus* and *Zingiber officinale*, with branches of *Cinnamomum cassia*, fruit of *Pachyma hoelen* and *Citrus aurantium* plants[CR076].

Hypocholesterolemic activity. Fermented dried tuber, at a dose of 5.0 ml/day in the ration of rats, was active. Rats were given the SKV Indian herbal formula for 3–4 months vs rats fed alcohol for 6 months[CR133].

Hypoglycemic activity. Water extract, at a dose of 0.5% in the drinking water of mice, was inactive. Strain SLN × C3H/HE F₁ obese mice, treated with extract in drinking water between ages 3 and 32 weeks, showed no lessening of obesity or decrease in glucose tolerance[CR046]. Fermented dried tuber, at a dose of 5.0 ml/day in the ration of rats, was active. Rats were given the SKV Indian herbal formula for 3–4 months vs rats alcohol for 6 months[CR133].

Hypotensive activity. Ethanol/water (1:1) extract of dried rhizome, at variable dosage levels administered intravenously to dogs, produced weak activity[CR144]. Water extract of rhizome, administered intravenously to cats, was active[CR020].

Hypothermic activity. Methanol extract of dried root, at a dose of 5.0 mg/kg administered to mice intraperitoneally, was active vs aconitine-induced writhing[CR016].

Inotropic effect (positive). Water extract of rhizome was active on frog's heart[CR020].

Insect repellent activity. The essential oil was active on *Bruchus chinensis* and *Sitophilus oryzae*[CR093]. At a concentration of 0.24%, the essential oil was active on *Stegobium paniceum*[CR093]. A 0.78% concentration was active on *Rhizopertha dominica*[CR093].

Juvenile hormone activity. The essential oil was active on *Dysdercus koenigii*[CR097].

Molluscicidal activity. Ethanol (95%) and petroleum ether extracts of dried root, at a concentration of 250.0 ppm, were inactive on *Biomphalaria pfeifferi* and *Bulinus truncatus*[CR108].

Molting activity (insect). The essential oil was active on *Dysdercus koenigii*[CR097].

Mutagenic activity. Water and methanol extracts of commercial sample of rhizome, at concentrations of 100.0 mg/ml on agar plate, were inactive on *Bacillus subtilis* H-17(Rec+) and *Salmonella typhimurium* TA100 and TA98. Metabolic activation had no effect on the results[CR022].

Nitrous oxide inhibition. Methanol extract of the rhizome showed inhibition of nitrous oxide production by murine macrophage cell line, RAW 264.7 cells, due to the suppression of iNOS protein, as well as iNOS mRNA expression, determined by Western blotting analyses, respectively[CR153].

Plant germination inhibition. Protoplasts were active[CR007].

Plant growth inhibitor. Essential oil of root, at a concentration of 400.0 ppm, inhibited the germination and hypocotyl elongation of lettuce and white clover[CR094]. Water extract of tuber was active on white clover, *Digitaria sanguinalis* and *rumex*[CR008,CR100].

Plasma protein concentration. Fermented dried tuber, at a dose of 5.0 ml/day in the ration of rats, increased the plasma protein concentration. Rats were fed the SKV Indian herbal formula for 3–4 months vs rats fed alcohol for 6 months[CR133].

Platelet activating factor binding inhibition. Hot water extract, at a concentration of 10.0 mg/ml, was equivocal on rabbit platelets; 15% inhibition[CR056].

Platelet aggregation stimulation. Hexane extract of dried leaves and stem was inactive[CR072].

Prostaglandin inhibition. Chloroform and hot water extracts of dried rhizome produced strongly active and active inhibition, respectively[CR085].

Prostaglandin synthetase inhibition. Hot water extract of a commercial sample of rhizome, at a concentration of 750.0 mg/ml, was active on rabbit microsomes. Hot water extract of dried rhizome, at a concentration of 750.0 mg/ml, was active on rabbit microsomes[CR112].

Smooth muscle relaxant activity. Methanol extract of rhizome, at a concentration of 1.0 mg/ml, was inactive on rat ileum. The extract's smooth muscle stimulant activity was also inactive on rat ileum. However, uterine relaxation effect on rat uterus was strongly active vs oxytocin-induced contractions. No uterine stimulant effect was shown on rat uterus[CR044].

Superoxide production inhibition. Methanol extract of the rhizome inhibited the production of oxygen by phorbol ester-stimulated by murine macrophage cell line, RAW 264.7 cells, in dose- and time-dependent manners[CR153].

Toxic effect (general). Ethanol/water (1:1) extract of dried rhizome, at a dose of 10.0 gm/kg administered to mice by gastric intubation and subcutaneously, was inactive. Dose expressed as dry weight of plant[CR144].

Toxicity assessment (quantitative). Ethanol (95%) extract of root, administered intraperitoneally to mice, produced LD_{50} 90.0 gm/kg[CR015]. Ethanol (defatted with petroleum ether) extract of dried tuber, administered intraperitoneally to mice, produced LD_{50} > 0.5 gm/kg[CR099]. Ethanol/water (1:1) extract of dried rhizome, administered intraperitoneally to both sexes of mice, produced LD_{50} 681.0 mg/kg[CR091].

Uric acid decrease. Fermented dried tuber, at a dose of 5.0 ml/day in the ration of rats, was active. Rats were fed the SKV Indian herbal formula for 3–4 months vs rats fed alcohol for 6 months[CR133].

Weight Loss. Dried root, taken by human adults orally at a dose of 2.0 gm/day, was active. Sixty-four obese patients were given this drug twice daily for 2 months. There was a significant reduction in weight. Blood pressure was lowered in hypertensive patients, but not in normotensive patients. Side effects were mild, with some nausea initially and appetite suppression in 12 subjects[CR123].

REFERENCES

CR001 Suwal, P. N. Medicinal plants of Nepal. Ministry of Forests, Department of Medicinal Plants, Thapathali, Kathmandu, Nepal, 1970.

CR002 Quisumbing, E. Medicinal plants of the Philippines. Tech Bull 16, Rep Philippines, Dept Agr Nat Resources, Manilla 1951; 1.

CR003 Couvee. Compilation of herbs, plants, crops supposed to be effective in various complaints and illnesses. **J Sci Res** 1952; 1s.

CR004 Han, B. H., H. J. Chi, Y. N. Han and K. S. Ryu. Screening of the anti-inflammatory activity of crude drugs. **Korean J Pharmacog** 1972; 4(3): 205–209.

CR005 Meguro, M. and M. V. Bonomi. Inhibitory action of *Cyperus rotundus* rhizome extracts on the developemnt of some fungi. **Univ Sao Paulo Fac Fil Cienc Let Bol Bot** 1969; 24: 145.

CR006 Meguro, M. Growth-regulating substances in *Cyperus rotundus* rhizome. 1. Effect of rhizome extract on germination and growth of higher plants. **Univ Sao Paulo Fac Fil Cienc Let Bol Bot** 1969; 24: 127.

CR007 Meguro, M. Growth-regulating substances in *Cyperus rotundus* rhizome. ll. Nature and properties of the inhibitor. **Univ Sao Paulo Fac Fil Cienc Let Bol Bot** 1969; 24: 145.

CR008 Singh, S. P. Presence of a growth inhibitor in the tubers of nutgrass. **Proc Indian Acad Sci Ser** 1968; 67B: 18.

CR009 Hikino, H., K. Aota, Y. Maebayashi and T. Takemoto. Structure of absolute configuration of cyperolone. **Chem Pharm Bull** 1967; 15: 349.

CR010 Kapadia, V. H., V. G. Naik, M. S. Wadia and S. Dev. Sesquiterpenoids from the essential oil of *Cyperus rotundus*. **Tetrahedron Lett** 1967; 1967: 4661.

CR011 Hikino, H., K. Aota and T. Takemoto. Structure and absolute configuration of cyperol, and isocyperol. **Chem Pharm Bull** 1967; 15: 1929.

CR012 Kapadia, V. H., B. A. Nagasampagi, V. G. Naik and S. Dev. Studies in sesquiterpenes. XXII. Structure of mustakone and copaene. **Tetrahedron** 1965; 21: 607.

CR013 Hikino, H., K. Aota, D. Kuwano and T. Takemoto. Structure and absolute configuration of alpha-rotunol and beta rotunaol, sesquiterpenoids of *Cyperus rotundus*. **Tetrahedron** 1971; 27: 4831.

CR014 Hikino, H., K. Aota and T. Takemoto. Structure and absolute configuration of sugeonol. **Chem Pharm Bull** 1968; 16: 52.

CR015 Akperbekova, B. A. and R. A. Abdullaev. Diuretic effect of drug form and galenicals from the roots of *Cyperus rotundus* growing in Azerbaidzhan. **Izv Akad Nauk Az Ssr Ser Biol Nauk** 1966; 4: 98.

CR016 Gupta, M. B., T. K. Palit and K. P. Bhargava. Pharmacological studies to isolate the active constituents from *Cyperus rotundus* processing anti-inflammatory, anti-pyretic and analgesic activities. **Indian J Med Res** 1971; 59: 76.

CR017 Hikino, H., K. Aota and T. Takemoto. Structure of sugetriol. **Chem Pharm Bull** 1967; 15: 1433.

CR018 Anon. The atlas of commonly used Chinese traditional drugs, revolutionary committee of the Inst Materia Medica, Chinese Acad Sci, Peking, 1970.

CR019 Khalmatov, K. K. and E. D. Bazhenova. The diuretic action of some wild plants of Uzbekistan. **Tr Tashk Farm Inst** 1966; 4: 5.

CR020 Akperbekova, B. A. and D. Y. Guseinov. Studies on the influence of pharmaceutic preparations from rhizomes of *Cyperus rotundus* growing in Azerbaizhan on the heart and vascular system. **Azerb Med Zh** 1966; 43:12.

CR021 Hikino, H., K. Aota and T. Takemoto. Structure and absolute configuration of cyperotundone. **Chem Pharm Bull** 1966; 14: 890.

CR022 Morimoto, I., F. Watanabe, T. Osawa, T. Okitsu and T. Kada. Mutagenicity screening of crude drugs with *Bacillus subtilis* rec-assay and salmonella/microsome reversion assay. **Mutat Res** 1982; 97: 81–102.

CR023 Rageau, J. Les Plantes Medicinales De La Nouvelle-Cal edonie. Trav & Doc De Lorstom No. 23. Paris, 1973.

CR024 Jochle, W. Menses-inducing drugs: their role in antique, medieval and renaissance gynecology and birth control. **Contraception** 1974; 10: 425–439.

CR025 Stuart, G. A. Chinese Materia Medica. Vegetable Kingdom. American Presbyterian Mission Press, Shanghai, 1911.

CR026 Ichimura, T. Important medicinal plants of Japan. Kanazawa city, Tokyo, 1932.

CR027 Petelot, A. Les Plantes Medicinales du Cambodge, du Laos et du Vietnam, Vol. 1–4. Archives des Recherches Agronomiques et Pastorales au Vietnam No. 23, 1954.

CR028 Kalsi, P. S., M. L. Gandhi and I. S. Bhatia. Chemical studies on the essential oil from *Cyperus rotundus*. **J Res Punjab Agr Univ** 1969; 6: 383.

CR029 Wills, G. D. Sugars, phosphorus and iron in purple nutsedge. **Weed Sci** 1972; 20: 348.

CR030 Trivedi, V. P. and A. S. Mann. Vegetable drugs regulating fat metabolism in Caraka (Lekhaniya Dravyas). **Q J Crude Drug Res** 1972; 12: 1988.

CR031 Watt, J. M. and M. G. Breyer-Brandwijk. The medicinal and poisonous plants of Southern and Eastern Africa. 2nd Ed, E. S. Livingstone, Ltd., London, 1962.

CR032 Burkhill, I. H. Dictionary of the economic products of the Malay peninsula. Ministry of Agriculture and Co-operatives, Kuala Lumpur, Malaysia. Vol. 1, 1966.

CR033 Clifford, H. T. and J. B. Harborne. Flavonoid pigmentation in the sedges (Cyperaceae). **Phytochemistry** 1969; 8: 123–126.

CR034 Rizk, A. F. M. The Phytochemistry of the Flora of Qatar. Scientific and Applied Research Centre, University of Qatar, Kingprint, Richmond, UK. 1986; 582pp.

CR035 Hsu, H. Y. The Chemical Constituents of Oriental Herbs. Oriental Healing Arts Institute. Long Beach , CA 1986; 932pp.

CR036 Chen, H. C. and S. M. Lin. Determination of mineral elements in certain crude drugs (Part 1). **Kaohsiung J Med Sci**, 1988; 4: 259–272.

CR037 List, P. H. and L. Horhammer. Hager's Handbuck der Pharmazeutischen Praxis, Vols. 2–6, Springer-Verlag, Berlin, 1969–1979.

CR038 Thebtaranonth, C., Y. Thebtaranonth, S. Wanauppathamkul and Y. Yuthavong. Antimalarial sesquiterpenes from tubers of *Cyperus rotundus*. Structure of 10,12-Peroxycalamenene, a sesquiterpene endoperoxide. **Phytochemistry** 1995; 40(1): 125–128.

CR039 Hikino, H., C. Konno, Y. Ikeda, N. Izumi and T. Takemoto. Stereo-selectivity in microbiological transformation of stereoisomers of alpha-cyperone and dihydro-alpha-cyperone with colletotrichum phomoides. **Chem Pharm Bull** 1975; 23: 1231.

CR040 Misra, L. P., L. D. Kapoor and R. S. Choudhri. Effect of herbicides on the chlorophyll content of nutgrass (*Cyperus rotundus* L.). **Photosynthetica** (Prague) 1974; 8: 302.

CR041 Hikino, H. and K. Aota. Sesquiterpenoids. Part 52. 4A,5A-oxideudesm-11-En-3A-Ol, sesquitterpenoid of *Cyperus rotundus*. **Phytochemistry** 1976; 15: 1265–1266.

CR042 Singhal, K. C. Anthelmintic activity of berberine hydrochloride against *Syphacia obvelata* in mice. **Indian J Exp Biol** 1976; 14: 345–347.

CR043 Kong, Y. C., S. Y. Hu, F. K. Lau, C. T. Che, H. W. Yeung, S. Cheung and J. C. C. Hwang. Potential anti-fertility plants from Chinese medicine. **Amer J Chin Med** 1976; 4: 105–128.

CR044 Woo, W. S. and E. B. Lee. The screening of biological active plants in Korea using isolated organ preparations. I. Anticholinergic and oxytocic actions in the ileum and uterus. **Annu Rept Nat Prod Res Inst Seoul Natl Univ** 1976; 15: 138.

CR045 Keys, J. D. Chinese Herbs, Botany, Chemistry and Pharmacodynamics. Charles E. Tuttle Co., Rutland, Vermont, USA, 1976.

CR046 Nagasawa, H., T. Iwabuchi and H. Inatomi. Protection by tree-peony (Paeonia suffruticosa Andr.) of obesity in (SLN × C3H/HE) F_1 obese mice. **In Vitro** 1991; 5(2): 115–118.

CR047 Shin, K. H., M. S. Chung, Y. I. Chae, K. Y. Yoon and T. S. Cho. A survey for aldose reductase inhibition of herbal medicines. **Fitoterapia** 1993; 64(2): 130–133.

CR048 Kurokawa, M., H, Ochiai, K. Nagasaka, M. Neki, H. X. Xu, S. Kadota, S. Sutardio, T. Matsumoto, T. Namba and K. Shiraki. Antiviral traditional medicines against Herpes Simplex Virus (HSV-1), Poliovirus, and Measles virus In Vitro and their therapeutic efficacies for HSV-1 infection in mice. **Antiviral Res** 1993; 22(2/3): 175–188.

CR049 Gupta, S., J. N. S. Yadava and J. S. Tandon. Antisecretory (antidiarrheal) activity of Indian medicinal plants against *Escherichia coli* enterotoxin-induced secretion in rabbit and guinea pig ileal loop models. **Int J Pharmacog** 1993; 31(3): 198–204.

CR050 Vu, V. D. and T. T. Mai. Study on analgesic effect of *Cyperus stoloniferus* **Retz. Tap Chi Duoc Hoc** 1994; 1: 16–17.

CR051 Tanira, M. O. M., A. K. Bashir, R. Dib, C. S. Goodwin, I. A. Wasfi and N. R. Banna. Antimicrobial and phytochemical screening of medicinal plants. **Ethnopharmacol** 1994; 41(3): 201–205.

CR052 Komai, K., M. Shimizu, C. S. Tang and H. Tsutsui. Sesquiterpenoids of *Cyperus bulbosus, Cyperus tuberosus* and *Cyperus rotundus*. **Kinki Daigaku Nogakubu Kiyo** 1994; 27: 39–45.

CR052   Komai, K., M. Shimizu, C. S. Tang and H. Tsutsui. Sesquiterpenoids of *Cyperus bulbosus, Cyperus tuberosus* and *Cyperus rotundus*. **Kinki Daigaku Nogakubu Kiyo** 1994, 27: 39–45.

CR053   Dhilon, R. S., S. Singh, S. Kundra and A. S. Basra. Studies on the chemical composition and biological activity of essential oil from *Cyperus rotundus* Linn. **Plant Growth Regul** 1993; 13(1): 89–93.

CR054   Holdsworth, D. K. Traditional medicinal plants of Rarotonga, Cook Islands Part 1. **Int J Crude Drug Res** 1990; 28(3): 209–218.

CR055   Kalsi, P. S., A. Sharma, A. Singh, I. P. Singh and B. R. Chabra. Biogenetically important sesquiterpenes from *Cyperus rotundus*. **Fitoterapia** 1995; 66(1): 94.

CR056   Han, B. H., O. K. Yang, Y. C. Kim and Y. N. Han. Screening of the platelet activating factor (PAF) antagonistic activities on herbal medicines. **Yakhak Hoe Chi** 1994; 38(4): 462–468.

CR057   Park, S. Y. and J. W. Kim. Screening and isolation of the antitumor agents from medicinal plants. (1). **Korean J Pharmacog** 1992; 23(4): 264–267.

CR058   Paknikar, S. K., O. Motl and K. K. Chakravarti. Structures of rotundene and rotundenol. **Tetrahedron Lett** 1977; 1977: 2121.

CR059   Iwamura, J., M. Kameda, K. Kamai and N. Hirao. The constituents of essential oils of *Cyperus serotinus* Rottb. and *Cyperus rotundus* L. **Nippon Kagaku Kaishi** 1977; 7: 1018–1020.

CR060   Komai, K., J. Iwamura and K. Ueki. Isolation, identification and physiological activities of sesquiterpenes in purple nutsedge tubers. **Zasso Kenkyu** 1977; 22(1): 14.

CR061   Sing, N. B and P. N. Singh. A new flavonol glycoside from the mature tubers of *Cyperus rotundus* L. **J Indian Chem Soc** 1986: 63(4): 450.

CR062   Shinde, S., S. Phadke and A. W. Bhagwat. Effect of Nagarmotha (*Cyperus rotundus* Linn.) on reserpine-induced emesis in pigeons. **Indian J Physiol Pharmacol** 1988; 32(3): 229–230.

CR063   Itokawa, H. Research on the antineoplastic drugs from natural sources, especially from higher plants. **Yakugaku Zasshi** 1988; 108(9): 824–841.

CR064   Han, B. H., Y. N. Han and M. H. Park. Chemical and Biochemical Studies on Antioxidant Components of Ginseng. Advances in Chinese Medicinal Materials Research. World Scientific Press Philadelphia, PA. 1984; 485–498.

CR065   Yu, L. A. and Q. L. Xu. Treatment of infectious hepatitis with an herbal decoction. **Phytother Res** 1989; 3(3): 13,14.

CR066   Komai, K. and C. S. Tang. A chemotype of *Cyperus rotundus* in Hawaii. **Phytochemistry** 1989; 28(7): 1883–1886.

CR067   Choe, T. Y. Antibacterial activities of some herb drugs. **Korean J Pharmacog** 1986; 17(4): 302-307.

CR068   Mohsin, A., A. H. Shah, M. A. Al-Yahya, M. Tariq, M. O. M. Tanira and A. M. Ageel. Analgesic antipyretic activity and phytochemical screening of some plants used in traditional Arab system of medicine. **Fitoterapia** 1989; 60(2): 174–177.

CR069   Chen, C. P., C. C. Lin and T. Namba. Screening of Taiwanese crude drugs for antibacterial activity against *Streptococcus mutans*. **J Ethnopharmacol** 1989; 27(3): 285–295.

CR070   Shah, G. L. and G. V. Gopal. Ethnomedical notes from the tribal inhabitants of the North Gujarat (India). **J Econ Taxon Botany** 1985; 6(1): 193–201.

CR071   Reddy, M. B., K. R. Reddy and M. N. Reddy. A survey of medicinal plants of Chenchu Tribes of Andhra Pradesh, India. **Int J Crude Drugs Res** 1988; 26(4): 189–196.

CR072   Triratana, T., P. Pariyakanok, R. Suwannuraks and W. Naengchomnog. The study of medicinal herbs on coagulatin mechanism. **J Dent Assoc Thailand** 1988; 38(1): 25–30.

CR073   Weenen, H., M. H. H. Nkumya, D. H. Bray, L. B. Mwasumb, L. S. Kinabo, V. A. E. B. Kilimali and J. B. P. A. Wijnberg. Antimalarial activity of Tanzanian medicinal plants. **Planta Med** 1990; 56(4): 371–373.

CR074 Weenen, H., M. H. H. Nkunya, D. H. Bray, et al. Antimalarial compounds containing an unsaturated carbonyl moiety from Tanzanian medicinal plants. **Planta Med** 1990; 56(4): 368–370.

CR075 Lee, J. S. and J. W. Kim. Screening of biological activity of crude drugs using brine shrimp bioassay. **Korean J Pharmacog** 1990; 21(1): 100–102.

CR076 Moon, Y. N., M. H. Chung, H. K. Jhoo, D. Y. Lim and H. J. Yoo. Influence of Sopung-tang on the blood pressure response of the rat. **Korean J Pharmacog** 1990; 21(2): 173–178.

CR077 Nagaraju, N. and K. N. Rao. A survey of plant crude drugs of Rayalaseema, Andhra Pradesh, India. **J Ethnopharmacol** 1990; 29(2): 137–158.

CR078 Sato, A. Cancer chemotherapy with Oriental medicine. l. Antitumor activity of crude drugs with human tissue cultures in In vitro screening. **Int J Orient Med** 1990: 15(4): 171–183.

CR079 Masood, A.and K. S. Ranjan. The effect of aqueous plant extracts on growth and aflatoxin production by *Aspergillus flavus*. **Lett Appl Microbiol** 1991; 13(1): 32–34.

CR080 Misra, P., N. L. Pal, P. Y. Guru, J. C. Katiyar and J. S. Tandon. Antimalarial activity of traditional plants against erythrocytic stages of *Plasmodium berghei*. **Int J Pharmacog** 1991; 29(1): 19–23.

CR081 Vadavathy, S. and K. N. Rao. Antipyretic activity of six indigenous medicinal plants of Tirumala Hills, Andhra Pradesh, India. **J Ethnopharmacol** 1991; 33(1/2): 193–196.

CR082 Ekundayo, O., R. Oderinde, M. Ogundeyin and E. Stahl-Biskup. Essential oil constituents of *Cyperus tuberosus* Rottb. rhizomes. **Flavour Fragrance J** 1991; 6(4): 261–264.

CR083 Gupta, M., R. Nath, A. Srivastava, K. Shanker, K. Kishor and K. B. Bhargava. Anti-inflammatory and antipyretic activities of beta-sitosterol. **Planta Med** 1980; 39: 157–163.

CR084 Avirutnant, W. and A. Pongpan. The antimicrobial activity of some Thai flowers and plants. **Mahidol Univ J Pharm Sci** 1983; 10(3): 81–86.

CR085 Sankawa, U. Modulators of Arachidonate cascade contained in medicinal plants used in traditional medicine. (Abstract). **Abstr 3rd Congress of the Federation of Asian Oceanian Biochemists**, Bangkok, Thailand 1983; 28.

CR086 Yun, H. S. and I. M. Chang. Plants with liver protective activities (1). **Korean J Pharmacog** 1977; 8: 125–129.

CR087 Woo, W. S., K. H. Shin, I. C. Kim and C. K. Lee. A survey of the reponse of Korean medicinal plants on drug metabolism. **Arch Pharm Res** 1978; 1: 13–19.

CR088 Chow, S. Y., S. M. Chen and C. M. Yang. Pharmacological studies on Chinese herb medicine. III. Analgesic effect of 27 Chinese herb medicine. **J Formosa Med Assoc** 1979; 75: 349–357.

CR089 Wang, D. X. Treatment of generalized scleroderma with combined traditional Chinese and Western medicine. **Chung-Hua l Hsueh Tsa Chih** (Engl Ed) 1979; 92: 427–430.

CR090 Singh, P. N. and S. B. Singh. A new saponin from mature tubers of *Cyperus rotundus*. **Phytochemistry** 1980; 19: 2056.

CR091 Dhawan, B. N., M. P. Dubey, B. N. Mehrotra, R. P. Rastogi and J. S. Tandon. Screening of Indian plants for biological activity. Part IX. **Indian J Exp Biol** 1980; 18: 594–606.

CR092 Khan, M. R., G. Ndaalio, M. H. Nkunya, H. Wevers and A. N. Sawhney. Studies on African medicinal plants. Part I. Preliminary screening of medicinal plants for antibacterial activity. **Planta Med Suppl** 1980; 40: 91–97.

CR093 Kokate, C. K., H. P. Tipnis, L. X. Gonsalves and J. L. D'Cruz. Anti-insect and juvenile hormone mimicking activities of essential oils of *Adhatoda vasica*, *Piper longum* and *Cyperus rotundus*. (Abstract). **Abstr 4th Asian Symp Med Plants Spices**, Bangkok, Thailand, 1980; 154.

CR094 Komai, K. and K. Ueki. Plant growth inhibitors in purple nutsedge (*Cyperus rotundus* L.). **Zasso Kenkyu** 1980; 25(1): 42–47.

CR095   Chang, I. M. and H. S. Yun. Evaluation of medicinal plants with potential hepatonic activities and study on hepatonic activities of *Plantago semen*. (Abstract). **Abstr 4th Asian Symp Med Plants Spices**, Bangkok, Thailand 1980; 69.

CR096   Anon. A Barefoot Doctor's Manual, Revised Edition, Cloudburst Press of America, 2116 Western Ave., Seattle, Washington, USA. (ISBN-0-88930-012-7). 1977; 372pp.

CR097   Gonsalves, L. X., C. K. Kokate and H. P. Tipnis. Anti-insect and juvenile hormone mimicking activities of *Cyperus rotundus* and *Lantana camara*. **Indian J Pharm Sci** 1979; 41: 250A.

CR098   Wu, D. Y. Treatment of 136 cases of uterine mycoma with "Kung Ching Tang". **Chung I Tsa Chih** 1981; 22(1): 34,35.

CR099   Woo, W. S., E. B. Lee and I. Chang. Biological evaluation of Korean medicinal plants II. **Yakhak Hoe Chi** 1977; 21: 177–183.

CR100   Komai, K. and K. Ueki. Secondary metabolic compounds in purple nutsedge (*Cyperus rotundus* L.) and their plant growth inhibition. **Shokubutsu No Kagaku Chosetsu** 1981; 16: 32–37.

CR101   Kapoor, S. L. and L. D. Kapoor. Medicinal plant wealth of the Karimnagar District of Andhra Pradesh. **Bull Med Ethnobot Res** 1980; 1: 120–144.

CR102   Adesina, S. K. Studies on some plants used as anticonvulsants in Amerindian and African traditional medicine. **Fitoterapia** 1982; 53: 147–162.

CR103   Tanaka, S., M. Saito and M. Tabata. Bioassay of crude drugs for hair growth promoting activity in mice by a new simple method. **Planta Med Suppl** 1980; 40: 84–90.

CR104   Harborne, J. B., C. A. Williams and K. L. Wilson. Flavonoids in leaves and inflorescences of Australian *Cyperus* species. **Phytochemistry** 1982; 21: 2491–2507.

CR105   Saxena, R. C. *Cyperus rotundus* in conjunctivitis. **J Res Ayur Siddha** 1980; 1(1): 115–120.

CR106   Pushpangadan, P. and C. K. Atal. Ethno-medico-botanical investigations on Kerala I. Some primitive tribals of Western Ghats and their herbal medicine. **J Ethnopharmacol** 1984; 11(1): 59–77.

CR107   Yousif, G., G. M. Iskander and D. El Beit. Investigation of the alkaloidal components in the Sudan flora. III. **Fitoterapia** 1983; 54(6): 269–272.

CR108   Ahmed, E. M., A. K. Bashir and Y. M. El Kheir. Investigations of molluscicidal activity of certain Sudanese plants used in folk medicine. Part IV. **Planta Med** 1984; 1: 74–77.

CR109   Itokawa, H., S. Mihashi, K. Watanabe, H. Natsumoto and T. Hamanaka. Studies on the constituents of crude drugs having inhibitory activity against contraction of the ileum caused by histamine or barium chloride (1). Screening test for the activity of commercially available crude drugs and the related plant materials. **Shoyakugaku Zasshi** 1983; 37(3): 223–228.

CR110   John, D. One hundred useful raw drugs of the Kani Tribes of Trivandrum Forest Division, Kerala, India. **Int J Crude Drug Res** 1984; 22(1): 17–39.

CR111   Akbar, S., M. Nisa and M. Tariq. Effects of aqueous extract of *Cyperus rotundus* Linn. on Carrageenin-induced oedema in rats. **Nagarjun** 1982; 25(11): 253–255.

CR112   Kiuchi, F., M. Shibuya, T. Kinoshita and U. Sankawa. Inhibition of prostaglandin biosynthesis by the constituents of medicinal plants. **Chem Pharm Bull** 1983; 31(10): 3391–3396.

CR113   Singh, N., R. Nath, D. R. Singh, M. L. Gupta and R. P. Kohli. An experimental evaluation of the protective effects of some indigenous drugs on carbon tetrachloride-induced hepatotoxicity in mice and rats. **Q J Crude Drug Res** 1978; 16(1): 8–16.

CR114   Sircar, N. N. Pharmaco-therapeutics of Dasemani drugs. **Ancient Sci Life** 1984; 3(3): 132–135.

CR115   Choi, S. Y. and I. M. Chang. Plants with liver protective activities. **Ann Rep Nat Prod Res Inst Seoul Natl Univ** 1982; 21: 49–53.

CR116   Sahu, T. R. Less known uses of weeds as medicinal plants. **Ancient Sci Life** 1984; 3(4): 245–249.

CR117 Jaysweera, D. M. A. Medicinal plants (indigenous and exotic) used in Ceylon. Part II. Cactaceae-Fagaceae. National Science Council of Sri Lanka, Colombo. 1980; 160pp.

CR118 Woo, W. S., E. B. Lee, K. H. Shin, S. S. Kang and H. J. Chi. A review of research on plants for fertility regulation in Korea. **Korean J Pharmacog** 1981; 12(3): 153–170.

CR119 Khan, M. R., G. Ndaalio, M. H. H. Nkunya and H. Wevers. Studies on the rationale of African traditional medicine. Part II. Preliminary screening of medicinal plants for anti-gonoccoci activity. **Pak J Sci Ind Res** 1978; 27(5/6): 189–192.

CR120 Shin, K. H. and W. S. Woo. A survey of the response of medicinal plants on drug metabolism. **Korean J Pharmacog** 1980; 11: 109–122.

CR121 Chang, I. M. and H. S. Yun. Plants with liver-protective activities, pharmacology and toxicology of aucubin. Advances in Chinese Medicinal Materials Research World Scientific Press, Philadelphia, PA. 1984; 269–285.

CR122 Almagboul, A. Z., A. K. Bashir, A. Farouk and A. K. M. Salih. Antimicrobial activity of certain Sudanese plants used in folkloric medicine. Screening for antibacterial activity (IV). **Fitoterapia** 1985; 56(6): 331–337.

CR123 Bambhole, V. D. and G. G. Jiddewar. Evaluation of *Cyperus rotundus* in the management of obesity and high blood pressure of human subjects. **Nagarjun** 1984; 27(5): 110–113.

CR124 Yun, H. S. and I. M. Chang. Liver protective activities of Korean medicinal plants. **Korean J Pharmacog** 1980; 11: 149–152.

CR125 Liu, X. L. Twelve cases of aplastic anemia treated mainly by ready made Chinese drugs. **Chung I Tsa Chih** 1984; 25(10): 759–760.

CR126 Ohta, S., N. Sakurai, T. Inoue and M. Shinoda. Studies on chemical protectors against radiation. XXV. Radioprotective activities of various crude drugs. **Yakugaku Zasshi** 1987; 107(1): 70–75.

CR127 Lama, S. and S. C. Santra. Development of Tibetan plant medicine. **Sci Cult** 1979; 45: 262–265.

CR128 Yang, L. L., K. Y. Yen, Y. Kiso and H. Kikino. Antihepatotoxic actions of Formosan plant drugs. **J Ethnopharmacol** 1987; 19(1): 103–110.

CR129 Chen, C. P., C. C. Lin and T. Namba. Development of natural crude drug resources from Taiwan. (VI). In vitro studies of the inhibitory effect on 12 microorganisms. **Shoyakugaku Zasshi** 1987; 41(3): 215–225.

CR130 Gonzalez, F and M. Silva. A survey of plants with antifertility properties described in the South American folk medicine. Abstr Princess Congress 1 Thailand, Dec. 1987; 20pp.

CR131 Sakai, T., K. Kobashi, M. Tsunezuka, M. Hattori and T. Namba. Studies on dental caries prevention by traditional Chinese medicines (Part VI). on the fluoride contents in crude drugs. **Shoyakugaku Zasshi** 1985; 39(2): 165–169.

CR132 Shanmugasundaram, E. R. B., U. Subramaniam, R. Santhini and K. R. Shanmugasundaram. Studies on brain structure and neurological function in alcoholic rats controlled by an Indian medicinal formula (SKV). **J Ethnopharmacol** 1986; 17(3): 225–245.

CR133 Shanmugasundaram, E. R. B. and K. Radah Shanmugasundar. An Indian herbal formula (SKV) for controlling voluntary ethanol intake in rats with chronic alcoholism. **J Ethnopharmacol** 1986; 17(2): 171–182.

CR134 Lee, E. B., H. S. Yun and W. S. Woo. Plants and animals used for fertility regulation in Korea. **Korean J Pharmacog** 1977; 8: 81–87.

CR135 Pan. P. C. The application of Chinese traditional medicine in the treatment of vaginal cancer. **Chin J Obstet Gynecol** 1960; 8: 156–162.

CR136 Hikino, H., K. Aota and T. Takemoto. Sesquiterpenoids. Part XXXIII. Structure and absolute configuration of kobusone and isokobusone. **Chem Pharm Bull** 1969; 17: 1390–1394.

CR137 Hikino, H., K. Aota, D. Kuwano and T. Takemoto. Structure of alpha-rotunol and beta-rotunol. **Tetrahedron Lett** 1969; 2741–2742.

CR138 Chopra, R. N. Indigenous Drugs of India. Their Medical and Economic

Aspects. The Art Press, Calcutta, India, 1933; 550pp.

CR139   Indira, M., M. Sirsi, S. Randomir and S. Dev. Occurrence of estrogenic substances in plants. I. Estrogenic activity of *Cyperus rotundus*. **J Sci Ind Res** 1956; 15C: 202–204.

CR140   Radomir, S., S. Devi and M. Sirsi. Chemistry and antibacterial activity of nut grass. **Curr Sci** (India) 1956; 25: 118–119.

CR141   Narasimhan, P. T. and R. Senich. Infrared investigations of the hydrocarbon cyprene II. **Proc Indian Acad Sci Ser A** 1956; 43: 156–162.

CR142   Hegde, B. J. and B. S. Rao. Essential oil from the rhizomes of *Cyperus rotundus*, Linn. **J Soc Chem Ind** 1935; 54: 387–389.

CR143   Neville, G. A., I. C. Nigam and J. L. Holmes. Identification of ketones in Cyperus. NMR and mass-spectral examination of the 2,4-dinitrophenylhydrazones. **Tetrahedron** 1968; 24(10): 3891–3897.

CR144   Mokkhasmit, M., K. Swasdimongkol, W. Ngarmwathana and U. Permphiphat. Study on toxicity of Thai medicinal plants. (Continued). **J Med Assoc Thailand** 1971; 54(7): 490–504.

CR145   Rivera, G. Preliminary chemical and pharmacological studies on "cundeamor," *Momordica charantia* L. (Part I). **Amer J Pharm** 1941; 113(7): 281–297.

CR146   Moore, B. D., E. Isidoro and J. R. Seeman. Distribution of 2-Carboxyarabinitol among plants. **Phytochemistry** 1993; 34(3): 703–707.

CR147   Kimura, Y. and M. Ohtani. Essential oil of root of *Cyperus rotundus* L. of Japan. I. **J Pharm Soc Japan** 1928; 48: 971–977.

CR148   Hikino, H., K. Aota and T. Takemoto. Structure and absolute configuration of sugetriol. **Chem Pharm Bull** 1968; 16: 1900–1906.

CR149   Nene, Y. L., P. N. Thapliyal and K. Kumar. Screening of some plant extracts for antifungal properties. **Labdev J Sci Tech B** 1968; 6(4): 226–228.

CR150   Chang, I. M. and H. S. Yun. Liver-protective activities of *Plantago asiatica* seeds. **Planta Med** 1980; 39: 246A.

CR151   Sonwa, M. M and W. A. Konig. Chemical study of the essential oil of *Cyperus rotundus*. **Phytochemisty** 2001; 58(5): 799–810.

CR152   Jeong, S. J., T. Miyamoto, M. Inagaki, Y. C. Kim and R. Higuchi. Rotundines A-C, three novel sesquiterpene alkaloids from *Cyperus rotundus*. **J Nat Prod** 2000; 63(5): 673–675.

CR153   Seo, W. G., H. O. Pa, G. S. Oh, K. Y. Chai, T. O. Kwon, Y. G. Yun, N. Y. Kim and H. T. Chung. Inhibitory effects of methanol extract of *Cyperus rotundus* rhizomes on nitric oxide and superoxide productions by murine macrophage cell line, RAW 264.7 cells. **J Ethnopharmacol** 2001; 76(1): 59–64.

CR154   Ha, J. H., K. Y. Lee, H. C. Choi, J. Cho, B. S. Kang, J. C. Lim and D. U. Lee. Modulation of radioligand binding to the GABA(A)-benzodiazepine receptor complex by a new component from *Cyperus rotundus*. **Biol Pharm Bull** 2002; 25(1): 128–130.

11 | *Curcuma longa*
L.

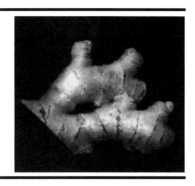

Common Names

Acafrao	Brazil	Rajani	India
Ango	Brazil	Rame	Indonesia
Ango hina	Brazil	Renga	Cook Islands
Asabi-e-safr	Arabic Countries	Rerega	Cook Islands
Avea	Arabic Countries	Saffran vert	Mauritius
Besar	Nepal	Safran	Mauritius
Cago	Nepal	Safran	Rodrigues Islands
Curcuma	Nepal	Tale'a	Rodrigues Islands
Curcuma	Iran	Temoe lawak	Rodrigues Islands
Dilau	India	Temu kunyit	Malaysia
Dilaw	Philippines	Temu-lawak	Indonesia
Goeratji	Indonesia	Tumeric	Japan
Haldi	Fiji	Tumeric	Nepal
Haldi	India	Tumeric	Thailand
Haledo	Nepal	Turmeric	Brazil
Halodhi	India	Turmeric	India
Hardi	Fiji	Turmeric	Iran
Haridra	Malaysia	Turmeric	Japan
Huang chiang	Malaysia	Turmeric	Malaysia
Javanese turmeric	Indonesia	Turmeric	Marquesas Islands
Kakoenji	Indonesia	Turmeric	Mauritius
Kalo haledo	Nepal	Turmeric	Nepal
Kerqum	Morocco	Turmeric	Sri Lanka
Khamin chan	Thailand	Turmeric	Taiwan
Kiko eka	Marquesas Islands	Turmeric	Thailand
Koening	Indonesia	Turmeric	USA
Koenir	Indonesia	Ukon	India
Koenjet	Indonesia	Ukon	Japan
Kondin	Indonesia	Ukon	Taiwan
Kurcum	Oman	Ul Gum	South Korea
Mena	Rotuma	Warse	Oman
Nghe	Vietnam	Wong keong	Malaysia
Nisha	India	Wong keung	Malaysia
Oendre	Indonesia	Zardchoobeh	Iran
Pasupu	India		

From: *Medicinal Plants of the World, vol. 1: Chemical Constituents, Traditional and Modern Medicinal Uses, 2nd ed.*
By: Ivan A. Ross © Humana Press Inc., Totowa, NJ

BOTANICAL DESCRIPTION

A stemless, rhizomatous herb of the ZINGIBERACEAE family with fleshy rhizome, branched, with bright orange to yellow within. Leaves are large, elongated and borne at the top of the non-woody underground stem, with overlapping petioles. Leaves are light green, 30–40 cm long and 8–12 cm wide with thin ellipse-shaped or elongate lance-shaped blades. The pale yellow cylindrical inflorescence, 10–15 by 6–8 cm, develops in the center of the leaves. It consists of curved bracts, each with at least 2 yellow flowers, except in the upper part, where the bracts are white or pink. A stamen with short filament, broad and constricted at the apex is found in the floret. The anther is versatile and usually spurred at the base. The ovaries consist of three-locules, each containing 2 ovules. The capsules are ellipsoid. Seeds are rare.

ORIGIN AND DISTRIBUTION

Native to India but is cultivated in the tropics.

TRADITIONAL MEDICINAL USES

Arabic countries. Hot water extract of dried rhizome is taken orally and in the form of a pessary in Unani medicine, as an abortifacient[CL131].

Brazil. Dried rhizome is used to protect against snakebite[CL037].

China. Hot water extract of dried tuber is taken orally in traditional medicine to improve circulation and to dissolve blood clots[CL132]. Oils of dried fruit, together with oils of *Zingiber officinale*, *Saussurea lappa*, *Sansevieria roxburghiana* and *Rubia cordifolia* are mixed with salt, buttermilk and rice, and massaged onto patient during fever. The mixture is also taken orally for cough. Essential oil of dried fruit is taken orally to bring unconscious patients to consciousness, mixed with honey and leaf of "patola"[CL168].

Cook Islands. Decoction of dried rhizome is taken orally for urinary tract ailments. Skin of *Pandanus tectorius* fruit, combined with *Ocimum basilicum* leaves or grated rhizome of *Curcuma longa*, is boiled and then taken. Grated rhizome is used externally to treat septic puncture wounds[CL152]. Three dried roots are covered by a leaf of *Syzygium malaccensis*, crushed and squeezed into the water of six green coconuts, the solution is taken orally daily for 3 days. Urinary infection is treated by drinking a mixture of two dried roots with 12 leaves and a piece of *Syzygium malaccensis* bark squeezed into the juice of coconut. After 3 days of treatment and purge, a dose is taken with coconut or castor oil[CL057].

England. Dried rhizome, together with *Curcuma aromatica*, licorice, sulfur and ferrous sulfate, is taken orally for amenorrhea[CL184].

Fiji. Poultice of dried rhizome and boiled rice is applied to boils to bring to a head, it is applied externally to aid healing of sprains, bruises and open wounds, and ophthalmically for eye diseases[CL158].

Haiti. Extract of dried rhizome is taken to treat liver complaints[CL062].

Hawaii. Water extract of the bulb is taken orally for asthma[CL054]. Hot water extract of dried entire plant is taken orally for renal or urinary calculi[CL166].

India. Fresh rhizome, ground with cow milk and castor oil, is applied externally to treat paronychia[CL042]. To prevent stomach disorders, 3 to 5 ml of fresh juice is taken regularly on an empty stomach[CL145]. Hot water extract of dried rhizome is taken orally for slow lactation[CL001], to regulate fat metabolism[CL013] and for diabetes[CL016], as a tonic and carminative, for diarrhea, dropsy, jaundice and liver diseases[CL145]. Externally, the dried rhizome is used on fresh wounds, as a counter-irritant on insect stings and to facilitate the scabbing process in chickenpox and smallpox. The dried rhizome is taken orally as an anthelmintic, for urinary diseases, for liver diseases and jaundice and as a cancer remedy[CL019]. Dried rhizome, mixed with latex of *Carthamus tinctorius*, is taken orally for tonsillitis[CL042]. Dried rhizome powder, mixed with the juice of *Aloe vera*, is used externally to treat wounds. The powder, mixed with *Murraya paniculata* paste, is used externally for fractured bones. Powder, mixed with *Helicteres isora* and turmeric powder, is used externally for cuts and wounds[CL091]. Hot water extract of powder is taken orally as a tonic[CL114]. *Curcuma longa* rhizome and *Calotropis procera* root are kept together for 20 days, ground up and a pinch is taken in the morning with milk cream for 3 days to obtain relief from headache[CL126]. *Curcuma longa* rhizome and leaves of *Aristolochia indica* leaves are made into a paste and applied to the forehead, 2 applications per day heals headache quickly[CL137]. A paste of rhizome and leaves of *Zornia diphylla* is applied to dislocated limb joints for relief. A paste of *Ocimum sanctum* leaf and *Curcuma longa* rhizome is applied externally to snakebite and other bites or stings. *Aristolochia indica* root, ground with *Curcuma longa* rhizome is applied externally to snakebite and skin diseases[CL142]. *Datura stramonium* and *Curcuma longa* rhizome are made into a paste and used externally for pimples. For sprains, *Cissampelos pareira* roots and *Curcuma longa* rhizome are made into a paste and applied on the affected area[CL149]. One handful of *Leucas linifolia* plants, 50 grams of *Brassica campestris* seed, and 1 average *Curcuma longa* rhizome are ground into a paste and applied to the forehead daily at sunrise for 7 days for migraine[CL157]. Root, ground with *Oroxylum indicum* stem bark, is made into pills. Five grams are taken twice a day for 10 days for jaundice[CL165]. Rhizome is used externally as an insect repellent[CL187]. Hot water extract of rhizome is taken orally as an emmenagogue[CL002], and externally[CL070] and orally[CL011] as an antivenin. Water extract of dried root,

mixed with *Alangium salvifolium* powder, is used externally for wounds and vaginal discharge[CL091]. Hot water extract of dried root is taken orally as an anti-inflammatory agent in Ayurvedic medicine[CL148].

Indonesia. Hot water extract of rhizome is taken orally by female adults to promote menses[CL003]. Tuber is taken orally as a laxative after menses, leukorrhea of postpartum recovery. Tuber is used externally for scabies. Water extract of tuber, mixed with *Acorus calamus* and vinegar, is taken orally for postpartum recovery. Tuber, ground with water, is used externally for swellings and rheumatism[CL130].

Iran. Powder of dried rhizome is taken orally as a digestant and an antiflatulant[CL027].

Japan. Hot water extract of dried rhizome is taken orally as an aromatic stomachic, diuretic, and for jaundice and menstrual pain in Oriental medicine[CL104]. In Chinese medicine, it is used to inhibit blood coagulation (Oketsu)[CL151]. Hot water extract of fresh rhizome is taken orally as a cholagogue[CL078].

Malaysia. Dried rhizome, mixed with camphor in a paste form, is worn externally as an abortifacient[CL009]. Hot water extract of the dried rhizome is taken orally for amenorrhea[CL012].

Marquesas Island. Root, mixed with other plants, is burnt and the vagina exposed to the smoke to treat prolonged menstruation[CL007]. Decoction of dried root is taken orally for hepatitis and liver troubles[CL164].

Mauritius. Hot water extract of dried root is taken orally for 3 days as an emmenagogue[CL109]. Hot water extract of rhizome is used as an emmenagogue[CL015].

Nepal. Hot water extract of dried rhizome is used externally for skin diseases[CL108]. Hot water extract of rhizome is taken orally as an anthelmintic[CL066]. Dried rhizome is used for fistula. Surgical thread is dipped in solution of ash of *Achyranthes aspera*, then in latex of *Euphorbia antiquorum*, and then coated with powder of *Curcuma longa*. Thread is pierced through the fistula and healing occurs[CL020].

Philippines. Decoction of fresh root is taken orally to treat fever in infants and to treat bleeding during pregnancy. Fresh root juice is taken orally to decrease the pain of early labor[CL155].

South Korea. Hot water extract of dried rhizome is taken orally, as a contraceptive, abortifacient, and emmenagogue[CL156], and to induce menstruation[CL182].

Taiwan. Hot water extract of dried rhizome is taken orally as a diuretic and aromatic stomachic, and for jaundice[CL021].

USA. Dried rhizome, in a proprietary product called "pseudo hard-on pills" contains *Albus simila* (25%), *Curcuma longa* (50%), *Purus saccharum*, and *Zingiber officinale* (10%) each, is taken orally as an aphrodisiac[CL106].

Vietnam. Hot water extract of dried rhizome is taken orally as a drug in traditional medicine. Listed in the Vietnamese pharmacopeia (1974 edition)[CL120].

CHEMICAL CONSTITUENTS

(ppm unless otherwise indicated)

2-Hydroxy-methyl anthraquinone: Rh[CL075]
2-5-dihydroxy bisabola-3-10-diene: Rh 3.2[CL086]
4-Hydroxy bisabola-2-10-dien-9-one: Rh 5.1[CL086]
4-Hydroxy cinnamoyl-(feruloyl)-methane: Rh 180[CL154]
4-Hydroxy-cinnamoyl methane: Rh[CL046]
4-Hydroxy-feruloxyl methane: Rh[CL046]
4-Methoxy bisabola-3-10-dien-2-one: Rh 13.5[CL086]
5-Hydroxy bisabola-2-10-dien-9-one: Rh 0.3[CL086]
5-Hydroxy procurcumenol: Rh 0.6[CL086]
5'-Methoxy curcumin: Rh 20[CL025]
Alpha atlantone: Rt[CL121]
Alpha curcumene: Rh[CL100,CL040]
Alpha phellandrene: Rh EO[CL029], Rt Call[CL111], Rt[CL121]

Alpha pinene: Tu[CL141], Rh EO 0.53%[CL122]
Alpha turmerine: Rh 3.7%[CL086]
Alpha turmerone: Rh[CL133]
Beta bisabolene: Rh[CL100,CL040]
Beta pinene: Tu[CL141], Rh EO 0.27%[CL122]
Beta sesquiphellandrene: Rh[CL100]
Beta sitosterol: Rh[CL071]
Beta turmerone: Rh[CL100]
Bis-(4-hydroxy-cinnamoyl) methane: Rh[CL046]
Bis-(para-hydroxy-cinnamoyl) methane: Rh 0.136%[CL154]
Bis-demethoxy curcumin: Rh 6.6–7500[CL025,CL139], P|[CL072], Tu[CL141], Rt 400[CL139]
Bisabolene: Rt[CL121]
Bisacumol: Rh 2.1[CL086]
Bisacurone: Rh 9.3[CL086]
Borneol: Rt[CL121], Rh, Tuber[CL141]
Caffeic acid: Rh 5[CL119]
Campesterol: Rh[CL071]
Camphene: Rh, Tu[CL141]
Camphor: Tu[CL141], Rh EO 0.06%[CL122]
Caryophylene: Rh, Tu[CL141]
Cholesterol: Rh[CL071]
Cineol: Tu[CL141], Rh EO 2.92%[CL122]
Curcumene: Rh EO 12.17%[CL122], Tu[CL141]
Curcumenol: Rh 64.5[CL086], Rh EO 2.13%[CL122]
Curcumenone: Rh 26.3[CL086]
Curcumin: Rh 0.10–1.79%[CL153,CL139], Oleoresin 17.5%[CL159], Rt[CL061]
Curdione: Rh EO 1.19%[CL122], Tu, Rh[CL141]
Curlone: Rh 120[CL124]
Curzerenone C: Rh EO 2.04%[CL122]
Curzerenone: Tu, Rh[CL141]
Cyclocurcumin: Rh 13.3[CL026]
Dehydro curdione: Rh 4.5[CL086]
Demethoxy curcumin: Rh 0.0007%–1.11%[CL025,CL139], Rt 0.05%[CL139], P|[CL072]
Di-feruloyl methane: Rh[CL112]
Di-para-coumaroyl methane: Rh[CL112]
Epi-procurcumenol: Rh 1.3[CL086]
Eugenol: Tu[CL141], Rh EO 0.21%[CL122]
Feruloyl-para-coumaroyl methane: Rh[CL112]
Gamma atlantone: Rt[CL121]
Germacron-(4S',5S)-epoxide: Rh 0.7[CL086]
Germacron-13-al: Rh 0.6[CL086]
Germacrone: Rh[CL100]
Germacrone,4(S)-5(S)-epoxy: Rh[CL040]
Guaiacol: Rh[CL028]

Hepta-1-4-6-triene-3-one,1-7-bis-(4 ben-zenoid-hydroxy-phenyl): Rh 2.6[CL024]

Hepta-1-6-diene-3-5-dione,1-(4-hydroxy-3-methoxy-phenyl)-7-(3-4-dihydroxy-phenyl): Rh 3.9[CL024]

Iso-borneol: Rh EO 0.02%[CL122]

Iso-procurcumenol: Rh 1.6[CL086]

Limonene: Rh EO 0.23%[CL122], Tu[CL141]

Linalool: Rh EO 0.16%[CL122], Tu[CL141]

Mono-demethoxy curcumin: Rh[CL146], Rt[CL061], Tu[CL141]

Ortho coumaric acid: Lf[CL073]

Para coumaric acid: Rh 345[CL119]

Para cymene: Rh 2.5%[CL017]

Para-hydroxy-cinnamoyl feruloyl methane: Rh[CL160]

Para-tolyl-methyl-carbinol: Rh[CL004]

Penta-trans-1-trans-4-dien-3-one,1-5-bis-(4-hydroxy-3-methoxy-phenyl): Rh 26.6[CL025]

Penta-trans-4-dien-3-one,1(4-hydroxy-3-methoxy-phenyl)-5-(4-hydroxy-phenyl): Rh 13.3[CL025]

Procurcumenol: Rh 0.1[CL086]

Protocatechuic acid: Lf[CL073]

Sabinene: Rh EO[CL029], Rt[CL121]

Saturated fatty acids: Rh[CL071]

Stigmasterol: Rh[CL071]

Syringic acid: Lf[CL073]

Terpinene: Tu[CL141], Rh EO 2.72%[CL122]

Terpineol: Rh EO 0.05%[CL122]

Tolyl-methyl-carbinol: Rh[CL005]

Turmerin: Tu[CL004]

Turmerone AR: Rh[CL100]

Turmerone: Rt[CL121], Tu[CL141], Rh EO 24.07%[CL122]

Turmeronol A: Rh 282.1[CL022]

Turmeronol B: Rh 192.8[CL022]

Ukonan A: Rh 33–6600[CL081,CL021]

Ukonan B: Rh 47[CL081]

Ukonan C: Rh 52–315[CL081,CL088]

Ukonan D: Rh 40.8[CL023]

Unsaturated fatty acids: Rh[CL071]

Vanillic acid: Lf[CL073]

Zedoarondiol: Rh 35[CL086]

Zingiberene: Rh EO 8.14%[CL122], Rt[CL121]

PHARMACOLOGICAL ACTIVITIES AND CLINICAL TRIALS

Abortifacient effect. Hot water extract of dried root, taken orally by pregnant women, was inactive. A mixture of the following was given in the form of a decoction to a number of pregnant women. No toxic effects were noted. Dosing was 3 times daily for 3 days. The mixture contained *Angelica sinensis* (root), *Ligusticum wallichii* (root), *Prunus persica* (seed), *Carthamus tinctorius* (flowers), *Paeonia obvata* (root), *Achyranthes bidentata* (root), *Leonurus sibiricus* (aerial parts), *Lycopus lucidus* var. Hirta (leaf), *Curcuma longa* (root) and *Campsis grandiflora* (flowers)[CL183].

Adrenal hypertrophy effect. Water extract of dried rhizome, together with a mixture of *Levisticum officinale*, *Artemisia cappilaris* and *Chrysanthemum indicum*, was active when administered to mice[CL038].

Alkaline phosphatase inhibition. Water extract of fresh rhizome, administered intragastrically to ducklings at a concentration of 50.0 mg/day, was active vs aflatoxin B-1 hepatotoxicity. Enzyme was measured in the serum[CL047].

Alkaline phosphatase stimulation. Methanol extract of dried rhizome, administered intraperitoneally to rats at a dose of 100.0 mg/kg, was active vs alpha naphthylisothiocyanate-induced hepatotoxicity[CL093].

Allergenic activity. Commercial sample of rhizome powder was active on human adults. Reaction to patch tests occurred most commonly in patients who were regularly exposed to the substance, or who already had dermatitis on the fingertips. Previously unexposed patients had few reactions (i.e., not irritant reactions)[CL074].

Antiamoebic activity. Ethanol/water (1:1) extract of rhizome, at a concentration of 125.0 mcg/ml in broth culture, was active on *Entamoeba histolytica*[CL006].

Antiasthmatic activity. Dried rhizome, taken orally by human adults at a dose of 250.0 mg/person, was active. Administration was to 26 (11 male and 15 female) patients with bronchial asthma once daily for 3 weeks. No side effects were observed.

The preparation also contained *Glycyrrhiza glabra*[CL115]. A dose of 6–12 gm/person daily for 15–20 days was active. One hundred seven patients with "tamak swasa vatapradhan" (chronic bronchitis or asthma), ages 31–50, had fair to good response[CL114].

Antibacterial activity. Chloroform, ethanol (95%) water and petroleum ether extracts of dried rhizome, at a concentration of 250.0 mg/ml on agar plate, were active on *Bacillus subtilis*, *Escherichia coli*, *Pseudomonas aeruginosa*, and *Staphylococcus aureus*[CL055]. Ethanol (95%) extract, at a concentration of 10.0 mg/ml, was inactive on *Corynebacterium diptheriae*, *Diplococcus pneumoniae*, *Staphylococcus aureus*, *Streptococcus viridans*, and *Streptococcus pyogenes*[CL097]. Water extract, at a concentration of 10.0 mg/ml, was inactive on *Corynebacterium diptheriae* and *Diplococcus pneumoniae*, and produced weak activity on *Staphylococcus aureus*, *Streptococcus viridans*, and *Streptococcus pyogenes*[CL097]. Essential oil of rhizome, on agar plate, was inactive on *Bacillus cereus*, *Escherichia coli*, *Pseudomonas aeruginosa*, and *Staphylococcus aureus*[CL169]. Ethanol (95%) extract of rhizome, in broth culture, was active on *Lactobacillus acidophilus* and *Staphylococcus aureus*; equivocal on *Escherichia coli* and inactive on *Salmonella typhosa*[CL006]. Undiluted essential oil, on agar plate, was inactive on *Bacillus cereus*, *Escherichia coli*, *Pseudomonas aeruginosa*, and *Staphylococcus aureus*[CL129]. Water and hot water extracts of dried rhizome, on agar plate at a concentration of 0.5 ml/disc, was inactive on *Bacillus subtilis* H-17(REC+) and H-17(REC–). Rhizome, on agar plate at variable concentrations, was active on *Bacillus subtilis* H-17(REC+)[CL138].

Anticoagulant activity. Chromatographic fraction of dried rhizome, administered intraperitoneally to mice at a dose of 0.08 gm/kg, was active, results significant at $P < 0.05$ level. Ethyl acetate extract of dried rhizome, administered intraperitoneally to mice at a dose of 0.1 gm/kg, produced strong activity, results significant at $P < 0.01$ level. The water extract, at a dose of 0.1 gm/kg, was equivocal[CL151].

Anticomplement activity. Polysaccharide fraction of dried rhizome, administered intraperitoneally to guinea pigs at a dose of 100.0 mg/kg, was active[CL162].

Anticonvulsant activity. Ethanol/water (1:1) extract of rhizome, administered intraperitoneally to mice at a dose of 250.0 mg/kg, was inactive vs electroshock[CL006].

Anticrustacean activity. Ethanol (95%) extract of dried rhizome was inactive on *Artemia salina*. The assay system was intended to predict for antitumor activity[CL036].

Antiedema activity. Methanol extract of dried rhizome, administered to mice at a dose 2.0 mg/ear, was active vs 12-0-tetradecanoylphorbol-13-acetate(TPA)-induced ear inflammation. The inhibition ratio (IR) was 71[CL151].

Antifungal activity. Chloroform and ethanol (95%) extracts of dried rhizome, on agar plate, were active, and water extract produced weak activity on *Epidermophyton floccosum*, *Microsporum gypseum*, and *Trichophyton rubrum*[CL105]. Essential oil of dried rhizome, on agar plate at a concentration of 1:100, was active on *Trichoderma viride*, *Aspergillus flavus*, *Microsporum gypseum*, and *Trichophyton mentagrophytes*[CL128]. Water extract of dried rhizome, at a concentration of 10.0 mg/ml on agar plate, was inactive on *Microsporum canis*, *Microsporum gypseum*, *Phialophora jeanselmei* and *Piedraia hortae*, and weakly active on *Trichophyton mentagrophytes*[CL097]. Essential oil of dried rhizome, on agar plate at a concentration of 1:100, was active on *Curvularia oryzae*, *Helminthosporum oryzae*, *Penicillum corymbiferum*, *Penicillum javanicum*, and *Penicillum lilacinum*[CL128]. Essential oil, on agar plate, was equivocal on *Aspergillus aegypticus*; active on *Trichoderma viride* and inactive on *Penicillium cyclopium*[CL169]. A concentration of 3000 ppm, on agar plate, was active on *Aspergillus niger*[CL049]. Undiluted essential oil, on agar plate, was inactive on *Penicillium cyclopium*, *Trichoderma viride* and *Aspergillus aegyptiacus*[CL129]. Fresh leaf essential oil, at a concentration of 5000 ppm on agar plate, produced weak activity on *Aspergillus flavus*[CL174].

Antihepatotoxic activity. Ethanol/water (1:1) extract of dried rhizome, in rat-liver cell culture, and when administered intraperitoneally to mice, was active vs carbon tetrachloride-induced hepatotoxicity[CL104]. Methanol extract, administered intraperitoneally to mice at a dose of 100.0 mg/kg, produced weak activity vs carbon tetrachloride hepatotoxicity[CL053]. Hot water extract of the dried rhizome, in cell culture at a concentration of 1.0 mg/plate, was active on hepatocytes, as measured by leakage of LDH and ASAT[CL062]. Methanol extract of dried rhizome, administered intraperitoneally to rats of both sexes at a dose of 300.0 mg/kg, produced weak activity vs alpha-naphthylisothiocyanate-induced hepatotoxicity. Methanol extract, administered subcutaneously to rats of both sexes at a dose of 100.0 mg/kg, was inactive vs carbon tetrachloride-induced hepatotoxicity[CL179]. Methanol-insoluble fraction of dried rhizome, administered intragastrically to ducklings at a dose of 10.0 mg/animal, was active vs aflatoxin B1-induced hepatotoxicity. A mixture containing tumeric, fresh garlic, asafoetida, curcumin, ellagic acid, butylated hydroxy toluene and butylated hydroxy anisole were used[CL050].

Antihypercholesterolemic activity. Ethanol/water (1:1) extract of dried rhizome, administered intragastrically to rats at a dose of 30.0 mg/gm (dry weight of plant) every 6 hours for 48 hours, was active vs triton-induced hypercholesterolemia[CL080]. Ether and ethanol (95%) extracts of rhizome, administered by gastric intubation to rabbits at a dose of 1.0 gm/

animal, were inactive vs cholesterol-loaded animals[CL185].

Antihyperglyceridemic effect. Ethanol/water (1:1) extract of dried rhizome, administered intragastrically to rats at a dose of 30.0 mg/gm (dry weight of plant) every 6 hours for 48 hours, was active vs triton-induced hypercholesterolemia[CL080].

Antihyperlipemic activity. Ethanol/water (1:1) extract of dried rhizome, administered intragastrically to rats at a dose of 30.0 mg/gm (dry weight of plant) every 6 hours for 48 hours, was active vs triton-induced hypercholesterolemia[CL080]. Ether and ethanol (95%) extracts of rhizome, administered by gastric intubation to rabbits at a dose of 1.0 gm/animal, were inactive vs cholesterol-loaded animals[CL185].

Anti-implantation effect. Ethanol (95%) extract of dried rhizome, administered orally to rats at a dose of 100.0 mg/kg, was active. A 60.0% reduction in pregnancies (4/10) was observed. A dose of 200.0 mg/kg produced a 70.0% reduction. The petroleum ether and water extracts, at a dose of 100.0 mg/kg, produced 80.0% reduction and a dose of 200.0 mg/kg produced a 100.0% reduction[CL030].

Anti-inflammatory activity. Ethanol (95%) extract of dried rhizome, administered intraperitoneally to male rats at a dose of 100.0 mg/kg, was active vs granuloma pouch model. Doses of 200.0, 400.0, and 800.0 mg/kg, were active vs carrageenin-induced pedal edema. A dose of 50.0 mg/kg was inactive vs granuloma pouch model. Water extract, at doses of 5, 10, 20, 40 and 80 mg/kg, were active vs carrageenin-induced rat pedal edema. A dose of 10.0 mg/kg was inactive vs granuloma pouch model, and a dose of 20.0 mg/kg was active. Petroleum ether extract, at a dose of 12.5 mg/kg, was inactive vs granuloma pouch model; 25.0 mg/kg was active vs granuloma pouch model, but inactive vs carrageenin-induced rat pedal edema. A dose of 50.0 mg/kg was active vs carragee-nin-induced rat pedal edema[CL032]. Rhizome, taken orally by human adults at a dose of 50.0 mg/person, was active. The clinical efficacy of a herbomineral formulation containing roots of *Withania sonifera*, stems of *Boswellia serrata*, rhizomes of *Curcuma longa* and a zinc complex (Articulin-F) was evaluated in a randomized, double-blind, placebo-controlled, cross-over study in patients with osteoarthritis. After a 1 month single blind run-in period, 42 patients with osteoarthritis were randomly allocated to receive either a drug treatment or a matching placebo for a period of 3 months. After a 15-day wash-out period the patients were transferred to the other treatment for a further period of 3 months. Clinical efficacy was evaluated every 2 weeks on the basis of severity of pain, morning stiffness, Ritchie Articular Index, joint score, disability score and grip strength. Other parameters, like erythro-cyte sedimentation rate and radiological examination, were carried out on a monthly basis. Treatment with the herbo-mineral formation produced a significant drop in severity of pain and disability score. Radiological assessment, however, did not show any significant changes in either group. Side effects observed with this for-mulation did not necessitate withdrawal of treatment[CL094]. Polysaccharide fraction of dried rhizome, administered intraperito-neally to rats at a dose of 100.0 mg/kg, was active vs adjuvant-induced arthritis, results significant at $P < 0.01$ level[CL162]. Root essential oil, administered orally to rats at a dose of 0.1 ml/kg, was active vs carragee-nin-induced pedal edema[CL014].

Anti-ischemic effect. Rhizome, adminis-tered intragastrically to rats at a dose of 5.0 gm/kg, was active on the heart. The dose also contained nicotinic acid. The dose was given daily for 7 days, during the last 2 of which isoproterenol was also given. Isoprot-erenol-induced ischemic effects on the heart were prevented[CL087].

Antimutagenic activity. Hot water extract of dried rhizome, on agar plate at concentra-tions of 40.0 mg/plate and at the minimum toxic dose, were inactive on *Salmonella typhimurium* TA100 vs aflatoxin-B1-induced mutagenesis. Metabolic activation had no effect on the results. Dried rhizome extract, on agar plate at a concentration of 50.0 mg/ml, was inactive on *Salmonella typhimurium* TA1535 vs aflatoxin- and mitomycin-induced mutagenesis[CL095]. Water extract of rhizome, at a concentration of 0.33 mg/ml, was active on rat liver microsomes. The for-mation of labeled benzo[a]pyrene-DNA adducts was inhib-ited[CL063]. The infusion, at a concentration of 25.0 mcg/plate on agar plate, was active on *Salmonella typhimurium* TA100. 1-methyl-3-nitro-1-nitrosoguani-dine-induced mutagenesis was inhibited by 25%. There was a 38% inhibition of 4-nitro-D-phenylenediamine-induced mutagenesis of *Salmonella typhimurium* TA98. Infusion of rhizome, administered intragastrically to mice at a dose of 3.0 mg/animal, was active. The incidence of benzo[a]pyrene-induced forestomach tumors was reduced by 53% by pretreatment with the extract. Intraperito-neal administration of the infusion was active. The formation of benzo[a]pyrene-induced bone marrow micronucleated cells was decreased 40% by pretreatment with the extract[CL033]. Powdered rhizome, at a concen-tration of 0.033 mg/ml, was active on rat liver microsomes. Formation of labeled benzo[a]pyrene-DNA adducts was inhib-ited[CL063]. Powdered rhizome, administered intragastrically to rats at a dose of 0.5% of the diet, was active. Animals fed the diet for 1 month before being given 3-methyl-cholanthrene intraperitoneally produced urine with reduced mutagenicity on *Salmo-nella typhimurium* TA100 and TA98, with or without activation with S9, as assessed by Ames test[CL177].

Antimycobacterial activity. Ethanol (95%) extract of entire plant, in broth culture, was active on *Mycobacterium tuberculosis* H37RVTMC 102. The extract was used in a dilution of 1:80[CL090]. Leaf juice, on agar plate, produced weak activity on Mycobacterium tuberculosis, MIC < 1:40[CL010].

Antinematodal activity. Water extract of rhizome, at a concentration of 10.0 mg/ml, produced weak activity, and the methanol extract, at a concentration of 1.0 mg/ml, was active on *Toxacara canis*[CL096].

Antioxidant activity. Hexane and methanol extracts of rhizome, at concentrations of 0.1%, were active[CL154]. Hexane extract of dried rhizome, at a concentration of 0.06%, was inactive when tested on lard. The methanol extract was active[CL143]. Hot water extract of a commercial sample of tuber, at a concentration of 100.0 ng/ml, was active vs protection of DNA against peroxidative injury[CL076]. Water extract of rhizome was active on rat brain vs Fe^{2+}/scorbate-Fe^{2+}/TBH-induced lipid peroxidation. The biological activity was highly dose-dependent, IC_{50} 100.0 mcg/ml. The extract was also active vs lipid peroxidation induced by TBARS, IC_{50} 50.0 mcg/ml[CL060].

Antispasmodic activity. Ethanol/water (1:1) extract of rhizome was active on guinea pig ileum[CL006].

Antispermatogenic effect. Root, in the ration of male mice at a concentration of 0.5%, and of male rats at a concentration of 0.15% of the diet, was inactive[CL113].

Antitumor activity. Ethanol (95%) extract, administered intraperitoneally to mice at a dose of 100.0 mg/kg, was inactive on Sarcoma 180(ASC); the water extract was active[CL084]. Hot water extract of dried root, administered intraperitoneally to mice at variable dosage levels, was active on CA-Ehrlich-ascites. A mixture of *Bufo bufo*, *Solanum nigrum*, *Solanum lyratum*, *Duchesnea indica*, *Angelica sinensis*, *Curcuma longa* and *Salvia miltiorrhiza* was used[CL135]. Methanol extract of dried rhizome, administered intraperitoneally to mice at a dose of 0.03 gm/kg, was inactive on LEUK-SN36. A dose of 0.1 gm/kg was active[CL116]. Polysaccharide fraction of dried rhizome, administered intraperitoneally to mice at a dose of 100.0 mg/kg, was active on Sarcoma 180 (solid)[CL162]. Water and methanol extracts, administered intraperitoneally to mice at doses of 150.0 mg/kg on days 5, 6 and 7, were inactive on CA-Ehrlich-Ascites[CL018]. Water extract of dried rhizome, administered to mice at a dose of 100.0 mg/kg, was active on Sarcoma (ASC)[CL077].

Antiulcer activity. Ethanol (95%) extract of dried rhizome, administered intragastrically to rats at a dose of 500.0 mg/kg, was active vs hydrochloric acid-, sodium chloride-, sodium hydroxide-, hypothermic-resistant stress-, ethanol-, pylorus ligation-, indomethacin-, reserpine-, and cysteamine-induced ulcers[CL083]. Powdered dried rhizome, taken orally by human adults of both sexes at a dose of 250.0 mg/day, produced weak activity. In a clinical study in Thailand with 60 patients, the control group received an antacid. The treatment was given before meals and at bedtime for 2 weeks[CL052].

Antiviral activity. Hot water extract of dried rhizome, in cell culture, was active on vesicular stomatitis virus. The prescription included 10 gm each of *Curcuma longa* rhizome, *Rheum officinale* root, *Cimicifuga foetida* rhizome, *Anemarrhena asaphodeloides* rhizome, *Areca catechu* seed, *Magnolia officinalis* bark and *Scutellaria baicalensis* root; also included were 5 gm *Amomum tsao-ko* fruit and the insects *Bombyx mori* and *Cryptotympana pustulata*[CL085]. Water extract of dried rhizome, in cell culture at a concentration of 10.0%, was inactive on Herpes virus Type 2, Influenza virus A2(Manheim 57), Poliovirus ll and Vaccinia virus[CL150].

Antiyeast activity. Chloroform, ethanol (95%) and water extracts of dried rhizome, on agar plate were inactive on *Candida albicans*, *Cryptococcus neoformans* and *Sac-*

charomyces cerevisae[CL105]. Dried oleoresin, at a concentration of 500.0 ppm on agar plate, was active on *Debaryomyces hansenii* vs ascospore production. Inactive on: *Candida lipolytica* vs pseudomycelium production; *Hansenula anomala* vs pseudomycelium and ascospore production; *Lodderomyces elongisporus* vs pseudomycelium production; *Rhodotorula rubra* vs pseudomycelium production; *Saccharomyces cerevisiae* vs pseudomycelium and ascospore production; *Torulopsis glabrata* vs pseudomycelium production. In broth culture, the oleoresin, was inactive on *Candida lipolytica*, *Debaryomyces hansenii*, *Hansenula anomala*, *Kloeckera apiculata*, *Lodderomyces elongisporus*, *Rhodotorula rubra*, *Saccharomyces cerevisiae* and *Torulopsis glabrata* vs biomass production[CL170]. Water extract of rhizome, on agar plate at a concentration of 10.0 mg/ml, was inactive on *Candida albicans* and *Candida tropicalis*[CL097].

Apoptosis induction. Hexane extract of rhizome, in cell culture, was active on LEUK-HL60[CL069].

Arachidonate metabolism inhibition. Ether extract of dried tuber, at a concentration of 100.0 mcg/ml, was inactive on platelets vs AA incorporation into platelet phospholipids[CL172].

Ascaricidal activity. Root essential oil, at a concentration of 0.2%, was active. Forty-five minutes of exposure killed all the worms. A 0.2% piperazine citrate solution required 50 minutes of exposure to kill all the worms[CL107].

Carcinogenesis inhibition. Dried rhizome powder, in the ration of female mice at a dose of 2.0% of the diet/day, produced weak activity. Animals were 12 months of age at start of experiment vs DMBA-induced carcinogenesis. A dose of 5.0% of the diet/day was active at 8, 12 and 2 months of age to start the experiment, and strongly active at 6 months of age to start the experiment vs DMBA-induced carcinogenesis[CL064]. Ethanol

(95%) extract of dried rhizome, in the ration of female mice at a dose of 5.0% of the diet, was active vs benzo(a)pyrene-induced carcinogenesis; and on female hamster (Syrian) vs methylnitrosamine-induced carcinogenesis. A dose of 2.0% was inactive in mice vs benzo(a)pyrene-induced carcinogenesis[CL051]. Ethanol (95%) extract of rhizome, at a dose of 5.0% of the diet in the ration of Syrian hamster, was active vs methyl(acetoxymethyl) nitrosamine (DMN-OAC)-induced oral carcinogenesis, synergism with *Piper betel*[CL058]. Powdered root, in the ration of mice at a dose of 2.0% of the diet, was active vs Benzo(a)pyrene-induced tumorgenesis[CL098]. Rhizome in the ration of hamsters (Syrian), at a dose of 5.0% of the diet, was active vs DMN-OAC-induced oral carcinogenesis. When a combination of treatments of betel-leaf extract and tumeric, Beta-carotene and tumeric, or alpha-tocopherol and tumeric were used, the doses were active vs methyl nitrosamine-induced carcino-genesis[CL043]. A dose of 160.0 mg/per gm of diet was active vs 3'-methyl-4-dimethyl-aminoazobenzene-induced carcinogenesis[CL039]. Rhizome, in the ration of rats at a concentration of 0.1% of the diet, was active vs benzo[a]pyrene-induced carcinogenesis[CL041].

Cardiotonic activity. Ethanol/water (1:1) extract of rhizome, administered by perfusion, was inactive on the guinea pig heart[CL006].

Catalase stimulation. Rhizome, in the ration of rats at a concentration of 1.0% of the diet, produced weak activity[CL048].

Choleretic activity. Essential oil of fresh rhizome, administered intragastrically to rats at a dose of 300.0 mg/kg, was active[CL078].

Chromosomal aberration induction. Hot water extract of dried rhizome, administered intraperitoneally to mice, was inactive on bone marrow vs cyclophosphamide-induced damage[CL099]. Water extract of fresh tuber, at a concentration of 4.0%, was active. Assay was done on the root of *Allium cepa*; chromosome breakage was observed[CL045].

Clastogenic activity. Hot water extract of dried rhizome, administered intraperitoneally to mice, was inactive on bone marrow vs cyclophosphamide-induced damage[CL099]. Methanol extract of root, administered intraperitoneally to mice at a dose of 500 mg/kg, was active[CL167].

CNS depressant activity. Ethanol/water (1:1) extract of rhizome, administered intraperitoneally to mice at a dose of 250.0 mg/kg, was active[CL006].

Cytochrome B-5 increase. Powdered rhizome, administered intragastrically to mice at a dose of 4.0 gm/kg, was active. Assay was done in pups, presuming translactational exposure[CL065].

Cytochrome B-5 inhibition. Powdered root, in the ration of mice at a dose of 5.0% of the diet, was active[CL098].

Cytochrome P-450 induction. Powdered rhizome, administered intragastrically to mice at a dose of 4.0 gm/kg, was active. Assay was done in pups, presuming translactational exposure[CL065].

Cytochrome P-450 inhibition. Powdered root, in the ration of mice at a dose of 5.0% of the diet, was active[CL098]. Water extract of rhizome, at a concentration of 3.0 mg/ml, was active on rat liver microsomes[CL063].

Cytotoxic activity. Ethanol/water (1:1) extract of rhizome, in cell culture at a concentration of 1.0 mg/ml, was active on human lymphocytes, human leukemic lymphocytes and Dalton's lymphoma[CL019]. Ethanol/water (1:1) extract of rhizome, in cell culture, was inactive on CA-9KB, $ED_{50} >$ 20.0 mcg/ml[CL006]. Ether and petroleum ether extract of rhizome, in cell culture, were active on LEUK-L1210, ED_{50} 10.0 and 5.0 mcg/ml, respectively[CL163]. Ether extract of dried rhizome, in cell culture, was active on hepatoma HTC[CL112]. Water extract, at a concentration of 500.0 mcg/ml, produced weak activity on CA-Mammary-Micro-

alveolar[CL089]. Petroleum ether extract of dried rhizome, in cell culture, was active on LEUK-L1210, ED_{50} 1.8 mcg/ml[CL082]. Water extract of dried rhizome, in cell culture at a concentration of 0.1 mg/ml, was inactive on HELA cells. Methanol extract produced strong activity[CL018].

Desaturase-Delta-5 inhibition. Ethanol (95%) extract of fresh rhizome, at a concentration of 0.1%, was active. The effect was assayed by looking at the ratio of Dihomo-gamma-linolenic acid to arachidonic acid in cell-free preparations of *Mortierella alpina* IS-4[CL035].

Diuretic activity. Rhizome, in the ration of rats that were fed a low thiamine diet, showed no change in urinary or fecal excretion[CL188].

Embryotoxic effect. Ethanol (95%) extract of rhizome, administered orally to rats at doses of 100.0 and 200.0 mg/kg, produced 70% and 80% inhibition of pregnancy, respectively. Water extract produced 80% and 100% inhibition, respectively, and petroleum ether extract produced 80% and 100% inhibition, respectively[CL103]. Ethanol (95%), water and petroleum ether extracts of rhizome, administered orally to rats at doses of 100.0 mg/kg, were active[CL181].

Food consumption reduction. Powdered rhizome, administered intragastrically to rats at a dose of 10.0% of the diet, was inactive[CL177].

Gastric secretory inhibition. Water extracts, at a dose of 132.0 mg/kg, and methanol extract of the entire plant, at a dose of 155.0 mg/kg, administered intragastrically to rabbits, were active. Gastric juice was collected by catheter[CL079].

Gastrointestinal disorders. Powdered dried rhizome, taken orally by human adults at a dose of 500.0 mg/person, was active. A randomized double-blind study was conducted to examine the efficacy of treating dyspepsia with given extract. Patients were given the dose 4 times per day, after meals and before bed, for 7 days. Eighty patients were assigned to control or treatment groups. A statistically significant 87% of the treatment and 53% of the control group showed improvement, though patient satisfaction ran only 50% and 47%[CL176].

Genotoxicity activity. Rhizome, administered by gastric intubation to mice at doses of 2.5, 5.0 and 7.5 gm/kg, was inactive[CL136].

Glutamate oxaloacetate transaminase inhibition. Hot water extract of dried rhizome, administered subcutaneously to mice at a dose of 20.0 gm/kg, was active vs carbon tetrachloride-induced hepatotoxicity. The dose represents the amount of crude drug equivalent, results significant at P < 0.01 level[CL140].

Glutamate oxaloacetate transaminase stimulation. Methanol extract of dried rhizome, administered intraperitoneally to rats at a dose of 100.0 mg/kg, was active vs Alpha-naphthylisothiocyanate-induced hepatotoxicity[CL093].

Glutamate pyruvate transaminase inhibition. Hot water extract of dried rhizome, administered subcutaneously to mice at a dose of 20.0 gm/kg (the amount of crude drug equivalent), was active vs carbon tetrachloride-induced hepatotoxicity, results significant at P < 0.01 level[CL140]. Water extract of fresh rhizome, in the ration of ducklings at a concentration of 50.0 mg/day, was active vs aflatoxin B-1 hepatotoxicity. Enzyme was measured in the serum[CL047].

Glutamate pyruvate transaminase stimulation. Methanol extract of dried rhizome, administered intraperitoneally to rats at a dose of 100.0 mg/kg, was active vs Alpha-naphthylisothiocyanate-induced hepatotoxicity[CL093]. Water extract of fresh rhizome, in the ration of ducklings at a concentration of 50.0 mg/day, was active vs aflatoxin B-1 hepatotoxicity. Enzyme was measured in the serum[CL047].

Glutathione formation induction. Powdered root, in the ration of mice at a dose of 5.0% of the diet, was active[CL098].

Glutathione peroxidase stimulation. Rhizome, in the ration of rats at a concentration of 1.0% of the diet, produced weak activity[CL048].

Glutathione-S-Transferase induction. Powdered rhizome, administered intragastrically to mice at a dose of 4.0 gm/kg, was active. Assay was done in pups, presuming translactational exposure[CL065]. Powdered root, in the ration of mice at a dose of 5.0% of the diet, was active[CL098]. Rhizome, administered intragastrically to mice at a concentration of 4.0 gm/kg, was active. Progeny's liver looked at after translactational exposure; other significant enzyme included soluble sulfhydryl cytochrome B5 and cytochrome P450[CL065].

GRAS status. Rhizome and root (Sect. 582.10) and essential oil (Sect. 582.20) obtained GRAS status by United States of America Food and Drug Administration in 1976 as flavoring agents[CL031].

Hyaluronidase inhibition. Root essential oil, administered orally to male mice at a dose of 0.1 ml/kg, was active[CL014].

Hypoglycemic activity. Water extract of rhizome, administered orally to rabbits at a dose of 10.0 mg/kg, was inactive[CL016]. Drop in blood sugar of 15 mg relative to inert-treated control indicated positive results[CL016].

Hypothermic activity. Ethanol/water (1:1) extract of rhizome, administered intraperitoneally to mice at a dose of 250.0 mg/kg, was inactive[CL006].

Immunostimulant activity. Polysaccharide fraction of dried rhizome administered intraperitoneally to mice at a dose of 100.0 mg/kg for 5 days was inactive vs SRBC challenge. A dose of 200.0 mg/kg was active, results significant at P < 0.01 level[CL162].

Immunosuppressant activity. Water extract of rhizome, administered by gastric intubation to rats at a dose of 100.0 mg/kg, was active. Daily dosing for 10 days to typhoid bacillus, RBC-stimulated sheep showed the antibody titer to be significantly inhibited[CL125]. Hot water extract of rhizome, administered intraperitoneally to rats, was active[CL118].

Insect repellent activity. Petroleum ether extract of dried rhizome, at variable concentrations, was active on *Rhyzopertha dominica*, *Sitophilus granarius* and *Tribolium castaneum*[CL134]. Petroleum ether extract of root, at a concentration of 680.0 mcg/sq. cm, was active on *Tribolium castaneum*[CL121]. Root essential oil was active on *Aedes aegypti*[CL180].

Insecticide activity. Methanol extract of dried rhizome was active on *Spodoptera litura* larvae[CL147]. Powdered rhizome, applied externally to human adults, was active. *Azadirachta indica* leaves and *Curcuma longa* root were ground to form a paste, 4:1 by weight. This was spread over the entire body daily. Ninety seven percent of 814 cases of scabies were cured within 15 days of treatment[CL034]. Water extract of dried root, at variable concentrations, was inactive on *Blatella germanica* and *Oncopelatus fasciatus*. Intravenous dose of 40.0 ml/kg produced weak activity on *Periplaneta americana*[CL186].

Interferon induction stimulation. Hot water extract of dried rhizome, administered intragastrically to mice at a dose of 0.4 ml/animal for 7 days, was active. The prescription also included 10 gm each of *Curcuma longa* rhizome, *Rheum officinale* root, *Cimicifuga foetida* rhizome, *Anemarrhena asaphodeloides* rhizome, *Areca catechu* seed, *Magnolia officinalis* bark and *Scutellaria baicalensis* root, also included are 5 gm *Amomum tsaoko* fruit, and the insects *Bombyx mori* and *Cryptotympana pustulata*. A dose of 0.6 ml/animal, administered intraperitoneally, was also active[CL085].

Intestinal absorption inhibition. Water extract of dried rhizome, at a concentration of 1.0% administered by perfusion, produced weak activity in rats vs absorption of sulfaguanidine. Methanol and water extracts at a concentration of 0.1% were inactive[CL173].

Lactate dehydrogenase stimulation. Methanol extract of dried rhizome, administered intraperitoneally to rats at a dose of 100.0 mg/kg, was active vs Alpha-naphthyl-isothiocyanate-induced hepatotoxicity[CL093].

Leukopenic activity. Water extract of rhizome, administered intragastrically to mice at a dose of 100.0 mg/kg, was active[CL101].

Lipid peroxide formation inhibition. Hot water extract of a commercial sample of tuber was active, IC_{50} 200.0 ng/ml[CL076]. Hot water extract of dried rhizome, in cell culture at a concentration of 1.0 mg/plate, was inactive on hepatocytes monitored by production of malonaldehyde[CL062].

Liver regeneration stimulation. Commercial sample of oleoresin, at a concentration of 0.6% of the diet in the ration of male rats, was inactive. Partially hepatectomized animals were dosed daily for 7 days[CL123].

Mutagenic activity. Bulb, on agar plate at a concentration of 50.0 mcg/plate, was active on *Salmonella typhimurium* TA1535, and inactive on *Salmonella typhimurium* TA1537 and TA1538[CL175]. Infusion, on agar plate at a concentration of 200.0 mcg/plate, was inactive on *Salmonella typhimurium* TA100 and TA98. Metabolic activation had no effect on the results[CL033]. Chloroform/methanol (2:1) extract of rhizome, on agar plate at a concentration of 10.0 mg/plate, produced complete growth inhibition of the Pig-Kidney LLC-PK1 and Trophoblastic-Placenta cells, thus, it was impossible to interpret the results. Effect was the same with or without metabolic activation. Water extract of rhizome, on agar plate at a concentration of 100.0 mg/plate, was inactive on Pig-Kidney-LLC-PK-1 and Trophoblastic-Placenta cells. The effect was the same with or without metabolic activation[CL117]. Ethanol (95%) extract of dried rhizome, on agar plate at a concentration of 10.0 mg/plate, was active on *Salmonella typhimurium* TA102, and inactive on *Salmonella typhimurium*

TA98[CL036]. Ethanol (95%) extract of dried rhizome, on agar plate at a concentration of 250.0 mcg/plate, was inactive on *Salmonella typhimurium* TA98, TA100 and TA1535. Metabolic activation had no effect on the results[CL044]. Ethanol (95%) extract of fresh rhizome, on agar plate at a concentration of 360.0 mcg/plate, was inactive on *Salmonella typhimurium* TA100, TA98, TA1535 and TA1538. Metabolic activation had no effect on the results[CL044]. Ethanol (95%) extract of root, on agar plate at a concentration of 15.0 mg/plate, was active on *Salmonella typhimurium* TA98. Streptomycin dependent strains of TA98 were tested. Metabolic activation had no effect on the results[CL161]. Hot water and methanol extracts of rhizome, on agar plate at concentrations of 50.0 mg/disc (expressed as dry weight of plant), were inactive on *Salmonella typhimurium* TA98 and TA100. Effect was the same with or without metabolic activation. Histidine was removed from the extract prior to testing[CL127]. Resin, on agar plate at a concentration of 160.0 mcg/plate, was inactive on *Salmonella typhimurium* TA100, TA98, and TA1535[CL144]. Water extract of dried rhizome, at a concentration of 50.0 mg/ml on agar plate, was inactive on *Salmonella typhimurium* TA1535. Mutagenicity was assayed by SOS UMU test. Metabolic activation had no effect on the results[CL095]. Water and hot water extracts of dried rhizome, on agar plate at a concentration of 0.5 ml/disc, and rhizome, at variable concentrations, were inactive on *Bacillus subtilis* M-45(REC-) and H-17(REC+)[CL138].

Myocardial uptake of 86-RB enhanced. Hot water extract of dried tuber, administered intraperitoneally to mice at variable dosage levels, was inactive, as evidenced by uptake of 86-RB by the myocardium[CL132].

Necrotic effect. Ethanol (95%) extract of rhizome, on agar plate at a concentration of 250.0 mcg/plate, was inactive on *Salmonella typhimurium* TA1538. Metabolic activation had no effect on the results[CL044].

Nematocidal activity. Hexane extract of dried rhizome was active on *Toxacara canis*[CL026].

Nitrosation inhibition. Rhizome, at variable concentrations was active on *Salmonella typhimurium* TA100 and TA1535 vs nitrosation of methylurea[CL171].

Ovulation inhibition effect. Ethanol (95%), water and petroleum ether extracts of rhizome, administered orally to rabbits at doses of 100.0 and 200.0 mg/kg, were inactive[CL030]. Water and petroleum ether extracts of rhizome, administered orally to rabbits at doses of 100.0 mg/kg, were inactive[CL181].

Phagocytosis capacity increased. Polysaccharide fraction of dried rhizome, administered intraperitoneally to mice at a dose of 100.0 mg/kg, was active vs clearance of colloidal carbon, results significant at $P < 0.01$ level[CL162]. Plant extract, on agar plate at a concentration of 0.5%, was inactive and stimulated acid production on *Escherichia coli*, *Streptococcus faecalis*, *Streptococcus lactis*, and active on *Lactobacillus acidophilus* and *Lactobacillus plantarum*[CL102].

Plasma bilirubin decrease. Methanol extract of dried rhizome, administered intraperitoneally to rats at a dose of 100.0 mg/kg, was inactive vs Alpha-naphthylisothiocyanate-induced hepatotoxicity[CL093].

Platelet aggregation inhibition. Ether extract of dried tuber, at a concentration of 100.0 mcg/ml, was inactive vs collagen- and ADP-induced aggregation, and A23187 used as ionophore vs calcium ionophore-induced aggregation. A concentration of 50.0 mcg/ml was active vs arachidonic acid-induced aggregation[CL172]. Water extract of dried rhizome was active on the platelets of human adults and rabbits. The dose consisted of a mixture of *Levisticum officinale*, *Artemisia cappilaris*, *Curcuma longa* and *Chrysanthemum indicum*[CL038].

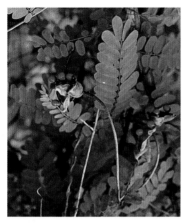

Plate 1. *Abrus precatorius* (*see* full discussion in Chapter 2).

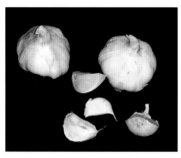

Plate 2. *Allium sativum* (*see* full discussion in Chapter 3).

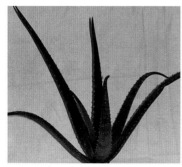

Plate 3. *Aloe vera* (*see* full discussion in Chapter 4).

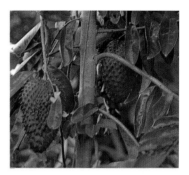

Plate 4. *Annona muricata* (*see* full discussion in Chapter 5).

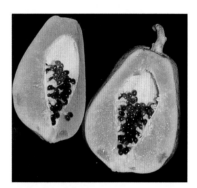

Plate 5. *Carica papaya* (*see* full discussion in Chapter 6).

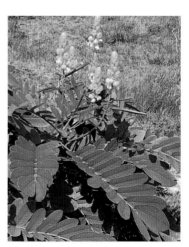

Plate 6. *Cassia alata* (*see* full discussion in Chapter 7).

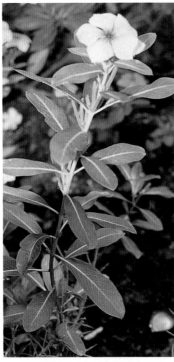

Plate 7. *Catharanthus roseus*
(*see* **full discussion**
in Chapter 8).

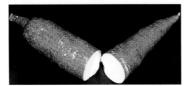

Plate 8. *Manihot esculenta*
(*see* **full discussion**
in Chapter 18).

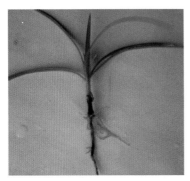

Plate 9. *Cyperus rotundus* (*see*
full discussion in Chapter 10).

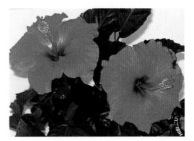

Plate 10. *Hibiscus rosa-sinensis*
(*see* **full discussion**
in Chapter 12).

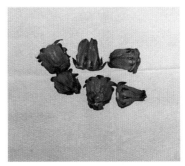

Plate 11. *Hibiscus sabdariffa*
(*see* **full discussion in Chapter 13).**

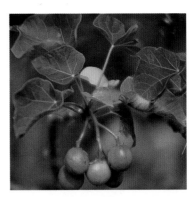

Plate 12. *Jatropha curcas* (*see*
full discussion in Chapter 14).

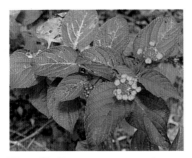

Plate 13. *Lantana camara* (*see* full discussion in Chapter 15).

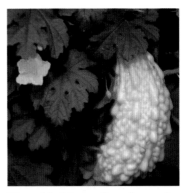

Plate 16. *Momordica charantia* (*see* full discussion in Chapter 19).

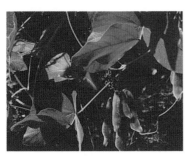

Plate 14. *Macuna pruriens* (*see* full discussion in Chapter 16).

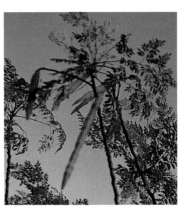

Plate 17. *Moringa pterygosperma* (*see* full discussion in Chapter 20).

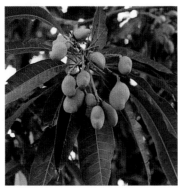

Plate 15. *Mangifera indica* (*see* full discussion in Chapter 17).

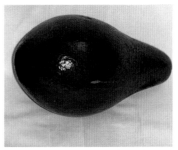

Plate 18. *Persea americana* (*see* full discussion in Chapter 21).

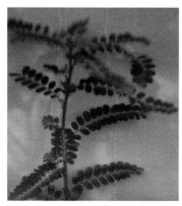

Plate 19. *Phyllanthus niruri*
(*see* **full discussion
in Chapter 22).**

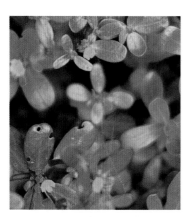

Plate 20. *Portulaca oleracea* (*see*
full discussion in Chapter 23).

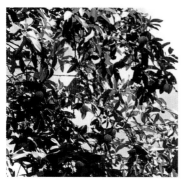

Plate 21. *Psidium guajava* (*see*
full discussion in Chapter 24).

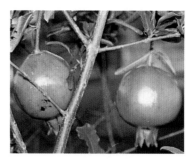

Plate 22. *Punica granatum* (*see*
full discussion in Chapter 25).

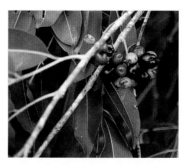

Plate 23. *Syzygium cumini* (*see*
full discussion in Chapter 26).

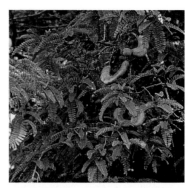

Plate 24. *Tamarindus indica* (*see*
full discussion in Chapter 27).

Protease (HIV) inhibition. Water extract of rhizome, at a concentration of 200.0 mcg/ml, was equivocal[CL059].

Radical scavenging effect. Hot water extract of dried rhizome, at a concentration of 250.0 mg/liter, was inactive when measured by decolorization of diphenylpicryl hydroxyl radical solution. There was 6 % decoloration[CL062].

RBC synthesis antagonist. Water extract of rhizome, administered intragastrically to mice at a dose of 100.0 mg/kg, was active[CL101].

Spasmogenic activity. Methanol extract of dried rhizome, at a concentration of 5.0 mg/ml, was inactive on the rat ileum[CL178].

Spasmolytic activity. Methanol extract of dried rhizome, at a concentration of 5.0 mg/ml, was inactive on the rat ileum vs ACh-induced contractions[CL178].

Sulfhydryl-containing compound increase. Powdered rhizome, administered intragastrically to mice at a dose of 4.0 gm/kg, was active. Assay was done on pups, presuming translactational exposure[CL065]. Water extract of rhizome, at a concentration of 50.0 mcg/ml, was active on rat brain. There was a decrease in the depletion of sulfhydryl-containing compounds induced by promoters of lipid peroxidation[CL060].

Superoxide dismutase stimulation. Rhizome, in the ration of rats at a concentration of 1.0% of the diet, produced weak activity[CL048].

Taenicide activity. Root essential oil, at a concentration of 0.2%, was active on *Taenia saginata*. Forty-two minutes of exposure was required to kill all the worms. A 0.2% piperazine citrate solution required 60 minutes of exposure to kill all the worms[CL107].

Teratogenic activity. Ethanol (95%), water and petroleum ether extracts of rhizome, administered orally to female rabbits at doses of 200.0 mg/kg, were inactive[CL030]. Root, in the ration of female mice and rats at a concentration of 0.5% of the diet for 7 days, was inactive[CL113].

Thromboxane B-2 synthesis inhibition. Ether extract of dried tuber, at a concentration of 100.0 mcg/ml, was active on platelets vs calcium ionophore A23187 stimulation of platelets. A concentration of 62.5 mcg/ml was active, 12-HETE synthesis was stimulated[CL172].

Toxic effect (general). Ethanol (95%) extract of rhizome, administered intragastrically to mice at a dose of 100.0 mg/kg, was inactive[CL101]. Ethanol (95%) extract of rhizome, in the ration of male guinea pigs and female monkeys at variable dosage levels for 3 weeks, was inactive. No toxic effects or abnormal morphological or histological results were observed. Doses of 300.0 mg/kg and 2.5 gm/kg, in the ration of Rhesus monkeys and rats of both sexes, were inactive. Dosing was only on the first day, followed by control diet for 3 weeks[CL110].

Toxic effect. Commercial sample of oleoresin, at variable dosage levels in the ration of pigs, was active. Animals were fed dietary levels of the oleoresin equal to 60, 296 and 1551 mg/kg/day for 102–109 days. All dose levels showed a significant dose-dependent increase in liver and thyroid weight. A reduction in weight gain and feed conversion efficiency was observed in the high dose group. The 2 higher dose groups showed evidence of thyroidal hyperplasia, epithelial changes in the urinary bladder and kidney and pericholangitis[CL159].

Toxicity assessment (quantitative). Ethanol (95%) extract of rhizome, administered intraperitoneally to mice, produced LD_{50} 3.98 gm/kg; water extract, LD_{50} 430.0 mg/kg and petroleum ether extract, LD_{50} 525.0 mg/kg[CL032]. Ethanol/water (1:1) extract of rhizome, administered intraperitoneally to mice, produced LD_{50} 500.0 mg/kg[CL006].

Tyrosinase inhibition. Methanol extract of dried rhizome, at a concentration of 167.0 mcg/ml, was active[CL056]. An extract of skin-lightening cosmetics contained extracts of *Syzygium aromaticum*, *Curcuma longa*, *Areca* *catechu*, and/or *Sauesurea lappa* (comprising melanin inhibitors), in addition to base materials showed tyrosinase-inhibiting activity[CL068].

Uterine stimulant effect. Methanol extract of dried rhizome, at a concentration of 5.0 mg/ml, was inactive on the uterus of rats[CL178]. Methanol/water (1:1) extract of leaves, at a dose of 10.0 mcg/ml, was active on the hamster uterus[CL008].

WBC-macrophage stimulant. Water extract of freeze-dried rhizome, at a concentration of 2.0 mg/ml, was inactive. Nitrite formation was used as an index of the macrophage-stimulating activity to screen effective foods[CL092].

Weight gain inhibition. Powdered rhizome, administered intragastrically to rats at a dose of 10.0% of the diet, was inactive[CL177].

REFERENCES

CL001   Jain, S. K. and C. R. Tarafder. Medicinal plant-lore of the Santals. **Econ Bot** 1970; 24: 241-278.

CL002   Quisumbing, E. Medicinal plants of the Philippines. **Tech Bull** 16, Rep Philippines, Dept Agr Nat Resources, Manilla 1951; 1.

CL003   Couvee. Compilation of herbs, plants, crops supposed to be effective in various complaints and illnesses. **J Sci Res** 1952; 1s: 1.

CL004   Grabe, F. The choleretic action of *Curcuma domestica*. Naunyn-Schmiedeberg's **Arch Exp Pathol Pharmakol** 1934; 176: 673.

CL005   Supniewski, J. V. and J. Hano. The pharmacological action of phenylethylcarbinol and p-toluylmethylcarbinol. **Bull Int Acad Pol Sci Lett Cl Med** 1935; 573.

CL006   Dhar, M. L., M. M. Dhar, B. N. Mehrotra and C. Ray. Screening of Indian plants for biological activity. Part I. **Indian J Exp Biol.** 1968; 6: 232-247.

CL007   Suggs, R. C. Marquesan Sexual Behavior. Harcourt, Brace and World, Inc., New York, 1966.

CL008   Goto, M., T. Noguchi, T. Watanabe, I. Ishikawa, M. Komatsu and Y.

CL009   Aramaki. Uterus-contracting ingredients in plants. **Takeda Kenkyusho Nempo** 1957; 16: 21.

Gimlette, J. D. Malay Poisons and Charm Cures. J & A Churchill, London, 3rd Edition, 1929.

CL010   Fitzpatrick, F. K. Plant substances active against *Mycobacterium tuberculosis*. **Antibiot Chemother** 1954; 4: 528.

CL011   Saha, J. C., E. C. Savini and S. Kasinathan. Ecbolic properties of Indian medicinal plants. Part I. **Indian J Med Res** 1961; 49: 130–151.

CL012   Hooper, D. On Chinese medicine. Drugs of Chinese pharmacies in Malaya. **Gard Bull STR Settlm** 1929; 6: 1.

CL013   Trivedi, V. P. and A. S. Mann. Vegetable drugs regulating fat metabolism in Caraka (Lekhaniya Dravyas). **Q J Crude Drug Res** 1972; 12: 1988.

CL014   Gupta, S. S., D. Chandra and N. Mishra. Anti-inflammatory and anti-hyaluronidase activity of volatile oil of *Curcuma longa*. **Indian J Physiol Pharmacol** 1972; 16: 263A.

CL015   Watt, J. M. and M. G. Breyer-Brandwijk. The Medicinal and Poisonous Plants of Southern and Eastern Africa. 2nd Ed, E. S. Livingstone, Ltd., London, 1962.

CL016   Jain, S. R. and S. N. Sharma. Hypoglycaemic drugs of Indian indigenous origin. **Planta Med** 1967; 15(4): 439–442.

CL017   Ratanasonthorn, S. Studies of volatile oil from *Curcuma longa*. **Undergraduate Special Project Report** 1952; 11pp.

CL018   Kosuge, T., M. Yokota, K. Sugiyama, T. Yamamoto, M. Y. Ni and S. C. Yan. Studies on antitumor activities and antitumor principles of Chinese herbs. I. Antitumor activities of Chinese herbs. **Yakugaku Zasshi** 1985; 105(8): 791–795.

CL019   Kuttan, R., P. Bhanumathy, K. Nirmala and M. C. George. Potential anticancer activity of turmeric (*Curcuma longa*). **Cancer Lett** 1985; 29(2): 197–202.

CL020   Gewali, M. B., M. Hattori, Y. Tezuka, T. Kikuchi and T. Namba. Four ingol type diterpenes from *Euphorbia antiquorum* L. **Chem Pharm Bull** 1989; 37(6): 1547–1549.

CL021 Tomoda, M., R. Gonda, N. Shimizu, M. Kanari and M. Kimura. A reticuloendothelial system activating glycan from the rhizomes of *Curcuma longa*. **Phytochemistry** 1990; 29(4): 1083–1086.

CL022 Imai, S., M. Morikiyo, K. Furihata, Y. Hayakawa and H. Seto. Turmeronol A and turmeronol B, new inhibitors of soybean lipoxygenase. **Agr Biol Chem** 1990; 54(9): 2367–2371.

CL023 Gonda, R., K. Takeda, N. Shimizu and M. Tomoda. Characterization of a neutral polysaccharide activity on the reticuloendothelial system from the rhizome of *Curcuma longa*. **Chem Pharm Bull** 1992; 40(1): 185–188.

CL024 Nakayama, R., Y. Tamura, H. Yamanaka, H. Kikuzaki and N. Nakatani. Two curcuminoid pigments from *Curcuma domestica*. **Phytochemistry** 1993; 33(2): 501–502.

CL025 Masuda, T., A. Jitoe, J. Isobe, N. Nakatani and S. Yonemori. Anti-oxidative and anti-inflammatory curcumin-related phenolics from rhizomes of *Curcuma domestica*. **Phytochemistry** 1993; 32(6): 1557–1560.

CL026 Kiuchi, F., Y. Goto, N. Sugimoto, N. Akao, K. Kondo and Y. Tsuda. Nematocidal activity of turmeric: Synergistic action of curcuminoids. **Chem Pharm Bull** 1993; 41(9): 1640–1643.

CL027 Zagari, A. Medicinal Plants. Vol 4, 5th Ed., Tehran University Publications, No 1810/4, Tehran, Iran, 1992; 4: 969pp.

CL028 Karig, F. Rapid identification of curcuma rhizomes with the TAS (thermomicroseparation and application) process. **Dtsch Apoth Ztg** 1975; 115: 325.

CL029 Mitra, C. R. Important Indian spices. I. *Curcuma longa* (Zingiberaceae). Riechst **Aromen Koerperpflegem** 1975; 25: 15.

CL030 Garg, S. K. Effect of *Curcuma longa* (rhizomes) on fertility in experimental animals. **Planta Med** 1974; 26: 225–227.

CL031 GRAS status of foods and food additives. **Fed Regist** 1976; 41: 38,644.

CL032 Yegnanarayana, R., A. P. Saraf and J. H. Balwani. Comparison of anti-inflammatory activity of various extracts of *Curcuma longa*. **Indian J Med Res** 1976; 64: 601.

CL033 Azuine, M. A., J. J. Kayal and S. B. Bhide. Protective role of aqueous turmeric extract against mutagenicity of direct-acting carcinogens as well as benzo(a)pyrene-induced genotoxicity and carcinogenicity. **J Cancer Res Clin Oncol** 1992; 118(6): 447–452.

CL034 Charles, V. and S. X. Charles. The use and efficacy of *Azadirachta indica* (neem) and *Curcuma longa* (turmeric) in scabies. **Trop Geogr Med** 1992; 44: 178–181.

CL035 Shimizu, S., S. Jareonkitmongkol, H. Kawashima, K. Akimoto and H. Yamada. Inhibitory effect of curcumin on fatty acid desaturation in *Mortierella alpina* 1S-4 and rat liver microsomes. **Lipids** 1992; 27(7): 509–512.

CL036 Mahmoud, I., A. Alkofahi and A. Abdelaziz. Mutagenic and toxic activities of several spices and some Jordanian medicinal plants. **Int J Pharmacog** 1992; 30(2): 81–85.

CL037 Ferriera, L. A. F., O. B. Henriques, A. A. S. Anderoni, G. R. F. Vital, M. M. C. Campos, G. G. Habermehl and Y. L. G. De Morales. Antivenom and biological effects of Arturmerone isolated from *Curcuma longa* (Zingiberaceae). **Toxicon** 1992; 30(10): 1211–1218.

CL038 Liu, Y. G. Hypolipemics and blood platelet aggregation inhibitors comprising fish oil and plant extracts. **Patent-US**-4,842,859: 1989; 6pp.

CL039 Aruna, K. and V. M. Sivaramakrishnan. Anticarcinogenic effects of some Indian plant products. **Food Chem Toxicol** 1992; 30(11): 953–956.

CL040 Uehara, S. I., I. Yasuda, K. Takeya and H. Itokawa. Terpenoids and curcuminoids of the rhizoma of *Curcuma xanthorrhiza* Roxb. **Yakugaku Zasshi** 1992; 112(11): 817–823.

CL041 Mukundan, M. A., M. C. Chacko, V. V. Annapurna and K. Krishnaswamy. Effect of turmeric and curcumin on BP-DNA adducts. **Carcinogenesis** 1993; 14(3): 493–496.

CL042   Reddy, M. B., K. R. Reddy and M. N. Reddy. A survey of plant crude drugs of Anantapur District, Andhra Pradesh, India. **Int J Crude Drug Res** 1989; 27(3): 145–155.

CL043   Azuine, M. A. and S. V. Bhide. Protective single/combined treatment with betel leaf and turmeric against methyl (acetoxymethyl) nitrosamine-induced hamster oral carcinogenesis. **Int J Cancer** 1992; 51: 412–415.

CL044   Nagabhushan, M. and S. V. Bhide. Nonmutagenicity of curcumin and its antimutagenic action versus chili and capsaicin. **Nutr Cancer** 1986; 8(3): 201–210.

CL045   Abraham, S., S. K. Abraham and G. Radhamony. Mutagenic potential of the condiments, ginger and turmeric. **Cytologia** 1976; 41(3/4): 591–595.

CL046   Park, S. N. and Y. C. Boo. Cell protection from damage by active oxygen with curcuminoids. **Patent-Fr Demande-** 2,655,054 1991; 13pp.

CL047   Soni, K. B., A. Rajan and R. Kuttan. Reversal of aflatoxin induced liver damage by turmeric and curcumin. **Cancer Lett** 1992; 66(2): 115–121.

CL048   Reddy, A. C. P. and B. R. Lokesh. Effect of dietary turmeric (Curcuma longa) on iron-induced lipid peroxidation in the rat liver. **Food Chem Toxicol** 1994; 32(3): 279–283.

CL049   Mishra, A. and N. Dubey. Evaluation of some essential oils for their toxicity against fungi causing deterioration of stored food commodities. **Appl Environ Microbiol** 1994; 60(4): 1101–1105.

CL050   Soni, K. B., A. Rajan, R. Kuttan. Inhibition of aflatoxin-induced liver damage in ducklings by food additives. **Mycotoxin Res** 1993; 9(1): 22–27.

CL051   Azuine, M. A. and S. V. Bhide. Ajuvant chemoprevention of experimental cancer: catechin and dietary turmeric in forestomach and oral cancer models. **J Ethnopharmacol** 1994; 44(3): 211–217.

CL052   Kositchaiwat, C., S. Kositchaiwat and J. Havanondha. Ulcer comparison to liquid antacid: A controlled clinical trial. **J Med Assoc Thailand** 1993; 76(1): 601–605.

CL053   Kumazawa, N., S. Ohto, O. Ishizuka, N. Sakurai, A. Kamogawa and M. Shinoda. Protective effects of various methanol extracts of crude drugs on experimental hepatic injury induced by carbon tetrachloride in rats. **Yakugaku Zasshi** 1990; 110(12): 950–957.

CL054   Hope, B. E., D. G. Massey and G. Fournier-Massey. Hawaiian materia medica for Asthma. **Hawaii Med J** 1993; 52(6): 160–166.

CL055   Sankaranarayanan, J. and C. I. Jolly. Phytochemical, antibacterial and pharmacological investigation on Momordica charantia Linn., Emblica officinalis Gaertn. and Curcuma longa Linn. **Indian J Pharm** Sci 1993; 55(1): 6–13.

CL056   Shirota, S., K. Miyazaki, R. Aiyama, M. Ichioka and T. Yokikura. Tyrosinase inhibitors from crude drugs. **Biol Pharm Bull** 1994; 17(2): 266–269.

CL057   Holdsworth, D. K. Traditional medicinal plants of Rarotonga, Cook Islands Part I. **Int J Crude Drug Res** 1990; 28(3): 209–218.

CL058   Azuine, M. A. and S. V. Bhide. Protective single/combined treatment with betel leaf and turmeric against methyl (acetoxymethyl) nitrosamine-induced hamster oral carcinogenesis. **Int J Cancer** 1992; 51(3): 412–415.

CL059   Kusumoto, I. T., T. Nakabayashi, H. Kida, H. Miyashiro, M. Hattori, T. Namba and K. Shimotohno. Screening of various plant extracts used in Ayurvedic medicine for inhibitory effect on human immunodeficiency virus type 1 (HIV-1) protease. **Phytother Res** 1995; 9(3): 180–184.

CL060   Selvam, R., L. Subramanian, R. Gayathri and N. Angayarkanni. The antioxidant activity of turmeric (Curcuma longa). **J Ethnopharmacol** 1995; 47(2): 59–67.

CL061   Ruby, A. J., G. Kuttan, K. Dinesh Babu, K. N. Rajasekharan and R. Kuttan. Anti-tumor and antioxidant activity of natural curcuminoids. **Cancer Lett** 1995; 91(1): 79–83.

CL062   Joyeux, M., F. Mortier and J. Fleurentin. Screening of antiradical, antilipoperoxidant and hepatoprotective effects of nine plant extracts used in Caribbean folk medicine. **Phytother Res** 1995; 9(3): 228–230.

CL063 Deshpande, S. S. and G. B. Maru. Effects of curcumin on the formation of benzo(a)pyrene derived DNA adducts In Vitro. **Cancer Lett** 1995; 96(1): 71–80.

CL064 Bhide, S. V., D. Magnus, A. Azuine, M. Lahiri and N. T. Telang. Chemoprevention of mammary tumor virus-induced and chemical carcinogen-induced rodent mammary tumors by natural plant products. **Breast Cancer Res Treat** 1994; 30(3): 233–242.

CL065 Singh, A., S. P. Singh and R. Bamezai. Postnatal modulation of hepatic biotransformation system enzymes via translactational exposure of F1 mouse pups to turmeric and curcumin. **Chem Lett** 1995; 96: 87–93.

CL066 Bhattarai, N. K. Folk anthelmintic drugs of Central Nepal. **Int J Pharmacog** 1992; 30(2): 145–150.

CL067 Luper, S. A review of plants used in the treatment of liver diseases: part two. **Altern Med Rev** 1999; 493: 178–188.

CL068 Shirota, S., K. Myazaki, M. Ichioka and T. Yokokura. Skin-lightening cosmetics containing melanin inhibitors from plants. **Patent-Japan Kokai Tokkyo Koho**-06,227,960 1994; 4pp.

CL069 Paek, S. H., G. J. Kim, H. S. Jeong and S. K. Yum. AR-tumerone and B-atlantone induced internucleosomal DNA fragmentation associated with programmed cell death in human myeloid leukemia HL-60 cells. **Arch Pharm Res** 1996; 19(2): 91–94.

CL070 Selvanayahgam, Z. E., S. G. Gnanevendhan, K. Balakrishna and R. B. Rao. Antisnake venom botanicals from ethnomedicine. **J Herbs Spices Medicinal Plants** 1994; 2(4): 45–100.

CL071 Moon, C. K., N. S. Park and S. K. Koh. Studies on the lipid components of Curcuma longa. I. The composition of fatty acids and sterols. **Soul Taehakkyo Yakhak Nonmunjip** 1976; 1: 132.

CL072 Zhao, D. Y. and M. K. Yang. Separation and determination of curcuminoids in Curcuma longa L. and its

preparation by HPLC. **Yao Hsueh Hsueh Pao** 1986; 21(5): 382–385.

CL073 Merh, P. S., M. Daniel and S. D. Sabnis. Chemistry and taxonomy of some members of the Zingiberales. **Curr Sci** 1986; 55(17): 835–839.

CL074 Seetharam, K. A. and J. S. Pasricha. Condiments and contact dermatitis of the finger tips. **Indian J Dermatol Venereol Leprol** 1987; 53(6): 325–328.

CL075 Ogbeide, O. N., O. I. Eduaveguavoen and M. Parvez. Identification of 2-(hydroxymethyl) anthraquinone in Curcuma domestica. **Pak J Sci** 1985; 37(1/4): 15–17.

CL076 Shalini, V. K. and L. Srinivas. Lipid peroxide induced DNA damage: Protection by turmeric (Curcuma longa). **Mol Cell Biochem** 1987; 77(1): 3–10.

CL077 Itokawa, H. Research on antineoplastic drugs from natural sources, especially from higher plants. **Yakugaku Zasshi** 1988; 108(9): 824–841.

CL078 Ozaki, Y. and O. B. Liang. Cholagogic action of the essential oil obtained from Curcuma xanthorrhiza Roxb. **Shoyakugaku Zasshi** 1988; 42(4): 257–263.

CL079 Sakai, K., Y. Miyazaki, T. Yamane, Y. Saitoh, C. Ikwaw and T. Nishihata. Effect of extracts of Zingiberaceae herbs on gastric secretion in rabbits. **Chem Pharm Bull** 1989; 37(1): 215–217.

CL080 Dixit. V. P., P. Jain and S. C. Joshi. Hypolipidaemic effects of Curcuma longa L. and Nardostachys jatamansi DC. in triton-induced hyperlipidaemic rats. **Indian J Physiol Pharmacol** 1988; 32(4): 299–304.

CL081 Gonda, R., M. Tomoda, N. Shimizu and M. Kanari. Characterization of polysaccharides having activity on the reticuloendothelial system from the rhizome of Curcuma longa. **Chem Pharm Bull** 1990; 38(2): 482–486.

CL082 Ahn, B. Z. and J. H. Lee. Cytotoxic and cytotoxicity-potentiating effects of the curcuma root on L1210 cell. **Korean J Pharmacog** 1989; 20(4): 223–226.

CL083 Rafatullah, S., M. Tariq, M. A. Al-Yahya, J. S. Mossa and A. M. Ageel. Evaluation of turmeric (Curcuma longa) for gastric and duodenal antiulcer activity in rats. **J Ethnopharmacol** 1990; 29(1): 25–34.

CL084   Itokawa, H., F. Hirayama, S. Tsuruoka, K. Mizuno, K. Takeya and A. Nitta. Screening test for antitumor activity of crude drugs (III). Studies on antitumor activity of Indonesian medicinal plants. **Shoyakugaku Zasshi** 1990; 44(1): 58–62.

CL085   Cai, D. F., J. L. Wang, D. Z. Xun, X. J. Meng and J. Ma. Anti-viral and interferon-inducing effect of kangli powder. **Chung Hsi I Chieh Ho Tas Chih** 1988; 8(12): 731–733.

CL086   Ohshiro, M., M. Kuroyanagi and A. Ueno. Structures of sesquiterpenes from *Curcuma longa*. **Phytochemistry** 1990; 29(7): 2201–2205.

CL087   Arora, R. B., T. Khanna, M. Imran and D. K. Balani. Effect of lipotab on myocardial infarction induced by isoproterenol. **Fitoterapia** 1990; 61(4): 356–358.

CL088   Gonda, R. and M. Tomoda. Structural features of ukonan C, a reticuloendothelial system-activated polysaccharide from the rhizome of *Curcuma longa*. **Chem Pharm Bull** 1991; 39(2): 441–444.

CL089   Sato, A. Studies on anti-tumor activity of crude drugs. 1. The effects of aqueous extracts of some crude drugs in short-term screening test. **Yakugaku Zasshi** 1989; 109(6): 407–423.

CL090   Grange, M. and R. W. Davey. Detection of antituberculous activity in plant extracts. **J Appl Bacteriol** 1990; 68(6): 587–591.

CL091   Nagaraju, N. and K. N. Rao. A survey of plant crude drugs of Rayalaseema, Andhra Pradesh, India. **J Ethnopharmacol** 1990; 29(2): 137–158.

CL092   Miwa, M., Z. L. Kong, K. Shinohara and M. Watanabee. Macrophage stimulating activity of foods. **Agr Biol Chem** 1990; 54(7): 1863–1866.

CL093   Kumazawa, N., S. Ohta, S. H. Tu, A. Kamogawa amd M. Shinoda. Protective effects of various methanol extracts of crude drugs on experimental hepatic injury induced by Alpha-naphthylisothiocyanate in rats. **Yakugaku Zasshi** 1991; 11193): 199–204.

CL094   Kulkarni, R. R., P. S. Patki, V. P. Jog, S. G. Gandage and B. Patwardhan. Treatment of osteoarthritis with a herbomineral formulation: A double-blind, placebo-controlled, cross-over study. **J Ethnopharmacol** 1991; 33(1/2): 91–95.

CL095   Chang, I. M., I. C. Guest, J. Lee-Chang, N. W. Paik, and R. Y. Ryun. Assay of potential mutagenicity and antimutagenicity of Chinese herbal drugs by using SOS Chromotes (*E. coli* PQ37) and SOS UMU test (*S. typhimurium* TA1535/PSK 1002). **Proc First Korea-Japan Toxicology Symposium Safety Assessment of Chemicals In Vitro** 1989; 133–145.

CL096   Kiuchi, F., N. Nakamura, N. Miyashita, S. Nishizawa, Y. Tsuda and K. Kondo. Nematocidal activity of some anthelmintics, traditional medicines, and spices by a new assay method using larvae of *Toxocara canis*. **Shoyakugaku Zasshi** 1989; 43(4): 279–287.

CL097   Naovi, S. A. H., M. S. Y. Khan and S. B. Vohora. Anti-bacterial, anti-fungal and anthelmintic investigations on Indian medicinal plants. **Fitoterapia** 1991; 62(3): 221–228.

CL098   Azuine, M. A. and S. V. Bhide. Chemopreventive effect of turmeric against stomach and skin tumors induced by chemical carcinogens in Swiss mice. **Nutr Cancer** 1992; 17(1): 77–83.

CL099   Liu, D. X., X. J. Yin, H. C. Wang, Y. Zhou and Y. H. Zhang. Antimutagenicity screening of water extracts from 102 kinds of Chinese medicinal herbs. **Chung-Kuo Chung Yao Tsa Chi Li** 1990; 15(10): 617–622.

CL100   Uehara, S. I., I. Yasuda, K. Takeya and H. Itokawa. Comparison on the commercial turmeric and its cultivated plant by their constituents. **Shoyakugaku Zasshi** 1992; 46(1): 55–61.

CL101   Qureshi, S., A. H. Shah and A. M. Ageel. Toxicity studies on *Alpinia galanga* and *Curcuma longa*. **Planta Med** 1992; 58(2): 124–127.

CL102   Shankar, T. N. and V. S. Murthy. Effect of turmeric (*Curcuma longa*) on the growth of some intestinal bacteria In Vitro. **J Food Sci Technol** 1978; 15: 152.

CL103 Garg, S. K., V. S. Mathur and R. R. Chaudhury. Screening of Indian plants for antifertility activity. **Indian J Exp Biol** 1978; 16: 1077–1079.

CL104 Kiso, Y., Y. Suzuki, N. Watanabe, Y. Oshima and H. Hikino. Antihepatotoxic principles of *Curcuma longa* rhizomes. **Planta Med** 1983; 49(3): 185–187.

CL105 Achararit, C., W. Panyayong and E. Ruchatakomut. Inhibitory action of some Thai herbs to fungi. **Undergraduate Special Project Report** 1983; 13pp.

CL106 Czajka, P., D. Pharm, J. Field, P. Novak and J. Kunnecke. Accidental aphrodisiac ingestion. **J Tenn Med Assoc** 1978; 71: 747.

CL107 Bannerjee, A., and S. S. Nigam. In Vitro anthelmintic activity of the essential oils derived from the various species of the genus Curcuma Linn. **Sci Cult** 1978; 44: 503,504.

CL108 Singh, M. P., S. B. Malla, S. B. Rajbhandari and A. Manandhar. Medicinal plants of Nepal-retrospects and prospects. **Econ Bot** 1979; 33(2): 185–198.

CL109 Sussman, L. K. Herbal medicine on Mauritius. **J Ethnopharmacol** 1980; 2(3): 259–278.

CL110 Bhavani Shankar, T. N., N. V. Shantha, H. P. Ramesh, I. A. S. Murthy and V. S. Murthy. Toxicity studies in turmeric (*Curcuma longa*). Acute toxicity studies in rats, guinea pigs and monkeys. **Indian J Exp Biol** 1979; 18: 73–75.

CL111 Opdyke, D. L. J. Monographs on fragrance raw materials. Alphaphellandrene. **Food Cosmet Toxicol** 1978; 16: 843–844.

CL112 Matthes, H. W. D., B. Luu and G. Ourisson. Chemistry and biochemistry of Chinese drugs. Part VI. Cytotoxic components of *Zingiber zerumbet*, *Curcuma zedoaria* and *C. domestica*. **Phytochemistry** 1980; 19: 2643–2650.

CL113 Vijayalaxmi. Genetic effects of turmeric and curcumin in mice and rats. **Mutat Res** 1980; 79: 125–132.

CL114 Jain, J. P., L. S. Bhatnager and M. R. Parsai. Clinical trials of haridra (*Curcuma longa*) in cases of tamak swasa & kasa. **J Res Indian Med Yoga Homeopathy** 1979; 14(2): 110–119.

CL115 Shankara, M. R., N. S. N. Murthy and L. N. Shastry. Method of manufacture and clinical efficacy of rasamanikya mishrana in tamaka shwasa (bronchial asthma). **Indian J Pharm Sci** 1979; 41: 267B.

CL116 Chang, I. M. and W. S. Woo. Screening of Korean medicinal plants for antitumor activity. **Arch Pharm Res** 1980; 3(2): 75–78.

CL117 Rockwell, P. and I. Raw. A mutagenic screening of various herbs, spices, and food additives. **Nutrition and Cancer** 1979; 1: 10–15.

CL118 Godhwani, J. L. and J. B. Gupta. Modification of immunological response by garlic, guggal and turmeric: An experimental study in animals. (Abstract). **Abstr 13th Annu Conf Indian Pharmacol Soc** Jammu-tawi India 1980; Abstr-12.

CL119 Schultz, J. M. and K. Herrmann. Occurrence of hydroxybenzoic acids and hydroxycinnamic acid in spices. IV. Phenolics of spices. **Z Lebensm-Unters Forsch** 1980; 171: 193–199.

CL120 Nguyen, Van Dan. List of simple drugs and medicinal plants of value in Vietnam. **Proc Seminar of the Use of Medicinal Plants in Healthcare**, Tokyo 13–17 September 1977, WHO Regional Office Manila 1977; 65–83.

CL121 Su, H. C. F., R. Horvat and G. Jilani. Isolation, purification, and characterization of insect repellents from *Curcuma longa* L. **J Agr Food Chem** 1982; 30: 290–292.

CL122 Fang, H. J., J. G. Yu, Y. H. Chen and Q. Hu. Studies on Chinese curcuma. II. Comparison of the chemical components of essential oils from rhizome of five species of medicinal curcuma plants. **Yao Hsueh Hsueh Pao** 1982; 17: 441–447.

CL123 Gershbein, L. L. Regeneration of rat liver in the presence of essential oils and their components. **Food Cosmet Toxicol** 1977; 15: 173–182.

CL124 Kiso, Y., Y. Suzuki, Y. Oshima and H. Hikino. Sesquiterpenoids. 59. Sterostructure of curlone, a sesquiterpenoid of *Curcuma longa* rhizomes. **Phytochemistry** 1983; 22(2): 596–597.

CL125 Godhwani, J. D., J. B. Gupta and A. P. Dadhich. Modification of immunological response by garlic, guggal and turmeric: An experimental study in albino rats. **Proc Indian Pharmacol Soc** 1980; Abstract-I2.

CL126 Lal, S. D. and B. K. Yadav. Folk medicine of Kurukshetra district (Haryana), India. **Econ Bot** 1983; 37(3): 299–305.

CL127 Yamamoto, H., T. Mizutani and H. Nomura. Studies on the mutagenicity of crude drug extracts. I. **Yakugaku Zasshi** 1982; 102: 596–601.

CL128 Banerjee, A. and S. S. Nigam. Antifungal efficacy of the essential oils derived from the various species of the genus Curcuma Linn. **J Res Indian Med Yoga Homeopathy** 1978; 13(2): 63–70.

CL129 Ross, S. A., N. E. El-Keltawi and S. E. Megalla. Antimicrobial activity of some Egyptian aromatic plants. **Fitoterapia** 1980; 51: 201–205.

CL130 Hirschhorn, H. H. Botanical remedies of the former Dutch East Indies (Indonesia). I: Eumycetes, Pteridophyta, Gymnospermae, Angiospermae, (Monocotylendones only). **J Ethnopharmacol** 1983; 7(2): 123–156.

CL131 Razzack, H. M. A. The concept of birth controls in Unani medical literature. **Unpublished Manuscript** 1980; 64pp.

CL132 Pong, J. J., W. F. Wang, T. F. Lee and W. Liu. Effect of 28 herbal drugs on the uptake of 86-RU by mouse heart muscle. **Chung Ts'ao Yao** 1981; 12(1): 33,34.

CL133 Golding, B. T., E. Pombo and C. J. Samuel. Turmerones: Isolation from turmeric and their structure. **Chem Commun** 1982; 1982: 363–364.

CL134 Jilani, G. and H. C. F. Su. Laboratory studies on several plant materials as insect repellents for protection of cereal grains. **J Econ Entomol** 1983; 76(1): 154–157.

CL135 Wang, K. R., Y. L. Zhao, D. S. Wang and M. L. Zhao. Effects of traditional Chinese herbs, toad tincture and adenosine 3',5' camp on Ehrlich ascites tumor cells in mice. **Chin Med J** 1982; 95(7): 527–532.

CL136 Abraham, S. K. and P. C. Kesavan. Genotoxicity of garlic, turmeric and asafoetida in mice. **Mutat Res** 1984; 136(1): 85–88.

CL137 Dixit, R. S. and H. C. Pandey. Plants used as folk-medicine in Jhansi and Lalitpur sections of Bundelkhand, Uttar Pradesh. **Int J Crude Drug Res** 1984; 22(1): 47–51.

CL138 Ungsurungsie, M., O. Suthienkul and C. Paovalo. Mutagenicity screening of popular Thai spices. **Food Chem Toxicol** 1982; 20: 527–530.

CL139 Chen, J. M., Y. H. Chen and J. G. Yu. Studies on Chinese curcuma. 4. Quantitative determination of curcuminoids in the root and tuber. **Chung Ts'ao Yao** 1983; 14(2): 59–63.

CL140 Kiso, Y., Y. Suzuki, C. Konno, H. Hikino, I, Hashimoto and Y. Yagi. Liver-protective drugs. 3. The validity of the Oriental medicines. 38. Application of carbon tetrachloride-induced liver lesion in mice for screening of liver protective crude drugs. **Shoyakugaku Zasshi** 1982; 36: 144–238.

CL141 Chen, Y. H., J. G. Yu and H. J. Fang. Studies in Chinese curcuma. III. Comparison of the volatile oil and phenolic constituents from the rhizome and the tuber of Curcuma longa. **Chung Yao T'ung Pao** 1983; 8(1): 27–29.

CL142 John, D. One hundred useful raw drugs of the Kani Tribes of Trivandrum Forest Division, Kerala, India. **Int J Crude Drug Res** 1984; 22(1): 17–39.

CL143 Lee, C. Y., J. W. Chiou and W. H. Chang. Studies on the antioxidative activities of spices grown in Taiwan. **Chung-Kuo Nung Yeh Hua Hsueh Hui Chih** 1982; 20(1/2): 61–66.

CL144 Jensen, N. J. Lack of mutagenic effect of turmeric oleoresin and curcumin in the salmonella/mammalian microsome test. **Mutat Res** 1982; 105(6): 393–396.

CL145 Deka, L., R. Majumdar and A. M. Dutta. Some Ayurvedic important plants from district Kamrup (Assam). **Ancient Sci Life** 1983; 3(2): 108–115.

CL146 Gorchakova, N. K., N. I. Grinkevich and A. N. Fogel. Curcuma longa L. as a source of bile-expelling drugs. **Farmatsiya** (Moscow) 1984; 33(3): 12–13.

CL147 Rukachaisirikul, N., L. Benchapornkullanij, V. Rukachaisirikul, S. Permkan, P. Dampawan and P. Wiriyachitra. Extraction of substances toxic to

Spodoptera litura Fabr. from some readily available plants. **Warasan Songkhia Nakkharin** 1983; 5(4): 359–362.

CL148 Sircar, N. N. Pharmaco-therapeutics of Dasemani Drugs. **Ancient Sci Life** 1984; 3(3): 132–135.

CL149 Jain, S. P. and H. S. Puri. Ethnomedicinal plants of Jaunsar-Bawar Hills, Uttar Pradesh, India. **J Ethnopharmacol** 1984; 12(2): 213–222.

CL150 May, G. and G. Willuhn. Antiviral activity of aqueous extracts from medicinal plants in tissue cultures. **Arzneim-Forsch** 1978; 28(1): 1–7.

CL151 Kosuge, T., H. Ishida, H. Yamazaki and M. Ishii. Studies on active substances in the herbs used for oketsu, blood coagulation, in Chinese medicine. I. On anticoagulative activities of the herbs for oketsu. **Yakugaku Zasshi** 1984; 104(4): 1050–1053.

CL152 Whistler, W. A. Traditional and herbal medicine in the Cook Islands. **J Ethnopharmacol** 1985; 13(3): 239–280.

CL153 Kosuge, T., H. Ishida and H. Yamazaki. Studies on active substances in the herbs used for oketsu ("stagnant blood") in Chinese medicine. III. On the anticoagulative principles in *Curcumae rhizoma*. **Chem Pharm Bull** 1985; 33(4): 1499–1502.

CL154 Todd, S., T. Miyase, H. Arichi, H. Tanizawa and Y. Takino. Natural antioxidants. III. Antioxidative components isolated form rhizome of *Curcuma longa* L. **Chem Pharm Bull** 1985; 33(4): 1725–1728.

CL155 Velazco, E. A. Herbal and traditional practices related to maternal and child health care. **Rural Reconstruction Review** 1980; 35–39.

CL156 Woo, W. S., E. B. Lee, K. H. Shin, S. S. Kang and H. J. Chi. A review of research on plants for fertility regulation in Korea. **Korean J Pharmacog** 1981; 12(3): 153–170.

CL157 Tiwari, K. C., R. Majumder and S. Bhattacharjee. Folklore medicines from Assam and Arunachal Pradesh (District Tirap). **Int J Crude Res** 1979; 17(2): 61–67.

CL158 Singh, Y. N. Traditional medicine in Fiji. Some herbal folk cures used by Fiji Indians. **J Ethnopharmacol** 1986; 15(1): 57–88.

CL159 Bille, N., J. C. Larsen, E. V. Hansen and G. Wurtzen. Subchronic oral toxicity of turmeric oleoresin in pigs. **Food Chem Toxicol** 1985; 23(11): 967–973.

CL160 Rao, T. S., N. Basu and H. H. Siddiqui. Anti-inflammatory activity of curcumin analogues. **Indian J Med Res** 1982; 75(April): 574–578.

CL161 Shashikanth, K. N. and A. Hosono. In vitro mutagenicity of tropical spices to streptomycin dependent strains of *Salmonella typhimurium* TA98. **Agr Biol Chem** 1986; 50(11): 2947–2948.

CL162 Kinoshita, G., F. Nakamura and T. Maruyama. Immunological studies on polysaccharide fractions from crude drugs. **Shoyakugaku Zasshi** 1986; 40(3): 325–332.

CL163 Lee, J. H., S. K. Kang, and B. Z. Ahn. Antineoplastic natural products and the analogues. XI. Cytotoxic activity against L1210 cell of some raw drugs from the Oriental medicine and folklore. **Korean J Pharmacog** 1986; 17(4): 286–291.

CL164 Weniger, B., M. Rouzier, R. Daguilh, D. Henrys, J. H. Henrys and R. Anton. Popular medicine of the Central Plateau of Haiti. 2. Ethnopharmacological inventory. **J Ethnopharmacol** 1986; 17(1): 13–30.

CL165 Hemadri, K. and S. S. Rao. Jaundice: Tribal medicine. **Ancient Sci Life** 1984; 3(4): 209–212.

CL166 Mukerjee, T., N. Bhalla, G. Singh Aulakh and H. C. Jain. Herbal drugs for urinary stones. Literature appraisal. **Indian Drugs** 1984; 21(6): 224–228.

CL167 Jain, A. K., H. Tezuka, T. Kada and I. Tomita. Evaluation of genotoxic effects of turmeric in mice. **Curr Sci** 1987; 56(19): 1005–1006.

CL168 Lama, S. and S. C. Santra. Development of Tibetan plant medicine. **Sci Cult** 1979; 45: 262–265.

CL169 El-Keltawi, N. E. M., S. E. Megalla and S. A. Ross. Antimicrobial activity of some Egyptian aromatic plants. **Herba Pol** 1980; 26(4): 245–250.

CL170 Conner, D. E. and L. R. Beuchat. Inhibitory effects of plant oleoresins on yeasts. **Interact Food Proc Int IUMS-ICFMH Symp.**, 12th 1983; 1984: 447–451.

CL171   Nagabhushan, M., U. J. Nair, A. J. Amonkar, A. V. D'Souza and S. V. Bhide. Curcumins as inhibitors of nitrosation In vitro. **Mutat Res** 1988; 202(1): 163–169.

CL172   Srivastava, K. C. Extracts from two frequently consumed spices-cumin (*Cuminum cyminum*) and turmeric (*Curcuma longa*)- inhibit platelet aggregation and alter eicosanoid biosynthesis in human blood platelets. Prostaglandins **Leukotrienes Essent Fatty Acids** 1989; 37(1): 57–64.

CL173   Sakai, K., N. Oshima, T. Kutsuna, Y. Miyazaki, H. Nakajima, T. Muraoka, K. Okuma and T. Nishino. Pharmaceutical studies on crude drugs. I. Effect of the Zingiberaceae crude drug extracts on sulfaguanidine absorption from rat small intestine. **Yakugaku Zasshi** 1986; 106(10): 947–950.

CL174   Mishra, A. K. and N. K. Dubey. Fungitoxicity of essential oil of *Amomum subulatum* against *Aspergillus flavus*. **Econ Bot** 1990; 44(4): 530–532.

CL175   Sivaswamy, S. N., B. Balchandran, S. Balanehru and V. M. Sivaramakrishnan. Mutagenic activity of South Indian food items. **Indian J Exp Biol** 1991; 29(8): 730–737.

CL176   Thamlikitkul, V., T. Dechatiwongse, C. Chantrakul, S. Nimitnon, W. Punkrut, S. Wongkonkatape, N. Boontaeng, S. Taechaiya, A. Riewpaiboon, S. Timsard, et al., Randomized double-blind study of *Curcuma domestica* Val. for dyspepsia. **J Med Assoc Thailand** 1989; 72(11): 613–620.

CL177   Polasa, K., B. Sesikaran, T. P. Krishna and K. Krishnaswamy. Turmeric (*Curcuma longa*)-induced reduction in urinary mutagens. **Food Chem Toxicol** 1991; 29(10): 699–706.

CL178   Lee, E. B. and Y. S. Lee. The screening of biologically active plants in Korea using isolated organ preparations. (V). Anticholinergic and oxytocic actions in rat's ileum and uterus. **Korean J Pharmacog** 1991; 22(4): 246–248.

CL179   Ohta, S., N. Sato, S. H. Tu and M. Shinoda. Protective effects of Taiwan crude drugs on experimental liver injuries. **Yakugaku Zasshi** 1992; 113(12): 870–880.

CL180   Dixit, R. S., S. L. Perti and R. N. Agarwal. New repellents. **Lab Dev** 1965; 3: 273.

CL181   Garg, S. K. Effect of *Curcuma longa* on fertility in female albino rats. **Bull P. G. I.** 1971; 5: 178.

CL182   Lee, E. B., H. S. Yun and W. S. Woo. Plants and animals used for fertility regulation in Korea. **Korean J Pharmacog** 1977; 8: 81–87.

CL183   Li, F. K. Problems concerning artificial abortion through oral administration of traditional drugs. **Ha-Erh-Pin Chung-I** 1965; 1: 11–14.

CL184   Anon. More Secret Remedies. What They Cost and What They Contain. British Medical Association, London. 1912; 185–209.

CL185   Pachauri, S. P. and S. K. Makherjee. Effect of *Curcuma longa* (Haridra) and *Curcuma amada* (Amragandhi) on the cholesterol level in experimental hypercholesterolemia of rabbits. **J Res Indian Med** 1970; 5: 27–31.

CL186   Heal, R. E., E. F. Rogers, R. T. Wallace and O. Starnes. A survey of plants for insecticidal activity. **Lloydia** 1950; 13: 89–162.

CL187   Nayar, S. L. Vegetable insecticides. **Bull Natl Inst Sci India** 1955; 4: 137–145.

CL188   Meghal, S. K. and M. C. Nath. Effect of spice diet on the intestinal synthesis of thiamine in rats. **Ann Biochem Exp Med** 1962; 22: 99–104.

CL189   Pal, S., T. Choudhuri, S. Chattopadhyay, A. Bhattacharya, G. K. Datta, T. Das and G. Sa. Mechanisms of curcumin-induced apoptosis of Ehrlich's ascites carcinoma cells. **Biochem Biophys Res Commun** 2001; 283(3): 658–665.

CL190   Zhang, W., D. Liu, X. Wo, Y. Zhang, M. Jin and Z. Ding. Effects of *Curcuma longa* on proliferation of cultured bovine smooth muscle cells and on expression of low-density lipoprotein receptor in cells. **Chin Med J (Engl)** 1999; 112(4): 308–311.

CL191   Prucksunand, C., B. Indrasukhsri, M. Leethochawalit and K. Hungspreugs.

Phase II clinical trial on effect of the long turmeric (*Curcuma longa* Linn) on healing of peptic ulcer. **Southeast Asian J Trop Med Public Health** 2001; 32(1): 208–215.

CL192   Tawatsin, A., S. D. Wratten, R. R. Scott, U. Thavara and Y. Techadam-rongsin. Repellency of volatile oils from plants against three mosquito vectors. **J Vector Ecol** 2001; 26(1): 76–82.

CL193   Wuthi-udomler, M., W. Grisanapan, O. Luanratana and W. Caichompoo. Antifungal activity of *Curcuma longa* grown in Thailand. **Southeast Asian J Trop Med Public Health** 2000; 31 Suppl 1: 178–182.

CL194   Collett, G. P., C. N. Robson, J. C. Mathers and F. C. Campbell. Curcumin modifies Apc(min) apoptosos resistance and inhibits 2-amino 1-methyl-6-phenylimidazo[4,5-b]pyridine (PhIP) induced tumor formation in Apc9min mice. **Carcinogenesis** 2001; 22(5): 821–825.

CL195   Kim, D. S., S. Y. Park and J. K. Kim. Curcuminoids from *Curcuma longa* L. (Zingiberaceae) that protect PC12 rat pheochromocytoma and normal human umbilical vein endothelial cells from beta A(I-42) insult. **Neurosci Lett** 2001; 303(1): 57–61.

CL196   Jayadeep, V. R., O. S. Arun, P. R. Sudhakaran and V. P. Menon. Changes in the prostaglandin levels in alcohol toxicity: effect of curcumin and N-acetylcysteine. Department of Biochemistry, University of Kerala, Kariavattom campus, Trivandrum, India 2000.

CL197   Ramirez-Bosca, A., A. Soler, M. A. Carrion, J. Diaz-Alperi, A. Bernd, C. Quintanilla, E. Quintanilla Almagro and J. Miquel. An hydroalcoholic extract *Curcuma longa* lowers the apo B/apo A ratio. Implications for athero-genesis prevention. **Mech Ageing Dev** 2000; 119(1-2): 41–47.

CL198   Chuang, S. E., A. L. Cheng, J. K. Lin and M. L. Kuo. Inhibition by curcumin of diethylnitrosamine-induced hepatic hyperplasia, inflammation, cellular gene products and cell-cycle-related proteins in rats. **Food Chem Toxicol** 2000; 38(11): 991–995.

CL199   Bhaumik, S., M. D. Jyothi and A. Khar. Differential modulation of nitric oxide production by curcumin in host macrophages and NK cells. **FEBS Lett** 2000; 483(1): 78–82.

CL200   Skrzypczak-Jankun, E., N. P. McCabe, S. H. Selman and J. Jankun. Curcumin inhibits lipoxygenase by binding to its central cavity: theoretical and X-ray evidence. **Int J Mol Med** 2000; 6(5): 521–526.

CL201   Ushida, J., S. Sugie, K. Kawabata, Q. V. Pham, T. Tanaka, K. Fujii, H. Takeuchi, Y. Ito and H. Mori. Chemo-protective effect of curcumin on N-nitrosomethylbenzylamine-induced esophageal carcinogenesis in rats. **Jpn J Cancer Res** 2000; 91(9): 893–898.

CL202   Ramsewak, R. S., D. L. DeWitt and M. G. Nair. Cytotoxicity, antioxidant and anti-inflammatory activities of cur-cumins I-III from *Curcuma longa*. **Phytomedicine** 2000; 7(4): 303–308.

CL203   Singh, R. and B. Rai. Antifungal po-tential of some higher plants against *Fusarium udum* causing wilt disease of *Cajanus cajan*. **Microbios** 2000; 102(403): 165–173.

CL204   Rasmussen, H. B., S. B. Christensen, L. P. Kvist and A. Karazmi. A simple and efficient separation of the curcumins, the antiprotozoal constitu-ents of *Curcuma longa*. **Planta Med** 2000; 66(4): 396–398.

CL205   Deters, M., C. Siegers, P. Muhl and W. Hansel. Choleretic effects of cur-cuminoids on an acute cyclosporin-induced cholestasis in the rat. **Planta Med** 1999; 65(7): 610–613.

CL206   Antony, S., R. Kuttan and G. Kuttan. Immunomodulatory activity of cur-cumin. **Immunol Invest** 1999; 28(5-6): 291–303.

CL207   Ramirez-Tortosa, M. C., M. D. Mesa, M. C. Aguilera, J. L. Quiles, L. Baro, C. L. Ramirez-Tortosa, E. Martinez-Victoria and A. Gil. Oral administra-tion of turmeric extract inhibits LDL oxidation and has hypocholester-olemic effects in rabbits with experi-mental atherosclerosis. **Atherosclerosis** 1999; 147(2): 371–378.

CL208   Sidhu, G. S., H. Mani, J. P. Gaddipatti, A. K. Singh, P. Seth, K. K. Banaudha,

G. K. Patnaik and R. K. Maheshwari. Curcumin enhances wound healing in streptozotocin in-duced diabetic rats and genetically diabetic mice. **Wound Repair Regen** 1999; 7(5): 362–374.

CL209   Rajakrishnan, V., P. Viswanathan, K. N. Rajasekharan and V. P. Menon. Neuroprotective role of curcumin from *Curcuma longa* in ethanol-induced brain damage. **Phytother Res** 1999; 13(7): 571–574.

CL210   Singhal, S. S., S. Awasthi, U. Pandya, J. T. Piper, M. K. Saini, J. Z. Cheng and Y. C. Awasthi. The effect of curcumin on glutathione-linked enzymes in K562 human leukemia cells. **Toxicol Lett** 1999; 109(1-2): 87–95.

CL211   Kang, B. Y., Y. J. Song, K. M. Kim, Y. K. Choe, S. Y. Hwang and T. S. Kim. Curcumin inhibits Th1 cytokine pro-file in CD4+ T cells by suppressing interleukin-12 production in macroph-ages. **Br J Pharmacol** 1999; 128(2): 380–384.

CL212   Bhaumik, S., R. Anjum, N. Rangaraj, B. V. Pardhasaradhi and A. Khar. Curcumin mediated apoptosis in AK-5 tumor cells involves the production of reactive oxygen intermediates. **FEBS Lett** 1999; 456(2): 311–314.

CL213   Lal, B., A. K. Kapoor, O. P. Asthana, P. K. Agrawal, R. Prasad, P. Kumar and R. C. Srimal. Efficacy of curcumin in the management of chronic anterior uveitis. **Phytother Res** 1999; 13(4): 318–322.

CL214   Navis, I., P. Sriganth and B. Premalatha. Dietarty curcumin with cisplatin administration modulates tumor marker indices in experimental fibrosarcoma. **Pharmacol Res** 1999; 39(3): 175–179.

CL215   Kawamori, T., R. Lubet, V. E. Steele, G. J. Keloff, R, B. Kaskey, C. V. Rao and B. S. Reddy. Chemopreventive effect of curcumin, a naturally occur-ring anti-inflammatory agent, during the promotion/progression stages of colon cancer. **Cancer Res** 1999; 59(3): 597–601.

12 | Hibiscus rosa-sinensis

L.

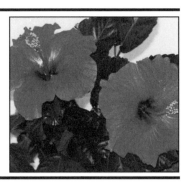

Common Names

Ampolo	Nicaragua	Gwo waz baya	Trinidad
Antolanagan	Philippines	Hibiscus	Easter Island
Ardhol	Fiji	Hibiscus	Guyana
Aroganan	China	Hibiscus	Vietnam
Avispa	Nicaragua	Hindu-ma-pangi	Bangladesh
Banban	Papua-New Guinea	Hong can	Vietnam
Bunga raya	Malaysia	Jaba	India
Chemparathy	India	Jabaphool	India
China rosa	Kuwait	Japa	India
China rose	India	Japa puspi	Nepal
China rose plant	India	Japakusum	India
Chinese hibiscus	Nepal	Jasum	Fiji
Choon kin phee	Malaysia	Jasum	India
Chou blak	Haiti	Jasunt	India
Chuan chin pi	Malaysia	Jaswand	India
Chuan chin pi	Vietnam	Jia pushpa	India
Chuen kan pi	Malaysia	Joba	India
Cucarda	Peru	Kaute	India
Dam but	Vietnam	Kaute'enua	Cook Islands
Dasani	India	Kaute'enua	Rarotonga
Dok mai	Vietnam	Kauti	Rarotonga
Double hibiscus	Trinidad	Kayaga	China
Fencing flower	Trinidad	Kembang sepatu	Indonesia
Fla baya	Trinidad	Koute	Indonesia
Fleur barriere	Trinidad	Lagitua	New Britain
Flores rosa	Guam	Lelegurua	New Britain
Foulsepatte	Rodrigues Islands	Loloru	New Britain
Fu-yong-pi	China	Mandaar	India
Ghanti phul	Nepal	Mandara	India
Gros rose	French Guiana	Rose de chine	Vietnam
Gudhal	India	Rose of China	China
Gumamila	Philippines	Rose-cayenne	Guadeloupe
Gurhal	India	Roz kaiyen	Guadeloupe
Gwo fla bays	Trinidad	Sadaphool	India
Gwo fle baye	Trinidad	Sambathoochedi	India

From: *Medicinal Plants of the World, vol. 1: Chemical Constituents, Traditional and Modern Medicinal Uses, 2nd ed.*
By: Ivan A. Ross © Humana Press Inc., Totowa, NJ

Senicikobia	India	Takuragan	China
Senitoa yaloyalo	India	Tapulaga	China
Shoe black	Nicaragua	Tiare kalova kalova	Papua-New Guinea
Shoe flower	Indonesia	Tulipan	Mexico
Shoe flower	Nepal	Wavu wavu	Indonesia
Shoe flower plant	Kuwait	Woz baya	Trinidad

BOTANICAL DESCRIPTION

A shrub of the MALVACEAE family with long slender branches up to about 6 meters tall. The branches are arranged spirally on the stem, are ovate, have long stalks and measure up to 15 cm long and 10 cm wide. Flowers are borne singly in the axils of the upper leaves, usually on rather long stalks. They have an epicalyx of 5–7 bracteoles about 1 cm long and cupular calyx about 2.5 cm long. The corolla is short-lived of 5 very showy, contorted-overlapping petals. Many varieties exist differing in size and color corolla, in single or double forms. The fruit (very rarely formed) is a capsule about 3 cm long.

ORIGIN AND DISTRIBUTION

A native of southeastern Asia. Very commonly cultivated and relict by old habitations and cultivation in a wide range of situations. Now commonly found throughout the tropics, and as a houseplant throughout the world. Most ornamental varieties are hybrids, many of them resulting from crosses with the African *H. schizopetalus*.

TRADITIONAL MEDICINAL USES

Bangladesh. A decoction of the flower with green betel nut is given to regulate the menstrual cycle[HR033].

China. Hot water extract of flowers is taken orally as an emmenagogue and a tonic[HR092]. Hot water extract of the bark is taken orally as an emmenagogue[HR022,HR008].

Cook Islands. Hot water extract of dried flowers and leaves is used for ailing infants. Flowers, or sometimes leaves with or without *Gardenia taitensis* leaves, are boiled or fried in coconut cream and taken internally or used as a massage. Hot water extract of dried leaves and flowers is taken orally for gonorrhea. Infusion is taken orally as an abortifacient[HR078].

East Indies. Hot water extract of flowers is taken orally to regulate menstruation and to produce abortion[HR022]. Leaf juice, in combination with *Vernonia cinerea*, is administered orally by midwives to stimulate expulsion of afterbirth[HR022].

Fiji. Fresh leaf juice is taken orally to enhance childbirth and for diarrhea[HR082]. Hot water extract of flowers and leaves is taken orally to ease childbirth[HR045]. Infusion of dried flowers is taken orally to aid digestion[HR082].

French Guiana. Hot water extract of flowers is taken orally for the grippe[HR026].

Ghana. Peeled twig is used as a chewstick[HR062].

Guadeloupe. Hot water extract of flowers is taken orally as a sodorific and antitussive. Syrup is made by boiling unopened flowers, and taken orally with sugar[HR074].

Guam. Leaves are applied to affected parts to promote draining of abscesses[HR006].

Haiti. Decoction of dried flowers is taken orally for flu and cough[HR086]. Decoction of dried leaves is taken orally for flu, cough, and stomach pain. For eye problems, macerated leaves are used in a bath for the head[HR086].

Hawaii. Flowers are eaten to produce lactation[HR089].

India. Decoction of dried flowers is taken orally for abortion[HR035]. Hot water extract is taken orally as an antifertility agent[HR059]. Hot water extract is used as a contraceptive in

Ayurvedic medicine. For this, the flowers with their sexual parts (pistil and stamens) are taken orally by the female patient. Four to 5 flowers make 1 dose, and 2–3 doses are taken per day at intervals of 5–6 hours[HR073]. Dried buds are eaten as a treatment for diabetes. One unopened flower (mature bud) is chewed and eaten per day early in the morning before taking meals, for up to 10 days or until the level of blood sugar is reduced to the tolerance limit. This treatment is said to be good in managing the disease but is not a permanent cure[HR049]. Fresh buds are taken orally by women to produce complete sterilization. Three flower buds are collected just before blooming and mixed with the water left after washing rice. One such bud makes 1 dose. The female is given 1 dose orally per day on the 4th, 5th and 6th days of the menses. The application is repeated for 3–4 months for permanent sterilization[HR073]. Flowers and leaves are taken orally for constipation and painful bowel motion. The leaves and flowers are churned into a mucilaginous juice with water and filtered. Half a cup of the filtrate is taken by mouth every day before going to bed[HR040]. Hot water extract of dried stems is taken orally as a diuretic[HR063]. Hot water extract of the flower is taken orally for menorrhagia, bronchitis[HR002] and as an emmenagogue[HR004]. For the treatment of menarche[HR034] and as a contraceptive[HR044] in Ayurvedic medicine, flower decoction along with "Jaggary" is taken orally. Hot water extract of aerial parts is taken orally as an aphrodisiac and emmenagogue[HR091]. Hot water extract of leaves is taken orally as an aperient, laxative and anodyne, and to expel the placenta after childbirth. Externally, in combination with juice of *Veronia cineria*, it is used as an emmolient[HR044]. Root juice is taken orally as an abortifacient. Five milliliters each of root juices of *Plumbago rosea* and *Hibiscus rosa-sinensis* are given on an empty stomach along with red-colored brain of a species of fresh water fish locally known as "Magur"[HR077]. Hot water extract of root is taken orally as a demulcent and for coughs[HR044].

Indonesia. Flowers are taken orally to regulate menstruation, to produce abortion[HR003], and as an emmenagogue[HR014]. Juice of leaves is taken orally by women in labor[HR003].

Japan. Decoction of fresh leaves is taken orally as an antidiarrheal[HR024].

Kuwait. Flowers are taken orally by females as an emmenagogue and by males as an aphrodisiac[HR043].

Malaysia. Hot water extract of roots is taken orally for fevers and venereal diseases[HR022]. Infusion of hot water extract of flowers is taken orally as an expectorant[HR022]. Water extract of the bark is taken orally as an emmenagogue[HR016].

Mexico. Infusions of bark, leaves or flowers are taken orally to treat dysentery[HR036].

Nepal. Hot water extract of roots is taken orally for coughs[HR001]. Powdered-dried flowers are administered intravaginally to accelerate parturition. Two to 4 teaspoonfuls are given during labor pains[HR039].

New Britain (East). Hot water extract of flowers is taken orally to regulate menstruation[HR045].

New Caledonia. Decoction of hot water extract of flowers is taken orally as an emmenagogue and abortifacient[HR015].

Northern Ireland. Water extract of fresh flowers and leaves is taken orally to induce labor. Flowers and young leaves are soaked in coconut water and the solution is taken orally to induce labor in the Northern Provinces[HR061].

Papau-New Guinea. Flowers are taken orally to relieve pain during labor[HR005]. Hot water extract of flowers and leaves is taken orally to induce labor. Leaves and flowers are soaked in coconut juice for several hours and taken orally[HR045].

Peru. Hot water extract of dried flowers is taken orally by males as a contraceptive and by females as an emmenagogue[HR087]. Hot water extract of dried stems is taken orally as a contraceptive and emmenagogue[HR087].

Philippines. Fresh flowers are bruised and applied to tumors and inflammations; water extract is taken orally in bronchial catarrh for a sodorific effect[HR008]. Hot water extracts of bark, roots and flower are used externally as emmolients[HR017]; paste of flowerbud is applied topically to cancerous swellings[HR020]. Leaf juice, together with leaves of *Vernonia cinerea*, is used to stimulate expulsion of the afterbirth[HR003] and the hot water extract is used externally as an emmolient[HR017].

Rarotonga. Decoction of fresh leaves is taken orally to treat women for irregular menstrual periods[HR032]. Infusion of fresh flowers is taken orally as an abortifacient[HR032].

Samoa. Hot water extract of flowers and leaves is taken orally to ease childbirth[HR045]. Water extract of fresh flowers and leaves is taken orally to induce labor[HR061].

South Africa. Leaves are cooked and eaten as spinach in Matabeleland and Nyasaland[HR020].

Trinidad. Decoction[HR029] and infusion[HR052] of hot water extract of flowers is taken orally for amenorrhea.

Vanuata. Decoction made from the petals is taken orally for amenorrhea and to induce abortion[HR037]. Decoction of leaves is taken orally to treat uterine hemorrhage. Eight leaves are squeezed with water then boiled for a few minutes. The preparation is taken orally as necessary. To induce sterility, a large handful of leaves are squeezed into 250 ml of water and all of it is taken orally during menstruation. The treatment is repeated during the following menstrual cycle[HR037]. Decoction of stem bark is taken orally for menorrhagia. Grate a handful of bark, prepare a decoction, cool it and drink of a maximum of 2 or 3 doses. Infusion of leaves is taken orally for menorrhagia. Six leaves are crushed in water, brought to a boil and taken orally[HR037].

Vietnam. Flowers are taken orally for dysmenorrhea[HR003] and as an abortive[HR018].

Hot water extract of dried leaves is used as a drug in traditional medicine[HR070]. Water extract of the bark is taken orally as an emmenagogue[HR018,HR003].

CHEMICAL CONSTITUENTS

(ppm unless otherwise indicated)

Apigenidin: Fl[HR068]
Arachidic acid: Lf[HR030]
Behenic acid: Lf[HR030]
Beta sitosterol: Lf, St[HR010], St Bk 40.8[HR023], Pl[HR047]
Campesterol: Pl[HR048]
Catalase: Petal, Lf[HR095]
Cholesterol: Pl[HR048]
Citric acid: Fl[HR096]
Cyanidin diglucoside: Fl[HR013]
Cyanidin: Fl[HR094,HR067]
Cyanin: Fl[HR094,HR012]
Dec-9-yn-1-oic acid methyl ester: St Bk[HR023]
Dec-9-yn-1-oic acid: St Bk[HR023]
Dec-9-ynoic acid methyl ester: St Bk 4.6[HR076], Rt Bk 0.8[HR025]
Dec-9-ynoic acid: St Bk 1.2[HR076]
Decanoic acid: Lf[HR030]
Docosan-1-ol: Lf[HR030]
Ergosterol: Pl[HR048]
Fructose: Fl[HR096]
Gentisic acid: Lf[HR021]
Glucose: Fl[HR096]
Heneicosan-1-ol: Lf[HR030]
Heneicosanoic acid: Lf[HR030]
Heptacosan-1-ol: Lf[HR030]
Heptacosanoic acid: Lf[HR030]
Heptadecanoic acid methyl ester, 9 methylene-8-oxo: St Bk 2.3–13.6[HR023,HR025]
Hexacosan-1-ol: Lf[HR030]
Hexacosanoic acid: Lf[HR030]
Hibiscus mucilage Rl: Lf 116.6[HR024]
Iso-octacosan-1-ol: Lf[HR030]
Iso-triacontan-1-ol: Lf[HR030]
Kaempferol-3-0-beta-D-xylosyl-glucoside: Petal[HR012]
Lauric acid: Lf[HR030]
Lignoceric acid: Lf[HR030]
Malvalic acid methyl ester: Rt Bk 54.4[HR030]
Malvalic acid: Lf[HR030]
Margaric acid: Lf[HR030]
Montanyl alcohol: Lf[HR030]
Myristic acid: Lf[HR030]

N-Docosane: Lf[HR030]
N-Dotriacontane: Lf[HR030]
N-Eicosane: Lf[HR030]
N-Heneicosane: Lf[HR030]
N-Hentriacontane: Fl 0.102%[HR094], Lf[HR030]
N-Heptacosane: Lf[HR030]
N-Heptadecane: Lf[HR030]
N-Hexacosane: Lf[HR030]
N-Hexadecane: Lf[HR030]
N-Nonacosane: Lf[HR030]
N-Nonadecane: Lf[HR030]
N-Octacosane: Lf[HR030]
N-Octadecane: Lf[HR030]
Non-8-yn-1-oic acid methyl ester:
    St Bk[HR023]
Non-8-yn-1-oic acid: St Bk[HR023]
Non-8-ynoic acid methyl ester: St Bk
    17.7[HR076], Rt Bk 1.2[HR025]
Non-8-ynoic acid: St Bk 4.6[HR076]
Nonadecanoic acid: Lf[HR030]
Nonadec-trans-10-enoic acid, 11-methoxy-
    9-oxo methyl ester: Rt Bk 3.5[HR025]
Nonanoic acid: Lf[HR030]
N-Pentacosane: Lf[HR030]
N-Triacontan-1-ol: Lf[HR030]
N-Triacontane: Lf[HR030]
N-Tricosane: Lf[HR030]
Octacosan-1-ol: Lf[HR030]
Octacosanoic acid: Lf[HR030]
Octadec-11-yn-1-oic acid methyl ester,
    10-oxo: Rt Bk 3.8[HR023]
Octadec-11-ynoic acid, 10-oxo methyl
    ester: Rt Bk[HR025]
Octadec-9-yn-1-oic acid methyl ester,
    8-oxo: St Bk 3.8[HR023]
Octadec-9-ynoic acid, 8-oxo methyl ester:
    Rt Bk[HR025]
Octadecadienoic acid: Lf[HR030]
Octadecanoic acid, 10-methylene-9-oxo
    methyl ester: Rt Bk 6.8[HR025]
Octadec-trans-9-enoic acid, 10-methoxy-
    8-oxo methyl ester: 3.6[HR025]
Octanoic acid: Lf[HR030]
Oxalic acid: Fl[HR096]
Palmitic acid: Lf[HR030]
Pelargonidin: Fl[HR068]
Pentacosan-1-ol: Lf[HR030]
Pentacosanoic acid: Lf[HR030]
Pentadencanoic acid: Lf[HR030]
Quercetin: Fl 300[HR094]
Quercetin-3-0-beta-D-sophorotrioside:
    Petal[HR012]

Quercetin-3-7-di-o-beta-D-glucoside:
    Petal[HR012]
Quercetin-3-di-o-beta-D-glucoside:
    Petal[HR012]
Stearic acid: Lf[HR030]
Sterculic acid methyl esther: Rt Bk 36.1[HR025]
Sterculic acid, 2-hydroxy methyl ester:
    Rt Bk 1.8[HR025,HR050]
Sterculic acid: Lf[HR030]
Stigmasterol: Pl[HR048]
Sucrose: Fl[HR096]
Taraxeryl acetate: Lf, St[HR010]
Tartaric acid: Fl[HR096]
Tetracosan-1-ol: Lf[HR030]
Triacontan-1-ol: Lf[HR030]
Tricosan-1-ol: Lf[HR030]
Tricosanoic acid: Lf[HR030]
Tridecanoic acid: Lf[HR030]
Undecanoic acid: Lf[HR030]

PHARMACOLOGICAL ACTIVITIES AND CLINICAL TRIALS

Abortifacient effect. Ethanol (95%), water and petroleum ether extracts of leaves, flowers and roots, administered orally, dried roots by gastric intubation and dried leaves subcutaneously to rats at doses of 200.0, 200.0, and 150.0 mg/kg, respectively, were inactive. Ethanol (95%), water and petroleum ether extracts of stem, administered orally, and of dried stem, administered by gastric intubation to rats at doses of 200.0 mg/kg, were inactive[HR090]. Ethanol/water (1:1) extract of the dried entire plant, administered by gastric intubation to rats at a dose of 200.0 mg/kg, was inactive[HR080]. Water-insoluble and ether-soluble fractions of a total benzene extract of dried flowers, administered by gastric intubation to rats at a dose of 186.0 mg/kg, were active[HR069]. Ether-soluble and water-insoluble fractions of a total benzene extract, at a dose of 73.0 mg/kg, were active[HR081]. Ethanol (90%), water and petroleum ether extracts of dried flowers, administered by gastric intubation at doses of 200.0, 200.0, and 150.0 mg/kg, respectively, were inactive[HR075].

Acid phosphatase stimulation. The effect of 50% ethanolic and benzene extracts of *Hibiscus rosa-sinensis* flowers on the estrogen dependent enzyme (acid and alkaline phosphatase) activity of rat uterus was studied. A significant increase in the acid phosphatase and decrease in alkaline phosphatase was reported with both the extracts, the effect being dose-related for both the enzymes. The antiestrogenic property of the ethanolic and benzene extracts was further confirmed in rats by a significant reduction in the fresh uterine content of protein, non-protein, nitrogen and total solid matter. Benzene and ethanol/water (1:1) extracts of flowers, administered orally to female rats daily for 12–18 days at doses of 75.0 mg/kg, were equivocal. At doses of 150.0 mg/kg and 300.0 mg/kg, both extracts were active[HR056].

Alkaline phosphatase inhibition. Benzene and ethanol/water (1:1) extracts of flowers, administered orally to rats daily for 12–18 days, were active at doses of 75.0 mg/kg, 150.0 mg/kg, and 300.0 mg/kg[HR056].

Analgesic activity. Ethanol (70%) extract of dried leaves, administered orally to mice at a dose of 125.0 mg/kg, was active vs inhibition of aconitine-induced writhing[HR058].

Androgenic effect. Benzene extract of dried flowers, administered by gastric intubation, and ethanol (95%) extract, administered orally to normal male[HR067] and castrated[HR057] rats at doses of 250.0 mg/kg, were inactive[HR009].

Anticonvulsive activity. The ethanol extract of flowers was active. The activity was present in the acetone soluble part of the ethanolic extract. The extract protected animals from maximum electro-shock, electrical kindling andpentylenetetrazole-induced convulsions in mice. It also inhibited convulsions induced by lithium-pilocarpine and electrical kindling. However, they failed to protect animals from strychnine-induced convulsions. The behavioral effects of D-amphetamine were antagonized and pentobarbitone-induced sleep was potentiated. The brain content of gamma-aminobutyric acid and sertonin were raised and the extract was found to be anxiogenic and general depressant of the central nervous system[HR101].

Anti-FSH activity. Ethanol (95%) extract of flowers, administered orally to rats at a dose of 150.0 mg/animal, was active[HR009].

Antiestrogenic effect. Benzene extract of dried flowers, administered by gastric intubation to rats at a dose of 200.0 mg/kg, was equivocal and active at a dose of 250.0 mg/kg. The extract was also active when administered orally to mice at a dose of 1 gm/kg, and subcutaneously at a dose of 250.0 mg/kg. The ethanol/water (1:1) extract was equivocal in rats when administered by gastric intubation at a dose of 200.0 mg/kg, and active when administered orally at a dose of 150.0 mg/kg[HR060]. Studies with the total benzene extract of *H. rosa-sinensis* flowers revealed antiestrogenic activity in bilaterally ovariectomized immature albino rats. It disrupts the estrous cycle in rats, depending on the dose and duration of treatment. The extract led to a reduction in the weights of the ovary, uterus and pituitary. Ovaries showed follicular atresia and uterine atrophic changes. These effects could be reversed 30 days after withdrawal of the plant extract. In guinea pigs, the benzene and ethanolic extract of the flowers produced an increase in the ovarian weight, as well as in the weight and diameter of the corpora lutea, indicating an anti-estrogenic activity. Benzene extract of the flowers, administered orally to ovariectomized rats at doses of 50.0, 100.0, 150.0, 200.0, and 250.0 mg/kg, were active. Ethanol (95%) extract of the flowers, administered orally to ovariectomized rats, was inactive at a dose of 100.0 mg/kg and active at doses of 150.0, 200.0, and 250.0 mg/kg[HR054]. Ethanol/water (1:1) extract was active at a dose of 75.0 mg/kg;

reduction of glycogen content in uterus of treated animals is claimed indicative of antiestrogenic activity[HR053].

Antifertility effect. Ethanol (95%) extract of dried flowers, taken orally by human females at a dose of 750.0 mg/person, was active. The dose was divided and taken 3 times daily from the 7th to the 22nd day of the menstrual cycle. Twenty-one women, 15 to 35 years of age, were in the test group. Seven of the women discontinued the treatment. Three of the 7 women discontinued treatment due to non-associated illness. No pregnancies have developed in the 14 women after up to 20 months[HR065]. In another trial, women between the ages of 18 and 45 were given Vidangadi yoga, and herbal medicine consisting of *Embelia ribes* seeds, *Hibiscus rosa-sinensis* flowers and *Ferula foetida* oleoresin mixed in equal amounts. Eight hundred-milligram tablets were given 3 times per day with water or milk during menstruation for 6 days. Of the 1083 patients enrolled in the study, 83.1% did not become pregnant. Five hundred continued treatment for 36 cycles or more. No toxic effect was observed[HR083].

Antifungal activity. Ethanol/water (50%) extract of dried leaves was active on *Rhizoctonia solani*. Mycelial inhibition was 34.50%[HR088].

Antigonadotropin effect. Benzene extract of dried flowers, administered by gastric intubation to male and female rats at a dose of 250.0 mg/kg, was active[HR067].

Anti-implantation effect. Benzene extract of dried flowers, administered by gastric intubation to mice at a dose of 1.0 gm/kg, was active. Dosing was done on days 1–4 of gestation, in the morning[HR079]. The extract was inactive at a dose of 250.0 mg/kg, with dosing on days 1–3[HR067], and at 750.0 mg/kg administered orally to mice[HR085]. Benzene extract of leaves and stem bark, administered by gastric intubation to rats at a dose of 250.0 mg/kg, produced 12.5% activity[HR042]. Benzene

extract of petals, administered orally to rats at a dose of 100.0 mg/kg, was active[HR007]. Ethanol/water (1:1) extract of the aerial parts, administered orally to mice at a dose of 100.0 mg/kg, was inactive[HR019]. Hibiscus has been investigated extensively for its antifertility effect. Different parts of the plant have been screened for their effect on the reproductive system. The benzene extract of *H. rosa-sinensis* flowers (100 mg/kg) revealed post-coital antifertility effect in female albino rats, leading to 80% reduction in the implantation site on the 10th day of pregnancy. The fetal loss in the rats was within the normal range, indicating the absence of any abortifacient effect in the benzene extract. The petroleum ether extract was devoid of antifertility effect, whereas with the ether and ethanolic extracts of the flower petals, a change in the sex ratio of the pups born was observed, the incidence of male:female pups born being higher in the extract-treated rats. Benzene extract of the flower, administered orally to rats at doses of 50.0 and 250.0 mg/kg, was active[HR027,HR028,HR046]. Ethanol (95%) extract of flowers, administered orally to rats at a dose of 250.0 mg/kg, produced weak activity. Water and petroleum ether extracts of flowers, administered orally to rats at doses of 250.0 mg/kg, were inactive[HR028].

Anti-inflammatory activity. Ethanol (70%) extract of dried leaves, administered intraperitoneally to rats at a dose of 100.0 mg/kg, was active vs carrageenin-induced pedal edema[HR058].

Antiovulatory effect. Benzene extract of the flower, administered intraperitoneally to adult mice at doses of 125 and 250 mg/kg body weight, produced an increase in atretic follicles and the absence of corpora lutea. This effect may be due to an imbalance in the hormonal environment, as there may be an increase in the endogenous secretion of estrogen by the atretic follicles and to the estrogenicity of the extract[HR099].

Antipyretic activity. Ethanol (70%) extract of dried leaves, administered intraperitoneally to rats at a dose of 100.0 mg/kg, was active vs brewer's yeast-induced pyrexia[HR058]. Ethanol/water (1:1) extract of the aerial parts, administered intraperitoneally to mice at a dose of 500.0 mg/kg, was active[HR019].

Antispasmodic activity. Ethanol/water (1:1) extract of the aerial parts was active on guinea pig ileum vs ACh and histamine-induced spasms[HR019].

Antispermatogenic effect. Benzene extract of dried flowers, administered by gastric intubation to rats at a dose of 250.0 mg/kg, was active. The animals were dosed daily for 30 days. Spermatogenesis was arrested at the early spermatid stage. The tubules showed disquamation of genital elements in the lumen. The tubules consisted of spermatogonia, sertoli cells, and spermatocytes, and degenerated spermatids. The Leydig cells were atrophic. After 45 days of treatment, a general derangement in the tubules was observed. The spermatocytes were darkly stained, and between them empty spaces were seen, suggesting disappearance of tubular elements. After 60 days of treatment, marked degenerative changes were noticed in the seminiferous tubules. Hypoplasia of all germinal elements, excluding spermatogonia, was observed. Reduction in weight of testes, epididymis, seminal vesicles, prostate and pituitary was noted after treatment[HR067]. Ethanol (95%) extract of the dried flowers, administered by gastric intubation to rats at doses of 50.0 mg/animal and 150.0 mg/animal with daily dosing for 30 days, was inactive. With daily dosing for 15 days of 250.0 mg/animal, cells in seminiferous tubules showed degranulation and vacuolization, absence of sperm and decrease in tubular diameter; interstitial cells were not affected. Daily dosing for 30 days caused a complete disorganization of the testicular architecture, shrinkage of the seminiferous tubules and complete destruction of spermatogonial cells. Germinal epithelium was affected and the Leydig cells were absent. Cells of sertoli were the least affected[HR093]. Ethanol (95%) extract of the flower, administered orally to rams and rats at doses of 250.0 mg/animal and 150.0 mg/animal, respectively, was active[HR009]. Benzene, chloroform, and alcoholic extracts of the flower, administered intraperitoneally to male albino mice at doses of 125 and 250 mg/kg body weight, produced a decrease in the spermatogenic elements of testis and epididymal sperm count. High content of testicular cholesterol may be due to lowered androgen synthesis. The increase in the weight of the accessory reproductive organs indicates the androgenicity of the plant extract[HR100].

Antiviral activity. Ethanol (80%) extract of freeze-dried plant, in cell culture at variable concentrations, was equivocal on coxsackie B2 virus, measles virus and poliovirus I, and inactive on adenovirus, Herpes virus type 1 and Semlicki-forest virus vs plaque inhibition[HR072].

Barbiturate potentiation. Ethanol/water (1:1) extract of the aerial parts, administered intraperitoneally to mice at a dose of 500.0 mg/kg, was active[HR019].

Beta-glucuronidase inhibition. Benzene and ethanol/water (1:1) extracts of dried flowers, administered by gastric intubation to normal and ovariectomized female rats at doses of 200.0 mg/kg, with dosing on days 1–5, were active[HR084].

Beta-glucuronidase stimulation. Benzene and ethanol/water (1:1) extract of dried flowers, administered by gastric intubation to ovariectomized rats at doses of 200.0 mg/kg with dosing on days 1–5, produced weak activity[HR084].

CNS depressant activity. Ethanol/water (1:1) extract of the aerial parts, administered intraperitoneally to mice at a dose of 500.0 mg/kg, was active[HR019].

Embryotoxic effect. Benzene extract of dried flowers, administered by gastric intubation to pregnant rats at doses of 100.0, 150.0 and 186.0 mg/kg with dosing on days 1–10, was active. The ether-soluble and water insoluble fractions of the total benzene extracts were also active[HR069]. Water extract, at doses of 200.0 and 270.0 mg/kg[HR075] and ethanol (95%) extract at 200.0 mg/kg[HR035], administered by gastric intubation to pregnant rats, were inactive. Petroleum ether extract of dried flowers, administered by gastric intubation to pregnant rats at a dose of 150.0 mg/kg, was inactive[HR075]. Benzene extract of flowers, administered by gastric intubation to rats at a dose of 250.0 mg/kg, was active; ethanol (95%), water and petroleum ether extracts at doses of 200.0, 200.0 and 150.0 mg/kg, administered orally to rats, respectively, were inactive[HR090]. Ethanol (95%), water and petroleum ether extracts of leaves and roots, administered orally, and dried roots and dried leaves by gastric intubation to rats at doses of 200.0, 200.0 and 150.0 mg/kg respectively, were inactive. Ethanol (90%), water and petroleum ether extracts of stem, administered orally and dried stem by gastric intubation to rats, were inactive[HR090].

Estrogenic effect. Benzene extract of dried flowers, administered subcutaneously to infant mice[HR057] and by gastric intubation to female rats[HR067] at doses of 250.0 mg/kg, was inactive.

Estrous cycle disruption effect. Benzene extract of the flower, administered orally to rats at a dose of 50.0 mg/kg, was active[HR031]. Benzene extract of the flower, administered intraperitoneally to adult mice at doses of 125 and 250 mg/kg body weight, produced an irregular estrous cycle with prolonged estrus and metestrus. The treatment also indicated estrogenic effect immature mice by early opening of the vagina, premature cornification of the

vaginal epithelium and an increase in uterine weight[HR099].

Gonadotropin synthesis inhibition. Benzene extract of the flower, administered orally to rats at a dose of 250.0 mg/kg, was active[HR041].

Hypoglycemic effect. The water extract, administered orally to rats at a dose of 250 mg/kg daily for 7 days, significantly improved glucose tolerance in rats. The peak blood glucose level was obtained at 30 min of glucose load (2 gm/kg), thereafter a decreasing trend was recorded up to 2 hours. In streptozotocin diabetic rats, no significant effect was observed with the extract, while glibenclamide significantly lowered the glucose level up to 7 hours[HR097]. The alcoholic extract of the leaf, administered orally to rats at a dose of 250 mg/k daily for 7 days, showed significant improvements in the ability to utilize the external glucose load. Average blood glucose lowering was 39%[HR098].

Hypotensive activity. Ethanol/ water (1:1) extract of the aerial parts, administered intravenously to dogs at a dose of 50.0 mg/kg, was active[HR019].

Hypothermic activity. Ethanol/water (1:1) extract of the aerial parts, administered intraperitoneally to mice at a dose of 500.0 mg/kg, was active[HR019].

Inotropic effect positive. Hot water extract of dried leaves, at a concentration of 320.0 microliters, was inactive on guinea pig atrium[HR051].

Juvenile hormone activity. Acetone extract of dried stem produced weak activity on *Dysdercus cingulatus*[HR055].

Lactate-dehydrogenase-X inhibition. Benzene extract of dried flowers, administered subcutaneously to male *Rhinopoma kinneari* at a dose of 7.5 mg/animal, was equivocal[HR066], and the hot water extract was active[HR064]. Enzyme levels were measured in testes daily, after a single injection of the extract.

Luteotropic effect. Benzene extract of dried flowers, administered by gastric intubation to guinea pigs at doses of 150.0 and 300.0 mg/kg, was active, results significant at $P < 0.005$ level. At a dose of 75.0 mg/kg, the extract was inactive. The ethanol/water (1:1) extract, at doses of 150.0 and 300.0 mg/kg, was inactive[HR071].

Menstruation induction effect. Water extract of leaves was active on the non-pregnant uterus of rabbits, and inactive on the non-pregnant uterus of rats[HR011].

Ovulation inhibition effect. Ethanol/water (1:1) extract of the aerial parts, administered orally to rabbits at a dose of 50.0 mg/kg, was inactive vs copper acetate-induced ovulation[HR091].

Plant germination inhibition. Methanol extract of fresh stem bark was active on lettuce seeds[HR023].

Radical scavenging effect. Ethanol/water (1:1) extract of dried entire plant, at a concentration of 5.0 mcg/ml, was inactive vs superoxide anion, estimated by the neo-tetrazolium method[HR038].

Teratogenic activity. Ethanol (95%) extract of dried flowers, administered by gastric intubation to pregnant rats at a dose of 270.0 mg/kg, was inactive[HR035]. Benzene extract of petals, administered orally to rats at a dose of 100.0 mg, was inactive[HR007].

Toxicity assessment (quantitative). Ethanol (70%) extract of dried leaves, administered intraperitoneally to mice, produced LD_{50} 1.533 gm/kg[HR058]. Ethanol/water (1:1) extract of the aerial parts, administered intraperitoneally to both sexes of mice, produced LD_{50} 1.0 gm/kg[HR019].

REFERENCES

HR001 Suwal, P. N. Medicinal Plants of Nepal. Ministry of Forests, Department of Medicinal Plants, Thapathali, Kathmandu, Nepal, 1970.

HR002 Jain, S. K. and C. R. Tarafder. Medicinal plant-lore of the Santals. **Econ Bot** 1970; 24: 178–241.

HR003 Quisumbing, E. Medicinal plants of the Philippines. **Tech Bull 16**, Rep Philippines, Dept Agr Nat Resources, Manila 1951; 1.

HR004 Malhi, B. S. and V. P. Trivedi. Vegetable antifertility drugs of India. **Q J Crude Drug Res** 1972; 12: 19–22.

HR005 Paijmans, K. P. New Guinea Vegetation. Elsevier Scientific Publ. Co., New York, 1976.

HR006 Haddock, R. L. Some medicinal plants of Guam including English and Guamanian common names. **Report Regional Tech Mtg Med Plants**, Papeete, Tahiti, Nov, 1973, South Pacific Commissioner, Noumea, New Caledonia 1974; 79.

HR007 Batta, S. K. and G. Santhakumari. The antifertility effect of *Ocimum santum* and *Hibiscus rosa-sinensis*. **Indian J Med Res** 1970; 59: 777.

HR008 Pardo De Tavera, T. H. Medicinal Plants of the Philippines. Blakiston, Philadelphia, 1901.

HR009 Kholkute, S. D., S. Chatterjee, D. N. Srivastava and K. N. Udupa. Effect of *Hibiscus rosa-sinensis* on the reproductive organs of male rats. **J Reprod Fertil** 1974; 38: 233–234.

HR010 Agarwal, S. K. and P. R. Rastogi. Triterpenoids of *Hibiscus rosa-sinensis*. **Indian J Pharmacy** 1971; 33: 41.

HR011 Agarwal, S. L. and S. Shinde. Studies on *Hibiscus rosa-sinensis*. II. Preliminary Pharmacological Investigations. **Indian J Med Res** 1967; 55: 1007–1010.

HR012 Subramanian, S. S. and A. G. R. Nair. Flavonoids of four malvaceous plants. **Phytochemistry** 1972; 11: 15,188.

HR013 Hayashi, K. Anthocyanins. XIII. Several anthocyanins containing cyanidin as the aglycone. **Acta Phytochim** 1944; 14: 55.

HR014 Steenis-Kruseman, M. J. Van. Select Indonesian medicinal plants. **Organiz Sci Res Indonesia Bull** 1953; 18: 1.

HR015 Rageau, J. Les Plantes Medicinales de la Nouvelle-Caledonie. Trav & Doc De Lorstom No. 23. Paris, 1973.

HR016 Hooper, D. On Chinese medicine. Drugs of Chinese pharmacies in Malaya. **Gard Bull STR Settlm** 1929; 6: 1.

HR017 ANON, Description of the Philippines. Part I., Bureau of Public Printing, Manila, 1903.

HR018 Petelot, A. Les Plantes Medicinales du Cambodge, du Laos et du Vietnam, Vol. 1–4. Archives Des Recherches Agronomiques Et Pastorales Au Vietnam No. 23, 1954.

HR019 Bhakuni, O. S., M. L. Dhar, M. M. Dhar, B. N. Dhawan and B. N. Mehrotra. Screening of Indian plants for biological activity. Part II. **Indian J Exp Biol** 1969; 7: 250–262.

HR020 Watt, J. M. and M. G. Breyer-Brandwijk. The Medicinal and Poisonous Plants of Southern and Eastern Africa. 2nd Ed, E. S. Livingstone, Ltd., London, 1962.

HR021 Griffiths, L. A. On the distribution of gentisic acid in green plants. **J Exp Biol** 1959; 10: 437.

HR022 Burkhill, I. H. Dictionary of the Economic Products of the Malay Peninsula. Ministry of Agriculture and Cooperatives, Kuala Lumpur, Malaysia. Vol. 1, 1966.

HR023 Nakatani, M., Y. Fukunaga and T. Hase. Aliphatic compounds from *Hibiscus rosa-sinensis*. **Phytochemistry** 1986; 25(2): 449–452.

HR024 Shimizu, N., M. Tomoda, I. Suzuki and K. Takada. Plant mucilages. XLIII. A representative mucilage with biological activity from the leaves of *Hibiscus rosa-sinensis*. **Biol Pharm Bull** 1993; 16(8): 735–739.

HR025 Nakatani, M., K. Matsouka, Y. Uchio and T. Hase. Two aliphatic enone ethers from *Hibiscus rosa-sinensis*. **Phytochemistry** 1994; 35(5): 1245–1247.

HR026 Luu, C. Notes on the traditional pharmacopoeia of French Guyana. **Plant Med Phytother** 1975; 9: 125–135.

HR027 Kholkute, S. D. and K. N. Udupa. Effects of *Hibiscus rosa-sinensis* on pregnancy of rats. **Planta Med** 1976; 29: 321–329.

HR028 Kholkute, S. D., V. Mudgal and P. J. Deshpande. Screening of indigenous medicinal plants for antifertility potentiality. **Planta Med** 1976; 29: 151–155.

HR029 Wong, W. Some folk medicinal plants from Trinidad. **Econ Bot** 1976; 30: 103–142.

HR030 Srivastava, D. N., S. K. Bhatt and K. N. Udupa. Gas chromatographic iden-tification of fatty acids, fatty alcohols, and hydrocarbons of *Hibiscus rosa-sinensis* leaves. **J Amer Oil Chem Soc** 1976; 53: 607.

HR031 Kholkute, S. D., S. Chatterjee and K. N. Udupa. Effect of *Hibiscus rosa-sinensis* on estrous cycle and reproductive organs in rats. **Indian J Exp Biol** 1976; 14: 703–704.

HR032 Holdsworth, D. K. Traditional medicinal plants of Rarotonga, Cook Islands. Part II. **Int J Pharmacog** 1991; 29(1): 71–79.

HR033 Alam, M. K. Medicinal ethnobotany of the Marma Tribe of Bangladesh. **Econ Bot** 1992; 46(3): 330–335.

HR034 Reddy, M. B., K. R. Reddy and M. N. Reddy. A survey of plant crude drugs of Anantapur District, Andhra Pradesh, India. **Int J Crude Drug Res** 1989; 27(3): 145–155.

HR035 Nath, D., N. Sethi, R. K. Singh and A. K. Jain. Commonly used Indian aborti-facient plants with special reference to their teratologic effects in rats. **J Ethnopharmacol** 1992; 36(2): 147–154.

HR036 Zamora-Martinez, M. C. and C. N. P. Pola. Medicinal plants used in some rural populations of Oaxaca, Puebla and Veracruz, Mexico. **J Ethnopharmacol** 1992; 35(3) 229–257.

HR037 Bourdy, G. and A. Walter. Maternity and medicinal plants in Vanuatu. I. The cycle of reproduction. **J Ethnopharmacol** 1992; 37(3): 179–196.

HR038 Masaki, H., S. Sakaki, T. Atsumi and H. Sakurai. Active-oxygen scavenging activity of plant extracts. **Biol Pharm Bull** 1995; 18(1): 162–166.

HR039 Bhattarai, N. K. Folk herbal remedies for gynecological complaints in central Nepal. **Int J Pharmacog** 1994; 32(1): 13–26.

HR040 Bhandary, M. J., K. R. Chandrashekar and K. M. Kaveriappa. Medical ethnobotany of the Siddis of Uttar Kannada District, Karnataka, India. **J Ethnopharmacol** 1995; 47(3): 149–158.

HR041 Kholkute, S. D. Effect of *Hibiscus rosa-sinensis* on spermatogenesis and accessory reproductive organs in rats. **Planta Med** 1977; 127–135.

HR042 Kholkute, S. D., V. Mudgal and K. N. Udupa. Studies on the antifertility potentiality of *Hibiscus rosa-sinensis*. Parts of medicinal value: Selection of species and seasonal variation. **Planta Med** 1977; 31–35.

HR043   Alami, R., A. Macksad and A. R. El-Gindy. Medicinal Plants in Kuwait. Al-Assiriya Printing Press, Kuwait, 1976.

HR044   Dixit, V. P. Effects of chronically administered Malvaviscus flower extract on the female genital tract. **Indian J Exp Biol** 1977; 15: 650–652.

HR045   Holdsworth, D. K. Medicinal plants of Papua-New Guinea, Technical Paper No. 175, South Pacific Commission, Noumea, New Caledonia, 1977.

HR046   Kholkute, S. D., D. N. Srivastava, S, Chatterjee and K. N. Udupa. Effects of some compounds isolated from *Hibiscus rosa-sinensis* on pregnancy in rats. **J Res Indian Med Yoga Homeopathy** 1976; 11: 106–108.

HR047   Chouhan, U. K. and R. N. Skukla. Sterols of some Malvaceae with particular emphasis on cholesterol occurrence. **J Sci Res (Bhopal)** 1984; 6(1): 49–50.

HR048   Chauhan, U. K. Sterols of some malvaceous plants with particular emphasis on cholesterol occurrence. **Proc Nat Acad Sci India Ser B** 1984; 54(3): 236–239.

HR049   Alam, M. M., M. B. Siddiqui and W. Husain. Treatment of diabetes through herbal drugs in rural India. **Fitoterapia** 1990; 61(3): 240–242.

HR050   Nakatani, M. and T. Hase. Sterochemistry of methyl 2-hydroxysterculate from *Hibiscus rosa-sinensis*. **Chem Lett** 1991; 1991(1): 47–48.

HR051   Carbajal, D., A. Casaco, L. Arruzazabala, R. Gonzalez and V. Fuentes. Pharmacological screening of plant decoctions commonly used in Cuban folk medicine. **J Ethnopharmacol** 1991; 33(1/2): 21–24.

HR052   Ayensu, E. S. Medicinal plants of the West Indies. **Unpublished Manuscript** 1978; 110 pp.

HR053   Prakash, A. O. Glycogen contents in the rat uterus. Response to *Hibiscus rosa-sinensis* extracts. **Experientia** 1979; 35: 1122,1123.

HR054   Kholkute, S. D. and K. N. Udupa. Antiestrogenic activity of *Hibiscus*

rosa-sinensis flowers. **Indian J Exp Biol** 1976; 14: 175-176.

HR055   Gopakumar, B., B. Ambika and V. K. K. Prabhu. Juvenomimetic activity in some South Indian plants and the probable cause of this activity in *Morus alba*. **Entomon** 1977; 2: 259–261.

HR056   Prakash, A. O. Acid and alkaline phosphatase activity in the uterus of rat treated with *Hibiscus rosa-sinensis* Linn. extracts. **Curr Sci** 1979; 48: 501–503.

HR057   Kholkute, S. D. and K. N. Udupa. Biological profile of total benzene extract of *Hibiscus rosa-sinensis* flowers. **J Res Indian Med Yoga Homeopathy** 1978; 13(3): 107–109.

HR058   Singh, N., R. Nath, A. K. Agarwal and R. P. Kohli. A pharmacological investigation of some indigenous drugs of plant origin for evaluation of their antipyretic, analgesic and anti-inflammatory activities. **J Res Indian Med Yoga Homeopathy** 1978; 13: 58–62.

HR059   Krishnamurthy, V. No easy way to new pill. **Indian Express**, September 17, 1980.

HR060   Prakash, A. O. Protein concentration in rat uterus under the influence of *Hibiscus rosa-sinensis* Linn. extracts. **Proc Indian Acad Sci Ser** 1979; B 45: 327–331.

HR061   Holdsworth, D. K., C. L. Hurley and S. E. Rayner. Traditional medicinal plants of New Ireland, Papua, New Guinea. **Q J Crude Drug Res** 1980; 18(3): 131–139.

HR062   Adu-Tutu, M., Y. Afful, K. Asante-Appiah, D. Lieberman, J. B. Hall and M. Elvin-Lewis. Chewing stick usage in Southern Ghana. **Econ Bot** 1979; 33: 320–328.

HR063   Maheswari, J. K., K. K. Singh and S. Saha. Ethno-medicinal uses of plants by the Tharus of Kheri District, U. P. **Bull Med Ethnobot Res** 1980; 1: 318–337.

HR064   Singwi, M. S. and S. B. Lall. Effect of *Hibiscus rosa-sinensis* on testicular lactate dehydrogenases of *Rhinopoma kinneari* Wroughton. (Microchiroptera. Mammalia). **Curr Sci** 1981; 50: 360–362.

HR065   Tiwari, P. V. Preliminary clinical trial on flowers of *Hibiscus rosa-sinensis* as an oral contraceptive agent. **J Res Indian**

Med Yoga Homeopathy 1974; 9(4): 96–98.

HR066 Singwi, M. S. and S. B. Lall. Effect of flower extract of *Hibiscus rosa-sinensis* on testicular lactate dehydrogenases of a non-scrotal bat *Rhinopoma kinneari* Wroughton. **Indian J Exp Biol** 1981; 19: 359–362.

HR067 Kholkute, S. D. and K. N. Udupa. Antifertility properties of *Hibiscus rosa-sinensis*. **J Res Indian Med Yoga Homeopathy** 1974; 9(4): 99–102.

HR068 Meditsch, J. D. O. and E. C. Barros. Hibiscus dyes as acid-base indicators. **An Assoc Bras Quim** 1978; 29(1): 89.

HR069 Singh, M. P., R. H. Singh and K. N. Udupa. Antifertility activity of a benzene extract of *Hibiscus rosa-sinensis* flowers in female albino rats. **Planta Med** 1982; 44: 171–174.

HR070 Nguyen, Van Dan. List of simple drugs and medicinal plants of value in Vietnam. **Proc Seminar of the Use of Medicinal Plants in Healthcare**, Tokyo 13–17 September 1977, WHO Regional Office Manila. 65–83.

HR071 Prakash, A. O. Effect of *Hibiscus rosa-sinensis* Linn. extracts on corpora lutea of cyclic guinea pigs. **Sci Cult** 1980; 46: 330,331.

HR072 Van Den Berghe, D. A., M. Ieven, F. Mertens, A. J. Vlietinck and E. Lammens. Screening of higher plants for biological activities. II. Antiviral activity. **J Nat Prod** 1978; 41: 463–467.

HR073 Tiwari, K. C., R. Majumder and S. Bhattacharjee. Folklore information from Assam for family planning and birth control. **Int J Crude Drug Res** 1982; 20: 133–137.

HR074 Vitalyos, D. Phytotherapy in domestic traditional medicine in Matouba-Papaye (Guadeloupe). **Dissertation-Ph.D.-Univ Paris** 1979; 110 pp.

HR075 Prakash, A. O. and R. Mathur. Effect of oral administration of *Hibiscus rosa-sinensis* Linn. extract on early and late pregnancy in albino rats. **J Jiwaji Univ** 1976; 4: 79–82.

HR076 Nakatani, M., T. Yamachika, T. Tanoue and T. Hase. Structures and synthesis of seed-germination inhibitors from *Hibiscus rosa-sinensis*. **Phytochemistry** 1985; 24(1): 39–42.

HR077 Hemadri, K. and S. Sasibhushana Rao. Antifertility, abortifacient and fertility promoting drugs from Dandakaranya. **Ancient Sci Life** 1983; 3(2): 103–107.

HR078 Whistler, W. A. Traditional and herbal medicine in Cook Islands. **J Ethnopharmacol** 1985; 13(3): 239–280.

HR079 Pal, A. K., K. Bhattacharya, S. N. Kabir and A. Pakrashi. Flowers of *Hibiscus rosa-sinensis*, a potential source of contragestative agent. II. Possible mode of action with reference to anti-implantation effect of the benzene extract. **Contraception** 1985; 32(5): 517–529.

HR080 Aswal, B. S., D. S. Bhakuni, A. K. Goel, K. Kar, B. N. Mehrotra and K. C. Mukherjee. Screening of Indian plants for biological activity. Part X. **Indian J Exp Biol** 1984; 22(6): 312–332.

HR081 Bhattacharya, K., S. N. Kabir, A. K. Pal and A. Pakrashi. Effect of benzene extract of *Hibiscus rosa-sinensis* flowers on facultative delayed implantation and uterine uptake of estrogen in mice. **IRCS Med Sci** 1984; 12(9): 841–842.

HR082 Singh, Y. N. Traditional medicine in Fiji. Some herbal folk cures used by Fiji Indians. **J Ethnopharmacol** 1986; 15(1): 57–88.

HR083 Trivedi, V. P. and K. Shukla. A study of effects of an indigenous compound drug on reproductive physiology. **J Sci Res Pl Med** 1980; 1(3/4): 41–47.

HR084 Prakash, A. O., S. Shukla, R. Mathur. *Hibiscus rosa-sinensis* Linn.: Its effect on beta-glucuronidase in the uterus of ovariectomized rats. **Curr Sci** 1985; 54(15): 734–736.

HR085 Kabir, S. N., K. Bhattacharya, A. K. Pal and A. Pakrashi. Flowers of *Hibiscus rosa-sinensis*, a potential source of contragestive agent: I. Effect of benzene extract on implantation of mouse. **Contraception** 1984; 29(4): 385–397.

HR086 Weniger, B., M. Rouzier, R. Daguilh, D. Henrys, J. H. Henrys and R. Anthon. Popular medicine of the Central Plateau of Haiti. 2. Ethnopharmacological inventory. **J Ethnopharmacol** 1986; 17(1): 13–30.

HR087 Ramirez, V. R., L. J. Mostacero, A. E. Garcia, C. F. Mejia, P. F. Pelaez, C. D. Medina and C. H. Miranda.

Vegetales empleados en medicina tradicional Norperuana. **Banco Agrario Del Peru & NACL Univ Trujillo**, Trujillo, Peru, June 1988; 54pp.

HR088 Renu. Fungitoxicity of leaf extracts of some higher plants against *Rhizoctonia* · *solani* Kuehn. **Nat Acad Sci Lett** 1983; 6(8): 245–246.

HR089 Kobayashi, J. Early Hawaiian uses of medicinal plants in pregnancy and childbirth. **J Trop Pediatr Environ Child Health** 1976; 22: 260.

HR090 Prakash, A. O. and R. Mathur. Screening of Indian plants for antifertility activity. **Indian J Exp Biol** 1976; 14: 623–626.

HR091 Gupta, M. L., T. K. Gupta and K. P. Bhargava. A study of antifertility effects of some indigenous drugs. **J Res Indian Med** 1971; 6: 112–116.

HR092 Dragendorff, G. Die Heilpflanzen Der Verschiedenen Volker Und Zeiten, F. Enke, Stuttgart, 1898; 885 pp.

HR093 Kholkute, S. D., S. Chatterjee, D. N. Srivas Ava and K. N. Udupa. Antifertility effect of the alcoholic extract of Japa (*Hibiscus rosa-sinensis*). **J Res Indian Med** 1972; 7: 72–73.

HR094 Shrivastava, D. N. Phytochemical analysis of japaksum. **J Res Indian Med Yoga Homeopathy** 1974; 9(4): 103–104.

HR095 Pattanaik, S. A comparative study of the catalase activity of the petals and leaves of *Hibiscus rosa-sinensis*. **Curr Sci** 1949; 18: 212–213.

HR096 Lin, Y. C. The study of red pigments on Taiwan plants. **Proc Natl Sci Counc Part I (Taiwan)** 1975(8): 133–137.

HR097 Sachdewa, A., R. Nigam and L. D. Khemani. Hypoglycemic effect of *Hibiscus rosa-sinensis* L. leaf extract in glucose and streptozotocin induced hyperglycemic rats. **Indian J Exp Biol** 2001; 39(3): 284–286.

HR098 Sachdewa, A., D. Raina, A. K. Srivastava and L. D. Khemani. Effect of *Aegle marmelos* and *Hibiscus rosa-sinensis* leaf extract on glucose tolerance in glucose induced hyperglycemic rats (Charles foster). **J Environ Biol** 2001; 22(1): 53–57.

HR099 Murthy, D. R., C. M. Reddy and S. B. Patil. Effect of benzene extract of *Hibiscus rosa-sinensis* on the estrous cycle and ovarian activity in albino mice. **Biol Pharm Bull** 1997; 20(7): 756–758.

HR100 Reddy, C. M., D. R. Murthy and S. B. Patil. Antispermatogenic and androgenic activities of various extracts of *Hibiscus rosa-sinensis* in albine rats. **Indian J Exp Biol** 1997; 35(11): 1170–1174.

HR101 Kasture, V. S., C. T. Chopde and V. K. Deshmukh. Anticonvulsive activity of *Albizzia lebbeck*, *Hibiscus rosa-sinensis* and *Butea monosperma* in experimental animals. **J Ethnopharmacol** 71(1–2): 65–75.

13 | Hibiscus sabdariffa

Gaertn.

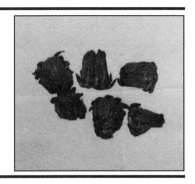

Common Names

Abuya	Congo-Brazzaville	Mesta	Bangladesh
Baquitche	Guinea-Bissau	Nsa	Congo-Brazzaville
Basap	Senegal	Otesse	Guinea-Bissau
Bisap	Senegal	Patwa	India
Bondio	Senegal	Red roselle	India
Cutcha	Guinea-Bissau	Red sorrel	Egypt
Dakouma	Senegal	Red sorrel	Germany
Fasab	Senegal	Red sorrel	India
Folere	Guinea-Bissau	Red sorrel	Senegal
Gogu	India	Rosa de Jamaica	Guatemala
Hamaiga	Nicaragua	Rosella	Egypt
Ibuya	Congo-Brazzaville	Roselle	Egypt
Indian sorrel	Senegal	Roselle	India
Inkulu	Congo-Brazzaville	Roselle	Iraq
Jericho rose	Germany	Roselle	Japan
Karkade	Egypt	Roselle	Mexico
Karkade	Germany	Roselle	Senegal
Karkade	Italy	Roselle hemp	Senegal
Karkade	Somaliland	Roxella-red sorrel	Thailand
Karkadeh	Sudan	Satui	Sierra Leone
Karkadesh	Egypt	Sawa sawa	Sierra Leone
Krachiap daeng	Thailand	Senegal bisap	Senegal
Kuges	Senegal	Sudan tea	East Africa
Lal ambari	India	Susur	Indonesia

BOTANICAL DESCRIPTION

The plant is an erect annual herb of the MALVACEAE family with a reddish cylindrical stem, nearly glabrous. Leaves are simple, having petiole, blade 3–5 lobed or parted, the lobes serrated or obtusely toothed. Flowers are solitary, axial, nearly sessile, 5 to 7 cm in diameter; consisting of epicalyx–segments 8–12, distinct, lanceolate to linear, adnate at base of the calyx; calyx is thick, red, and fleshy, cup-like, deeply parted, prominently 10-nerved; petals 5, yellow, twice as long as calyx. Stamens are numerous; the filaments united into a

From: *Medicinal Plants of the World, vol. 1: Chemical Constituents, Traditional and Modern Medicinal Uses, 2nd ed.*
By: Ivan A. Ross © Humana Press Inc., Totowa, NJ

staminal column; style single, 5-branched near summit, stigma capitate. The fruit is capsule, ovoid, pointed, 1 to 2 cm long, shorter than the calyx, having densely sharp and stiff hairs.

ORIGIN AND DISTRIBUTION

A native to the tropics, it is extensively cultivated for its succulent fleshy, edible calyx, and the stem yields a fairly strong fiber.

TRADITIONAL MEDICINAL USES

Africa. Hot water extract of seeds is taken as a diuretic and tonic. Seed oil is used externally to heal sores on camels[HS018].

Brazil. Hot water extract of root is taken orally as a stomachic and externally as an emollient[HS018].

Cameroon. Hot water extract of dried leaves is taken orally as an anthelmintic[HS049].

Congo. Hot water extract of leaves is taken orally to expedite delivery[HS009].

East Africa. Hot water extract of leaves is taken orally to relieve coughs[HS018]. Unripe fruit juice is taken orally with salt, pepper, asafetida and molasses as a remedy for biliousness. Hot water extract of leaves is used as a flavoring agent, diuretic, choleretic, febrifuge and hypotensive, to decrease viscosity of blood and to stimulate intestinal peristalsis. Externally, the extract is used for sores and wounds[HS018].

Egypt. Decoction of hot water extract of the calyx is taken with sugar 3 times daily for high blood pressure[HS036]. Hot water extract of the entire plant is taken orally for heart and nerve diseases, as a laxative, to reduce weight, as a diuretic, to activate and neutralize hepatic secretion, to activate gastric secretion, as a digestive, for arteriosclerosis, as a diaphoretic, to give a euphoric impression and as an intestinal antiseptic[HS008]. Leaf essential oil is taken orally to treat cancer[HS015].

Guatemala. Hot water extract of dried calyx is taken orally as a diuretic and for renal inflammation[HS050].

Guinea–Bissau. Seeds are taken orally by males as an aphrodisiac[HS018].

India. Hot water extract of leaves is taken orally as a diuretic, choleretic, febrifuge and hypotensive, to decrease blood viscosity and to stimulate intestinal peristalsis[HS018]. Water extract of seed is taken orally to relieve dysuria and strangury, for mild cases of dyspepsia and to relieve debility[HS018].

Mexico. Hot water extract of leaves is taken orally as a diuretic, choleretic and febrifuge, for hypotension, to decrease viscosity of the blood and to stimulate intestinal peristalsis[HS018].

Senegal. Hot water extract of leaves is used externally on wounds[HS013], and orally to lower blood pressure[HS018]. Hot water extract of flowers is taken orally to combat fatigue, for indigestion and as a diaphoretic, cholagogue and diuretic[HS013].

Sierra Leone. Decoction of dried leaves is taken orally to treat postpartum hemorrhage, to initiate contractions and as a diuretic during pregnancy (mixed with leaves of *Dialium guineensis*)[HS044].

Sudan. Hot water extract of flowers is taken orally as a blood purifier[HS010]. Hot water extract of the dried flowers is taken orally for coughs[HS041].

Thailand. Decoction of dried calyx is taken orally for high blood pressure[HS054].

CHEMICAL CONSTITUENTS
(ppm unless otherwise indicated)

3-Methyl-1-butanol: Lf, Fr[HS018]
Acetic acid: Fr, Sd[HS018]
Alpha terpenyl acetate: Fr, Lf, Sd[HS018]
Anisaldehyde: EO[HS024] Lf, Sd[HS018]
Ascorbic acid: Fl 0.01–0.11%[HS018]
Ascorbic acid: Fr 0.054–0.375%[HS018]
Behenic acid: Sd[HS018]
Benzyl alcohol: Fr, Lf[HS018]
Beta carotene: Fl[HS018]
Beta sitosterol: Sd (61.3% Sterols)[HS037]
Beta sitosterol-beta-D-galactoside: Lf[HS016]
Campesterol: Sd (16.5% Sterols)[HS037]
Caprylic acid: Fr, Lf[HS015]
Cholesterol: Sd (5.1% Sterols)[HS037]

Chrysanthemin: Fl[HS017]
Citric acid: Fl[HS005], Fr[HS007]
Cyanidin-3-sambubioside: Fl[HS017]
Cyanin: Fl[HS042]
Delphinidin: Cx[HS027]
Delphinidin-3-glucoside: Fl[HS042]
Delphinidin–3–sambubioside: Fl[HS017]
Ergosterol: Sd (3.2% Sterols)[HS037]
Ethanol: Lf, Sd[HS015]
Eugenol: EO[HS024]
Formic acid: Fr, Sd[HS015]
Furfural: EO[HS024]
Gossypetin: Fr[HS007], Fl[HS008]
Gossypol: Sd 25.2%[HS051]
Hexadecanoic acid: Sd[HS033]
Hibiscetin: Fl[HS012]
Hibiscic acid: Fl[HS012]
Hibiscin: Fl[HS019]
Hibiscitrin: Pe[HS004]
Lauric acid: Sd[HS021]
Levulinic acid methyl ester: EO[HS024]
Linoleic acid: Sd (14.6% Lipids)[HS038]
Linolenic acid: Sd[HS033]
Malic acid: Fl[HS005,HS003]
Malvalic acid: Sd (1.3% Lipids)[HS038]
Malvin: Fl[HS020]
Methanol: Lf, Fr, Sd[HS015]
Myristic acid: Sd (2.1% Lipids)[HS038]
Myrtillin: Fl[HS017]
Oleic acid: Sd (34.0% Lipids)[HS038]
Oxalic acid: Fl[HS002]
Palmitic acid: Sd (35.2% Lipids)[HS038]
Palmitoleic acid: Sd (2.0% Lipids)[HS038]
Pelargonic acid: Fr, Sd[HS015]
Propionic acid: Lf, Sd[HS015]
Protein: Sd[HS021]
Protocatechuic acid: Fl[HS011]
Quercetin: Fr[HS029]
Sabdaretin: Pe[HS004], Fl[HS012]
Starch: Sd 2.25%[HS021]
Stearic acid: Sd (3.4% Lipids)[HS038]
Sterculic acid: Sd (2.9% Lipids)[HS038]
Stigmasterol: Sd[HS037]
Sucrose: Cx[HS055]
Tannic acid: Fr[HS007]
Tartaric acid: Fl[HS005], Fr[HS007]

PHARMACOLOGICAL ACTIVITIES AND CLINICAL TRIALS

Acid phosphatase inhibition. Dried calyx, at a concentration of 10.0% of the diet of rats, produced weak activity vs cholesterol-loaded animals[HS022].

Acidifying activity. Decoction of dried fruit juice, administered orally to male human adults at a dose of 24.0 gm/day, was inactive[HS026].

Alkaline phosphatase inhibition. Dried calyx, at a concentration of 10.0% of the diet of rats, produced weak activity vs cholesterol-loaded animals[HS022].

Anthelmintic activity. Ethanol (95%) extract of dried leaves, at a concentration of 50.0 mg/ml, was inactive on *Lumbricus terrestris*[HS049].

Alpha amylase inhibition. Ethanol and acetone (50%) extracts of the tea were found to have high inhibitory activity against porcine pancreatic alpha-amylase[HS056].

Antibacterial activity. Seed oil, on agar plate, was active on *Bacillus anthracis* and *Staphylococcus albus*, and inactive on *Proteus vulgaris* and *Pseudomonas aeruginosa*[HS039].

Antiedema activity. Methanol extract of the flower, applied externally to mice at a dose of 2.0 mg/ear, was active. Inhibition ratio (IR) was 17 vs 12-0-tetradecanoyl-phorbol-13-acetate (TPA)-induced ear inflammation[HS023].

Antifungal activity. Ethanol/water (1:1) extract of dried leaves, at a concentration of 250.0 mg/ml on agar plate, was active on *Aspergillus fumigatus*, *Aspergillus niger*, *Botrytis cinerea*, *Penicillium digitatum*, *Rhizopus nigricans* and *Trichophyton mentagrophytes*, and inactive on *Aspergillus niger*. Dose expressed as dry weight of plant[HS053]. The flower, at a dose of 10.0 gm/liter in broth culture, was inactive on *Aspergillus flavus*. Aflatoxin formation was decreased [HS043]. Water extract of dried flowers, at a concentration of 500 mg/ml on agar plate, was active on *Aspergillus fumigatus*, *Botrytis cinerea*, *Fusarium oxysporum*, *Penicillium digitatum*, *Rhizopus nigricans* and *Trichophyton mentagrophytes* and inactive on *Aspergillus niger*. Dose expressed as dry weight of plant[HS047]. The 50% ethanol and acetone extracts of the tea produced high inhibitory activity against porcine pancreatic alpha-amylase. The activity was compared to that of structurally related citric acid, a known inhibitor of fungal alpha-amylase[HS056].

Antihypercholesterolemic activity. Dried calyx, at a concentration of 5.0% of the diet in the ration of rats, was active vs cholesterol-loaded animals[HS022].

Antihyperlipemic activity. Dried calyx, at a concentration of 5.0% of the diet in the ration of rats, was active vs cholesterol-loaded animals[HS022].

Antihypertensive effect. Infusion of the calyx, administered orally to spontaneously hypertensive and normotensive rats at doses of 500 and 1000 mg/kg body weight, significantly lowered both systolic and diastolic pressures. The reduction in blood pressure in both groups was positively correlated with weight. Continuous consumption of the infusion at 1000 mg/kg was discovered to lead to sudden death in spontaneously hypertensive rats[HS060]. *Hibiscus sabdariffa* tea administered orally to patients with moderate essential hypertension produced an 11.2% lowering of the systolic blood pressure and a 10.7% decrease of diastolic pressure 12 days after beginning the treatment as compared with the first day. Three days after stopping the treatment, systolic blood pressure was elevated by 7.9%, and diastolic pressure was elevated by 5.6% in the experimental and control groups[HS061].

Antihypertriglyceridemia effect. Dried calyx, at a concentration of 5.0% of the diet of rats, was active vs cholesterol-loaded animals[HS022].

Anti-inflammatory activity. Decoction of dried fruit, administered orally to human adults at a dose of 3.0 gm/person, was active. In this clinical trial, 50 patients with kidney stones were treated with extract 3 times a day for 7 days to 1 year. The extract showed anti-inflammatory action after operation. Dose expressed as dry weight of plant[HS034].

Antimutagenic activity. Ethanol (80%) extract of the flower, at a concentration of 12.5 mg/plate, educed about 60–90% of the mutagenicity induced by 2-amino-1-methyl-6-phenylimidazo[4,5-b]pyridine (PhIP) and other heterocyclic amines. Mutagenicity of methylazoxymethanol acetate, which like PhIP, is a colon carcinogen, was also efficiently inhibited by the extract[HS059].

Antischistosomal activity. Water extract of dried seeds, at a concentration of 10,000 ppm, was inactive on *Schistosoma mansoni*[HS030]. Water extract of dried sepals, at a concentration of 100.0 ppm, was active on *Schistosoma mansoni*[HS030].

Antitoxic activity. The flower, at a dose of 1.0 gm/liter in broth culture, was active on *Aspergillus flavus*. The production of aflatoxin was inhibited[HS043].

Antiviral activity. Water extract of the dried flower, at a concentration of 10% in cell culture, was active on Herpes virus type 2 and vaccinia virus, and inactive on influenza virus and poliovirus II[HS045].

Antiyeast activity. Ethanol/water (1:1) extract of dried leaves, at a concentration of 250.0 mg/ml on agar plate, was inactive on *Candida albicans* and active on *Saccharomyces pastorianus*. Dose expressed as dry weight of plant[HS053]. Water extract of the dried flower, at a concentration of 500 mg/ml on agar plate, was inactive on *Candida albicans* and active on *Saccharomyces pastorianus*. Dose expressed as dry weight of plant[HS047].

Chemopreventive activity. Ethanol (80%) extract of the flower, administered to rats, significantly inhibited aberrant crypt focus formation induced by azomethane and by 2-amino-1-methyl-6-phenylimidazo[4,5-b]pyridine[HS059].

Choleretic activity. Water extract of the flower, taken orally by human adults, was active[HS001].

Creatinine level decrease. Decoction of dried fruit juice, administered orally to male adults at a dose of 24.0 gm/day, was active[HS026].

Cytotoxic activity. Ethanol (70%) extract of the flower, in cell culture, was active on CA–Erlich–ascites. Greatest effect was observed only after 24 hours exposure[HS035]. Water extract of the dried flower, at a concentration of 10.0% in cell culture, produced weak activity on HELA cells[HS045].

Diuretic activity. Decoction of the dried calyx, administered by gastric intubation to rats at a dose of 1.0 gm/kg, produced strong activity[HS050]. Water extract of the flower, taken orally by human adults, was active[HS001].

Estrogenic effect. Water extract of the dried calyx, administered intraperitoneally to female rats at a dose of 500.0 mg/kg, was active, results significant at $P < 0.001$ level[HS052].

Feeding deterrent (insect). Acetone extract of dried shoots, undiluted, was active on *Diacrisia obliqua*[HS046].

Genitourinary effect. Decoction of dried fruit juice, administered orally to male adults at a dose of 24.0 gm/day, was active. Decreased urinary levels of sodium, potassium, phosphate, uric acid and calcium were demonstrated[HS026].

Glutamate-oxaloacetate-transaminase inhibition. Dried calyx, at a concentration of 10.0% of the diet in the ration of rats, was active vs cholesterol-loaded animals[HS022].

Glutamate-pyruvate-transaminase inhibition. Dried calyx, at a concentration of 10.0% of the diet in the ration of rats, produced weak activity vs cholesterol-loaded animals[HS022].

Hypotensive activity. Ethanol (95%) extract of dried calyx, administered intravenously to dogs at a dose of 200.0 mg/kg, produced weak activity[HS040]. Water extract of dried calyx, administered intravenously to cats at a dose of 25.0 mg/animal, was active. Animals were anesthetized with alpha-chlo-ralose. Effect blocked by atropine[HS031]. Water extract of the flower, taken orally by human adults, was active[HS001]. Water extract of the flower, administered intravenously to dogs, produced weak activity[HS006].

Intestinal motility inhibition. Water extract of dried calyx, administered to dogs at a dose of 5.0%, was active. Oral transit time assayed by first detection of phthalyl-sulphasalazine in blood. This dose was also active in rats when assayed by transit of graphite-agar suspension[HS032].

Laxative effect. Water extract of the flower, taken orally by human adults, was active[HS001].

Mutagenic activity. Dried fruit, on agar plate at a concentration of 50.0 mcg/plate, was active on *Salmonella typhimurium* TA100 and TA98. Metabolic activation required was required for positive results[HS029]. Seed oil was active on *Salmonella typhimurium* TA100 and TA98. Metabolic activation was not required for activity[HS048].

Smooth muscle relaxant activity. Hot water extract of dried petals was active on the rat aorta, IC_{50} 0.53 mg/ml vs ACh-induced contractions and IC_{50} 2.53 mg/ml when de-endothelialized muscle strips were used[HS025]. Water extract of dried calyx, at a concentration of 2.0%, was active on the rabbit ileum. The effect was not influenced by phentolamine, propanolol, haloperidol, and guanethidine[HS032].

Spasmogenic activity. Water extract of dried calyx, at a concentration of 0.4 mg/ml, was active on frog rectus abdominus muscle. The effect was slightly antagonized by tubocurarine. A concentration of 1.0 mg/ml was active on rabbit uterus. The effect was blocked by indomethacin and hydrocortisone, but not by atropine or cyperoheptadine[HS031]. The extract, at a concentration of 0.16%, was active on the rabbit ileum. The effect was blocked by atropine[HS032].

Spasmolytic activity. Water extract of dried calyx, at a concentration of 0.4

mg/ml, was active on frog rectus abdominus muscle. The effect was antagonized by tub-ocurarine vs ACh-induced contractions. The extract was also active on the rat uterus vs rhythmic contractions. The effect was not antagonized by rantidine or propanolol. At a concentration of 5.0 mg/ml, the extract was active on the guinea pig tracheal chain vs ACh-, histamine- and serotonin-induced contractions and also active on rabbit aorta. The effect was not antagonized by atropine, propanolol or ranitidine vs norepinephrine-induced contractions[HS031]. At 10.0 mg/ml, the extract was active on rat diaphragm. Physostigine and suxamethonium enhanced the effect vs electrically induced con-tractions[HS031]. Water extract of dried petals, at a concentration of 0.6 mg/ml, was active on the rat aorta vs norepinephrine-induced contractions, and inactive vs K+-induced contractions[HS028].

Toxicity assessment. Hot water extract of dried calyx, administered by gastric intubation to rabbits, produced LD_{50} 129.1 gm/kg[HS040].

Uricosuric activity. Decoction of dried calyx, administered to rats at a dose of 1.0 gm/kg, was active[HS050].

Uterine relaxation effect. Water extract of the flower was active on the rat uterus[HS006].

REFERENCES

HS001 Leclerc, H. Sida Sabdariffa (*Hibiscus sabdariffa*). **Presse Med** 1938; 46: 1060.

HS002 Leupin, K. Karkade. **Pharma Acta Helv** 1935; 10: 138.

HS003 Buogo, G. and D. Picchinenna. Chemical constituents of *Roselle hemp*. **Ann Chim Appl** 1937; 27: 577.

HS004 Rao, P. S. and T. R. Seshadri. Pigments of the flowers of *Hibiscus sabdariffa* – Isolation of sabdaretin, a new hydro-xyflavene. **Proc Indian Acad Sci Ser A** 1942; 16: 323.

HS005 Indovina, R. and G. Capotummino. Chemical investigation of some prod-ucts which can be obtained from *Hibiscus sabdariffa*. **Boll Studi Informas** (Palermo) 1938; 15:1.

HS006 Sharaf, A. The pharmacological char-acteristics of *Hibiscus sabdariffa*. **Planta Med** 1962; 10: 48–52.

HS007 Reaubourg, G. and R. H. Monceaux. The chemical, botanical and pharmaco-logical characteristics of the karkade (rosella) *Hibiscus sabdariffa* (Glossy-pifolius). **J Pharm Chim** 1940; 1(9): 292.

HS008 Rovesti, P. Therapeutic and dietetic properties of "Karkade" (*Hibiscus sabdariffa*), a new colonial pink tea. **Farmacista Ital** 1936; 3(1): 13.

HS009 Bouquet, A. Feticheurs et Medecines Traditionelles du Congo (Brazzaville). **Mem Orstom** No. 36,282 P. Paris, 1969.

HS010 El-Hamid, A. Drug plants of the Sudan Republic in native medicine. **Planta Med** 1970; 18: 278.

HS011 Perkin, A. G. Coloring matters of the flowers of *Hibiscus sabdariffa* and *Thespesia lampas*. **Proc Chem Soc** 1909; 1090: 248.

HS012 Kerharo, J. Senegal bisap (*Hibiscus sabdariffa*) or Guinea sorrel or red sor-rel. **Plant Med Phytother** 1971; 5: 277.

HS013 Kerharo, J. Le pisap du Senegal (*Hibis-cus sabdariffa* L.) ou oseille de Guinee, ou karkade de L'erythree. **Planta Med Phytother** 1971; 4: 227.

HS014 Rao, C. N. True vitamin A value of some vegetables. **J Nutr Diet** 1967; 4: 10.

HS015 Osman, A. M., M. El-Garby Younes and A. Mokhtar. Chemical examination of local plants. VIII. Comparative studies between constituents of different parts of Egyptian *Hibiscus sabdariffa*. **Indian J Chem** 1975; 13: 198.

HS016 Osman, A. M., M. El-Garby Younes and A. Mokhtar. Sitosterol-beta-D-galactoside from *Hibiscus sabdariffa*. **Phytochemistry** 1975; 14: 829–830.

HS017 Du, C. T. and F. J. Francis. Anthocya-nins of roselle (*Hibiscus sabdariffa*). **J Food Sci** 1974; 38: 810.

HS018 Morton, J. F. Renewed interest in roselle (*Hibiscus sabdariffa*), the long-forgotten "Florida Cranberry". **Proc Fla State Hort Soc** 1974; 87: 415.

HS019 Karawya, M. S., M. G. Ghourab and I. M. El-Shami. Study of anthocyanin content of karkadeh, "*Hibiscus sab-dariffa*". **Egypt J Pharm Sci** 1976; 16: 345.

HS020 Schilcher, H. Proposal for the valuation of hibiscus flowers calyx (*Hibiscus sabdariffa*) Part 2. Application possibilities of the TSS process. Part 14. Quality testing of commercial drugs and their value. **Dtsch Apoth Ztg** 1976; 116: 1155.

HS021 Al-Wandawi, H., K. Al-Shaikhly and M. Abdul-Rahman. Roselle seeds: A new protein source. **J Agr Food Chem** 1984; 32: 510–512.

HS022 El-Saadany, S. S., M. Z. Sithoy, S. M. Labib and R. El-Massry. Biochemical dynamics and hypocholesterolemic action of *Hibiscus sabdariffa* (karkade). **Nahrung** 1991; 35(6): 567–576.

HS023 Yasukawa, K., A. Yamaguchi, J. Arita, S. Sakurai, A. Ikeda and M. Takido. Inhibitory effect of edible plant extracts on 12-0-Tetradecanoylphorbol-13-acetate-induced ear oedema in mice. **Phytother Res** 1993; 7(2): 185–189.

HS024 Hyomi, M. and W. Miura. Hibiscus. **Koryo** 1992; 176: 97–102.

HS025 Obiefuna, P., O. Owolabi, B. Adegunloye, I. Obiefuna and O. Sofola. The petal extract of *Hibiscus sabdariffa* produces relaxation of isolated rat aorta. **Int J Pharmacog** 1994; 32(1): 69–74.

HS026 Kirdpon, S., S. N. Nakorn and W. Kirdpon. Changes in urinary chemical composition in healthy volunteers after consuming roselle (*Hibiscus sabdariffa* Linn.) juice. **J Med Assoc Thailand** 1994; 77(6): 314–321.

HS027 Sato, K., Y. Goda, K. Yoshihira and H. Noguchi. Structure and contents of main coloring constituents in the calyces of *Hibiscus sabdariffa* and commercial roselle color. **Shokuhin Eiseigaku Zasshi** 1991; 32(4): 301–307.

HS028 Owolabi, O. A., B. J. Adegunloye, O. P. Ajagbona, O. A. Sofola and P. C. M. Obiefuna. Mechanism of relaxant effect mediated by an aqueous extract of *Hibiscus sabdariffa* petals in isolated rat aorta. **Int J Pharmacog** 1995; 33(3): 210–214.

HS029 Takeda, N. and Y. Yasui. Identification of mutagenic substances in roselle color, elderberry color and safflower yellow. **Agr Biol Chem** 1985; 49(6): 1851,1852.

HS030 Elsheikh, S. H., A. K. Bashir, S. M. Suliman and M. E. Wassila. Toxicity of certain Sudanese plant extracts on Cercariae and Miracidia of *Schistosoma mansoni*. **Int J Crude Drug Res** 1990; 28(4): 241–245.

HS031 Ali, M. B., W. M. Salih, A. H. Mohamed and A. M. Homeida. Investigation of the antispasmodic potential of *Hibiscus sabdariffa* calyces. **J Ethnopharmacol** 1991; 31(2): 249–257.

HS032 Ali, M. B., A. H. Mohamed, W. M. Salih and A. H. Homeida. Effect of an aqueous extract of *Hibiscus sabdariffa* calyces on the gastrointestinal tract. **Fitoterapia** 1991; 62(6): 475–479.

HS033 Bishay, D. W. and C. S. Gomaa. Comparative chromatographic studies of oils of some medicinal seeds. **Egypt J Pharm Sci** 1976; 17: 249.

HS034 Anon. Verasing Mungmum (1982). The use of medicinal herbs for the treatment of kidney stone in the urinary system. **Abstr Seminar on the Development of Drugs from Medicinal Plants**, Bangkok, Thailand 1982; 117.

HS035 El-Merzabani, M. M., A. A. El-Aaser, M. A. Attia, A. K. El-Duweini and A. M. Ghazal. Screening system for Egyptian plants with potential antitumor activity. **Planta Med** 1979; 36: 150–155.

HS036 Salah Ahmed, M., G. Honda and W. Miki. Herb Drugs and Herbalists in the Middle East. Institute for the Study of Languages and Cultures of Asia and Africa. **Studia Culturae Islamicae** No. 8, 1979; 1–208.

HS037 Salama, R. B. and S. A. Ibrahim. Ergosterol in *Hibiscus sabdariffa* seed oil. **Planta Med** 1979; 36: 221.

HS038 Ahmad, M. U., S. K. Husain, I. Ahmad and S. M. Osman. *Hibiscus sabdariffa* seed oil: A re-investigation. **J Sci Food Agr** 1979; 30: 424–428.

HS039 Gangrade, H., S. H. Mishra and R. Kaushal. Antimicrobial activity of the oil and unsaponifiable matter of red roselle. **Indian Drugs** 1979; 16: 147–148.

HS040 Zhung, Y. L., J. R. Yeh, D. J. Lin, J. C. Yuan, R. L. Zhou and P. Q. Wang. Antihypertensive effect of *Hibiscus sabdariffa*. **Yao Hsueh T'Ung Pao** 1981; 16(5): 60C.

HS041　Hussein Ayoub, S. M. and A. Baerheim-Suendsen. Medicinal and aromatic plants in the Sudan. Usage and exploration. **Fitoterapia** 1981; 52: 243–246.

HS042　Anon. Food coloring agents from Hibiscus flowers. **Patent-Japan Kokai Tokkyo Koho**-81 1981; 141,358 5pp.

HS043　El-Shayeb, N. M. A. and S. S. Mabrouk. Utilization of some edible and medicinal plants to inhibit aflatoxin formation. **Nutr Rep Int** 1984; 29(2): 273–282.

HS044　Kargbo, T. K. Traditional practices affecting the health of women and children in Africa. **Unpublished Manuscript** 1984.

HS045　May, G. and G. Willuhn. Antiviral activity of aqueous extracts from medicinal plants in tissue cultures. **Arzneim-Forsch** 1978; 28(1): 1–7.

HS046　Tripathi, A. K. and S. M. A. Rizvi. Antifeedant activity of indigenous plants against *Diacrisia obliqua* Walker. **Curr Sci** 1985; 54(13): 630–631.

HS047　Guerin, J. C. and H. P. Reveillere. Antifungal activity of plant extracts used in therapy. I. Study of 41 plant extracts against 9 fungi species. **Ann Pharm Fr** 1984; 42(6): 553–559.

HS048　Polasa, K. and C. Rukmini. Mutagenicity tests of cashew nut shell liquid, rice-bran oil and other vegetable oils using the *Salmonella typhimurium*/microsome system. **Food Chem Toxicol** 1987; 25(10): 763–766.

HS049　Boum, B., L. Kamdem, P. Mbganga, N. Atangana and Y. Sabry. Contribution to the pharmacologic study of two plants used in traditional medicine against worms. **Rev Sci Technol (Health Sci Ser)** 1985; 2(3/4): 83–86.

HS050　Caceres, A., L. M. Giron and A. M. Martinez. Diuretic activity of plants used for treatment of urinary aliments in Guatemala. **J Ethnopharmacol** 1987; 19(3): 233–245.

HS051　Al-Wandawi, H., K. Al-Shaikhly and M. Abdul-Rahman. Roselle seeds: A new protein source. **J Agr Food Chem** 1984; 32(3): 510–512.

HS052　Ali, M. B., W. M. Salih and A. M. Humida. An oestrogen-like activity of *Hibiscus sabdariffa*. **Fitoterapia** 1989; 60(6): 547–548.

HS053　Guerin, J. C. and H. P. Reveillere. Antifungal activity of plant extracts used in therapy. l. Study of 41 plant extracts against 9 fungi species. **Ann Pharm Fr** 1984; 42(6): 553–559.

HS054　Panthong, A., D. Kanjanapothi and W. C. Taylor. Ethnobotanical review of medicinal plants from Thai traditional books. Part 1. Plants with anti-inflammatory, anti-asthmatic and antihypertensive properties. **J Ethnopharmacol** 1986; 18(3): 213–228.

HS055　Lin, Y. C. The study of red pigments in Taiwan plants. **Proc Natl Sci Counc Part I (Taiwan)** 1975 (8): 133–137.

HS056　Hansawasdi, C., J. Kawabata and T. Kasai. Alpha-amylase inhibitors from roselle (*Hibiscus sabdariffa* Linn.) tea. **Biosci Biotechnol Biochem** 2000; 64(5): 1041–1043.

HS057　Tseng, T. H., T. W. Kao, C. Y. Chu, F. P. Chou, W. L. Lin and C. J. Wang. Induction of apoptosis by hibiscus protocatechuic acid in human leukemia cells via reduction of retinoblastoma (RB) phosphorylation and Bcl-2 expression. **Bichem Pharmacol** 2000; 60(3): 307–315.

HS058　Wang, C. J., J. M. Wang, W. L. Lin, C. Y. Chu, F. P. Chou and T. H. Tseng. Protective effects of Hibiscus anthocyanins against tert-butyl hydroperoxide-induced hepatic toxicity in rats. **Food Chem Toxicol** 2000; 38(5): 411–416.

HS059　Chenonarin, T., T. Kinouchi, K. Kataoka, H. Arimochi, T. Kuwahara, U. Vinitketkumnuen and Y. Ohnishi. Effects of roselle (*Hibiscus sabdariffa* Linn.), a Thai medicinal plant, on the mutagenicity of various known mutagens in *Salmonella typhimurium* and on formation of aberrant crypt foci induced by the colon carcinogens azoxymethane and 2-amino-1-methyl-6-phenylimidazo[4,5-b]pyridine in F344 rats. **Food Chem Toxicol** 1999; 37(6): 591–601.

HS060　Onyenekwe, P. C., E. O. Ajani, D. A. Ameh and K. S. Gamaniel. Antihypertensive effect of roselle (*Hibiscus sabdariffa*) calyx infusion in spontaneously hypertensive rats and a comparison of its toxicity with that in Wistar rats. **Cell Biochem Funct** 1999; 17(3): 199–206.

HS061 Haji Faraji, M and A. Haji Tarkhani. The effect of sour tea (*Hibiscus sabdariffa*) on essential hypertension. **J Ethnopharmacol** 1999; 65(3): 231–236.

14 | Jatropha curcas

Miers.

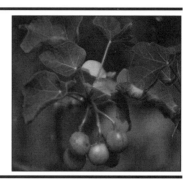

Common Names

American purging nut	South Africa	Physic nut	South Africa
Ba dau me	Vietnam	Physic nut	Thailand
Bagbherenda	Fiji	Physic nut	Virgin Islands
Barbados purging nut	South Africa	Physic nut bush	Fiji
Bi ni da zugu	Nigeria	Piao branco	Brazil
Big purge nut	South Africa	Pignon d'inde	Rodrigues Islands
Black vomit nut	South Africa	Pindi	India
Botuje	Nigeria	Pinnao de purga	Brazil
Cantal–muluung	Somalia	Pinon botija	Cape Verde Islands
Cuta	Mexico	Pinon	Guatemala
Datiwan	Nepal	Pinon	Mexico
Dinon	Puerto Rico	Pinon	Peru
Eso botuje	Nigeria	Pinoncillo	Mexico
Etamanane	Senegal	Punnetang	India
Fiki	Tonga	Purge nut bush	West Indies
Habb el meluk	Sudan	Purging nut	South Africa
Habb–el–meluk	Mexico	Purging nut	Thailand
Jarak pagar	Indonesia	Purging physic	Nicaragua
Kananeranda	India	Purgueira	Guinea–Bissau
Kasla	Philippines	Ram jyoti	Nepal
Lapalapa	Nigeria	Ramjeevan	Nepal
Lohong	Vietnam	Ratanjyot	India
Ma feng shu	Indonesia	Sabuu dam	Thailand
Medisiyen blen	West Indies	Saimal	Nepal
Mupfure–donga	Venda	Sajiba	Nepal
Nepalamu	India	Sajiwa	Nepal
Owulo idu	Nigeria	Sajiwan	Nepal
Pe–fo–tze	Vietnam	Sajiyon	Nepal
Perchnut	West Indies	Satiman–G	Nepal
Physic nut	Ghana	Sdatiwan	Nepal
Physic nut	Guam	Seemanepaalam	India
Physic nut	Guyana	Tartago	Puerto Rico
Physic nut	Nepal	Tong–chou	Vietnam
Physic nut	Nigeria	Tubaang–bakod	Cape Verde Islands

From: *Medicinal Plants of the World, vol. 1: Chemical Constituents, Traditional and Modern Medicinal Uses, 2nd ed.*
By: Ivan A. Ross © Humana Press Inc., Totowa, NJ

Tubang–bakod	Philippines	Wedsiyen	Haiti
Tubatuba	Guam	White physic nut	West Indies
Udukaju	Thailand	Wiriwiri	Fiji
Ungume	Guinea–Bissau		

BOTANICAL DESCRIPTION

A glabrous erect branched shrub of the EUPHORBIACEAE family, 2 to 5 meters high with stout, cylindrical green branches with viscid, milky or reddish sap. Leaves are orbicular-ovate, angular or somewhat 3 or 5-lobed, 10 to 15 cm long, acuminate and base cordate with long petioles. Cymes are axillary, peduncled. The flowers are greenish or greenish–white, 6 to 8 mm in diameter. The male and female bear at different times in the same inflorescence; petals 6 to 7 mm long. The petals are reflexed, stamens 10, the filaments of the inner 5, connate. Capsules at first fleshy, becoming dry, of 2 or 3 cocci, subspherical, 2.5 to 4 cm diameters with seeds blackish, about 2 cm long.

The 2 species commonly found in the tropics, *J. curcas*, Linn., (physic nut) and *J. gossypifolia* L. (bellyache bush), are the most widely used species in traditional medicine. No chemotaxonomic delimitation has been reported, and the species appear to have similar uses in folk medicine, same chemical constituents and similar pharmacological activity. This profile mainly concerns *J. curcas*, but references are made on *J. gossypifolia*.

ORIGIN AND DISTRIBUTION

Native to tropical America it is now widespread. Rather common, particularly near habitations.

TRADITIONAL MEDICINAL USES

Brazil. Dried entire plant is taken orally for sinusitis. *Luffa operculata* fruit and *Jatropha curcas* latex are mixed; practitioners advise caution in use because the latex is caustic[JC058]. Hot water extract of root is taken orally, as an anthelmintic[JC076]. Infu-

sion of dried leaf, seed or stem orally, is used for toothache, fever and headache[JC023].

Cambodia. Seed extract is taken orally as an abortifacient[JC002].

Cape Verde Islands. Hot water extract of the leaf is used to induce the secretion of milk especially in women who have recently given birth[JC080].

Colombia. Leaf decoction is used orally as a febrifuge[JC022].

Egypt. Hot water extract of seed is taken orally for jaundice[JC028].

Fiji. Fresh leaf juice is taken orally for diarrhea, fever and as a hemostatic. Fresh stem juice is used externally for sores and sprains. The stem juice is mixed in bath water[JC063].

Guam. Seeds, when taken orally, have been reported to be toxic. As few as 3 fruits may be fatal. In other cases, 1 to 4 seeds acted as a purgative. Symptoms include irritation of the throat and intense abdominal pain. Also included are vomiting, dizziness, restlessness, muscular spasms, drowsiness and even collapse (skin clammy, slow pulse). Smoke victims show mydriasis[JC007].

Guatemala. Hot water extract of the leaf is taken orally as a treatment for dysentery[JC078].

Guinea-Bissau. Hot water extract of the leaf is administered orally to accelerate secretion of milk in postpartum women[JC003].

Haiti. Dried leaf decoction is taken orally for edema, flu and cough. Fresh latex is rubbed on the tongue for buccal thrush. It is also used for burns and cutaneous infections. In the treatment of bruises, the leaves are applied in sequence until 1 of them sticks onto the skin. This is allowed to dry, and then replaced with another leaf until the bruise is healed[JC066].

India. Dried branches are applied externally for joint pains. Young branches are warmed in the fire then placed on the affected joint[JC061]. Dried entire plant is taken orally as a purgative[JC020]. Fresh latex is used for toothache. Teeth are cleaned with the stem, or leaf juice is applied to the painful tooth[JC062]. Fresh leaf juice is taken orally for epilepsy. Leaf juice is mixed with garlic powder and camphor and taken twice a day for 4 days[JC034]. Fresh leaves are used for guinea worms. Leaves are warmed and tied locally over the swelling to promote suppuration[JC041]. Hot water extract of seeds is taken orally as an abortifacient. The extract is also used for intestinal parasites. One seed is ground and soaked in water and a small amount of the extract is taken orally[JC088].

Indonesia. Hot water extract of stem is taken orally to treat matrix cancer and stomach cancer. Mixed with *Ageratum conyzoides*, *Eclipta alba* and *Spilanthes acmella*, the extract is taken after meals in the morning and evening[JC008].

Ivory Coast. Fresh leaves are used as a hemostatic[JC070].

Mexico. Fresh sap is taken orally for mouth sores. The sap is rubbed on the sore. The sap is also taken orally for whooping cough[JC055]. Latex is used to treat mouth infections[JC024].

Nepal. Hot water extract of leaf is taken orally as a lactagogue[JC001].

Nigeria. Decoction of root is taken orally to treat venereal disease. Dried leaf juice is used externally to treat ringworm. Juice from the leaves is applied to the affected part with cotton. Fresh latex is applied to the tongue to treat coated tongues. Hot water extract of dried leaf is taken orally to treat diarrhea. Ten to 15 leaves are crushed with potash and added to 1–2 glasses of water. The liquid can be stored and taken when required. Decoction made from young leaves is taken orally, as treatment for fever. Decoction prepared from the leaves is administered as a rectal injection to treat jaundice[JC014]. Hot water extract of dried seed is taken orally to treat arthritis[JC052]. Hot water extract of fresh root is taken orally for jaundice, as an anti-rheumatic and for dysentery. Infusion of fresh leaf and root is used externally as a treatment for ringworm. The infusion is used orally as an antipyretic and anticonvulsant[JC054].

Peru. Hot water extract of dried seed is taken orally as a purgative[JC069].

Philippines. Fresh leaves are pasted on the temples or the forehead to treat fever. The fresh bark is used to treat fractures and sprains. Strips of bark are blanched over steam or rolled over a low flame then secured with a bandage over the affected area[JC042].

Senegal. Fresh leaf juice is used as eyewash for eye diseases. The juice is also used externally for wounds and sores[JC056]. Hot water extract of dried entire plant is taken orally as a treatment for leprosy. Hot water extract of dried exudate is used for open sores. Hot water extract of dried leaves is taken orally as a treatment for odontalgia, syphilis and lung diseases. The extract is used externally for sores and for abscesses. Hot water extract of dried seed is administered orally as a treatment for enteralgia[JC033]. The seed is taken orally for stomachache[JC036].

Somalia. Infusion of dried seed is administered orally to treat constipation. Three seeds are roasted, the peel is removed, and the kernel is crushed and added to a cup of tea. The tea is taken and followed by 1–2 liters of milk. Purgation follows in 1–3 hours[JC007].

South Africa. Decoction of dried seed is taken orally as a purgative[JC038].

Sudan. Seeds are used as an oral contraceptive[JC005] and anthelmintic[JC045].

Thailand. Seed oil, mixed with a little chili, is administered orally as a laxative[JC064]. The entire plant is taken orally as a purgative[JC065].

Tonga. Infusion of dried leaves is taken orally to treat vaginal bleeding[JC057].

Venda. Decoction of dried root is used to rinse the oral cavity as a treatment for toothache. The decoction is also taken orally for sore throat[JC059].

Vietnam. Seed oil is taken orally as an abortive[JC004] and emmenagogue[JC006].

Virgin Islands. Hot water extract of the entire plant is administered orally as a treatment for the common cold, either alone or in combination with other plants[JC077].

West Africa. Hot water extract of dried leaves is used externally for guinea worm. Hot water extract of the seed oil is used externally as a rubefacient for parasitic skin diseases[JC035].

West Indies. Hot water extract of the leaf is taken orally for heart troubles[JC046].

Zaire. Infusion of dried leaf is taken orally for diarrhea, chest pains, coughs, anemia, urinary tract infections, diabetes, dental caries and infected wounds. Externally, the infusion is used on infected wounds and for skin diseases[JC025].

CHEMICAL CONSTITUENTS

(ppm unless otherwise indicated)

7-Keto-beta sitosterol: Sd[JC029]
Alpha amyrin: Lf 67[JC029]
Apigenin: Lf[JC079]
Arachidic acid: Sd 0.180–0.288%[JC016]
Beta sitosterol: Lf[JC028]
Campesterol: Lf[JC029]
Curcain: Lx[JC037]
Curcin: Sd[JC019]
Curculathyrane A: Pl[JC011]
Curculathyrane B: Pl[JC011]
Curcusone A: Rt 0.0132%[JC010]
Curcusone B: Rt 0.0127%[JC010]
Curcusone C: Rt 0.001%[JC010]
Curcusone D: Rt 0.004%[JC010]
Daucosterol: Lf 0.014%[JC029]
Friedelin: St 8[JC013]
Friedelinol: St 0.001%[JC013]
Ikshusterol: Lf 27[JC029]
J curcas flavonoid I: Lf 0.065%[JC028]
J. curcas flavonoid II: Lf 0.04%[JC028]
J. curcas triterpene: Lf 0.05%[JC028]
Jatropha factor C-1: Sd 65[JC044]
Jatropha factor C-2: Sd 65[JC044]
Jatrophin: Rt[JC012]

Jatrophol: Rt[JC012]
Jatropholone A: Rt[JC012]
Jatropholone B: Rt[JC012]
Jatropholone: Rt[JC010]
Lignoceric acid: Sd oil[JC016]
Linoleic acid: Sd 8.796–16.224%[JC009]
Linolenic acid: Sd 0.330–0.528%[JC016]
Myristic acid: Sd 0.540–0.864%[JC016]
Oleic acid: Sd 10.944–19.968%[JC009]
Palmitic acid: Sd 3.9900–6.5325%[JC016]
Palmitoleic acid: Sd 0.420–0.672%[JC016]
Phorbol, 12-deoxy-16-hydroxy: Sd oil[JC067]
Protein: Sd 16.2–18.6%[JC073]
Scoparone: St 10[JC013]
Stearic acid: Sd 2.640–8.736%[JC009]
Stigast-5-ene-3-beta, 7-alpha-diol: Lf 8[JC029]
Stigmasterol: Lf 0.025%[JC028]
Tomentin: Rt[JC012]
Triacontan-1-ol: Lf 36[JC029]
Vitexin: Lf [JC079]

PHARMACOLOGICAL ACTIVITIES AND CLINICAL TRIALS

Analgesic activity. Ethanol/water (1:1) extract of the aerial parts, administered to mice intraperitoneally at a dose of 0.25 mg/kg, was inactive vs tail pressure method[JC075].

Antibacterial activity. Ethanol/water (1:1) extract of the aerial parts, at a concentration of 25 mcg/ml on agar plate, was inactive against *Bacillus subtilis*, *E. coli*, *Salmonella typhosa*, and *Agrobacterium tumefaciens*[JC075]. Ethyl acetate extract of dried aerial parts, at a concentration of 1.0 mg/disk on agar plate, was inactive against *E. coli* and *Staphylococcus aureus*. Water extract of the dried aerial parts, at a concentration of 1.0 mg/disk on agar plate, was inactive against *E. coli* and *Staphylococcus aureus*[JC072]. Methanol extract of dried leaves, at a concentration of 10 mg/ml on agar plate, was inactive against *Escherichia coli*, *Klebsiella pneumoniae*, *Salmonella typhimurium*, *Pseudomonas aeruginosa*, and *Streptococcus mutans*. The extract was also active on *Staphylococcus aureus*, MIC 125.0 mcg/ml[JC025]. A 95% ethanol extract of sun-dried leaves, at a concentration of 50.0 mg/ml on agar plate, was active against *Sta-*

phylococcus aureus and inactive on *Bacillus subtilis*. Extract of 10 ml/gm plant material was used. An aliquot of 0.1 ml extract was placed in well on the plate[JC068]. Ethanol (95%) extract of dried root and stem, at a concentration of 10.0 mg/ml on agar plate, was inactive on *Corynebacterium diptheriae* and *Diplococcus pneumoniae* and weakly active on *Staphylococcus aureus, Streptococcus pyogenes*, and *Streptococcus viridans*. Water extract of dried root and stem, at a concentration of 10.0 mg/ml on agar plate, was inactive on *Corynebacterium diptheriae* and *Diplococcus pneumoniae*, and weakly active on *Staphylococcus aureus, Streptococcus pyogenes*, and *Streptococcus viridans*[JC048]. Methanol extract of dried seeds, at a concentration of 2.0 mg/ml on agar plate, was active on *Corynebacterium diptheriae* and *Pseudomonas aeruginosa* and inactive on *Neisseria* species, *Salmonella* species, *Staphylococcus aureus, Streptobacillus* species, and *Streptococcus* species[JC040].

Anticonvulsant activity. Ethanol/water extract (1:1) of the aerial parts, at a concentration of 0.25 mg/kg administered intraperitoneally to mice, was inactive vs electroshock-induced convulsions[JC075]. Ethanol (70%) extract of fresh root, administered intraperitoneally to mice of both sexes, was active vs metrazole-induced convulsions and weakly active vs strychnine-induced convulsions[JC054].

Anticrustacean activity. Ethanol extract of dried seeds (defatted with petroleum ether) was inactive on *Artemia salina*, LD_{50} > 1.0 mg/ml[JC051].

Antidiarrheal activity. Petroleum ether and methanol extracts of the root were active against castor oil induced diarrhea and intraluminal accumulation of fluid. It also reduced gastrointestinal motility after charcoal meal administration in albino mice[JC085].

Antifertility effects. The fruits and seeds, administered to female rats in the ration at a dose of 3.3% of the diet, were 100% effective[JC005].

Antifungal activity. Ethanol/water (1:1) extract of the aerial parts, at a concentration of 25 mcg/ml on agar plate, was inactive on *Microsporum canis, Trichophyton mentagrophytes*, and *Aspergillus niger*[JC075]. Ethyl acetate extract of the dried aerial parts, at a concentration of 0.13 mg/ml on agar plate, was active on *Microsporum canis*, and inactive on *Microsporum fulvum, M. gypseum*, and *Trichophyton gallinae*. Water extract of the dried aerial parts, on agar plate, was inactive against *M. canis, M. fulvum, M. gypseum* and *Trichophyton gallinae*[JC072]. Acetone/water (50:50) extract of fresh latex, on agar plate, was inactive against *Microsporum gypseum* and *Trichophyton mentagrophytes*[JC032]. Methanol extract of dried leaves, at a concentration of 10.0 mcg/ml on agar plate, was inactive on *Candida albicans*. Methanol extract of dried leaves, at a concentration of 10.0 mg/ml on agar plate, was inactive against *Aspergillus niger* and *Microsporum gypseum*[JC025]. Ethanol (95%) extract of sun-dried leaves, at a concentration of 50 mg/ml on agar plate, was inactive on *Aspergillus niger*. Extract of 10 ml/gm plant material was used. An aliquot of 0.1 ml extract was placed in well on the plate[JC068].

Anti-inflammatory activity. Ethanol/water (1:1) extract of the aerial parts, administered orally to male rats at a dose of 0.25 mg/kg, was inactive vs carrageenin-induced pedal edema. The animals were dosed 1 hour before carrageenin injections[JC075].

Antimolluscicidal activity. Extracts of the seeds were active against both *Bullinus globosus* and *Oncomelania hupensis*, the latter being the more sensitive snail. The activity was associated with phorbol esters extracted from the oil. Of the pure phorbol esters tested, 4 beta-phorbol-13-decanoate killed both snail species at a concentration of 0.001% (10 ppm)[JC083].

Antiparasitic activity. Sap exhibited germicidal actions on the growth of *Staphylococcus, Bacillus*, and *Micrococcus* species on contact and retained the effects on treated bench surface for close to 6 hours after the initial application. Ova of *Ascaris lumbricoides* and *Necator americanus*, incubated in 50 and 100% concentrations of the sap at room temperature, showed no evidence of embryonation after 21 days in the case of *A. lumbricoides*, negative on hatchability in hookworm, or complete distortion in both. The sap also exhibited strong inhibitory effect on normal larval growth of mosquito, but was highly toxic to mice when administered through oral or intraperitoneal routes[JC084].

Antischistosomal activity. Ethanol (95%) extract of the plant, at a concentration of 2000 mg/ml, was inactive on Schistosoma, *Hematobium cercariae*, *H. Miracida* and *H. ova*[JC060].

Antispasmodic activity. Ethanol/water (1:1) extract of the aerial parts, administered to guinea pigs, was inactive vs ACh- and histamine-induced spasms[JC075].

Antitumor activity. Chloroform extract of leaves and twigs, administered intraperitoneally to mice at a dose of 12.5 mg/kg, was active, 40% ILS; a dose of 25.0 mg/kg, 32% ILS and 50.0 mg/kg, 57% ILS on LEUK-P388. Ethanol (95%) extract of leaves and twigs, administered intraperitoneally to mice at a dose of 100.0 mg/kg, was active, 35% ILS; a dose 25.0 mg/kg, 41% ILS and 50.0 mg/kg, 33% ILS on LEUK-P388. Petroleum ether extract of leaves and twigs, administered intraperitoneally to mice, was inactive on LEUK-P388[JC029]. Ethanol (defatted with petroleum ether) extract of dried seeds, administered intraperitoneally to mice, was inactive on LEUK–P388[JC053].

Antiviral activity. Ethyl acetate extract of the dried aerial parts, in cell culture, was active on Cytomegalovirus, LC_{50} 7.0 mcg/ml. The virus was exposed to the extract before infecting the host cells[JC042]. The LC_{50} was greater than 100 mcg/ml (inactive) when infected host cells were exposed to the extract[JC072]. Ethyl acetate extract of the dried aerial parts, in cell culture, was active on Sindbis virus; LC_{50} 88.0 mcg/ml. Infected host cells were exposed to the extract[JC042]. The $LC_{50} < 1.0$ mcg/ml when the virus was exposed to the extract before infecting host cells. Water extract of the dried aerial parts, in cell culture, was active against Cytomegalovirus, LC_{50} 22.0 mcg/ml, when virus was exposed to extract before infecting host cells. When infected host cells were exposed to extract, a LC_{50} greater than 100 mcg/ml was obtained (inactive). Water extract of the dried aerial parts, in cells culture, was active on Sindbis virus, LC_{50} 32.0 mcg/ml, when infected host cells were exposed to the extract. The extract was active, $LC_{50} < 1.0$ mcg/ml, when the virus was exposed to the extract before infecting the host cells[JC072]. Methanol extract of dried leaves, at a concentration of 100 mcg/ml in cell culture, was weakly active against HIV virus[JC027]. Water extract of fresh leaves, in cell culture, was active against Tobacco Mosaic virus. The viral inhibitory activity was 40%[JC015]. Water extract of the branches strongly inhibited the HIV-induced cytopathic effects with low cytotoxicity[JC082].

Antiyeast activity. Ethanol/water (1:1) extract, at a concentration of 25 mcg/ml on agar plate, was inactive on *Candida albicans* and *Cryptococcus neoformans*[JC075]. Ethyl acetate extract of the dried aerial parts, at a concentration of 1.0 mg/disk on agar plate, was inactive against *Candida albicans* and *Saccharomyces cerevisiae*. The water extract was also inactive[JC072].

Barbiturate potentiation. Ethanol/water (1:1) extract of the aerial parts, administered intraperitoneally to mice at a dose of 0.25 mg/kg, was positive[JC075].

Cardiac effect. Methanol extract of dried seeds exhibited a negative chronotropic effect and a negative inotropic effect on guinea pig atrium[JC056].

Crown gall inhibition. Ethyl acetate extract of the dried aerial parts, in cell culture, produced LC_{50} 1.4 mcg/ml (active). The assay system was intended to predict for antitumor activity. Water extract was also active, $LC_{50} > 3.0$ mcg/ml[JC072]. Ethanol (defatted with petroleum ether) extract of dried seeds, at a concentration of 2.0 mg/ml on potato disk, was inactive on *Agrobacterium tumefaciens*. The hexane extract was inactive. The assay system was intended to predict for antitumor activity[JC053].

Cytotoxic activity. Ethanol/water (1:1) extract of leaves, in cell culture, was active against CA–9KB, $ED_{50} < 20.0$ mcg/ml[JC060]. Methanol extract of dried leaves, at a concentration of 100.0 mcg/ml in cell culture, was inactive against several human tumors[JC027]. Chloroform extract of leaves and twigs, in cell culture, was active on LEUK–P388, ED_{50} 1.1 mcg/ml and inactive on CA–9KB, $ED_{50} > 20.0$ mcg/ml[JC029]. Ethanol (95%) extract of leaves and twigs, in cell culture, was active on LEUK-P388, ED_{50} 2.4 mcg/ml, and inactive on CA-9KB, $ED_{50} > 20.0$ mcg/ml. Petroleum ether extract of leaves and twigs, in cell culture, was inactive on CA-9KB, $ED_{50} > 20.0$ mcg/ml, and inactive on LEUK-P388, $ED_{50} > 20.0$ mcg/ml[JC029]. Ethanol (defatted with petroleum ether) extract of dried seeds, in cell culture, was active on LEUK-P388, ED_{50} 9.0 mcg/ml[JC063,JC034]. The extract was inactive on CA–9KB, $ED_{50} > 30.0$ mcg/ml[JC051,JC053].

Diuretic activity. Ethanol/water (1:1) extract of the aerial parts, administered intraperitoneally to male rats at a dose of 0.125 mg/kg, was positive. Saline-loaded animals were used and urine was collected for 4 hours after dosing[JC075].

Glutamate dehydrogenase stimulation. Dried seeds, in the ration of chicken at a concentration of 0.5% of the diet, were active. Sorbitol-dehydrogenase was stimulated[JC017].

Hemolytic activity. Seed oil, in cell culture, was active on rabbit RBC, ED_{100} 0.1 mg/ml[JC026].

Hemostatic activity. Fresh leaf extract, at a concentration of 50%, was active on human whole blood[JC070].

Hypoglycemic activity. Ethanol/water (1:1) extract of the aerial parts, administered orally to rats at a dose of 250 mg/kg, was inactive. There was less than 30% drop in blood sugar level[JC075].

Hypothermic activity. Ethanol/water (1:1) extract of the aerial parts, administered intraperitoneally to mice at a dose of 0.25 mg/kg, was inactive[JC075].

Irritant activity. Acetone extract of a commercial sample of seeds, at a dose of 1.8 mcg/ear in mice was active, ID_{50} (24 hours). Seed oil, at a dose of 25.0 mcg/ear, produced weak activity, ID_{50} (24 hours)[JC044].

Larvicidal activity. Ethanol (95%) extract of dried fruits and leaves, at a concentration of 100 ppm, was weakly active on *Aedes fluviatilis*[JC021].

Molluscicidal activity. Aqueous slurry (homogenate) of fresh entire plant was inactive on *Lymnaea columella*, $LD_{100} > 1$ M ppm. Aqueous slurry of the fruits, roots and leaves was inactive on *Lymnaea cubensis*, $LD_{100} > 1$ M ppm[JC049]. Methanol extract of dried leaves, at a concentration of 100 ppm, was inactive on *Bulinus globosus*[JC047]. Ethanol (95%) extract of dried fruits and leaves, at a concentration of 100 ppm, was inactive on *Biomphalaria glabrata*.. Hexane extract of the dried fruits and leaves, at a concentration of 100 ppm, was inactive on *Biomphalaria glabrata*[JC031]. Benzene extract of fresh fruit pulp was active on *Oncomelania hupensis*, LD_{50} 40 ppm. Butanol extract of fresh fruit pulp was active on *Oncomelania hupensis*, LD_{50} 45 ppm. Methyl chloride extract of fresh fruit pulp was active on *Oncomelania hupensis quadrasi*, LD_{50} 65 ppm. Water extract of fresh fruit pulp was active on *Oncomelania hupensis*, LD_{50} 50 ppm. Water extract of fresh fruit pulp was active on *Oncomelania hupensis quadrasi*, LD_{50} 18–25 ppm and LD_{90} 27–48 ppm. Methanol extract of fresh fruit pulp was active on *Oncomelania hupensis quadrasi*, LD_{50} 6.7 ppm[JC048]. Ethanol (95%) extract of dried root, at a concentration of 100.0 ppm, was active on *Bulinus truncatus* with 65% mortality. The water extract, at a concentration of 160 ppm, was weakly active, with 50% mortality[JC050]. Methanol extract of dried seedpods, at a concentration of 100.0 ppm, was inactive on *Bulinus globosus*[JC047]. Methanol extract of dried stembark, at a concentration of 100.0 ppm, was inactive on *Bulinus globosus*[JC047].

Semen coagulation. Ethanol/water (1:1) extract of the aerial parts, at a concentration of 2%, was inactive on rats[JC075].

Spasmolytic activity. Butanol extract of dried leaves, at a concentration of 0.2 mg/ml, was active on guinea pig ileum. A 90.45% reduction in contraction was seen, vs ACh-induced contractions. A 28.49% reduction was seen vs KCl-induced contractions. Methanol extract of dried leaves, at a concentration of 0.2 mg/ml, was inactive on guinea pig ileum vs ACh- and KCl-induced contractions[JC039].

Spermicidal effect. Ethanol/water (1:1) extract of the aerial parts was inactive on rats[JC075].

Toxicity assessment (quantitative). Ethanol/water (1:1) extract of the aerial parts, administered intraperitoneally to mice, LD_{50} at 0.5 gm/kg[JC075]. Seed oil, administered intragastrically to rats produced severe diarrhea and gastrointestinal inflammation, LD_{50} 6.0 ml/kg[JC026]. Fresh fruit pulp, administered by gastric intubation at a dose of 10 gm/kg per day for 3 consecutive days, produced 100% mortality. Ten gm/kg, given as a single dose was inactive[JC048]. Water extract of seeds, administered subcutaneously to mice, produced MLD_{50} 300.0 mcg/animal[JC074]. Seed oil, administered subcutaneously to mice, was active, LD_{100} 1.0 ml/animal. The toxic element is destroyed by heat[JC081]. Ethanol (95%),

methanol (70%) and water extracts of dried seeds, administered intraperitoneally to mice at doses of 500.0 mg/kg, produced weak activity and some depression. Seed oil, in the ration of rats at a dose of 15.0% of the diet, was inactive. Roasted seeds, in the ration of rats at a dose of 48.0% of the diet, were active[JC056]. Seeds taken by children mistaken for edible nuts exhibited marked nausea, abdominal pain and vomiting with diarrhea in some patients. Recovery was rapid[JC071]. Dried seeds, fed to chicken in the ration at a concentration of 0.5% of the diet, produced death. Toxic signs included poor growth, locomotor disturbances and dullness. Animals also had hepatic, intestinal and renal lesions and significant increases in serum GOT, SHD, GDH and total protein levels. Other signs included congested heart and blood vessels, intestine and renal cortex, hepatocytes necrosis, erosion of intestinal mucous membranes, degeneration of renal tubular cells and an increase in hepatic and cardiac lipid levels[JC017,JC018]. Water extract of fresh seeds, administered intraperitoneally to mice at a dose of 5.0 mg/kg, produced death within 3 days. Fresh seeds, in the ration of mice at a dose of 25% of the diet, produced death within 11 days[JC030].

REFERENCES

JC001   Suwal, P. N. Medicinal Plants of Nepal. Ministry of Forests, Department of Medicinal Plants, Thapathali, Kathmandu, Nepal, 1970.

JC002   Quisumbing, E. Medicinal plants of the Philippines. **Tech Bull 16**, Rep Philippines, Dept Agr Nat Resources, Manilla 1951; 1.

JC003   Alvaro Viera, R. Subsidio para o Estudo da Flora Medicinal da Guinea Portuguesa. Agencia-Geral do Ultramar, Lisboa, 1959.

JC004   Petelot, A. Les Plantes Medicinales du Cambodge, du Laos et du Vietnam, Vol. 1–4. Archives des Recherches Agronomiques et Pastorales au Vietnam No. 23, 1954.

JC005 Mameesh, M. S., L. M. El-Hakim and A. Hassan. Reproductive failure in female rats fed the fruit or seed of *Jatropha curcas*. **Planta Med** 1963; 11: 98.

JC006 Perrot, E. and P. Hurrier. Matiere Medicale et Pharmacopee Sino-Annamites. Vigot Freres, Edit., Paris, 1907; 292pp.

JC007 Inman, N. Notes on some poisonous plants of Guam. **Micronesica** 1967; 3: 55.

JC008 Hsu, Y. T. Study on the Chinese drugs used as cancer remedy. **J Southeast Asian Res** 1967; 3: 63.

JC009 Jenwanichpanjakul, P., K. Sathapitanondha and S. Mansakul. Studies of chemical and physical properties of physic nut oil. **Science Thailand** 1981; 35(8): 820–823.

JC010 Naengchomnong, W., Y. Thebtaranonth, P. Wiriyachitra, K. T. Okamoto and J. Clardy. Isolation and structure determination of four novel diterpenes from *Jatropha curcas*. **Tetrahedron Lett** 1986; 27(22): 2439–2442.

JC011 Naengchomnong, W., Y. Thebtaranonth, P. Wiriyachitra, K. T. Okamoto and J. Clardy. Isolation and structure determination of two novel lathyranes from *Jatropha curcas*. **Tetrahedron Lett** 1986; 27(47): 5675–5678.

JC012 Chen, M., L. Hou and G. Zhang. The diterpenoids from *Jatropha curcas* L. Chih **Wu Hsueh Pao** 1988; 30(3): 308–311.

JC013 Talapatra, S. K., K. Mandal and B. Talapatra. Jatrocurin, a new tetracyclic triterpene from *Jatropha curcas*. **J Indian Chem Soc** 1993; 70(6): 543–548.

JC014 Bhat, R. B., E. O. Eterjere and V. T. Oladipo. Ethnobotanical studies from Central Nigeria. **Econ Bot** 1990; 44(3): 382–390.

JC015 Khan, M., D. C. Jain, R. S. Bhakuni, M. Zaim and R. S. Thakur. Occurrence of some antiviral sterols in *Artemisa annua*. **Plant Sci** 1991; 75: 161–165.

JC016 Asseleih, L. M. C. and C. H. Aponte. Pinoncillo, *Jatropha curcas*. El Pinoncillo, *Jatropha curcas* Recurso Biotico Silvestre del Tropico 1984: 5–16.

JC017 Badwi, S. M. A., H. M. Mousa, S. Adam and H. Hapke. Response of brown hisex chicks to low levels of *Jatropha curcas*, *Ricinus communis* or their mixture. **Vet Hum Toxicol** 1992; 34(4): 304.

JC018 Samia, M., E. Badwi, S. Adam and H. J. Hapke. Toxic effects of low levels of dietary *Jatropha curcas* seed on brown hisex chicks. **Vet Hum Toxicol** 1992; 34(2): 112–115.

JC019 Qureshi, A., A. Q. Saifi, N. T. Modi, S. S. Rao and N. A. Khan. Proteins and alkaloids of *Jatropha curcas* Linn. **Orient J Chem** 1990; 6(4): 275.

JC020 Reddy, M. B., K. R. Reddy and M. N. Reddy. A survey of plant crude drugs of Anantapur District, Andhra Pradesh, India. **Int J Crude Drug Res** 1989; 27(3): 145–155.

JC021 Consoli, R. A. G. B., N. M. Mendes, J. P. Pereira, B. D. S. Santos and M. A. Lamounier. Larvicidal properties of plant extracts against *Aedes fluviatilis* (Lutz) (Diptera: Culicidae) in the laboratory. **Mem Inst Oswaldo Cruz** (Rio De Janeiro) 1988; 83(1): 87–93.

JC022 Schultes, E. V. and R. F. Raffauf. De plantis toxicariis e mundo novo tropicale commentationes. XXXIX. Febrifuges of Northwest Amazonia. **Harvard Pap in Bot** 1994; 5: 50–68.

JC023 Elisabethsky, E. and Z. C. Castilhos. Plants used as analgesics by Amazonian Caboclos as a basis for selecting plants for investigation. **Int J Crude Drug Res** 1990; 28(4): 309–320.

JC024 Zamora-Martinez, M. C. and C. N. P. Pola. Medicinal plants used in some rural populations of Oaxaca, Puebla and Veracruz, Mexico. **J Ethnopharmacol** 1992; 35(3) 229–257.

JC025 Muanza, D. N., B. W. Kim, K. L. Euler and L. Williams. Antibacterial and antifungal activities of nine medicinal plants from Zaire. **Int J Pharmacog** 1994; 32(4): 337–345.

JC026 Gandhi, V. M., K. M. Cherian and M. J. Mulky. Toxicological studies on ratanjyot oil. **Food Chem Toxicol** 1995; 33(1): 39–42.

JC027 Muanza, D. N., K. L. Euler, L. Williams and D. J. Newman. Screening for anti-tumor and anti-HIV activities of nine medicinal plants from Zaire. **Int J Pharmacog** 1995; 33(2): 98–106.

JC028 Khafagy, S. M., Y. A. Mohamed, N. A. Abdel Salam and Z. F. Mahmoud. Phytochemical study of *Jatropha curcas*. **Planta Med** 1977; 31: 274–277.

JC029   Hufford, C. D. and B. O. Oguntimein. Non-polar constituents of *Jatropha curcas*. **Lloydia** 1978; 41: 161.

JC030   Abdu-Aguye, I., A. Sannusi, R. A. Alafiya-Tayo and S. R. Bhusnurmath. Acute toxicity studies with *Jatropha curcas* L. **Human Toxicol** 1986; 5(4): 269–274.

JC031   Mendes, N. M., N. M. Pereira, C. P. De Souza and M. L. Lima De Oliveira. Preliminary laboratory studies for the verification of molluscicidal activity of several species from the Brazilian flora. **Rev Saude Publ Sao Paulo** 1984; 18: 348–354.

JC032   Asthana, A., H. V. Mall, K. Dixit and S. Gupta. Fungitoxic properties of latex of plants with special reference to that of *Croton bonplandianus* Baill. **Int J Crude Drugs Res** 1989; 27(1): 25–58.

JC033   Le Grand, A. Anti-infectious phytotherapy of the tree-savannah, Senegal (Western Africa) III: A review of the phytochemical substances and antimicrobial activity of 43 species. **J Ethnopharmacol** 1989; 25(3): 315–338.

JC034   Reddy, M. B., K. R. Reddy and M. N. Reddy. A survey of medicinal plants of Chenchu tribes of Andhra Pradesh, India. **Int J Crude Drugs Res** 1988; 26(4): 189–196.

JC035   Comley, J. C. W. New macrofilaricidal leads from plants? **Trop Med Parasitol** 1990; 41(1): 1–9.

JC036   Le Grand, A. and P. A. Wondergem. Antiinfective phytotherapy of the savannah forests of Senegal (West Africa). 1. An inventory. **J Ethnopharmacol** 1987; 21(2): 109–125.

JC037   Nath, L. K. and S. K. Dutta. Extraction and purification of curcain, a protease from the latex of *Jatropha curcas* Linn. **J Pharm Pharmacol** 1991; 43(2): 111–114.

JC038   Nagaraju, N. and K. N. Rao. A survey of plant crude drugs of Rayalaseema, Andhra Pradesh, India. **J Ethnopharmacol** 1990; 29(2): 137–158.

JC039   Kambu, K., L. Tona, S. Kaba, K. Cimanga and N. Mukala. Antispasmodic activity of extracts proceeding of plant antidiarrheic traditional preparations used in Kinshasa, Zaire. **Ann Pharm Fr** 1990; 48(4): 200–208.

JC040   Hussain, H. S. N. and Y. Y. Deeni. Plants in Kano ethnomedicine: Screening for antimicrobial activity and alkaloids. **Int J Pharmacog** 1991; 29(1): 51–56.

JC041   Joshi, P. Herbal drugs used in Guinea worm disease by the tribals of Southern Rajasthan (India). **Int J Pharmacog** 1991; 29(1): 33–38.

JC042   Madulid, D. A., F. J. M. Gaerlan, E. M. Romero and E. M. G. Agoo. Ethnopharmacological study of the Ati tribe in Nagpana, Barotac Viejo, Iloilo. **Acta Manilana** 1989; 38(1): 25–40.

JC043   Naovi, S. A. H., M. S. Y. Khan and S. B. Vohora. Anti-bacterial, anti-fungal and anthelmintic investigations on Indian medicinal plants. **Fitoterapia** 1991; 62(3): 221–228.

JC044   Adolf, W., H. J. Operferkuch and E. Hecker. Irritant phorbol derivatives from four *Jatropha* species. **Phytochemistry** 1984; 23(1): 129–132.

JC045   Adam, S. E. I. Toxicity of indigenous plants and agricultural chemicals in farm animals. **Clin Toxicol** 1978; 13: 269–280.

JC046   Ayensu, E. S. Medicinal Plants of the West Indies. **Unpublished Manuscript** 1978; 110pp.

JC047   Adewunmi, C. O. and V. O. Marquis. Molluscicidal evaluation of some Jatropha species grown in Nigeria. **Q J Crude Drugs Res** 1980; 18: 141–145.

JC048   Yasuraoka, K., J. Hashiguchi and B. L. Blas. Laboratory assessment of the molluscicidal activity of the plant *Jatropha curcas* against *Oncomelania* snail. **Proc Philippine-Japan Joint Conf on Schistosomiasis Res & Control**, Manila, Japan Int Coop Agency 1980; 110–112.

JC049   Medina, F. R. and R. Woodbury. Terrestrial plants molluscicidal to Lymnaeid hosts of *Fasciliasis hepatica* in Puerto Rico. **J Agr Univ Puerto Rico** 1979; 63: 366–376.

JC050   El Kheir, Y. M. and M. S. El Tohami. Investigation of molluscicidal activity of certain Sudanese plants used in folk medicine. I. A preliminary biological screening for molluscicidal activity of certain Sudanese plants used in folk medicine. **J Trop Med Hyg** 1979; 82: 237–241.

JC051 Meyer, B. N., N. R. Ferrigni, J. E. Putnam, L. B. Jacobsen, D. E. Nichols and J. L. McLaughlin. Brine shrimp: A convenient general bioassay for active plant constituents. **Planta Med** 1982; 45: 31–34.

JC052 Iwu, M. M. and B. N. Anyanwu. Phytotherapeutic profile of Nigerian herbs. 1. Antiinflammatory and anti-arthritic agents. **J Ethnopharmacol** 1982; 6(3): 263–274.

JC053 Ferrigni, N. I., J. E. Putnam, B. Anderson, L. B. Jacobsen, D. E. Nichols, D. S. Moore, J. L. McLaughlin, R. G. Powell and C. R. Smith Jr. Modification and evaluation of the potato disc assay and antitumor screening of Euphorbiaceae seeds. **J Nat Prod** 1982; 45: 679–686.

JC054 Adesina, S. K. Studies on some plants used as anticonvulsants in Amerindian and African traditional medicine. **Fitoterapia** 1982; 53: 147–162.

JC055 Martinez, M. A. Medicinal plants used in a Totonac community of the Sierra Norte de Puebla. Tuzamapan de Galeana, Puebla, Mexico. **J Ethnopharmacol** 1984; 11(2): 203–221.

JC056 Panigrahi, S., B. J. Francis, L. A. Cano, M. B. Burbage. Toxicity of *Jatropha curcas* seeds from Mexico to rats and mice. **Nutr Rep Int** 1984. 29(5): 1089–1099.

JC057 Singh, Y. N., T. Ikahihifo, M. Panuve and C. Slatter. Folk medicine in Tonga. A study of the use of herbal medicines for obstetric and gynaecological conditions and disorders. **J Ethnopharmacol** 1984; 12(3): 305–329.

JC058 Van Den Berg, M. A. Ver-o-Peso: The ethnobotany of an Amazonian market. Advances in Economic Botany Ethnobotany in the Neotropics, G. T. Prance and J. A. Kallunki (Eds) New York Botanical Garden, Bronx, New York 1984; 1: 140–149.

JC059 Arnold, H. J. and M. Gulumian. Pharmacopoeia of traditional medicine in Venda. **J Ethnopharmacol** 1984; 12(1): 35–74.

JC060 Adewunmi, C. O. and V. O. Marquis. A rapid In Vitro screening method for detecting schistosomicidal activity of some Nigerian medicinal plants. **Int J Crude Drug Res** 1983; 21(4): 157–159.

JC061 Sahu, T. R. Less known uses of weeds as medicinal plants. **Ancient Sci Life** 1984; 3(4): 245–249.

JC062 Tiwari, K. C., R. Majumder and S. Bhattacharjee. Folklore medicines from Assam and Arunachal Pradesh (District Tirap). **Int J Crude Res** 1979; 17(2): 61–67.

JC063 Singh, Y. N. Traditional medicine in Fiji. Some herbal folk cures used by Fiji Indians. **J Ethnopharmacol** 1986; 15(1): 57–88.

JC064 Anderson, E. F. Ethnobotany of Hill Tribes of Northern Thailand. 1. Medicinal plants of Akha. **Econ Bot** 1986; 40(1): 38–53.

JC065 Anderson, E. F. Ethnobotany of Hill tribes of Northern Thailand. II. Lahu medicinal plants. **Econ Bot** 1986; 40(4): 442–450.

JC066 Weniger, B., M. Rouzier, R. Daguilh, D. Henrys, J. H. Henrys and R. Anthon. Popular medicine of the Central Plateau of Haiti. 2. Ethnopharmacological inventory. **J Ethnopharmacol** 1986; 17(1): 13–30.

JC067 Biehl. J. and E. Hecker. Irritant and antineoplastic principles of some species of the genus Jatropha (Euphorbiaceae). **34th Annual Congress on Medicinal Plant Research** Hamburg, Sept 22–27, 1986; 5: K31.

JC068 Le Grand, A., P. A. Wondergem, R. Verpoorte and J. L. Pousset. Anti-infectious phytotherapies of the tree-savannah of Senegal (West Africa). II. Antimicrobial activity of 33 species. **J Ethnophmarmacol** 1988; 22(1): 25–31.

JC069 Ramirez, V. R., L. J. Mostacero, A. E. Garcia, C. F. Mejia, P. F. Pelaez, C. D. Medina and C. H. Miranda. Vegetales empleados en medicina tradicional Norperuana. **Banco Agrario Del Peru & NACL Univ**, Trujillo, Peru, June 1988; 54pp.

JC070 Kone-Bamba, D., Y. Pelissier, Z. F. Ozoukou and D. Kouao. Hemostatic activity of 216 plants used in traditional medicine in the Ivory Coast. **Plant Med Phytother** 1987; 21(2): 122–130.

JC071 Mampane, K. J., P. H. Joubert and I. T. Hay. *Jatropha curcas*: Use as a traditional Tswana medicine and its role as a cause of acute poisoning. **Phytother Res** 1987; 1(1): 50,51.

JC072 Macrae, W. D., J. B. Hudson and G. H. N. Towers. Studies on the pharmacological activity of Amazonian Euphorbiaceae. **J Ethnopharmacol** 1988; 22(2): 143–172.

JC073 Padilla, S. P. and F. A. Soliven. Chemical analysis form possible sources of oils of forty-five species of oil-bearing seeds. **Philippine Agr** 1933; 22: 408–.

JC074 Mourgue, M., J. Delphaut, R. Baret and R. Kassab. Study of toxicity and localization of the toxalbumin (curcin) of the seeds of *Jatropha curcas*. **Bull Soc Chim Biol** 1961; 43: 517.

JC075 Dhawan, B. N., G. K. Patnaik, R. P. Rastogi, K. K. Singh and J. S. Tandon. Screening of Indian plants for biological activity. VI. **Indian J Exp Biol** 1977; 15: 208–219.

JC076 Friese, F. W. Certain little-known anthelmintics from Brazil. **Apoth ZTG** 1929; 44: 180.

JC077 Oakes, A. J. and M. P. Morris. The West Indian weedwoman of the United States Virgin Islands. **Bull Hist Med** 1958; 32: 164.

JC078 Logan, M. H. Digestive disorders and plant medicine in Highland Guatemala. **Anthropos** 1973; 68: 537–543.

JC079 Subramanian, S. S. , S. Nagarajan and N. Sulochana. Flavonoids of some euphorbiaceous plants. **Phytochemistry** 1971; 10: 2548–2549.

JC080 Roig y Mesa, J. T. Plantas Medicinales, Aromaticas o Venemosas de Cuba. Ministerio de Agricultura, Republica de Cuba, Havana. 1945: 872pp.

JC081 Heim, F and Rullier. The toxic principles of the seed and oil of the physic-nut tree (*Jatropha curcas* L.). **Bull Del Office Colonial** 1919; 12: 96–110.

JC082 Matsuse, I. T., Y. A. Lim, M. Hattori, M. Correa and M. P. Gupta. A search of anti-viral properties in Panamanian medicinal plants. The effects on HIV and its essential enzymes. **J Ethnopharmacol** 1999; 64(1): 15–22.

JC083 Liu, S. Y., F. Sporer, M. Wink, J. Jourdane, R. Henning, Y. L. Li and A. Ruppel. Anthraquinones in *Rheum palmatum* and *Rumex dentatus* (Polygonaceae), and phorbol esters in *Jatropa curcas* (Euphorbiaceae) with molluscicidal activity against the schistosome vector snails *Oncomelania*, Biophalaria and Bulinus. **Trop Med Int Health** 1997; 2(2): 179–188.

JC084 Fagbenro-Beyioku, A. F., W. A. Oyibo and B. C. Anuforom. Disinfectant/antiparasitic activities of *Jatropa curcas*. **East Afr Med J** 1998; 75(9): 508–511.

JC085 Mujumdar, A. M., A. S. Upadhye and A. V. Misar. Studies on antidiarrheal activity of *Jatropa curcas* root extract in albino mice. **J Ethnopharmacol** 2000; 70(2): 183–187.

15 | Lantana camara L.

Gaertn.

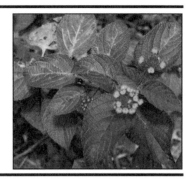

Common Names

Ach man	Guatemala	Mvuti	Tanzania
Aruppu	India	Orozus	Mexico
Big sage	West Indies	Orozuz	Mexico
Bonboye	West Indies	Panj phuli	India
Bunchberry	India	Pasarin	Panama
Bunga taya ayam	Guatemala	Pasarrion	Panama
Camara	Brazil	Pha-ka-krong	Guatemala
Camara	Canary Islands	Phakaa drong	Thailand
Cambara de espinto	Guatemala	Phakas krong	Thailand
Cariaquita	Colombia	Pink-edge red lantana	Australia
Cariaquito	West Indies	Prickly lantana	Guatemala
Carraquillo	Colombia	Ramtana	Guatemala
Cidreirarana	Brazil	Sanguinaria	Colombia
Common lantana	China	Siete negritos	Guatemala
Cuasquito	Guatemala	Skastajat stuki	Mexico
Cuencas de oro	Puerto Rico	Sweet sage	Guyana
Frutilla	Mexico	Talatala	Guatemala
Gandheriya	India	Tembelekan	Guatemala
Gurupacha	Colombia	Ti–plomb	West Indies
Hedge flower	Thailand	Tshidzimbambule	Venda
Kayakit	West Indies	Venturosa	Canary Islands
Kiwepe	Tanzania	Venturosa	Colombia
Lantana	Australia	Verveine	West Indies
Lantana	India	Vielle fille	Rodrigues Islands
Large leaf lantana	Guatemala	White sage	Guatemala
Latora moa	Guatemala	White sage	West Indies
Maviyakuku	Rwanda	Wild sage	India
Mille fleurs	West Indies	Yellow sage	Guatemala
Mkinda	Tanzania	Wild sage	West Indies

From: *Medicinal Plants of the World, vol. 1: Chemical Constituents, Traditional and Modern Medicinal Uses, 2nd ed.*
By: Ivan A. Ross © Humana Press Inc., Totowa, NJ

BOTANICAL DESCRIPTION

This is an erect, branching shrub of the VERBENACEAE family, 0.5 to 2 m high. Stems are 4-angled, armed with hooked prickles. Leaves opposite, blade ovate, 4 to 10 cm long, with coarse surfaces and toothed margins. Flowers are dense, long-stalked, flat-topped, head-like, axillary spikes about 2.5-cm across. The corolla is sympetalous, with a curved tube and a spreading limb about 8 mm wide; yellow, orange, red or pink in color. Fruit is a shiny, dark purple or black, globose drupe, 5 to 6 mm wide.

ORIGIN AND DISTRIBUTION

A native of tropical America, it is now a weed throughout the tropics, especially in coconut plantations, pastures and wastes areas. The natural distribution now extends northwards to Texas and South Carolina. It has become naturalized in many places, and forms impenetrable thickets in Ceylon and Indonesia.

TRADITIONAL MEDICINAL USES

Australia. Fresh fruit is eaten as a food. Mashed fresh leaves are applied to the skin to treat neurodermatitis, eczema, rashes, psoriasis, tinea, chicken pox, boils and bites, and to stop bleeding in traumatic injuries. Infusion is taken orally to treat whooping cough, catarrh, pulmonary problems and epidemic parotiditis, and to reduce fever. Decoction is used to treat aphids. Five hundred gm of leaves is boiled in 1 liter of water, strained and applied by spray[LC021].

Brazil. Decoction of dried aerial parts is used externally as a treatment for mange[LC087]. Decoction of dried leaves is taken orally for malaria, fevers, colds, and headache, and as a tonic and febrifuge[LC087,LC014,LC017]. Dried plant is given orally to cows to treat mange[LC020].

Canary Islands. Infusion of the dried aerial parts is taken orally by pregnant women as an abortifacient[LC075].

Colombia. Decoction of hot water extract of the entire plant is taken orally to facilitate childbirth. Infusion of the hot water extract is taken orally as an emmenagogue[LC001]. Hot water extract of dried entire plant is taken orally as an emmenagogue[LC083].

East Africa. Ash from dried leaves is mixed with salt and taken orally for sore throat, cough and toothache. Leaves are chewed for toothache. Vapor of boiling leaves is inhaled for headache and colds. Hot water extract of dried leaves is taken orally as a diaphoretic and stimulant and for jaundice, chest diseases and rheumatism. Fresh fruit is said to be toxic to children, although there is disagreement. Hot water extract of dried root is taken orally as a febrifuge and for malaria, including quinine-resistant cases. Toxicity has been reported in sheep and cattle[LC074].

Guatemala. Decoction of dried leaves is taken orally to treat rheumatism. A decoction of *Lantana camara* and *Slaix chilensis* is used. The decoction is also taken orally to treat constipation and eczema. Infusion of dried leaves is taken orally as a tonic and stimulant[LC021]. Hot water extract is used externally for wounds, ulcers, bruises, sores and infections of the skin and mucosa[LC084].

India. Ash of the entire plant is used externally for chronic ulcers[LC064]. Fresh leaves, when ingested, are reported to cause photodermatitis and possibly death in domestic animals[LC035]. Water extract of fresh leaves is applied to the eye for eye injuries[LC040].

Indonesia. Decoction of fresh root is taken orally to treat gonorrhea and leukorrhea. Pounded fresh leaves are applied to the skin to treat boils. Leaves are taken orally to treat intestinal spasm and as an emetic. Infusion is taken orally to treat rheumatism and as a diaphoretic. Tincture of fresh bark is taken orally as a tonic. Water extract of fresh flowers is given orally to children to treat cough[LC021]. Crushed leaves are applied on wounds[LC071]. Hot water extract of leaves is taken orally as a diaphoretic, carminative and antiseptic[LC085].

Kenya. Dried stem is used as toothbrush[LC037].

Mexico. Dried leaves, boiled with barley, are given orally to women in childbirth. The decoction is taken orally to relieve indigestion, to treat rheumatism, as a stomach tonic and to treat snakebite (poultice of crushed leaves is applied to the wound)[LC021]. The whole plant is rubbed with cold water to treat chills[LC018]. Water extract of fresh root is taken orally for dysentery, gastrointestinal pain, toothache, uterine hemorrhage and excess menstrual discharge. Water extract of fresh shoots is taken orally for rashes. The extract is used medicinally for "magical" illnesses comprising a variety of physiological illnesses and symptoms[LC070]. Infusion of dried fruits and leaves is taken orally for coughs[LC062]. Decoction of the leaf is taken orally as an appetizer and as a vomitive[LC018].

Nigeria. Infusion of fresh leaves and root is taken orally as an antiasthmatic, tonic and anticonvulsant. Hot water extract of the fresh leaves and root is taken orally as an anticonvulsant[LC059].

Panama. Decoction of dried leaves is taken orally to treat colds and stomach afflictions[LC021]. Extract of the entire plant is taken orally for digestive disorders. For skin diseases, decoction of the whole plant in warm water is applied to the affected skin areas[LC049].

Rwanda. Decoction of dried leaves is taken orally for malaria[LC045].

Southeast Asia. Pounded dried leaves are applied to the skin as a treatment for cuts and swelling. Lotion is prepared from pounded leaves to treat rheumatism. Infusion of the dried leaves is taken orally to treat bilious fevers (usually has emetic effect)[LC021].

Surinam. Infusion of dried entire plant is used as an herbal bath[LC021].

Tanzania. Decoction of dried root is taken orally for stomachache and vomiting. A grain of another plant species is added. Water extract is used externally for itching and rashes[LC074]. Fresh leaves are used in traditional medicine[LC072].

Thailand. Decoction of dried entire plant is taken orally for asthma. Crushed roasted leaves are used as a poultice for anti-inflammatory affections[LC088].

Tonga. Fresh leaf juice is applied to cuts to prevent infection[LC021].

USA. Extract of the plant is taken orally as a carminative[LC021].

Venda. Fresh leaves, macerated in cold water for several hours to 2 days, are used as an eye drop for eye injury[LC068].

Venezuela. Hot water extract of dried stem is taken orally as an emmenagogue[LC083].

Vietnam. Leaf tea is taken orally as an emmenagogue[LC005].

West Africa. Infusion of dried leaves is taken orally to treat coughs and colds, jaundice and chest pains, as a diaphoretic, stimulant and in bath for rheumatism[LC021].

West Indies. Hot water extract of leaves is taken orally as a common remedy for dysmenorrhea[LC002,LC048] and fever[LC048]. Decoction of dried leaves is taken orally for cough, flu and indigestion[LC078].

CHEMICAL CONSTITUENTS
(ppm unless otherwise indicated)

1-Triacontanol: Lf[LC097]

3-Ketoursolic acid: Lf[LC095]

8-Epi-loganin: Rt 70[LC007]

3-Beta,19-alpha dihydroxy ursan-28-oic acid: Rt[LC106]

21,22-Beta-epoxy-3-beta-hydroxy olean-12-en-28-oic acid: Rt[LC106]

22-Beta-hydroxyoleanonic acid: Lf[LC103]

Ajugose: Rt 0.19%[LC007]

Alpha amyrin: Lf, St[LC096]

Arachidic acid: Aer[LC097]

Beta sitosterol: Lf[LC097]

Camaric acid: Aer 0.119%[LC010]

Camarinic acid: Aer 11.6[LC010]

Camaroside: Lf 0.0181%[LC009]

Cineole: Lf[LC097]

Citral: Lf[LC097]
Diodantunezone: Rt[LC039]
Dipentene: Lf[LC097]
Eugenol: Lf[LC097]
Furfural: Lf[LC097]
Geniposide: Rt[LC007]
Geraniol: Lf[LC097]
Glucose: Aer[LC097]
Glycine: Lf[LC028]
Icterogenin: Lf[LC009]
Iso–diodantunezone: Rt[LC039]
Lamiridoside: Rt[LC007]
Lancamarone: Lf[LC094]
Lantadene A: Lf 0.3–0.7%[LC103,LC009,LC051]
Lantadene B: Lf 0.2%[LC103,LC093]
Lantadene C: Lf[LC100,LC103]
Lantadene D: Lf[LC103]
Lantaiursolic acid: Rt 24[LC008]
Lantanilic acid: Pl[LC010]
Lantanolic acid: Lf[LC099]
Lantanone: Aer[LC107]
Lantanoside: Aer[LC107]
Lantanose A: Rt 310[LC007]
Lantanose B: Rt 94[LC007]
Lantic acid: Lf[LC098]
Lantoic acid: Lf[LC006]
Leucine: Lf[LC028]
Linalool: Lf[LC097]
Linaroside: Aer[LC107]
Linoleic acid: Aer[LC097]
Maltose: Aer[LC097]
Methyl-3-oxo-ursolate: Lf[LC098]
Myristic acid: Aer[LC097]
Oleanolic acid: Aer 57[LC010]
Oleanonic acid: Lf 0.0241%[LC009]
Oleic acid: Aer[LC097]
Palmitic acid: Aer[LC097]
Phellandrene: Lf[LC097]
Phellandrone: Lf[LC097]
Pomolic acid: Aer 9.5[LC010]
Rhamnose: Aer[LC097]
Stachyose: Rt 0.0695[LC007]
Terpineol: Lf[LC097]
Theveside: Rt 14–900[LC007,LC023], Lf 800[LC023]
Theviridoside: Rt 320–500[LC023,LC007]
Tyrosine: Lf[LC028]
Valine: Lf[LC097]
Verbascose: Rt 0.081%[LC007]
Verbascoside: Pl[LC043]
Verbascotetracose: Rt 0.043%[LC007]

PHARMACOLOGICAL ACTIVITIES AND CLINICAL TRIALS

Acid phosphatase stimulation. Dried leaves, administered to guinea pigs by gastric intubation, were active[LC026].

Analgesic activity. Ethanol (95%) extract of leaves, administered intraperitoneally to rats, was only active with high doses[LC046].

Aniline hydroxylase induction. Dried leaves, administered to guinea pigs by gastric intubation at a dose of 2.0 gm/kg, were inactive[LC063].

Antibacterial activity. Decoction of dried leaves, in broth culture, was inactive on *Bacillus subtilis*, *Klebsiella pneumonia*, *Proteus vulgaris*, *Pseudomonas aeruginosa*, *Salmonella typhi*, *Sarcina lutea*, *Staphylococcus albus*, *Staphylococcus aureus*, and *Streptococcus mutans*[LC030]. Essential oil, on agar plate, was inactive on *Bacillus cereus*, *Escherichia coli*, *Pseudomonas aeruginosa*, and *Staphylococcus aureus*[LC081]. Ethanol (70%) extract of root, at a concentration of 100.0 mg/ml in broth culture, was inactive on *Bacillus subtilis* and *Escherichia coli*[LC047]. Fresh essential oil, at undiluted concentration on agar plate, was active on *Pseudomonas aeruginosa* and *Staphylococcus aureus*. The oil was inactive on *Bacillus cereus* and *Escherichia coli*[LC061]. Leaf essential oil, at undiluted concentration on agar plate, was active on *Bacillus subtilis*, zone of inhibition 13.0 mm; *Escherichia coli*, zone of inhibition 9.5 mm and *Sarcina lutea*, zone of inhibition 12.0 mm; and produced weak activity on *Staphylococcus aureus*, zone of inhibition 2.5 mm[LC050]. Petroleum ether extract of dried leaves, in broth culture, was active on *Salmonella typhi*, MIC 0.63 mg/ml; *Bacillus subtilis*, MIC 1.25 mg/ml and *Sarcina lutea*, MIC 1.25 mg/ml. The extract was inactive on *Klebsiella pneumoniae*, *Proteus vulgaris*, *Pseudomonas aeruginosa*, *Staphylococcus albus*, *Staphylococcus aureus*, and *Streptococcus mutans*[LC030]. Saline extract of leaves, at a concentration of 1:10 on agar plate, was active on *Staphylococcus aureus*[LC089]. Tincture of dried leaves (10 gm of leaves in 100 ml ethanol), at a concentration of 0.1 ml/disk on agar plate, was active on *Bacillus subtilis*. The tincture was inactive on *Proteus vulgaris*, *Pseudomonas aeruginosa*, *Salmonella typhi*, *Shigella flexneri*, *Staphylococcus aureus*, and *Streptococcus pyogenes*. At 30 ml/disk, the tincture was active on *Pseudomonas aeruginosa* and inactive on *Escherichia coli*[LC084]. Water extract of fresh leaves, at a concentration of 1.0% on agar plate, was inactive on *Neisseria gonorrhea*[LC072].

Anticonvulsant activity. Ethanol (70%) extract of fresh leaves, administered intraperitoneally to mice of both sexes at variable dosage levels, was active vs metrazole- and strychnine-induced convulsions[LC059].

Antifungal activity (plant pathogen). Ethanol (70%) extract of root, at a concentration of 100.0 mcg/ml in broth culture, was inactive on *Penicillium crustosum*[LC047]. Water extract of fresh leaves, at a concentration of 1.0%, was active on *Aspergillus niger* vs rot of tomato fruits caused by *Aspergillus niger* and aggravated by *Drosophila bucksii*[LC082]. Water extract of fresh shoots, at undiluted concentration on agar plate, was inactive on *Helminthosporium turcicum*[LC090].

Antifungal activity. Dried leaves, undiluted on agar plate, were active on *Aspergillus fumigatus* and *Aspergillus niger*[LC076]. Essential oil, at undiluted concentration on agar plate, was active on *Alternaria* species, *Aspergillus candidus*, *Aspergillus flavus*, *Aspergillus nidulans*, *Aspergillus niger*, *Cladosporium herbarum*, *Cunninghamella echinulata*, *Helminthosporium sacchariii*, *Microsporum gypseum*, *Mucor mucedo*, *Penicillum digitatum*, *Rhizopus nigricans*, *Trichophyton rubrum*, and *Trichothecium roseum*. No activity was observed for *Fusarium oxysporum* and *Aspergillus fumigatus*[LC015]. Essential oil, on agar plate, was inactive on *Trichoderma viride*, *Aspergillus aegyptiacus*, and *Penicillium cyclopium*[LC081]. Ethanol/water (1:1) extract

of dried seeds, at a concentration of 10%/disk on agar plate, was inactive on *Aspergillus niger*[LC066]. Fresh essential oil, at undiluted concentration on agar plate, was inactive on *Penicillium cyclopium*, *Trichoderma viride*, and *Aspergillus aegyptiacus*[LC061]. Methanol extract of dried leaves, at a concentration of 0.03% on agar plate, was inactive on *Trichophyton mentagrophytes*[LC058]. Water extract of fresh leaves, at a concentration of 1:1 on agar plate, was active on *Fusarium oxysporum* F. Sp. Lentis. The extract represented 1 gm dried leaf in 1.0 ml water[LC019].

Antihemorrhagic activity. Dried leaves, applied externally on wounds, as a paste, were effective on 80% of the cases. Leaves, taken orally by human adults, checked bleeding in 94% of the cases of rectal and 100% of nasal bleeding[LC077].

Antimalarial activity. Chloroform extract of dried root bark, produced weak activity on *Plasmodium falciparum*, IC_{50} 49.0 mcg/ml. The methanol extract was inactive, IC_{50} 499.0 mcg/ml and the petroleum ether extract was active, IC_{50} 10.0 mcg/ml vs hypoxanthine uptake by plasmodia[LC034].

Antimutagenic activity. Methanol extract of dried leaves, at a concentration of 50.0 microliters/disk on agar plate, was inactive on *Escherichia coli* B/R–WP2–TRP[LC069].

Antimycoplasmal activity. Petroleum ether extract and decoction of dried leaves, in broth culture, were inactive on *Mycoplasma hominis* and *Mycoplasma pneumoniae*[LC030].

Antitrichomonal activity. Methanol extract of dried leaves, at a concentration of 1.0 mg/ml, was inactive on *Trichomonas vaginalis*[LC045]. Dried leaves, undiluted on agar plate, were active on *Candida vaginalis*[LC076]. Ethanol (70%) extract of root, at a concentration of 100.0 mcg/ml in broth culture, was inactive on *Saccharomyces cerevisiae*[LC047]. Methanol extract of dried leaves, at a concentration of 0.03% on agar plate, was inactive on *Candida albicans*[LC058]. Petroleum ether extract and decoction of dried leaves, in broth culture, were inactive on *Candida albicans, Candida tropicalis,* and *Saccharomyces cerevisae*[LC030].

ATPase(mg++) stimulation. Dried leaves, administered by gastric intubation to guinea pigs at a dose of 2.0 gm/kg, were equivocal, results significant at $P < 0.001$ level[LC063]. At daily dosing for 3 days, the activity was positive[LC056].

ATPase(Na+/Ca++) stimulation. Dried leaves, administered to guinea pigs by gastric intubation at a dose of 2.0 gm/kg, were active, results significant at $P < 0.001$ level[LC063].

Bile lithogenic suppression. Leaves, administered orally to ewe at a dose of 100.0 gm/animal, were active[LC013].

Bronchodilator activity. Hot water extract of dried leaves, administered intravenously to guinea at a dose of 1.5 ml/animal, was inactive[LC042].

Cathepsin B induction. Dried leaves, administered by gastric intubation to guinea pigs, were active[LC026].

CNS depressant activity. Ethanol (70%) extract of fresh leaves, administered intraperitoneally to mice of both sexes at variable dosage levels, was active[LC059]. Ethanol (95%) extract of leaves, administered intraperitoneally to mice, was active[LC046].

Cholestatic effect. Powdered leaf, administered orally to guinea pigs at a dose of 6 gm/kg body weight, elicited cholestasis. Liver homogenate, bile, gall bladder, blood, urine, gastrointestinal tract content, and feces were analyzed for the principal hepatotoxin in the leaves (lantadene A), its congeners and biotransformation products. Lantadenes could not be detected but the reduced lantadenes A and B and 2 unidentified metabolites were detected in the contents of the lower gastrointestinal tract and feces[LC108].

Cytochrome C reductase inhibition. Dried leaves, administered to guinea pigs by gastric intubation at a dose of 2.0 gm/kg, were equivocal[LC063].

Cytochrome oxidase induction. Dried leaves, administered by gastric intubation to guinea pigs at a dose of 2.0 gm/kg, were active when dosed daily for 3 days[LC056].

Cytochrome P-450 induction. Dried leaves, administered by gastric intubation to guinea pigs at a dose of 2.0 gm/kg, were inactive[LC063].

Dermatitis producing effect. Dried leaves, applied externally on a 50-year-old patient with recurrent contact dermatitis, were active. The patient was patch tested to determine sensitivity[LC036]. Ethanol (95%) extract of fresh leaves, administered by gastric intubation to rats at a dose of 2.0 mg/kg, was active. The rats developed photodermatitis within 3 minutes of being exposed to sunlight[LC035]. Fresh leaves, used externally on human adults, was active vs patch test, 1.82% of 207 patients were sensitive[LC080].

Enzyme activity. Dried entire plant, administered to guinea pigs, was active on acid phosphatase stimulation, results significant at $P < 0.01$ levels The plant was inactive on alkaline phosphatase stimulation and inhibition; active on BUN raising effect and glutamate dehydrogenase stimulation, results significant at $P < 0.01$ level; glutamate oxaloacetate transaminase stimulation, results significant at $P < 0.01$ level; glutamate pyruvate transaminase inhibition, results significant at $P < 0.05$ level; lactate dehydrogenase stimulation, results significant at $P < 0.01$ level and sorbitol dehydrogenase stimulation, results significant at $P < 0.01$ level[LC073]. Dried leaves, administered by gastric intubation to guinea pigs at a dose of 2.0 gm/kg, were equivocal on NADH–ferricyanide reductase inhibition, results significant at $P < 0.001$ level[LC063]. There was an increase in the activity of glucokinase, and aldolase in the hepatic postmitochondrial fraction[LC026]. At daily dosing for three days, glutamate dehydrogenase stimulation was active[LC056]. The dose was active on glutathione-S-transferase induction[LC063].

Gall bladder paralysis. Entire plant, administered orally to ewe at a dose of 600.0 gm/animal, was active[LC024].

Glucose-6-Phosphatase inhibition. Dried leaves, administered by gastric intubation to guinea pigs at a dose of 2.0 gm/kg, were active[LC026].

Glutamate oxaloacetate transaminase stimulation. Dried leaves, administered by gastric intubation to cows at a dose of 6.0 gm/kg, were active[LC101].

Hair inhibition effect. Dried shoots, administered orally to guinea pigs at a dose of 20.0 gm/kg, were active. The animals developed alopecia[LC051].

Hematopoietic activity. Dried entire plant increased the number of erythrocytes and leukocytes, results significant at $P < 0.01$ level[LC073].

Hemotoxic activity. Dried leaves, administered by gastric intubation to ewe, were active. They decreased the blood's ability to coagulate[LC067].

Hepatotoxic activity. Dried aerial parts, administered orally to buffalo, cow, ewe and guinea pigs, produced obstructive jaundice, photosensitization and rise in serum glutamic oxaloacetic transaminase activity as well as histopathological changes in different organs of ewe, histopathological changes in liver and kidneys in cows and histopathological changes in various organs in guinea pigs[LC057]. Dried entire plant, in the ration of cow, was active[LC037]. Dried flowers, administered orally to guinea pigs at a dose of 20.0 gm/kg, were inactive[LC051]. Dried leaves, in the ration of cows, were active. The chief signs were photosensitization and jaundice. Dried leaves, administered by gastric intubation to cows at a dose of 6.0 gm/kg, were active. Serum bilirubin increased and au-

topsy showed liver damage[LC101]. A dose of 2.0 gm/kg, administered by gastric intubation to guinea pigs, produced a decrease in protein content of hepatic microsomes and in the ratios of phospho-lipid:protein and chol-esterol:protein[LC063]. Dosing guinea pigs daily for 3 days decreased the dry weights of DNA, RNA and protein content of liver at necropsy[LC053]. When administered orally to guinea pigs at a dose of 6.0 gm/kg, serum bilirubin increased markedly. Dried shoots, administered orally to guinea pigs at a dose of 20.0 gm/kg, were inactive[LC051]. Leaves, administered orally to ewe at a dose of 200.0 gm/animal, were active[LC025].

Hypertensive activity. Ethanol (95%) extract of leaves, administered intravenously to dogs, was active[LC046].

Hypotensive activity. Alkaloid fraction of dried leaves, administered intravenously to dogs, produced acceleration of respiration and "shivering"[LC092]. Ethanol (95%) extract of leaves, administered intraperitoneally to mice, was active[LC046].

Immunosuppressant activity. Powdered dried leaves, administered orally to sheep at a dose of 200.0 mg/kg, were active. Sheep showed suppression of both cellular and humoral immunity[LC041].

Insect repellent activity. Water extract of fresh leaves, at a concentration of 1.0%, was active vs rot of tomato fruits caused by *Aspergillus niger* and aggravated by *Drosophila bucksii*[LC082].

Insecticidal activity. Petroleum ether extract of dried leaves, at a concentration of 1.0 gm/liter, was inactive on *Lutzomyia longipalpis*[LC044]. Ethanol (95%) and petroleum ether extracts of dried plant, at concentrations of 50.0 mcg, were inactive on *Rhodnius neglectus*[LC020]. Petroleum ether extract of the entire plant, at a concentration of 100.0 ppm, was active on *Culex quinquefasciatus* producing 42% mortality[LC065]. The essential oil, at concentrations of 0.063, 0.125, 0.250 and 0.500% (v/w) on maize grain, was active.

Twenty 7-day old adult weevils (*Sitophilus zeamais*) were fed the grains treated with essential oil and with out as control. Significant insect mortality was obtained with the essential oil. The mortality increased with the concentration of the essential oil and the duration of exposure. The LD_{50} was 0.16%[LC105].

Juvenile hormone activity. Dried leaves were active on *Dysdercus koenigii*[LC054].

Lactate dehydrogenase stimulation. Dried leaves, administered by gastric intubation to guinea pigs, were active[LC026].

Lipid peroxide formation inhibition. Dried leaves, administered to guinea pigs in the ration, were active[LC060].

Liver effects. Ethanol (95%) extract of fresh leaves, administered to rats by gastric intubation at a dose of 1.0 gm/kg, was active. Bromosulphalein was injected into the rats and excretion by the liver into bile was measured. Excretion was affected indicating impaired liver function[LC035].

Molluscicidal activity. Aqueous homogenate of the fresh entire plant was inactive on *Lymnaea columella* and *Lymnaea cubensis*. Fruits, leaves and roots were tested[LC055]. Ethanol (80%) extract, at a concentration of 200.0 mg/liter, was inactive on *Biomphalaria pfeifferi* and *Bulinus truncatus*[LC038]. Ethanol (95%) and water extracts of dried stem bark, at concentrations of 1000 ppm, produced weak activities on *Biomphalaria glabrata* and *Biomphalaria straminea*[LC091]. Powdered dried leaves, at a concentration of 10,000 ppm, produced weak activity[LC079].

Molting activity (insect). Dried leaves were active on *Dysdercus koenigii*[LC054].

NADH reductase stimulation. Dried leaves, administered by gastric intubation to guinea pigs at a dose of 2.0 gm/kg, were active when dosed daily for 3 days[LC056].

NADPH-cytochrome C reductase stimulation. Dried leaves, administered by gastric intubation to guinea pigs at a dose of 2.0 gm/kg, were equivocal[LC063].

Nematicidal activity. Lantanoside, linaroside and Camarinic acid were tested against root knot nematode *Meloidogyne incognita* and showed 90, 85, and 100% mortality, respectively, at 1.0% concentration. The result was comparable to those obtained with the conventional nematicide furadan (100% mortality at 1.0% concentration)[LC107].

Nephrotoxic activity. Dried leaves, administered by gastric intubation to guinea pigs at a dose of 2.0 gm/kg daily for 3 days, decreased the dry weight of DNA, RNA and protein of kidneys at necropsy[LC053].

Nucleotidase inhibition. Dried leaves, administered by gastric intubation to guinea pigs at a dose of 2.0 gm/kg, were equivocal[LC063].

Pharmacokinetics. Dried aerial parts, administered to ewe intraruminally at a dose of 4.0 gm/kg, indicated that most of the toxin was retained in the rumen. It was readily absorbed in the small intestine, as well as the stomach and large intestine[LC027].

Pheromone (insect sex attractant). Ether extract of leaves and twigs was active on male Mediterranean fruit fly and equivocal on *Aspiculurus tetraptera*, male and female *Dacus dorsalis* and male and female melon fly[LC011].

Pheromone (insect sex attractant and signaling). Ether extract of the aerial parts was active on *Dacus dorsalis* (male) and equivocal on *Aspiculurus tetraptera*, *Dacus dorsalis* (female), Mediterranean fruit fly (male) and melon fly[LC011].

Pheromone (signaling). Ether extract of leaves and twigs was active on male Mediterranean fruit fly and equivocal on *Aspiculurus tetraptera*, *Dacus dorsalis* (females and males), and melon fly (males and females)[LC011].

Photosensitizer activity. Aerial parts, in the ration of livestock, were active[LC016]. Dried leaves, in the ration of cows, were active[LC102].

Plant germination inhibition. Chloroform extract of dried leaves was equivocal vs *Amaranthus spinosus* (13% inhibition)[LC052].

The water extract, at a concentration of 50.0%, was active. The effect was tested in spores of *Cyclosporum dentatus*. Methanol and water extracts of dried root, at a concentration of 50.0 ppm, were active on beans[LC070], and the spores of *Cyclosporum dentatus*[LC086], respectively. Water extract of dried inflorescence, at a concentration of 50.0%, was active on spores of *Cyclosporum dentatus*. Water extract of dried stem, at concentration of 50.0%, was active. The effect was tested in spores of *Cyclosporum dentatus*[LC086].

Plasma bilirubin increase. The dried entire plant fed to guinea pigs was active[LC073].

Protein synthesis inhibition. Dried leaves, administered orally to guinea pigs at a dose of 6.0 gm/kg, were active[LC051].

Respiratory depressant. Ethanol (95%) extract of leaves, administered intravenously to dogs, was active[LC046].

Smooth muscle relaxant activity. Ethanol (95%) extract of leaves was active on rat duodenum. Tissue becomes refractory at high concentrations[LC046].

Smooth muscle stimulant activity. Alkaloid fraction of dried leaves was active on rat intestine[LC092]. Ethanol (95%) and water extracts of bark and leaves, at a concentration of 0.1 mg/ml, were active on guinea pig ileum[LC032].

Succinate dehydrogenase stimulation. Dried leaves, administered by gastric intubation to guinea pigs at a dose of 2.0 gm/kg daily for 3 days, were active[LC056].

Toxic effect. Chromatographic fraction of dried leaves, administered by gastric intubation to guinea pigs at a dose of 125.0 mg/kg, was active. Treated animals became icterus, sedated and photosensitive. Bilirubin levels were generally elevated[LC029]. The ethanol (95%) extract, administered to rats, was also active[LC100]. The dried leaves, administered by gastric intubation to cows at a dose of 6.0 gm/kg, were active. Autopsy indicated liver damage and gastro-enteritis[LC101]. The

dried leaves, administered by gastric intubation to guinea pigs at a dose of 2.0 gm/kg, were active. The dose produced a decrease in hepatic mitochondrial protein content. The phospholipid-to-protein ratio did not change, but there was a marked increase in the cholesterol-to-protein ratio and the cholesterol-to-phospholipid ratio. Mitochondrial swelling, in the absence of or presence of ascorbic acid, decreased in hepatic mitochondria from Lantana intoxicated guinea pigs. Daily dosing for 3 days produced toxicity, including yellowness of conjunctiva and ears and photosensitization within 5 days[LC056]. The dried leaves, administered by gastric intubation to rabbits at a dose of 6.0% gm/kg, were active. Toxicity included ictericity, anorexia and decreased fecal output. Hepatotoxicity was observed histopathologically[LC031]. Dried entire plant, administered to buffalo by gastric intubation at a dose of 4.0 gm/animal, was active[LC050]. Fresh entire plant, administered to steer by gastric intubation at variable dosage levels, produced toxicities that included weakness, anorexia, icterus, constipation, dehydration, photosensitization, depression and hepatotoxicities. When administered orally, icterus, hydrothorax and dehydration were evident. Numerous hepatotoxicities and renal toxicities were seen[LC033]. Fresh leaves, in the ration of dogs, were active. Kidney and liver damage on a German Shepherd was reported. Other cases are reported on sheep, guinea pigs, horses, cattle and others. The leaves, in the ration of cattle at a dose of 350.0 mg/animal, produced photosensitization, dermatitis, liver and kidney damage, intestinal hemorrhage, paralysis of the gall bladder and death in 1–4 days[LC022]. Water extract of fruit, administered intraperitoneally to rats, was active with 2/2 deaths. The extract of unripe fruits produced 4/5 deaths[LC012].

Toxicity assessment (quantitative). Ethanol/water (1:1) extract of the entire plant, administered intraperitoneally to mice, produced LD_{50} > 1.0 gm/kg[LC004].

UDP-glucuronyl transferase inhibition.
Dried leaves, administered by gastric intubation to guinea pigs, were active, results significant at $P < 0.001$ level[LC063].

Uterine relaxation effect. Alkaloid fraction of dried leaves was active on rat uterus. There was inhibition of motility[LC092].

Uterine stimulant effect. Water extract of root was inactive on rat uterus[LC003].

Xanthine oxidase stimulation. Dried fruit, administered orally to guinea pigs at a dose of 20.0 gm/kg, was inactive. Enzymes were measured in the liver and kidneys. Dried leaves, administered orally to guinea pigs at a dose of 6.0 gm/kg, were active. Enzyme was measured in the liver and kidneys[LC051]. Dried shoots, administered orally to guinea pigs at a dose of 20.0 gm/kg, were inactive. Enzyme was measured in the liver and kidneys[LC051].

REFERENCES

LC001   Garcia-Barriga, H. Flora Medicinal de Colombia. Vol. 2/3 Universidad Nacional, Bogota, 1975.

LC002   Asprey, G. F. and P. Thornton. Medicinal plants of Jamaica. Part I. **West Indian Med J** 1953; 2(4): 233–252.

LC003   Barros, G. S. G., F. J. A. Mathos, J. E. V. Vieira, M. P. Sousa and M. C. Medeiros. Pharmacological screening of some Brazilian plants. **J Pharm Pharmacol** 1970; 22: 116.

LC004   Bhakuni, O. S., M. L. Dhar, M. M. Dhar, B. N. Dhawan and B. N. Mehrotra. Screening of Indian plants for biological activity. Part II. **Indian J Exp Biol** 1969; 7: 250–262.

LC005   Perrot, E. and P. Hurrier. Matiere Medicale et Pharmacopee Sino-Annamites. Vigot Freres, Edit., Paris, 1907; 292pp.

LC006   Roy, S. and A. K. Barua. The structure and stereochemistry of a triterpene acid from *Lantana camara*. **Phytochemistry** 1985; 24(7): 1607–1608.

LC007   Pan, W. D., Y. J. Li, L. T. Mai, K. Ohtani, R. Kasai and O. Tanaka. Studies on chemical constituents of the roots of *Lantana camara*. **Yao Hsueh Hsueh Pao** 1992; 27(7): 515–521.

LC008   Pan, W. D., Y. J. Li, L. T. Mai, K. H. Ohtani, R. T. Kasai, O. Tanaka and D. O. Yu. Studies on triterpenoid constituents of the roots of *Lantana camara*. **Yao Hsueh Hsueh Pao** 1993; 28(1): 40–44.

LC009   Pan, W. D., L. T. Mai, Y. J. Li, X. L. Xu and D. Q. Yu. Studies on the chemical constituents of the leaves of *Lantana camara*. **Yao Hsueh Hsueh Pao** 1993; 28(1): 35–39.

LC010   Siddiqui, B. S., S. M. Raza, S. Begum, S. Siddiqui and S. Firdous. Pentacyclic triterpenoids from *Lantana camara*. **Phytochemistry** 1995; 38(3): 681–685.

LC011   Keiser, I., E. J. Harris, D. H. Mayashita, M. Jacobson and R. E. Perdue. Attraction of ethyl ester extracts of 232 botanicals to Oriental fruit flies, melon flies and Mediterranean fruit flies. **Lloydia** 1975; 38(2): 141–152.

LC012   Der Marderosian, A. H., F. B. Giller and F. C. Roia. Phytochemical and toxicological screening of household ornamental plants potentially toxic to humans. 1. **J Toxicol Environ Health** 1976; 1: 939.

LC013   Pass, M. A., A. A. Seawright and T. Heath. Effect of ingestion of *Lantana camara* on bile formation in sheep. **Biochem Pharmacol** 1976; 25: 2101.

LC014   Brandao, M., M. Botelho and E. Krettli. Antimalarial experimental chemotherapy using natural products. **Cienc Cult** 1985; 37(7): 1152–1163.

LC015   Sharma, S. K. and V. P. Singh. The antifungal activity of some essential oils. **Ind Drugs Pharm Ind** 1979; 14(1): 3–6.

LC016   Apul, B. S. and J. K. Mali. Poisoning of livestock by some toxic plants. **Progressive Farming** 1982: 6–7.

LC017   Elisabethsky, E. and Z. C. Castilhos. Plants used as analgesics by Amazonian Caboclos as a basis for selecting plants for investigation. **Int J Crude Drug Res** 1990; 28(4): 309–320.

LC018   Zamora-Martinez, M. C. and C. N. P. Pola. Medicinal plants used in some rural populations of Oaxaca, Puebla and Veracruz, Mexico. **J Ethnopharmacol** 1992; 35(3) 229–257.

LC019   Singh, J., A. K. Dubey and N. N. Tripathi. Antifungal activity of *Mentha spicata*. **Int J Pharmacog** 1994; 32(4): 314–319.

LC020   Schmeda-Hirschmann, G. and A. Rojas de Arias. A screening method for natural products on Triatomine bugs. **Phytother Res** 1992; 6(2): 68–73.

LC021   Gladding, S. *Lantana camara*. **Aust J Med Herb** 1995; 7(1): 5–9.

LC022   Morton, J. F. Lantana, or Red Sage (*Lantana camara* L., Verbenaceae), notorious weed and popular garden flower: Some cases of poisoning in Florida. **Econ Bot** 1994; 48(3): 259–270.

LC023   Rimpler, H. and H. Sauerbier. Iridoid glucosides as taxonomic markers in the genera Lantana, Lippia, Aloysia and Phyla. **Biochem Syst Ecol** 1986; 14(3): 307–310.

LC024   Pass, M. A. and T. Heath. Gallbladder paralysis in sheep during Lantana poisoning. **J Comp Pathol** 1977; 87: 301.

LC025   Pass, M. A., R. T. Gemmell and T. J. Heath. Effect of Lantana on the ultrastructure of the liver of sheep. **Toxicol Appl Pharmacol** 1978; 43: 589.

LC026   Sharma, O. P., H. P. S. Makkar and R. K. Dawra. Effects of Lantana toxicity of lysosomal and cytosol enzymes in guinea pig liver. **Toxicol Lett** 1983; 16(1/2): 41–45.

LC027   Mc Sweeney, C. S. and M. A. Pass. The role of the rumen in absorption of Lantana toxins in sheep. **Toxicon Suppl** 1983; 3: 285–288.

LC028   Behari, M. and M. M. Goval. Amino acids in certain medicinal plants. **Acta Cienc Indica (Ser) Chem** 1984; 10(1): 10–11.

LC029   Sharma, O. P., R. K. Dawra and H. P. S. Makkar. Isolation and partial purification of Lantana (*Lantana camara* L.) toxins. **Toxicol Lett** 1987; 37(2): 165–172.

LC030   Forestieri, A. M., F. C. Pizzimenti, M. T. Monforte and G. Bisignano. Antibacterial activity of some African medicinal plants. **Pharmacol Res Commun Suppl** 1988; 20(5): 33–36.

LC031   Sharma, O. P., R. K. Dawra, L. Krishna and H. P. S. Makkar. Toxicity of Lantana (*Lantana camara* L.) leaves and isolated toxins to rabbits. **Vet Hum Toxicol** 1988; 30(3): 214–218.

LC032   Occhiuto, F., C. Circosta and R. Costa De Pasquale. Studies on some medicinal plants in Senegal: Effects on isolated guinea pig ileum. **J Ethnopharmacol** 1989; 26(2): 205–210.

LC033   Fourie, N., J. J. Van Der Lugt, S. J. Newsholme and P. W. Nel. Acute *Lantana camara* toxicity in cattle. **J South African Vet Assoc** 1990; 58(4): 173–178.

LC034   Weenen, H., M. H. H. Nkunya, D. H. Bray, L. B. Mwasumbi, L. S. Kinabo and V. A. E. B. Kilimali. Antimalarial activity of Tanzanian medicinal plants. **Planta Med** 1990; 56(4): 368–370.

LC035   Akhter, M. H., M. Mathur and N. K. Bhide. Skin and liver toxicity in experimental *Lantana camara* poisoning in albino rats. **Indian J Physiol Pharmacol** 1990; 34(1): 13–16.

LC036   Pasricha, J. S., P. Bhaumik and A. Agarwal. Contact dermatitis due to *Xanthium strumarium*. **Indian J Dermatol Venereol Leprol** 1990; 56(4): 319–321.

LC037   Johns, T., J. O. Kokwaro and E. K. Kimanani. Herbal remedies of the Luo of Siaya District, Kenya. Establishing quantitative criteria for consensus. **Econ Bot** 1990; 44(3): 369–381.

LC038   Abdel-Aziz, A., K. Brain and A. K. Bashir. Screening of Sudanese plants for molluscicidal activity and identification of leaves of *Tacca leontopetaloides* (L.) O Ktze (Tacaceae) as a potential new exploitable resource. **Phytother Res** 1990; 4(2): 62–65.

LC039   Abeygunawardena, C., V. Kumar, D. S. Marshall, R. H. Thomson and D. B. M. Wickramaratne. Furanonaphthoquinones from two Lantana species. **Phytochemistry** 1991; 30(3): 941–945.

LC040   Nagaraju, N. and K. N. Rao. A survey of plant crude drugs of Rayalaseema, Andhra Pradesh, India. **J Ethnopharmacol** 1990; 29(2): 137–158.

LC041   Ganai, G. N. and G. J. Jha. Immunosuppression due to chronic *Lantana camara*, L. toxicity in sheep. **Indian J Exp Biol** 1991; 29(8): 762–766.

LC042 Carbajal, D., A. Casaco, L. Arruzaza-bala, R. Gonzalez and V. Fuentes. Pharmacological screening of plant decoctions commonly used in Cuban folk medicine. **J Ethnopharmacol** 1991; 33(1/2): 21–24.

LC043 Herbert, J. M., J. P. Maffrand, K. Taoubi, J. M. Augereau, I. Fouraste and J. Gleye. Verbascoside isolated from *Lantana camara*, an inhibitor of protein kinase C. **J Nat Prod** 1991; 54(6): 1595–1600.

LC044 Arias, R. J., G. Schmeda-Hirschmann and A. Falcao. Feeding deterrency and insecticidal effects of plant extracts on *Lutzomyia longipalpis*. **Phytother Res** 1992; 6(2): 64–67.

LC045 Hakizamungu, E., L. Van Puyvelde and M. Wery. Screening of Rwandese medicinal plants for anti-trichomonas activity. **J Ethnopharmacol** 1992; 36(2): 143–146.

LC046 Nauriyal, M. M. and I. Gupta. Some pharmacological actions of *Lantana camara* leaves. **Indian J Anim Sci** 1977; 47: 844.

LC047 Taniguchi, M., A. Chapya, I. Kubo and K. Nakanishi. Screening of East African plants from antimicrobial activity. I. **Chem Pharm Bull** 1978; 26: 2910–2913.

LC048 Ayensu, E. S. Medicinal plants of the West Indies. **Unpublished Manuscript** 1978; 110pp.

LC049 Gupta, M. P., T. D. Arias, M. Correa and S. S. Lamba. Ethnopharma-cognostic observations on Panama-nian medicinal plants. Part 1. **Q J Crude Drug Res** 1979; 17(3/4): 115–130.

LC050 Avadhoot, Y. and K. C. Varma. Anti-microbial activity of essential oil of seeds of *Lantana camara* var. aculeata Linn. **Indian Drugs Pharm Ind** 1978; 13: 41–42.

LC051 Sharma, O. P., H. P. Makkar, R. N. Pal and S. S. Negi. Lantadene: A content and toxicity of the Lantana plant (*Lantana camara* Linn.) to guinea pigs. **Toxicon** 1980; 18: 485–488.

LC052 Rizvi, S. J. H., D. Mukerji and S. N. Mathur. A new report of possible source of natural herbicide. **Indian J Exp Biol** 1980; 18: 777–781.

LC053 Sharma, O. P., H. P. S. Makkar, R. K. Dawra and S. S. Negi. Hepatic and renal toxicity of Lantana in the guinea pig. **Toxicol Lett** 1980; 6: 347–351.

LC054 Gonsalves, L. X., C. K. Kokate and H. P. Tipnis. Anti-insect and juvenile hormone mimicking activities of *Cyperus rotundus* and *Lantana camara*. **Indian J Pharm Sci** 1979; 41: 250A.

LC055 Medina, F. R. and R. Woodbury. Ter-restrial plants molluscicidal to Lymnaeid hosts of *Fasciliasis hepatica* in Puerto Rico. **J Agr Univ Puerto Rico** 1979; 63: 366–376.

LC056 Sharma, O. P., H. P. S. Makkar and R. K. Dawra. Biochemical effects of the plant *Lantana camara* on guinea pig liver mitochondria. **Toxicon** 1982; 20: 783–786.

LC057 Sharma, O. P., P. S. Makkar, R. K. Dawra and S. S. Negi. A review of the toxicity of *Lantana camara* (Linn.) in animals. **Clin Toxicol** 1981; 18: 1077–1094.

LC058 Sawhney, A. N., M. R. Khan, G. Ndaalio, M. H. H. Nkunya and H. Wevers. Stud-ies on the rationale of African tradi-tional medicine. Part III. Preliminary screening for antifungal activity. **Pak J Sci Ind Res** 1978; 21: 193–196.

LC059 Adesina, S. K. Studies on some plants used as anticonvulsants in Amerindian and African traditional medicine. **Fitoterapia** 1982; 53: 147–162.

LC060 Sharma, O. P., R. K. Dawra and H. P. S. Makkar. Effect of *Lantana camara* toxic-ity on lipid peroxidation in guinea pig tissues. **Res Commun Chem Pathol Pharmacol** 1982; 38: 153–156.

LC061 Ross, S. A., N. E. El-Keltawi and S. E. Megalla. Antimicrobial activity of some Egyptian aromatic plants. **Fitoterapia** 1980; 51: 201–205.

LC062 Martinez, M. A. Medicinal plants used in a Totonac community of the Sierra Norte de Puebla: Tuzamapan de Galeana, Puebla, Mexico. **J Ethno-pharmacol** 1984; 11(2): 203–221.

LC063 Sharma, O. P., H. P. S. Makkar and R. K. Dawra. Biochemical changes in hepatic microsomes of guinea pig under Lantana toxicity. **Xenobiotica** 1982; 12(4): 265–269.

LC064 Sabnis, S. D. and S. J. Bedi. Ethnobo-tanical studies in Dadra-Nagar Haveli and Daman. **Indian J For** 1983; 6(1): 65–69.

LC065   Kalyanasundaram, M. and C. J. Babu. Biologically active plant extracts as mosquito larvicides. **Indian J Med Res** 1982; 76: 102–106.

LC066   Pandey, D. K., N. N. Tripathi, R. D. Tripathi and S. N. Dixit. Antifungal activity of some seed extracts with special reference to that of *Pimpinella diversifolia* DC. **Int J Crude Drug Res** 1983; 21(4): 177–182.

LC067   Uppal, R. P. and B. S. Paul. Haematological changes in experimental Lantana poisoning in sheep. **Indian Vet J** 1982; 59(1): 18–24.

LC068   Arnold, H. J. and M. Gulumian. Pharmacopoeia of traditional medicine in Venda. **J Ethnopharmacol** 1984; 12(1): 35–74.

LC069   Ishii, R., K. Yoshikawa, H. Minakata, H. Komura and T. Kada. Specificities of bioantimutagens in plant kingdom. **Agr Biol Chem** 1984; 48(10): 2587–2591.

LC070   Dominguez, X. A. and J. B. Alcorn. Screening of medicinal plants used by Huastec Mayans of Northeastern Mexico. **J Ethnopharmacol** 1985; 13(2): 139–156.

LC071   Sahu, T. R. Less known uses of weeds as medicinal plants. **Ancient Sci Life** 1984; 3(4): 245–249.

LC072   Khan, M. R., G. Ndaalio, M. H. H. Nkunya, H. Wevers. Studies on the rationale of African traditional medicine. Part II. Preliminary screening of medicinal plants for anti-gonoccoci activity. **Pak J Sci Ind Res** 1978; 27(5/6): 189–192.

LC073   Sharma, O. P., H. P. S. Makkar, R. K. Dawra and S. S. Negi. Changes in blood constituents of guinea pigs in Lantana toxicity. **Toxicol Lett** 1982; 11: 73–76.

LC074   Hedberg, I., O. Hedberg, P. J. Madati, K. E. Mshigeni, E. N. Mshiu and G. Samuelsson. Inventory of plants used in traditional medicine in Tanzania. Part III. Plants of the families Papilionaceae-Vitaceae. **J Ethnopharmacol** 1983; 9(2/3): 237–260.

LC075   Darias, V., L. Bravo, E. Barquin, D. M. Herrera and C. Fraile. Contribution to the ethnopharmacological study of the Canary Islands. **J Ethnopharmacol** 1986; 15(2): 169–193.

LC076   Saksena, N. and H. H. S. Tripathi. Plant volatiles in relation to fungistasis. **Fitoterapia** 1985; 56(4): 243–244.

LC077   Wanjari, D. G. Antihemorrhagic activity of *Lantana camara*. **Nagarjun** 1983; 27(2): 40,41.

LC078   Weniger, B., M. Rouzier, R. Daguilh, D. Henrys, J. H. Henrys and R. Anthon. Popular medicine of the Central Plateau of Haiti. 2. Ethnopharmacological inventory. **J Ethnopharmacol** 1986; 17(1): 13–30.

LC079   Bali, H. S., S. Singh and S. C. Pati. Preliminary screening of some plants for molluscicidal activity against two snail species. **Indian J Anim Sci** 1985; 55(5): 338–340.

LC080   Sharma, V. K. and S. Kaur. Contact dermatitis due to plants in Chandigarh. **Indian J Dermatol Venereol Leprol** 1987; 53(1): 26–30.

LC081   El-Keltawi, N. E. M., S. E. Megalla and S. A. Ross. Antimicrobial activity of some Egyptian aromatic plants. **Herba Pol** 1980; 26(4): 245–250.

LC082   Sinha, P. and S. K. Saxena. Effect of treating tomatoes with leaf extract of *Lantana camara* on development of fruit rot caused by *Aspergillus niger* in the presence of *Drosophila busckii*. **Indian J Exp Biol** 1987; 25(2): 143–144.

LC083   Gonzalez, F and M. Silva. A survey of plants with antifertility properties described in the South American folk medicine. (Abstract). **Abstr Princess Congress 1 Thailand**, Dec. 1987; 20pp.

LC084   Caceres, A., L. M. Giron, S. R. Alvarado, and M. F. Torres. Screening of antimicrobial activity of plants popularly used in Guatemala for the treatment of dermatomucosal diseases. **J Ethnopharmacol** 1987; 20(3): 223–237.

LC085   Singh, V. P., S. K. Sharma, and V. S. Khare. Medicinal plants from Ujjain District Madhya Pradesh. Part II. **Indian Drugs Pharm Ind** 1980; 5: 7–12.

LC086   Wadhwani, C. and T. N. Bhardwaja. Effect of *Lantana camara* L. extract on fern spore germination. **Experientia** 1981; 37(3): 245–246.

LC087   Hirschmann, G. S. and A. Rojas de Arias. A survey of medicinal plants of Minas Gerais, Brazil. **J Ethnopharmacol** 1990; 29(2): 159–172.

LC088   Panthong, A., D. Kanjanapothi and W. C. Taylor. Ethnobotanical review of medicinal plants from Thai traditional books, Part 1. Plants with anti-inflammatory, anti-asthmatic and antihypertensive properties. **J Ethnopharmacol** 1986; 18(3): 213–228.

LC089   Collier, W. A. and L. Van de Piji. The antibiotic action of plants, especially the higher plants, with results with Indonesian plants. **Chron Nat** 1949; 105: 8.

LC090   Nene, Y. L., P. N. Thapliyal and K. Kumar. Screening of some plant extracts for antifungal properties. **Labdev J Sci Tech** 1968; 6B(4): 226–228.

LC091   Pinheiro de Sousa, M. and M. Z. Rouquayrol. Molluscicidal activity of plants from Northeast Brazil. **Rev Bras Fpesq Med Biol** 1974; 7(4): 389–394.

LC092   Sharaf, A. and M. Naguib. A pharmacological study of the Egyptian plant, *Lantana camara*. **Egypt Pharm Bull** 1959; 41(6): 93–97.

LC093   Louw, P. G. J. Lantadene A, the active principle of *Lantana camara*. II. Isolation of lantadene B, and the oxygen functions of lantadene A and lantadene B. **Onderstepoort J Vet Sci Animal Ind** 1948; 23: 233–238.

LC094   Sharma, V. N. and K. N. Kaul. Lanacamarone. **Patent-Brit** 1959; 820,521.

LC095   Sundararamaiah, T. and V. V. Bai. Chemical examination of *Lantana camara*. **J Indian Chem Soc** 1973; 50(9): 620–.

LC096   Ahmed, Z. F., A. M. El-Moghazy Shoaib, G. M. Wassel and S. M. El-Sayyad. Phytochemical study of *Lantana camara*. Terpenes and lactones. II. **Planta Med** 1972; 22(1): 34–37.

LC097   Ahmed, Z. F., A. M. El-Moghazy Shoaib, G. M. Wassel and S. M. El-Sayyad. Phytochemical study of *Lantana camara*. I. **Planta Med** 1972; 21(3): 282–288.

LC098   Barua, A. K., P. Chakrabarti, P. K. Sanyal and B. Das. Triterpenoids. XXXII. Structure of lantic acid: A new triterpene from *Lantana camara*. **J Indian Chem Soc** 1969; 46(1): 100–101.

LC099   Barua, A. K., P. Chakrabarti, S. P. Dutta, D. K. Mukherjee and B. C. Das. Triterpenoids. XXXVII. Structure and stereochemistry of lantanolic acid. New triterpenoid from *Lantana camara*. **Tetrahedron** 1971; 27(6): 1141–1147.

LC100   Uppal, R. P. and B. S. Paul. Preliminary studies with crude lantadene, toxic principle of *Lantana camara* in albino rats. **Haryana Agr Univ J Res** 1971; 1(2): 98–102.

LC101   Dwivedi, S. K., G. A. Shivnani and H. C. Joshi. Clinical and biochemical studies in Lantana poisoning in ruminants. **Indian J Anim Sci** 1971; 41(10): 948–953.

LC102   Hunt, S. E. and P. J. McCosker. Serum adenosine deaminase activity in experimentally produced liver diseases of cattle and sheep. Yellow-wood, Lantana, carbon tetrachloride, and chronic copper poisoning. **Brit Vet J** 1970; 126(2): 74–81.

LC103   Sharma, O. P., A. Singh and S. Sharma. Levels of lantadenes, bioactive pentacyclic triterpenoids, in young and mature leaves of *Lantana camara* var. aculeate. **Fitoterapia** 2000; 71(5): 487–491.

LC104   Singh, A., O. P. Sharma, N. P. Kurade and S. Ojha. Detoxification of lantana hepatotoxin, lantadene A, using *Alcaligenes faecalis*. **J Appl Toxicol** 2001; 21(3): 225–228.

LC105   Bouda, H., L. A. Tapondjou, D. A. Fontem, and M. Y. Gumedzoe. Effect of essential oils from leaves of *Ageratum conyzoides*, *Lantana camara* and *Sitophilus zeamais* (Coleoptera, Curculionidae). **J Stored Prod** Res 2001; 37(2): 103–109.

LC106   Misra, L. and H. Laatsch. Triperpenoids, essential oil and photo-oxidative 28→ 13-lactonization of oleanolic acid from *Lantana camara*. **Phytochemistry** 2000; 54(8): 969–974.

LC107   Begum, S., A. Wahab, B. S. Siddiqui and F. Qamar. Nematicidal constituents of the aerial parts of *Lantana camara*. **J Nat Prod** 2000; 63(6): 765–767.

LC108   Sharma, S., O. P. Sharma, B. Singh and T. K. Bhat. Biotransformation of lantadenes, the pentacyclic triterpenoid hepatotoxins of lantana plant, in guinea pigs. **Toxicon** 2000; 38(9): 1191–1202.

16 | Mucuna pruriens

(L) DC.

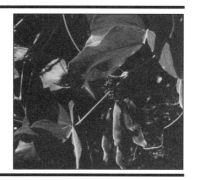

Common Names

Alkushi	Pakistan	Kawach	India
Alkusi	India	Kawanch	India
Atmagupta	India	Kawanch	Pakistan
Baidhok	India	Kawanh	India
Belki	India	Kerainch	India
Cigu	Thailand	Kewanch	India
Cowage	India	Konch	India
Cowhage	Nepal	Konchkari	Pakistan
Cowitch vine	Virgin Islands	Kowez	India
Cowitch	Guyana	Metaftum	Guinea–Bissau
Cowitch	Trinidad	Mijeh	Thailand
Cussu	India	Nipay	Philippines
Demar pirkok	Panama	Pois a gratter	Trinidad
Dulagondi	India	Poua grate	Guadeloupe
Ganhoma	Guinea–Bissau	Pwa grate	Haiti
Goncha	Pakistan	Pwa gwate	Trinidad
Horseeye bean	Thailand	Sijeh	Thailand
Kaocho	Nepal	Taingilotra	Madagascar
Kapikachchu	India	Tainkilotra	Madagascar
Kauso	Nepal	Talcodja	Guinea–Bissau
Kausva	Nepal	Vetvet bean	Japan
Kavach	India	Wanduru–me	Sri Lanka
Kavanch	India		

BOTANICAL DESCRIPTION

A vine of the PAPILIONACEAE family. The seeds of *Mucuna pruriens* are black in color with pale brown specks, uniform in shape, 9 to 12 mm long with funicular hilum and cellular pit growth around the hilum. The seed coat is hard, thick and glossy. The embryo completely fills the seed and is made up of 2 large fleshy cotyledons. Transverse section of seed shows an outer testa with a palisade epidermis made up of a rod-shaped macrosclereids with thickened anticlinal walls.

From: *Medicinal Plants of the World, vol. 1: Chemical Constituents, Traditional and Modern Medicinal Uses, 2nd ed.*
By: Ivan A. Ross © Humana Press Inc., Totowa, NJ

ORIGIN AND DISTRIBUTION

Originated in India, it is now commonly found throughout the tropics.

TRADITIONAL MEDICINAL USES

Brazil. Alcohol extract of dried seeds is taken orally as a nerve tonic. Alcohol and water extracts are taken orally as aphrodisiac[MP015].

Guadeloupe. Seeds, crushed and mixed with syrup, are given orally to infants as a vermifuge[MP046].

India. Hot water extract of dried fruit is administered orally to children in cases of stomach worms. Overdoses are fatal[MP045]. Water extract of leaves is taken orally as a nerve tonic, for dysentery, as an aphrodisiac and for scorpion stings[MP024]. Powdered pod trichomes are taken orally as an anthelmintic. About 4 to 5 pod hairs are taken along with milk or buttermilk[MP018]. Hot water extract of root is taken orally as an emmenagogue[MP007]. Dried root is used for rheumatism and gout. Roots of *Mucuna pruriens* and *Hymenodictyon excelsum* are heated in mustard oil, which is then rubbed on the affected area[MP022]. Hot water extract of dried root is taken orally for delirium in Ayurvedic and Unani medicine[MP042]. Dried powdered root is taken orally with honey as a blood purifier and diuretic, and to dissolve kidney stones[MP047]. Fresh root is taken orally to relieve dysmenorrhea, paving the way for effective conception in future menstrual cycles. Paste made from *Mucuna pruriens*, *Pygaeopremna herbacea*, *Tephrosia purpurea*, and *Gardenia turgida* roots, plus a few cloves of *Allium sativum* is given. Twenty grams of the paste is given on day 3 of menstruation[MP050]. Seeds are taken orally by male human adults to cure night dreams and impotency, to promote fertility and as an aphrodisiac to increase seminal fluid and manly vigor[MP008]. Hot water extract of boiled seeds is taken by male human adults as an aphrodisiac[MP010]. Powdered seeds, taken with milk (5 gm 3 times a day with sufficient quantity of milk), are used for diarrhea[MP017]. As an aphrodisiac, 2 seeds are powdered and taken with a cup of cow's milk[MP018]. Decoction of seed is taken orally for scorpion stings and snakebite[MP024]. Hot water extract of seeds is taken orally as a nervine[MP042]. Seeds are taken orally as an aphrodisiac in Ayurveda and Unani medicine[MP042]. Decoction of dried seeds is taken orally for abortion[MP014], as an aphrodisiac[MP037] and for sexual debility[MP038]. For persistent coughs, seeds are placed over a red hot plate or burning charcoal, and the fumes are inhaled through the mouth[MP048]. Decoction of dried seeds, together with *Terminalia arjuna* and *Sida retusa* is taken orally for pulmonary tuberculosis[MP059]. Fresh seeds, cooked in goat's milk, are taken orally as an aphrodisiac and for seminal weakness and impotence[MP047]. Hot water extract of dried seedpods is taken orally as an anthelmintic in Ayurvedic and Unani medicine[MP042].

Guinea–Bissau. Plant juice is taken orally as an emmenagogue. Seed is taken orally as an aphrodisiac[MP002].

Haiti. Decoction of dried fruit is taken orally for intestinal parasites[MP054].

Ivory Coast. Hot water extract of the entire plant is taken orally as an emmenagogue[MP004].

Madagascar. Decoction of water extract of seeds is taken orally as an aphrodisiac (120 gm/seeds in 1 liter of milk)[MP009].

Mozambique. Hot water extract of seeds is taken orally as an aphrodisiac[MP020].

Nepal. Hot water extract of seeds is taken orally as an aphrodisiac[MP001].

Nigeria. Dried leaf extract is used to treat snakebite[MP016].

Pakistan. Hot water extract of seeds is taken orally as an aphrodisiac[MP003].

Philippines. Fresh stem sap is used to treat sore and wind burns. A fresh stem is cut off on both ends, and the sap is blown from 1 end to the other over the mouth of the child[MP027].

Thailand. Dried leaves and stem are used for burns and cuts. *Oroxylum indicum* bark

and *Mucuna pruriens* leaves are pounded together and applied to burns and cuts[MP051].
Trinidad. Crushed seeds are taken orally with molasses for intestinal worms[MP033].
Virgin Islands. Hot water extract of the entire plant is taken orally for worms[MP062].

CHEMICAL CONSTITUENTS

(ppm unless otherwise indicated)

1-Methyl-3-carboxy-6,7-dihydroxy-1,2,3,4-Tetrahydroisoquinolone: Sd[MP031]
5-Hydroxytryptamine: Pod trich[MP005], Fr, Lf, St[MP019]
5-Methoxy tryptamine,N-N-dimethyl: Lf 25[MP005], St, Fr[MP019]
5-Methoxy-N,N-dimethyltryptamine-N-oxide: Lf[MP005], St, Fr[MP019]
5-Oxyindole-3-alkylamine: Sd[MP031]
6-Methoxyharman: Lf[MP030]
Alanine: Sd 0.55–1.16%[MP031]
Arachidic acid: Sd 65–1385[MP031]
Arginine: Sd 1.23–2.62%[MP031]
Aspartic acid: Sd1.99–4.21%[MP031]
Behenic acid: Sd 140–2265[MP031]
Beta carboline: Sd[MP029]
Beta sitosterol: Sd[MP029]
Bufotenine: St[MP019], Fr[MP019], Lf[MP005]
Calcium: Sd 1320–1600[MP031]
Carbohydrates: Sd 52.9–66.7%[MP031]
Choline: Lf[MP005]
Cis-12,13-epoxyoctadec–trans-9-cis-acid: Sd[MP030]
Cis–12,13–epoxyoctadec–trans-9-enoic-acid: Sd[MP030]
Cystine: Sd 1400–2965[MP031]
DOPA: Sd 0.24–4.80%[MP029]
Fat: Sd 0.7–6.3%[MP031]
Fiber: Sd 4.6–9.5%[MP031]
Gallic acid: Sd[MP029]
Glutamic acid: 1.91–4.04%[MP031]
Glutathione: Sd[MP029]
Glycine: Sd 0.72–1.53%[MP031]
Histidine: Sd 0.33–0.69%[MP031]
Indole-3-alkylamine: Sd[MP031]
Iron: Sd 200[MP029]
Isoleucine: Sd 0.75–1.59%[MP031]
Kilocalories: Sd 0.34–0.40%[MP031]
Lecithin: Sd[MP053]
Leucine: Sd 1.18–2.52%[MP031]
Linoleic acid: Sd 0.07–3.1%[MP031]
Linolenic acid: Sd 265–5800[MP031]
Lysine: Sd 0.97–2.10%[MP031]
Mucuna pruriens alkaloid P: Sd 27[MP063]
Mucuna pruriens alkaloid Q: Sd[MP063]
Mucuna pruriens alkaloid R: Sd 66[MP063]
Mucuna pruriens alkaloid S: Sd 33[MP063]
Mucuna pruriens alkaloid X: Sd[MP063]
Methionine: Sd 1875–3975[MP031]
Mucunadine: Sd[MP029]
Mucunain: Sd[MP029]
Mucunine: Sd[MP029]
Myristic acid: Sd 15–125[MP031]
N,N-Dimethyltryptamine: Sd[MP029]
N,N-Dimethyltryptamine-n-oxide: Sd[MP029]
Niacin: Sd 17–34[MP031]
Nicotine: Sd[MP029]
Oleic acid: Sd 735–11400[MP031]
Palmitic acid: Sd 0.14–3.38%[MP031]
Palmitoleic acid: Sd 35–630[MP031]
Phenylalanine: Sd 0.75–1.59%[MP031]
Phosphorus: Sd 0.32–0.47%[MP031]
Proline: Sd 0.92–1.96%[MP031]
Protein: Sd 15.5–33.1%[MP031]
Prurienidine: Sd 110[MP063]
Prurieninine: Sd 11[MP063]
Riboflavin: Sd 1.1–2.7[MP031]
Saponins: Sd 2.1%[MP031]
Serine: Sd 0.77–1.62%[MP031]
Serotonin: Sd[MP029]
Stearic acid: Sd 390–12475[MP031]
Thiamin: Sd 1.4–5.7[MP031]
Threonine: Sd 0.63–1.33%[MP031]
Trypsin: Sd 285–397[MP066]
Tryptamine: Sd[MP030]
Tyrosine: Sd 0.798–1.691%[MP031]
Valine: Sd 0.86–1.82%[MP031]
Vernolic acid: Sd oil 4.0%[MP032]

PHARMACOLOGICAL ACTIVITIES AND CLINICAL TRIALS

Anabolic activity. Plant, administered orally to castrated adult and young male mice at a dose of 7.70 mg/animal, was active. Animals were pretreated with testosterone over a period of 4 days. The plant was mixed with *Lactuca scariola*, *Hygrophila spinosa*, *Parmelia parlata*, *Argyreia speciosa*, *Tribulus terrestris*, and *Leptadenia reticulata*. When administered to infant mice at a dose of 22.0 mg/animal, the mixture was active. There was an increase in maltase activity of the dorsoventral prostate and increase in fructose content of seminal vesicles[MP061].

Analgesic activity. Ethanol (95%) extract of dried fruit trichomes, administered intragastrically to rats at a dose of 2.0 gm/kg, was active vs acetic acid-induced writhing. A dose of 1.0 gm/kg was active vs hot plate method. Ethanol (95%) extract of dried leaves, administered intragastrically to rats at a dose of 1.0 gm/kg, was active vs hot plate method and acetic acid-induced writhing[MP013].

Anticoagulant activity. Water extract of dried leaves, at a concentration of 1.0 mg/ml, was active on human whole blood[MP016].

Antidiabetic effect. Seed extract, administered orally to streptozotocin-diabetic mice for 40 days, reduced plasma glucose concentration by 9.07%; Urine volume was significantly higher in diabetic controls and the treatment prevented polyuria. After 10 days of administration urinary albumin levels were over 6 fold higher in diabetic controls. Renal hypertrophy was significantly higher in diabetic controls as compared to non-diabetic controls. The extract failed to modify renal hypertrophy[MP068].

Antigalactagogue effect. Seeds, taken orally by human adults at a dose of 15.0 gm/animal, were inactive. The subjects had hyperprolactinemia and galactorrhea. Both subjects had a history of secondary amenorrhea and primary sterility. Daily dosing (divided doses) for 24 weeks in 1 subject and 10 weeks in a second subject[MP036].

Antihypercholesterolemic activity. Decoction of dried leaves, administered intragastrically to rats at a dose of 5.0 gm/kg, was active vs diet- and triton-induced hypercholesterolemia[MP021].

Antihyperlipemic activity. Decoction of dried leaves, administered intragastrically to rats at a dose of 5.0 gm/kg, was active vs diet- and triton-induced hypercholesterolemia[MP021].

Anti-inflammatory activity. Ethanol (95%) extract of dried fruit trichomes, administered intragastrically to rats at a dose of 3.0 gm/kg, was active vs carrageenin-induced pedal edema. Ethanol (95%) extract of dried leaves, administered intragastrically to rats at a dose of 1.0 gm/kg, was active vs carrageenin-induced pedal edema[MP013].

Antiparkinson activity. Methanol extract of dried seeds, administered intraperitoneally to rats at a dose of 200.0 mg/kg, was active. An alcohol-insoluble methanol extract, free from L-DOPA was tested. Seeds, administered by gastric intubation to rats at a dose of 400.0 mg/kg, were active[MP043]. Seeds, taken orally by human adults at a dose of 15–40 gm/person, were active. L–DOPA content was about 4.5–5.5%. The study involved 33 patients with Parkinson's disease[MP039]. *Mucuna pruriens* and *Banisteria caapi* have been used in traditional therapies in the form of herbal preparations containing anticholinergics, levodopa, and monoamine oxidase inhibitors in the treatment of Parkinson's disease in the Amazon basin, India, and China[MP064]. In a clinical prospective study, the efficacy of a concoction in cow's milk of powdered *Mucuna pruriens* and *Hyscyamus reticulatus* seeds and *Withania somnifera* and *Sida cordifolia* roots was evaluated in 18 clinically diagnosed Parkinsonian patients (mean Hoen and Yahr value of 2.22). As per Ayurveda principles, 13 patients underwent cleansing for 28 days and palliative therapy for 56 days, 5 patients underwent palliative therapy alone for 84 days. The former group showed significant improvement in activities of daily living (ADL) and on motor examination as per UPDRS rating. Symptomatically, they exhibited better response in tremor, bradykinesia, stiffness and cramps as compared to the latter group. Excessive salivation worsened in both groups. Analyses of powdered samples in the milk, as administered in the patients, revealed about 200 mg of L-DOPA per dose[MP065].

Antipyretic activity. Ethanol (95%) extract of dried fruit trichomes, administered intragastrically to rats at a dose of 1.0 gm/kg, was active vs yeast-induced pyrexia. Ethanol (95%) extract of dried leaves, administered intragastrically to rats at a dose of 1.0 gm/kg, was active vs yeast-induced pyrexia[MP013].

Antiradiation effect. Methanol extract of dried prothallus, administered intraperitoneally to mice at a dose of 100 mg/kg, was inactive vs soft X-ray irradiation at lethal dose[MP055].

Antispasmodic activity. Ethanol/water (1:1) extract of fruit was active on guinea pig ileum vs ACh- and histamine-induced spasms. Ethanol/water (1:1) extract of root was active on guinea pig ileum vs ACh- and histamine-induced spasms[MP006].

Aphrodisiac activity. Plant, administered orally to male human adults, was active. A clinical trial involving 133 subjects ranging in age from 18–46 years presented cases of improper erection, night emissions, premature ejaculations, spermatorrhoea, functional impotence, and/or oligospermia. Of all patients, 71.4% claimed to be aided by the drug with no side effects[MP034]. Seeds, taken by male human adults at variable dosage levels, were active. The product known as "speman", contained a mixture of *Orchis mascula, Hygrophila spinosa, Lactuca scariola, Mucuna pruriens, Parmelia parlata, Argyreia speciosa, Tribulus terrestris* and *Leptadenia reticulata*. The study involved 21 infertile oligospermic patients in the age group of 25–35 years. Dosing with speman was 2 tablets 3 times daily for 4 weeks. Semen and blood samples were collected for analysis. Fifty percent of the subjects showed improvement of prostatic function as assessed by the activity of maltase and by the citric acid content, with increase in the activity of amylase and maltase and a decrease in post-treatment levels of glycogen in semi-

nal fluid. No marked change in seminal vesicular function was noted[MP041]. Ether and ethanol (95%) extracts of seeds, administered intraperitoneally to rats, were inactive. No effect on social behavior, including homosexual mounting, sniffing, lying over one another, and so forth, was observed[MP037]. *M. pruriens* is an ingredient of several commercial preparations claimed to have beneficial effects in the management of various sexual disorders. One such preparation is Tenex forte, which has other constituents like musk, saffron, yohimbine hydrochloride, nuxvomica pulvis, makardhwaj shilajeet, *Orchis mascula, Withania somnifera, Sida cordifolia, Bombax malabaricum, Argyreia speciosa,* and *Swarnamakshik bhasma*, as well as Mustong, which contains *M. pruriens, Glycyrrhiza glabra, Withania somnifera, Tribulus terrestris, Myristica fragrans,* and Tinospora. Some uncontrolled clinical studies have claimed to find these compound preparations effective in improving libido and performance in men[MP030].

Bronchodilator activity. Hot water extract of dried seeds, administered intravenously to guinea pigs at a dose of 1.5 ml/animal, was inactive[MP028].

Cholinesterase inhibition. Methanol extract of seeds, administered intraperitoneally to rats at a dose of 200.0 mg/kg, was inactive. An alcohol-insoluble methanol extract, free from L-DOPA, was tested[MP043].

Cytotoxic activity. Ethanol/water (1:1) extract of fruit, in cell culture, was inactive on CA-9KB, $ED_{50} > 20.0$ mcg/ml. Ethanol/water (1:1) extract of root, in cell culture, was inactive on CA-9KB, $ED_{50} > 20.0$ mcg/ml[MP006].

Embryotoxic effect. Water extract of seeds, administered intragastrically to pregnant rats at a dose of 175.0 mg/kg, was inactive[MP014].

Fertility promotion effect. Dried entire plant extract, taken orally by male human adults at a dose of 96.0 mg/day, was active.

Thirty-five patients with oligospermia were given 2 tablets 3 times per day for 3 months. Total sperm count and sperm motility improved[MP052].

FSH release inhibition. Seeds, taken orally by male human adults at variable dosage levels, were equivocal. The product contained a mixture of *Orchis mascula*, *Hygrophila spinosa*, *Lactuca scariola*, *Mucuna pruriens*, *Parmelia parlata*, *Argyreia speciosa*, *Tribulus terrestris*, and *Leptadenia reticulata* (known as speman). Dosing was 2 tablets 3 times daily for 4 days[MP041].

FSH synthesis stimulation. Seeds, taken orally by male human adults at variable dosage levels, were equivocal. The product contained a mixture of *Orchis mascula*, *Hygrophila spinosa*, *Lactuca scariola*, *Mucuna pruriens*, *Parmelia parlata*, *Argyreia speciosa*, *Tribulus terrestris*, and *Leptadenia reticulata* (known as speman). Dosing was 2 tablets 3 times daily for 4 days[MP041].

Genitourinary effect. Water extract of the entire plant, administered orally to mice at a dose of 5.0 mg/day, was active. The mice received a single dose of cadmium chloride (1 mg) plus test preparation of placebo for up to 60 days. The test group showed fewer toxic effects than the control group on the seminiferous tubules, epididymis, and spermatids. The test preparation contained *Orchis mascula*, *Lactuca serriola*, *Asteracantha longifolia*, *Mucuna pruriens*, *Parmelia perlata*, *Argyreia speciosa*, *Tribulus terrestris*, *Leptadenia reticulata*, and gold[MP057].

Gonadotropin release stimulation. Seeds, taken by male human adults orally at variable dosage levels, were equivocal. The product contained a mixture of *Orchis mascula*, *Hygrophila spinosa*, *Lactuca scariola*, *Mucuna pruriens*, *Parmelia parlata*, *Argyreia speciosa*, *Tribulus terrestris*, and *Leptadenia reticulata* (known as speman). Dosing was 2 tablets 3 times daily for 4 days[MP041].

Gonadotropin synthesis stimulation. Seeds, taken by male human adults orally

at variable dosage levels, were equivocal. The product contained a mixture of *Orchis mascula*, *Hygrophila spinosa*, *Lactuca scariola*, *Mucuna pruriens*, *Parmelia parlata*, *Argyreia speciosa*, *Tribulus terrestris*, and *Leptadenia reticulata* (known as speman). Dosing was 2 tablets 3 times daily for 4 days[MP941].

Hypocholesterolemic activity. Seeds, in the ration of rats, were active[MP011].

Hypoglycemic activity. Ethanol/water (1:1) extract of fruit, administered orally to rats at a dose of 250.0 mg/kg, was active. More than 30% drop in blood sugar level was observed. Ethanol/water (1:1) extract of root, administered orally to rats at a dose of 250.0 mg/kg, was active. More than 30% drop in blood sugar level was observed[MP006]. Ethanol/water (1:1) extract of seeds, administered orally to rats at a dose of 250.0 mg/kg, was inactive. Less than 30% drop in blood sugar level was observed[MP060]. Seeds, in the ration of rats, were active[MP011].

LH-release inhibition. Seeds, taken by male human adults orally at variable dosage levels, were equivocal. The product contained a mixture of *Orchis mascula*, *Hygrophila spinosa*, *Lactuca scariola*, *Mucuna pruriens*, *Parmelia parlata*, *Argyreia speciosa*, *Tribulus terrestris*, and *Leptadenia reticulata* (known as speman). Dosing was 2 tablets 3 times daily for 4 days[MP041].

LH-release stimulation. Seeds, taken orally by male human adults at variable dosage levels, were equivocal. The product contained a mixture of *Orchis mascula*, *Hygrophila spinosa*, *Lactuca scariola*, *Mucuna pruriens*, *Parmelia parlata*, *Argyreia speciosa*, *Tribulus terrestris*, and *Leptadenia reticulata* (known as speman). Dosing was 2 tablets 3 times daily for 4 days[MP041].

LH-synthesis stimulation. Seeds, taken by male human adults orally at variable dosage levels, were equivocal. The product used contained a mixture of *Orchis mascula*, *Hygrophila spinosa*, *Lactuca scariola*, *Mucuna* *pruriens, Parmelia parlata, Argyreia speciosa, Tribulus terrestris,* and *Leptadenia reticulata* (known as speman). Dosing was 2 tablets 3 times daily for 4 days[MP041].

Nematocidal activity. Decoction of a commercial sample of seeds, at a concentration of 10.0 mg/ml, was inactive on *Toxacara canis*[MP023]. Water extract of dried seeds, at a concentration of 10.0 mg/ml, was inactive on *Toxacara canis*; the methanol extract at a concentration of 1.0 mg/ml produced weak activity[MP026].

Penis erectile stimulant. Extract of dried seeds, taken orally by human adults, was active. Improvement in erection, duration of coitus and postcoital satisfaction has been observed in 56 cases treated for 4 weeks[MP056].

Plant growth inhibitor. Dried seeds exhibited allelopathic effect in field tests[MP012]. The acid fraction of ethanol (80%) extract inhibited the growth of *Lactuca sativa* seedlings[MP025].

Prolactin inhibition. Seeds, taken orally by female human adults at a dose of 15.0 gm/person, were inactive. Subjects had hyperprolactinemia and galactorrhea. Both subjects had a history of secondary amenorrhea and primary sterility. Daily dosing (divided doses) for 24 weeks in 1 subject and 10 weeks in a second subject. Inhibition of prolactin response to chlorpromazine injection in 5 subjects was positive[MP035].

Prostate treatment. Hot water extract of the entire plant, administered orally to human adults, was active. Forty-five patients with prostatitis were given the test preparation, and 10 more patients served as untreated controls. Of the 38 patients with benign hypertrophy in the test group, 28 improved and did not need surgery. All of the controls needed surgery. The test preparation contained *Orchis mascula, Lactuca serriola, Asteracantha longifolia, Mucuna pruriens, Parmelia perlata, Argyreia speciosa, Tribulus terrestris, Leptadenia reticulata,* and gold[MP058].

Prothrombin activity. *Echis carinatus* venom contains a mixture of proteins that affect the coagulative cascade, causing severe bleeding and hemorrhage. Seed extract, studied in prothrombin activation by *Echis carinatus* in vitro by clotting and chromogenic assay, produced an increase in procoagulant activity[MP067].

Spermatogenic effect. Seeds, taken orally by human adults at variable dosage levels, were equivocal. A group of 30 oligospermic infertilities in the age group of 24–46 years were studied over 4 months. Dosing was 3 times daily. Increases in magnesium content and in sperm count were reported. The product "speman" used, contained a mixture of *Orchis mascula, Hygrophila spinosa, Lactuca scariola, Mucuna pruriens, Parmelia parlata, Argyreia speciosa, Tribulus terrestris,* and *Leptadenia reticulata*[MP040]. Speman, used in a study involving 40 subjects to improve fertility, was active. Most of the patients claimed marked improvement relative to showing better semen profiles[MP038].

Taenicide activity. Ethanol (95%) and water extracts were active on *Taenia solium*[MP049].

Teratogenic activity. Water extract of seeds, administered intragastrically to pregnant rats at a dose of 175.0 mg/kg, was active[MP014].

Toxic effect. Water extract of seeds, in the ration of rats at variable dosage levels, was active. Feeding caused weight loss unless supplemented with L-methionine and L-tryptophan. The protein fraction of the seeds was incorporated into the experimental ration[MP044].

Toxicity assessment. Ethanol/water (1:1) extract of fruit and root, administered intraperitoneally to mice, produced a maximum tolerated dose of 1.0 gm/kg[MP006].

REFERENCES

MP001 Suwal, P. N. Medicinal Plants of Nepal. Ministry of Forests, Department of Medicinal Plants, Thapathali, Kathmandu, Nepal, 1970.

MP002   Alvaro Viera, R. Subsidio Para o Estudo da Flora Medicinal da Guinea Portuguesa. Agencia-Geral Do Ultramar, Lisboa, 1959.

MP003   Ahmad, Y. S. A Note on the Plants of Medicinal Value Found in Pakistan. Government of Pakistan Press, Karachi, 1957.

MP004   Bouquet, A. and M. Debray. Medicinal plants of the Ivory Coast. Trav Doc Orstom 1974; 32: 1.

MP005   Ghosal, S., S. Singh and S. K. Bhattachary. Alkaloids of Mucuna pruriens. Chemistry and pharmacology. Plant Med 1971; 19: 279

MP006   Dhar, M. L., M. M. Dhar, B. N. Mehrotra and C. Ray. Screening of Indian plants for biological activity. Part 1. Indian J Exp Biol 1968; 6: 232–247.

MP007   Saha, J. C., E. C. Savini and S. Kasinathan. Ecbolic properties of Indian medicinal plants. Part I. Indian J Med Res 1961; 49: 130–151.

MP008   Das, S. K. Medicinal, Economic and Useful Plants of India. Bally Seed Store, West Bengal, 1955.

MP009   Heckel, E. Les Plantes Medicinales et Toxiques de Madagascar. A. Challamel, Paris, 1903.

MP010   Burkhill, I. H. Dictionary of the Economic Products of the Malay Peninsula. Ministry of Agriculture and Cooperatives, Kuala Lumpur, Malaysia. Volume II, 1966.

MP011   Pant, M. C., I. Uddin, U. R. Bhardwaj and R. D. Tewari. Blood sugar and total cholesterol lowering effect of glycine soja (Sieb and Zucc.), Mucuna pruriens (D.C.) and Dolichos biflorus (Linn.) seed diets in normal fasting albino rats. Indian J Med Res 1968; 56 12: 1808–1812.

MP012   Fuiji, Y., T. Shibuya and T. Yasuda. Allelopathy of velvetbean: Its discrimination and identification of L-DOPA as a candidate of allelopathic substances. JARQ 1992; 25(4): 238–247.

MP013   Jauk, L., E. M. Galati, S. Kirjavainen, A. M. Forestieri and A. Trovato. Analgesic and antipyretic effect of Mucuna pruriens. Int J Pharmacog 1993; 31(3): 213–216.

MP014   Nath, D., N. Sethi, R. K. Singh and A. K. Jain. Commonly used Indian abortifacient plants with special reference to their teratologic effects in rats. J Ethnopharmacol 1992; 36(2): 147–154.

MP015   Elisabetsky, E., W. Figueiredo and G. Oliveria. Traditional Amazonian nerve tonics as antidepressant agents: Chaunochiton kappleri: A case study. J Herbs Spices Med Plants 1992; 1(1/2): 125–162.

MP016   Houghton, P. J. and K. P. Skari. The effect on blood clotting of some West African plants used against snakebite. J Ethnopharmacol 1994; 44(2): 99–108.

MP017   Girach, R. D., Aminuddin, P. A. Siddioui and S. A. Khan. Traditional plant remedies among the Kondh of District Dhenkanal (Orissa). Int J Pharmacog 1994; 32(3): 274–283.

MP018   Bhandary, M. J., K. R. Chandrashekar and K. M. Kaveriappa. Medical ethnobotany of the Siddis of Uttar Kannada District, Karnataka, India. J Ethnopharmacol 1995; 47(3): 149–158.

MP019   Smith, T. A. Tryptamine and related compounds in plants. Phytochemistry 1977; 16: 171–175.

MP020   Amico, A. Medicinal plants of Southern Zambesia. Fitoterapia 1977; 48: 101–139.

MP021   Iauk, L., E. M. Galati, A. M. Forestiri, S. Kirjavainen and A. Trovato. Mucuna pruriens decoction lowers cholesterol and total lipid plasma levels in the rat. Phytother Res 1989; 3(6): 263–264.

MP022   Jain, S. P. Tribal remedies from Saranda Forest, Bihar, India. I. Int J Crude Drug Res 1989; 27(1): 29–32.

MP023   Kiuchi, F., M. Hioki, N. Nakamura, N. Miyashita, Y. Tsuda and K. Kondo. Screening of crude drugs used in Sri Lanka for nematocidal activity on the larva of Toxacara canis. Shoyakugaku Zasshi 1989; 43(4): 288–293.

MP024   Nagaraju, N. and K. N. Rao. A survey of plant crude drugs of Rayalaseema, Andhra Pradesh, India. J Ethnopharmacol 1990; 29(2): 137–158.

MP025   Fuji, Y., T. Shibuya and T. Yasuda. L-3,4-Dihydroxyphenylalanine as an allelochemical candidate from Mucuna pruriens (L.) DC. Var. Utilis. Agr Biol Chem 1991; 55(2): 617–618.

MP026 Ali, M. A., M. Mikage, F. Kiuchi, Y. Tsuda and K. Kondo. Screening of crude drugs used in Bangladesh for nematocidal activity on the larva of *Toxacara canis*. **Shoyakugaku Zasshi** 1991; 45(3): 206–214.

MP027 Madulid, D. A., F. J. M. Gaerlan, E. M. Romero and E. M. G. Agoo. Ethnopharmacological study of the Ati tribe in Nagpana, Barotac Viejo, Iloilo. **Acta Manilana** 1989; 38(1): 25–40.

MP028 Carbajal, D., A. Casaco, L. Arruzaza-bala, R. Gonzalez and V. Fuentes. Pharmacological screening of plant decoctions commonly used in Cuban folk medicine. **J Ethnopharmacol** 1991; 33(1/2): 21–24.

MP029 List, P. H. and L. Horhammer. Hager's Handbuch der Pharmazeutischen Praxis, Vols. 2–6. Springer-Verlag, Berlin, 1969–1979.

MP030 Satyavati, G. V., et al. Medicinal Plants of India, Vols. 1–2. ICMR (Indian Council of Medical Research), New Delhi, 1976, 1987.

MP031 Duke, James A. Handbook of Phytochemical Constituents of GRAS Herbs. CRC Press, LLC 1992; 390–391.

MP032 Hasan, S. Q., M. R. K. Sherwani, I. Ahmad, F. Ahmad and S. M. Osman. Epoxy acids of *Mucuna prurita* seed oil. **J Indian Chem Soc** 1980; 57: 920–923.

MP033 Ayensu, E. S. Medicinal plants of the West Indies. **Unpublished Manuscript** 1978; 110pp.

MP034 Bhargava, N. C. and O. P. Singh. Fortege, and indigenous drugs in common sexual disorders in males. **Mediscope** 1978; 21(6): 140–144.

MP035 Vaidya, R. A., A. R. Sheth, S. D. Aloorkar, N. R. Rege, V. N. Bagadia, P. K. Devi and L. P. Shah. The inhibitory effect of the cowhage plant *Mucuna pruriens* and L-DOPA on chlorpromazine-induced hyperprolactinemia in man. **Neurology (India)** 1978; 26: 177,178.

MP036 Vaidya, R. A., S. D. Aloorkar, A. R. Sheth and S. K. Pandya. Activity of bromoergocryptine, *Mucuna pruriens* and L-DOPA in the control of hyperprolactinemia. **Neurology (India)** 1978; 26: 179–182.

MP037 Rao, M. R. R. and S. R. Parakh. Effect of some indigenous drugs on the sexual behavior of male rats. **Indian J Pharm Sci** 1978; 40: 236E.

MP038 Pardanani, D. S., R. J. Delima, R. V. Rao, A. Y. Vaze, P. G. Jayatilak and A. R. Sheth. Study of the effects of Speman on semen quality in oligospermic men. **Indian J Surg** 1976; 38: 34–39.

MP039 Vaidya, A. B., T. G. Rajagopalan, N. A. Mankodi, D. S. Amtarkar, P. S. Tathed, A. V. Purohit and N. H. Wadia. Treatment of Parkinson's Disease with cowhage plant-*Mucuna pruriens* Bak. **Neurology (India)** 1978; 26: 171–176.

MP040 Solepure, A. B., N. M .Joshi, B. V. Deshkar, S. R. Muzumdar and C. D. Shirole. The effect of "speman" on quality of semen in relation to magnesium concentration. **Indian Practitioner** 1979; 32: 663–668.

MP041 Jayatilak, P. G., A. R. Sheth, P. P. Mugatwala and D. S. Pardanani. Effect of an indigenous drug (Speman) on human accessory reproductive function. **Indian J Surg** 1976; 38: 12–15.

MP042 Kapoor, S. L. and L. D. Kapoor. Medicinal plant wealth of the Karimnagar District of Andhra Pradesh. **Bull Med Ethnobot Res** 1980; 1: 120–144.

MP043 Nath, C., G. P. Gupta, K. P. Bhargava, V. Lakshmi, S. Singh and S. P. Popli. Study of antiparkinsonian activity of seeds of *Mucuna prurita* hook. **Indian J Pharmacol** 1981; 13: 94–95.

MP044 Niranjan, G. S. and S. K. Katiyar. Chemical examination and biological evaluation of proteins isolated from some wild legumes. **J Indian Chem Soc** 1981; 58: 70–72.

MP045 Joshi, M. C., M. B. Patel and P. J. Mehta. Some folk medicines of Dangs, Gujarat State. **Bull Med Ethnobot Res** 1980; 1: 8–24.

MP046 Vitalyos, D. Phytotherapy in domestic traditional medicine in Matouba-Papaye (Guadeloupe). **Dissertation-Ph.D.-Univ Paris** 1979; 110pp.

MP047 Pushpangadan, P. and C. K. Atal. Ethno-medico-botanical investigations on Kerala 1. Some primitive tribals of Western Ghats and their herbal medicine. **J Ethnopharmacol** 1984; 11(1): 59–77.

MP048   Dixit, R. S. and H. C. Pandey. Plants used as folk-medicine in Jhansi and Lalitpur sections of Bundelkhand, Uttar Pradesh. **Int J Crude Drug Res** 1984; 22(1): 47–51.

MP049   Feroz, H., A. K. Khare and M. C. Srivastava. Review of scientific studies on anthelmintics from plants. **J Sci Res Pl Med** 1982; 3: 6–12.

MP050   Hemadri, K. and S. Sasibhushana Rao. Antifertility, abortifacient and fertility promoting drugs from Dandakaranya. **Ancient Sci Life** 1983; 3(2): 103–107.

MP051   Anderson, E. F. Ethnobotany of Hill Tribes of Northern Thailand. 1. Medicinal plants of Akha. **Econ Bot** 1986; 40(1): 38–53.

MP052   Madaan, S. Speman in oligospermia. **Probe** 1985; 115–117.

MP053   Panikkar, K. R., V. L. Majella and P. Madhavan Pillai. Lecithin from *Mucuna pruriens*. **Planta Med** 1987; 53(5): 503.

MP054   Weniger, B., M. Rouzier, R. Daguilh, D. Henrys, J. H. Henrys and R. Anthon. Popular medicine of the Central Plateau of Haiti. 2. Ethnopharmacological inventory. **J Ethnopharmacol** 1986; 17(1): 13–30.

MP055   Ohta, S., N. Sakurai, T. Inoue and M. Shinoda. Studies on chemical protectors against radiation. XXV. Radioprotective activities of various crude drugs. **Yakugaku Zasshi** 1987; 107(1): 70–75.

MP056   Sankaran, J. R. Problem of male virility – An Oriental therapy. **J Natl Integ Med Ass** 1984; 26(11): 315–317.

MP057   Rathore, H. S. and V. Saraswat. Protection of mouse testes, epididymis and adrenals with Speman against cadmium intoxication. **Probe** 1986; 25: 257–268.

MP058   Mukherjee, S., T. K. Ghosh and D. De. Effect of Speman on prostatism-A clinical study. **Probe** 1986; 25: 237–240.

MP059   Kumar, D. S. and Y. S. Prabhakar. On the ethnomedical significance of the Arjun tree, *Terminalia arjuna* (Roxb.) Wight & Arnot. **Indian J Homoeopath Med** 1984; 19(3): 114–120.

MP060   Dhawan, B. N., G. K. Patnaik, R. P. Rastogi, K. K. Singh and J. S. Tandon. Screening of Indian plants for biological activity. VI. **Indian J Exp Biol** 1977; 15: 208–219.

MP061   Jayatilak, P. G., D. S. Pardanani, B. D. Murty and A. R. Sheth. Effect of an indigenous drug (Speman) on accessory reproductive functions of mice. **Indian J Exp Biol** 1976; 14: 170.

MP062   Oakes, A. J. and M. P. Morris. The West Indian weedwoman of the United States Virgin Islands. **Bull Hist Med** 1958; 32: 164.

MP063   Rakhit, S. and D. N. Majumdar. *Mucuna pruriens* DC. Part V. Alkaloidal constituents and their characterization. **Indian J Pharmacy** 1956; 18: 285–287.

MP064   Manyam, B. V. and J. R. Sanchez-Ramos. Traditional and complementary therapies in Parkinson's disease. **Adv Neurol** 1999; 80: 565–574.

MP065   Nagashayana, N., P. Sankarankutty, M. R. Nampoothiri, P. K. Mohan and K. P. Mohanakumar. Association of L-DOPA with recovery following Ayurveda medication in Parkinson's disease. **J Neurol Sci** 2000; 176(2): 124–127.

MP066   Prakash, D., A. Niranjan and S. K. Tewari. Some nutritional properties of the seeds of three *Mucuna* species. **Int J Food Sci Nutr** 2001; 52(1): 79–82.

MP067   Guerranti, R., J. C. Aguiyi, E. Errico, R. Pagani and E. Marinello. Effects of *Mucuna pruriens* extract on activation of prothrombin by *Echis carinatus* venom. **J Ethnopharmacol** 2001; 75(2–3): 175–180.

MP068   Grover, J. K., V. Vats, S. S. Rathi and R. Dawar. Traditional Indian anti-diabetic plants attenuate progression of renal damage in streptozotocin induced diabetic mice. **J Ethnopharmacol** 2001; 76(3): 233–238.

17 | Mangifera indica

L.

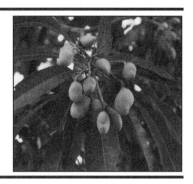

Common Names

Aam	Fiji	Mango	Guam
Aam	India	Mango	Guatemala
Aamp	Nepal	Mango	Guyana
Aanp	Nepal	Mango	Haiti
Alfonso mango	India	Mango	India
Am	India	Mango	Ivory Coast
Am	Pakistan	Mango	Mexico
Amba	Oman	Mango	Nepal
Amm	India	Mango	Nicaragua
Amp	Nepal	Mango	Pakistan
Amra	India	Mango	Peru
Amva	India	Mango	Puerto Rico
Andok–ntang	Guinea	Mango	Sudan
Asm	India	Mango	Tanzania
Bo–amb	India	Mango	Tonga
Bowen mango	USA	Mango	Venezuela
Bumango	Senegal	Mango dusa	Nicaragua
Chamorro	Guam	Mango tree	India
Embe	Tanzania	Mango fruit	India
Maamidi	India	Mangu	Nicaragua
Mam–maram	India	Mangue	Rodrigues Islands
Manga	Brazil	Mangueira	Brazil
Mangga	Guam	Mankro	Nicaragua
Mangguo	China	Mave	India
Mango	China	Mwembe	Tanzania
Mango	Brazil	Oegkoti–tong	India
Mango	Canary Islands	Ondwa	Guinea
Mango	Curacao	Pauh	Indonesia
Mango	Egypt	Skin mango	Brazil
Mango	Fiji	Vi papaa	Rarotonga

From: *Medicinal Plants of the World, vol. 1: Chemical Constituents, Traditional and Modern Medicinal Uses, 2nd ed.*
By: Ivan A. Ross © Humana Press Inc., Totowa, NJ

BOTANICAL DESCRIPTION

Trees of the ANACARDIACEAE family varying in size according to variety, and can be from 3 to 30 meters tall, typically heavy-branched from a stout trunk. Leaves spirally arranged on the branches, lanceolate-elliptical, pointed at both ends, the blades mostly up to about 25 cm long and 8 cm wide, sometimes much larger, reddish, and thinly flaccid when first formed (new flush). Inflorescences are large terminal pannicles of small polygamous, fragrant, yellow to pinkish flowers. Fruit is a drupe, variously shaped according to the variety, from ellipsoid to obliquely reniform, 5 to 15 cm long.

ORIGIN AND DISTRIBUTION

Records indicate that mango has been in cultivation on the Indian subcontinent for well over 4,000 years. It is a native of tropical Asia and introduced wherever the climate is sufficiently warm and damp. It is now completely naturalized in many parts of the tropics and subtropics, and here and there a component of mature secondary vegetation.

TRADITIONAL MEDICINAL USES

Brazil. Decoction of dried bark is used to treat scabies[MI029].

Canary Islands. Dried oleoresin is used for food. Hot water extract of dried bark is taken orally for diarrhea. Hot water extract of fresh fruit is taken orally as an anthelmintic[MI090].

Curacao. Decoction of hot water extract[MI006] or tea[MI007] of leaves is taken orally for high blood pressure; 3 cups a day, 3 days in succession. Some take the decoction every day.

Fiji. Fresh kernel is eaten for dysentery and asthma; juice is used as a nose drop for sinus trouble. Fresh leaf juice, in coconut oil, is used externally for heat rash and burns. Hot water extract of dried bark is taken orally for syphilis. Unripe, fresh fruit pulp, mixed with curd is used for indigestion and stomachache[MI083].

Guam. The fruit has been reported to cause rash called mango dermatitis on human adults[MI008].

Haiti. Water extract of dried bark is taken orally for liver trouble[MI085].

India. Decoction of dried bark is used for diabetes. Ten grams of dried leaves of *Zanthoxylum armatum* are boiled in 8 liters of water, together with 125 gm of a mixture containing equal parts of bark of *Acacia nilotica*, *Mangifera indica* and *Syzygium cumini*, until the quantity of water is reduced to 2 liters. Fifty milliliters of decoction is taken twice daily after meals[MI052]. Hot water extract of the dried bark is taken orally for leukorrhea, bleeding hemorrhoids and lung hemorrhage[MI080]. Decoction of the stem bark is taken orally with cow's milk to treat menarche[MI026]. The decoction is taken orally, and the vapor is inhaled to treat jaundice[MI034]. As a contraceptive, the stem bark of the young mango plant, which has not flowered even once, is used. Fifty grams of fine stem bark powder is taken with alcoholic wine. It is said to be effective enough to cause abortion safely for up to 6 months after conception[MI087,MI065]. Dried seed powder is applied to the head to remove dandruff. The kernel starch is eaten as a famine food[MI075]. Extract of flowers is used for diarrhea and dysentery[MI019]. Fresh leaf juice is used for treating inflammation of the eyes; it is applied on eyes (protecting the eyelids) twice daily[MI035]. For styes, petiole juice is applied to the stye during the time it is painful or irritated. For permanent cure, apply when pus has started oozing[MI082]. The fruit is used as a laxative, diuretic, diaphoretic, astringent, and refrigerant[MI019]. Hot water extract of dried leaves is taken orally for diabetes[MI013,MI080], diarrhea and hiccups[MI080]. Dried leaves are used to prevent tooth decay. Powder or decoction is applied to teeth with finger or brush[MI048]. Hot water extract of kernel is taken orally as an anthelmintic, aphrodisiac, laxative and tonic[MI092]. Hot water extract of the bark is used as an astringent, tonic[MI019] and for menorrhagia[MI097]. Water extract of leaves is taken orally for coughs, asthma, dysentery and diarrhea[MI019].

Malaysia. Hot water extract of seed is taken orally for menorrhagia[MI011].

Nepal. Hot water extract of fruit is administered intravaginally to humans for hemorrhages of the uterus. Hot water extract of seeds is taken orally for asthma[MI001].

Nicaragua. Phenol/water extract of inner bark is used externally for wounds[MI051].

Panama. The fruit is eaten as a laxative. Hot water extract of leaves is used to treat rheumatism. Decoction of 15–20 leaves in 1 liter of water is prepared. Leaves are chewed for toothache and gum disorders[MI064].

Peru. Hot water extract of dried fruit is ingested as a traditional medicine[MI089].

Rarotonga. Fresh fruit rind is eaten as a refreshing tonic[MI024].

Senegal. Hot water extract of dried bark is used orally for mouth sores, odontalgia, and as a mouthwash for toothache. The extract is taken orally for dysentery and diarrhea; it is used externally for cutaneous affections. Hot water extract of dried leaves is taken orally for bronchitis, toothache, angina and blennorrhagia. Hot water extract of oleoresin is taken orally for syphilis[MI050].

Sri Lanka. Bruised bark and leaves of *Ervatania dichotoma*, bark of *Mangifera indica* and *Ficus glomerata* are boiled in coconut oil and applied to abraded skin of ulcers and fistulae as an astringent and antiseptic[MI076].

Tanzania. Decoction of dried stem bark is used orally for toothache. Decoction of root is taken orally for malaria[MI091].

Tonga. Infusion of dried leaves is used for the syndrome locally called Kita Fa' ele, consisting of fever, chills, dizziness, and lower abdominal pain presumed to result from insufficient rest during puerperium. *Mangifera indica, Diospyros lateriflora, Bischofia javanica,* *Pittosporum arborescens,* and *Colubrina asiatica* are used in the preparation[MI077].

Zaire. Infusion of dried stem bark is taken orally for diarrhea, chest pains, coughs, anemia, urinary tract infections, and diabetes. Externally, the infusion is used for infected wounds and skin diseases, and as an oral application for dental caries[MI028].

Particular care should be taken in using the shoots and flowers, since they may be contaminated with fungal toxins. Mycotoxins are among the most important chemical hazards in the rural countryside.

CHEMICAL CONSTITUENTS
(ppm unless otherwise indicated)

1-3-5-6-7-Pentamethoxy xanthone: Sh[MI037]
1-3-6-7-Tetramethoxy xanthone: Sh[MI037]
2-Ethyl hexanol: Pan[MI019]
4-Phenyl-n-butyl gallate: Fl[MI049]
5-(12-Cis-heptadecenyl): Fr Pe[MI043]
5-Dehydro-avenasterol: Ker[MI041]
5-Heptadec-cis-2-enyl resorcinol: Lx[MI040]
5-Methyl furfur-2-al: Fr Pu[MI062]
5-Pentadecyl resorcinol: Fr Pe[MI043]
6-Phenyl-N-hexyl gallate: Fl[MI049]
7-Dehydro-avenosterol: Ker[MI041]
Acetaldehyde: Fr[MI042]
Acetic acid ethyl ester: Fr[MI042]
Acetic acid methyl ester: Fr[MI042]
Acetic acid N-butyl ester: Fr[MI042]
Acetophenone: Fr Pu[MI062]
Acetyl furan: Fr Pu[MI062]
Alanine: Fl[MI031]
Allo-aromadendrene: Lf EO[MI059]
Alpha amyrenone: Sd oil[MI060]
Alpha amyrin: Rt Bk 33.3[MI039], St Bk 43.7–100[MI015,MI014]
Alpha cubebene: Lf EO[MI059]
Alpha farnesene: Lf EO[MI059]
Alpha guaiene: Lf EO[MI059]
Alpha humulene: Fr Pu[MI062]
Alpha phellandrene: Fr Pu[MI062]
Alpha pinene: Fr Pu[MI062], Lf EO[MI059]
Alpha terpinolene: Lf EO[MI059]
Alpha thujene: Lf EO[MI096]
Alpha tocopherol: Fr[MI012]
Amentoflavone: Bk[MI027]
Arachidic acid: Ker[MI041]
Arachidonic acid: Sd oil[MI044]

Ascorbic acid: Fr[MI003]
Benzaldehyde: Fr Pu[MI062]
Beta amyrenone: Sd oil[MI060]
Beta amyrin: Rt Bk 50[MI039],
    St Bk 43.7–100[MI015,MI014]
Beta bulnesene: Lf EO[MI059]
Beta caryophyllene: Lf EO[MI059]
Beta elemene: Lf EO[MI059]
Beta myrcene: EO[MI036]
Beta ocimene: Lf EO[MI059]
Beta phellandrene: Fr Pu[MI062]
Beta pinene: Lf EO[MI059]
Beta selinene: Fr Pu[MI062]
Beta sitosterol: Rt Bk[MI039], Fr Pe[MI043],
    St Bk[MI015,MI014], Lf[MI068], Pn[MI019]
Bis-2-ethyl hexanyl-phthalate: Pn[MI019]
Campesterol: Ker[MI041]
Camphene: Lf EO[MI059,MI096]
Car-3-ene: Fr Pu[MI062], Lf EO[MI059,MI096]
Caryophyllene: Fr Pu[MI062]
Catechin oxidase: Fr[MI063]
Cholesterol: Ker[MI041]
Cis-ocimene: EO[MI036]
Cis-zeatin riboside: Sd[MI072]
Cis-zeatin: Sd[MI072]
Citrostadienol: Ker[MI041]
Cycloartenol: St Bk 0.07%[MI053]
Cycloartenone: Sd oil[MI060]
Cyclobranol: Ker[MI041]
Cyclosadol: Ker[MI041]
D-arabinose: Fl[MI031]
Dammaradienol: Ker[MI041]
Dammarendiol II: St Bk 20[MI014]
Daucosterol: St Bk 3.7[MI015]
Delta cadinene: Lf EO[MI059]
Delta elemene: Lf EO[MI059]
Dimethyl sulfide: Fr Pu[MI062]
Eicos-9-en-1-oic acid: Ker[MI041]
Elaidic acid: Ker[MI041]
Elemicin: Lf EO[MI059]
Ellagic acid: Pn[MI019]
EO: Lf[MI059,MI096]
Estragole: Lf EO[MI059]
Eugenol methyl ester: Lf EO[MI059]
Euxanthone: Lf[MI098]
Fatty acids: Sd oil[MI094]
Friedelan-3-beta-ol: Rt Bk[MI039]
Friedelin: Rt Bk[MI039]
Friedelinol: Ker[MI041]
Fructose, 1-6-phosphatase: Fr[MI021]
Furfural: Fr Pu[MI062]
Galactose: Fl[MI031], Pn[MI019]

Gallic acid: Fr Pu[MI022], Pn[MI019], Lf[MI067]
Gallicin: Pn[MI019]
Gamma terpinene: Lf EO[MI059], Fr Pu[MI062]
Gentisic acid: Lf[MI010]
Germanicol: Ker[MI041]
Glochidonol: Sh[MI037]
Glucose: Fr[MI061]
Gramisterol: Ker[MI041]
Heptadecan-1-oic acid: Ker[MI041]
Hexadec-7-en-1-oic acid: Ker[MI041]
Hexadec-9-en-1-oic acid: Ker[MI041]
Homo-mangiferin: Lf[MI067]
Hopane-1-beta-3-beta-22-triol: St Bk[MI053]
Humulene: Lf EO[MI059]
Indicene: Lf EO[MI096]
Indicoside A: St Bk[MI016]
Indicoside B: St Bk[MI016]
Iso-mangiferin: Lf[MI079]
Iso-quercitrin methyl ether: Sh[MI037]
Isomangiferolic acid: St Bk[MI015,MI053]
Kaempferol methyl ether: Sh[MI037]
Kaempferol: Lf[MI098]
Laccase: Fr[MI063]
Lauric acid: Ker[MI041]
Limonene: Fr Pu[MI062], Lf EO[MI059]
Linalool: Lf EO[MI059]
Linoleic acid: Fr[MI043], Sd oil[MI044]
Linolenic acid: Sd oil[MI044], Fr Pe[MI043]
Lophenol: Ker[MI041]
Lupenone: Sh[MI037], Sd oil[MI060]
Lupeol: Sh[MI037], Lf[MI068], Ker[MI041]
Mangiferin: Bk[MI023], Fr Pe[MI061], Lf[MI067],
    Rt Bk[MI039]
Mangiferene: Lf EO[MI096]
Mangiferolic acid: Rt Bk[MI039], St Bk[MI015]
Mangiferonic acid methyl ester:
    St Bk 20[MI014]
Mangiferonic acid: Rt Bk[MI039], St Bk[MI015]
Meso inositol: Fr Pe[MI061]
Methyl cyclohexane: Fr Pu[MI062]
Myrcene: Lf EO[MI059]
Myricetin methyl ester: Sh[MI037]
Myristic acid: Ke[MI041]
N-hentriacontane: Galls[MI005]
N-heptacosane: Galls[MI005]
N-nonacosane: Galls[MI005]
N-octadecane: Pn[MI019]
N-octane: Pr Pu[MI062]
N-octyl gallate: Fl[MI049]
N-pentacosane: Galls[MI005]
N-pentyl gallate: Fl[MI049]
N-propyl gallate: Fl[MI049]

N-texatriacontane: Galls[MI005]
Nonadecan-1-oic acid: Ker[MI041]
Obtusifoliol: Ker[MI041]
Ocimene: Lf EO[MI096]
Ocotillol: St Bk 12.5[MI015]
Octacosan-1-ol: Pn[MI019]
Octadeca-6-9-dien-1-oic acid: Ker[MI041]
Octadeca-cis-9-cis-15-dienoic acid: Fr[MI017]
Octdeca-3-6-9-trien-1-oic acid: Ker[MI041]
Octillol II: St Bk 50[MI014]
Oleic acid: Sd oil[MI044], Fr Pe[MI043]
Palmitic acid: Fr Pe[MI043], Sd oil[MI044]
Para cymene: Fr Pu[MI062]
Pentadecan-1-oic acid: Ker[MI041]
Peonidin-3-galactoside: Fr Pe[MI098]
Phenylacetaldehyde: Fr Pu[MI062]
Propionaldehyde: Fr[MI042]
Protein: Lf 9.5%[MI093]
Protocatechuic acid: Lf[MI067]
Quercetin methyl ether: Sh[MI037]
Quercetin: Pl[MI098]
Quercitrin methyl ether: Sh[MI037]
Rutin: Lf 5.2%[MI070]
Sabinene: Lf EO[MI096]
Stearic acid: Sd[MI018], Sd oil[MI044], Ker[MI041]
Stigmast-7-en-3-beta-ol: Ker[MI041]
Stigmasterol: Ker[MI041]
Taraxerol: Lf[MI068]
Taraxerone: Lf[MI068]
Terpinene: Lf EO[MI096]
Threonine: Fl[MI031]
Toluene: Fr Pu[MI062]
Trans-zeatin ribose: Sd[MI072]
Trans-zeatin: Sd[MI072]
Trichloro ethylene: Fr Pu[MI062]
Tridecan-1-oic acid: Ker[MI041]
Tryptophan: Fl[MI031]
Ursolic acid: Sh[MI037]
Valencene: Fr Pu[MI062]
Valine: Fl[MI031]

PHARMACOLOGICAL ACTIVITIES AND CLINICAL TRIALS

Allergenic activity. Fresh fruit, eaten by human adult was active. A male exhibited periorbital edema, facial erythema, widespread urticaria and dyspnea 20 minutes after eating a mango fruit. Pulse was 100 beats/min, blood pressure 104/72. Anaphylaxis was diagnosed. He was treated with intravenous hydrocortisone and chlor-

pheniramine maleate and recovered. Prick testing with mango juice produced a wheal within 5 minutes. The patient had a history of asthma, eczema, hay fever and drug allergy[MI056]. Powder commercial sample of fruits was active on human adults. Reactions to patch tests occurred most commonly in patients who were regularly exposed to the substance, or who already had dermatitis on the fingertips. Previously unexposed patients had reactions (i.e., non-irritant reactions)[MI045].

Alpha-amylase activity. Ethanol extract of the leaves produced significant inhibitory activity in vitro[MI103].

Alpha-glucosidase activity. The ethanol extract of the bark, tested in vitro, produced significant inhibitory activity, IC_{50} value was 314 gm/ml[MI101].

Anthelmintic activity. Hot water extract of kernel, at a concentration of 1:50, was active on *Haemonchus contortus*[MI092].

Antiamebic activity. The stem bark, at a concentration of 80 microgram/ml, inhibited *Entamoeba histolytica* growth with MAC < 10 micrograms/ml[MI108].

Antibacterial activity. Ethanol (95%) extract of dried leaves, on agar plate, was active on *Escherichia coli* and *Staphylococcus aureus*[MI099]. Water extract was active on *Actinomycete* species and plaque bacteria. Commercial dentifrices were tested alone and in combination with plant extracts against plaque bacteria in the paper disk assay. The addition of plant extracts significantly increased the zone of inhibition relative to that of the dentifrices[MI048]. The extract was active on *Bacteroides gingivalis* vs 2 clinical isolates; *Pseudomonas* and *Streptococcus salivarius* vs 5 clinical isolates and *Streptococcus viridans* vs 40 clinical isolates. Water extract, taken orally by human adults, was active. Fifty patients with chronic suppurative peridontitis were given leaf extracts of *Mangifera indica*, *Camellia sinensis*, *Murray koenigii*, *Ocimum basilicum*, or *Azadirachta* *indica.* Bacterial populations declined by 50%, and 40 patients showed improvement[MI048]. The hot water extract, undiluted on agar plate, was inactive on *Escherichia coli* and *Staphylococcus aureus*[MI099]. Ethanol (95%) extract of fresh kernel, on agar plate, was active on *Agrobacterium tumefaciens*, MIC 1.5 mg/ml; *Sarcina lutea*, MIC 2.0 mg/ml; *Staphylococcus aureus*, MIC 2.0 mg/ml; *Bacillus firmis*, MIC 3.0 mg/ml; *Escherichia coli*, MIC 3.0 mg/ml; *Proteus vulgaris*, MIC 3.0 mg/ml and *Pseudomonas aeruginosa*, MIC 4.0 mg/ml[MI047]. Hot water extract of dried leaves, on agar plate, was active on *Sarcina lutea* and *Staphylococcus aureus*[MI095]. Methanol extract of dried stem bark, at a concentration of 10.0 mg/ml on agar plate, was inactive on *Escherichia coli, Pseudomonas aeruginosa, Salmonella typhimurium,* and *Streptococcus mutans*. The extract was active on *Klebsiella pneumonia* and *Staphylococcus aureus*, MIC 125.0 mcg/ml. The tannin fraction of dried stem bark, on agar plate, was active on *Citrobacter diversus* at a dose of 110.0 mcg/ml; *Salmonella enteritidis* at a dose of 120.0 mg/ml; *Staphylococcus aureus* at a concentration of 145.0 mcg/ml; *Escherichia piracoli, Klebsiella pneumonia,* and *Shigella flexneri* at a concentration of 200.0 mcg/ml. Weak activity was shown on *Escherichia coli* at a concentration of 225.0 mcg/ml[MI033].

Antidiabetic activity. The aqueous extract of the leaves, administered orally to normoglycemic, glucose-induced hyperglycemia and streptozotocin induced diabetic mice, produced a reduction of blood glucose level in normoglycemic and glucose-induced hyperglycemia, but did not have any effect on the streptozotocin-induced diabetic mice[MI102].

Antifungal activity. Ethanol (95%) extract of fresh kernel, at a concentration of 5.0 mg/ml on agar plate, was active on *Trichophyton mentagrophytes*[MI047]. Hot water extract of dried leaves, on agar plate, was inactive on *Aspergillus niger*[MI095]. Methanol extract of dried stem bark, at a concentration of 10.0 mg/ml, was inactive on *Aspergillus niger* and *Microsporum gypseum*[MI028].

Antihyperglycemic effect. Aqueous extract of the leaves, administered orally at a dose of 1 gm/kg to normoglycemic, glucose-induced hyperglycemic and streptozotocin-induced diabetic rats, did not alter the blood glucose levels in either normoglycemic or streptozotocin-induced diabetic rats. In glucose-induced, however, antidiabetic activity was seen when the extract and glucose were administered simultaneously and when the extract was given to the rats 60 min before the glucose. The hypoglycemic effect was compared with that of an oral dose of clorpropamide (200 mg/kg) under the same conditions[MI110].

Anti-inflammatory activity. Ethanol (95%) extract of fresh kernel, administered by gastric intubation to rats at a dose of 50.0 mg/kg, was active vs carrageenin-induced pedal edema, 5-HT-induced pedal edema, bradykinin-induced pedal edema, turpentine-induced pleurisy, granuloma pouch, cotton pellet granuloma and adjuvant-induced arthritis. The extract was inactive vs dextran-induced pedal edema and prostaglandin-induced pedal edema and weakly active vs formaldehyde-induced arthritis[MI047]. The aqueous extract of the bark, administered orally at a dose of 50–1000 mg/kg, produced a potent and dose-dependent antinociceptive effect against acetic acid test in mice. The mean potency DE_{50} was 54.5 mg/kg and the maximal inhibition attained was 94.4%. Dose of 20–1000 mg/kg dose-dependently inhibited the second phase of formalin-induced pain but not the first phase. The DE_{50} of the second phase was 8.4 mg/kg and the maximal inhibition was 99.5%, being more potent than indomethacin at doses of 20 mg/kg. The extract also significantly inhibited edema formation ($P < 0.01$) of both carrageenan-

and formalin-induced edema in rat, guinea pig and mice (maximal inhibitions: 39.5, 45.0, and 48.6, respectively)[MI104].

Antimalarial activity. Water extract of bark, administered orally to chicken at a dose of 7.82 gm/kg, was inactive on *Plasmodium gallinaceum*[MI002].

Antimycobacterial activity. Hot water extract of dried leaves, on agar plate, was inactive on *Mycobacterium phlei*[MI095].

Antinematodal activity. Water extract of dried leaves, at variable concentrations, was active on *Meloidogyne incognita*[MI071].

Antioxidant activity. The stem bark extract (vimang) 50–250 mg/kg, mangiferin 50 mg/kg, vitamin C 100 mg/kg, vitamin E 100 mg/kg, and beta-carotene 50 mg/kg were evaluated for their protective abilities against the 12-O-tetradecanoylphorbol-13-acetate (TPA)-induced oxidative damage in serum, liver, brain as well as in the hyperproduction of reactive oxygen species (ROS) by peritoneal macrophages. The treatment of mice with vimang, vitamin E and mangiferin reduced the TPA-induced production of ROS by 70, 17, and 44%, respectively. Similarly, the H_2O_2 levels were reduced by 55–73, 37, and 44%, respectively. Vimang, mangiferin, vitamin C plus E and beta-carotene decreased TPA-induced DNA fragmentation by 46–52, 35, 42, and 17%, respectively, in hepatic tissues, and by 29-34, 22, 41, and 17%, in brain tissues. Similar results were observed in respect to lipid peroxidation in serum, in hepatic mitochondria and microsomes, and in brain homogenate supernatants[MI105]. Vimang when tested in vitro for its antioxidant activity, indicated a powerful scavenger activity of hydroxyl radicals and hypochlorous acid and acted as an iron chelator. The extract also showed significant inhibitory effect on the peroxidation of rat-brain phospholipids and inhibited DNA damage by bleomycin or copper-phenanthroline systems[MI106].

Antitumor activity. Ethanol/water (1:1) extract of dried aerial parts, administered intraperitoneally to mice at a dose of 250.0 mg/kg, was inactive on Leuk-P388[MI081].

Antiviral activity. Ethanol (80%) extract of freeze-dried leaves, in cell culture at variable dosages, was equivocal on Coxsackie B2 virus, measles virus and Poliovirus; inactive on adenovirus, Herpes virus type 1 and Semilicki-forest virus vs plaque-inhibition[MI069]. Methanol extract of dried stem bark, at a concentration of 100.0 mcg/ml in cell culture, showed weak activity on HIV virus[MI032]. Undiluted leaf juice was inactive on bean mosaic virus. Reduction of infectiousness was measured[MI078]. Mangiferin, as determined by plaque inhibition assay, contained both anti-HSV-1 and -2 activities. An inhibition of the production of infectious HSV-2 virions from infected Vero cells could also be demonstrated[MI109].

Antiyeast activity. Ethanol (60%) extract of dried leaves, on agar plate, was inactive on *Candida albicans*[MI058]. Ethanol (95%) extract of fresh kernel, on agar plate at a concentration of 5.0 mg/kg, was active on *Candida lunata* and inactive on *Candida albicans*[MI047]. Hot water extract of dried leaves, on agar plate, was inactive on *Saccharomyces cerevisiae*[MI095]. Methanol extract of dried stem bark, at a concentration of 10.0 mg/ml on agar plate, was inactive on *Candida albicans*[MI028].

Ascaricidal activity. Ethanol (95%) extract of dried seeds was active on *Ascaris lumbricoides*[MI074].

Cytotoxic activity. Ethanol/water (1:1) extract of dried aerial parts, at a concentration of 25.0 mg/ml, was inactive on CA-9KB[MI081]. Methanol extract of dried stem bark, at a concentration of 100.0 mcg/ml, was equivocal on CA-HS-578-T, CA-mammary-MF-7, CA-mammary-MF-7/ADR, human breast cancer cell lines BT-549, MDA-MB-231, MDA-MB-435, MDA-N, T47-D and leukemia cell line

CCRF-CEM. Inactive on RPMI-8226 cells, and weakly active on CA-colon-KM12, CA-HCT-15, CA-human-colon COLO-205, CA-human-colon-HCT116, CA-human-nonsmall-cell-lung HOP-62, CA-human-ovarian OVCAR-3, CA-human-ovarian OVCAR-4, CA-human-ovarian OVCAR-5, CA-human-ovarian-SKOV-3, cancer cell line-human CNS-SNB75, human CNS cancer cell lines SF-268, SF-295, SF-539, SNB-19 and U251, human colon cancer cell lines HCC-2998, HT29 and SW620, human leukemia cell lines HL-60-TB and MOLT-4, human melanoma cell lines MALME-3M, SK-MEL-2 and SK-MEL-5, human nonsmall cell lung cancer cell line A549(ATCC), human nonsmall cell lung cancer cell line EKVX, human nonsmall cell lung cancer cell lines HOP-92, NCI-H226, NCI-H23, NCI-H322M, NCI-H460 and NCI-H522, human ovarian adenocarcinoma IGROV-1, human ovarian cancer cell line OVCAR-8, human renal cancer cell line 786-0, human renal cancer cell lines A498, CAKI-1, SN-12C, TK-10 and UO-31, Leuk-K562, Leuk-SR, Melanoma-LOX IMVI, elanoma-M14, Melanoma-SK-MEL-28, Melanoma-UACC-257, Melanoma-UACC-62, and *Mycobacterium fortuitum*[MI032]. Water extract of freeze-dried fruit was active on Leuk-P815. Tumor-toxic activity was evaluated by culturing Mastocytoma P815 cells with macrophage cells and measuring the incorporation of 3H-Thimidine radio-activity[MI054].

Dermatitis producing effect. Fresh fruit, applied externally to male children, was active. Cross-sensitivity resulted from the presence of phenols with 15-C side chains[MI030].

Enzymatic degradation effect. Ripe mango puree was treated with fungal polysaccharidases containing pectinolytic, hemicellulolytic, and cellulolytic activities for 2 hour at 50°C. A loss of 30% of the cell wall material was observed. Cell wall material polysaccharides were hydrolyzed to varying degrees: 88, 65, and 65%, respectively, of galacturonic acid-, arabinose-, and rhamnose-containing polymers were hydrolyzed, whereas 50% of cellulose was degraded. After 30 min of treatment, the ethanol precipitation test on the serum was negative, indicating that pectic substances were rapidly hydrolyzed. A viscosity drop of 90% was observed after 2 hours, confirming the dominant role of pectic substances in puree viscosity[MI107].

Estrogenic effect. Methanol extract of leaves, administered subcutaneously to mice, was active[MI009].

Hypoglycemic activity. Fibers of fresh fruit, at a concentration of 9.0%, were active. Fibrous waste, from processing fruit, slowed the rate of activity of amylase in potato starch and slowed the diffusion of glucose in a dialysis experiment[MI025]. Water extract of dried leaves, administered orally to rabbits at a dose of 10.0 mg/kg, was active. Drop in blood sugar of 15 mg relative to inert-treated control indicated positive results[MI013].

Immunomodulatory activity. Alcohol extract of the stem bark (containing 2.6% mangiferin) produced an increase in humoral antibody titer and delayed type hypersensitivity in mice[MI100].

Insecticidal activity. Petroleum ether extract of dried bark, at a concentration of 50.0 mcg, was active on *Rhodinius neglectus*[MI029].

Interleukin induction. Water extract of freeze-dried fruits produced weak activity. IL-1 activity was measured by the IL-1 dependent growth of a T-helper cell line[MI054].

Juvenile hormone activity. Acetone extract of stem was active[MI020].

Larvicidal activity. Water extract of dried cotyledons, at a concentration of 0.03 gm/ml, was inactive on *Culex quinquefasciatus*. The concentrations given are in grams of fresh plant material per ml water[MI046].

Molluscicidal activity. Aqueous slurry (homogenate) of fresh entire plant was inactive on *Lymnaea columella* and *Lymnaea cubensis*, LD_{100} for both was more than 1 M ppm[MI066]. Water extract of oven-dried leaves produced weak activity on *Biophalaria pfeifferi*[MI086]. Water saturated with fresh leaf essential oil, at a concentration of 1:10, was inactive on *Biomphalaria glabrata*[MI073].

Mutagenic activity. Seed oil was inactive on *Salmonella typhimurium* TA100 and TA98. Metabolic activation had no effect on the results[MI084].

Nutritional value. Seed oil, in the ration of rats at a dose of 10.0% of the diet, was active. Animals showed good growth performance and feed efficiency. The oil is rich in stearic and oleic acids and low in linoleic acid. The experiment was carried out over 3 generations of rats[MI038].

Plant germination effect. Water extracts of dried bark, dried leaves and dried stem, at concentrations of 500 gm/liter, produced weak activity on the seeds of *Cuscuta reflexa* after 6 days of exposure to the extract[MI057].

Plant growth inhibitor. Water extracts of dried leaves, dried stem and dried bark, at concentrations of 500.0 gm/liter, produced weak activity. *Cuscuta reflexa* seedling length, weight and dry weight were measured after 6 days exposure to the extract[MI057].

Spasmolytic activity. Butanol extract of dried trunk bark, at a concentration of 0.2 mg/ml, was active on guinea pig ileum. A reduction of 45.12% in contractions was seen vs ACh-induced contractions and 37.43% reduction in contractions vs KCl-induced contractions. Isopentyl alcohol extract of trunk bark, at a concentration of 0.2 mg/ml, produced 87.34% reduction in contractions vs ACh-induced contractions and 76.54% reduction in contractions vs KCl-induced contractions. Methanol extract of dried trunk bark, at a concentration of 0.2 mg/ml, produced 34.00% reduction in contractions vs ACh-induced

contractions and 20.17% reduction in contractions vs KCl-induced contractions[MI055]. The stem bark, at a concentration of 80 micrograms/ml in an organ bath, exhibited more that 70% inhibition of acetylcholine and/or KCl solution-induced contractions on isolated guinea-pig ileum[MI108].

Teratogenic activity. Seed oil, in the ration of rats, at a dose of 10.0% of the diet, was inactive. The experiment was carried out over 3 generations. There was no difference in litter size, birth weight or weaning weight over controls fed cocoa butter fat[MI038].

Toxic effect (general). Seed oil, in the ration of rats at a dose of 10.0% of the diet, was inactive. There was no effect on organ weights, cholesterol, triglyceride and lipid content of serum and liver, mating behavior, litter size, birth weight or mortality over controls fed cocoa-butter fat. Experiments were carried out over 3 generations[MI038].

Toxicity assessment (quantitative). Ethanol/water (1:1) extract of dried aerial parts, administered intraperitoneally to mice, produced $LD_{50} > 1000$ mg/kg[MI081].

Tumor promotion inhibition. Methanol extract of fresh fruit, at a concentration of 200.0 mcg in cell culture, was inactive on Epstein-Barr virus vs 12-0-hexadecanoyl-phorbol-13-acetate-induced Epstein-Barr virus activation[MI088].

Uterine stimulant effect. Ethanol/water (1:1) extract of dried aerial parts was active on rat uterus[MI081]. Water extract of kernel was inactive on nonpregnant uterus of guinea pigs[MI004].

WBC-Macrophage stimulant. Water extract of freeze-dried fruits, at a concentration of 2.0 mg/ml, produced weak activity on macrophages. Nitrile formation was used as an index of the macrophage-stimulating activity to screen effective foods[MI054].

Weight increase. Seed oil, in the ration of rats at a dose of 10.0% of the diet, produced weak activity. The experiment was carried out over 3 generations. The first generation showed a slight weight increase over controls fed cocoa butter fat[MI038].

REFERENCES

MI001   Suwal, P. N. Medicinal Plants of Nepal. Ministry of Forests, Department of Medicinal Plants, Thapathali, Kathmandu, Nepal, 1970.

MI002   Spencer, C. F., F. R. Koniuszy, E. F. Rogers et al. Survey of plants for antimalarial activity. **Lloydia** 1947; 10: 145–174.

MI003   Hermano, A. J. and G. Sepulveda, Jr. The vitamin content of Philippine foods. II. Vitamin C in various fruits and vegetables. **Philippine J Sci** 1934; 53: 379.

MI004   Kapur, R. D. Action of some indigenous drugs on uterus. A preliminary note. **Indian J Med Res** 1948; 36: 47.

MI005   Khanna, S. S. and E. G. Perkins. Application of gas liquid chromatography-mass spectrometry to analysis of natural products. Waxes from *Mangifera indica* and *Sesbania grandiflora*. **J Agr Food Chem** 1970; 18: 253.

MI006   Morton, J. F. A survey of medicinal plants of Curacao. **Econ Bot** 1968; 22: 87.

MI007   Morton, J. F. Folk-remedy plants and esophageal cancer in Coro, Venezuela. **Morris Arboretum Bull** 1974; 25: 24–34.

MI008   Inman, N. Notes on some poisonous plants of Guam. **Micronesica** 1967; 3: 55.

MI009   Ray, B. N. and A. K. Pal. Estrogenic activity of tree leaves as animal feed. **Indian J Physiol Allied Sci** 1967; 20: 6.

MI010   Griffiths, L. A. On the distribution of gentisic acid in green plants. **J Exp Biol** 1959; 10: 437.

MI011   Burkhill, I. H. Dictionary of the Economic Products of the Malay Peninsula. Ministry of Agriculture and Cooperatives, Kuala Lumpur, Malaysia. Volume II, 1966.

MI012   Mannan, A. and K. Ahmad. Studies on vitamin E in foods of East Pakistan. **Pak J Biol Agr Sci** 1966; 9: 13.

MI013   Jain, S. R. and S. N. Sharma. Hypoglycaemic drugs of Indian indigenous origin. **Planta Med** 1967; 15(4): 439–442.

MI014   Anjaneyulu, V., K. Harischandra, P. K. Ravi and J. D. Connolly. Triterpenoids from *Mangifera indica*. **Phytochemistry** 1985; 24(10): 2359–2367.

MI015   Anjaneyulu, V., J. S. Babu, M. M. Krishna and J. D. Connolly. 3-Oxo-2os,24r,epoxy-dammarane-25zeta, 26-diol from *Mangifera indica*. **Phytochemistry** 1993; 32(2): 469–471.

MI016   Khan, M. N. I., S. S. Nizami, M. A. Khan and Z. Ahmed. New saponins from *Mangifera indica*. **J Nat Prod** 1993; 56(5): 767–770.

MI017   Shibahara, A., K. Yamamoto, K. Shinkai, T. Nakayama and G. Kajimoto. Cis-9, cis-15-octadecadienoic acid: A novel fatty acid found in higher plants. **Biochim Biophys Acta** 1993; 1170(3): 245–252.

MI018   Osman, A. M., M. El-Garby Younes and A. E. Sheta. Chemical examination of local plants: IV. Isolation of free stearic acid from the kernels of *Mangifera indica*. **U A R J Chem** 1971; 1496): 653–654.

MI019   Maheshwari, M. L. and S. K. Mukerjee. Lipids and phenolics of healthy and malformed panicles of *Mangifera indica*. **Phytochemistry** 1975; 14: 2083–2084.

MI020   Prabhu, V. K. K. and M. John. Juvenomimetic activity in some plants. **Experientia** 1975; 31: 913.

MI021   Rao, N. N. and V. V. Modi. Fructose-1,6-diphosphatase from *Mangifera indica*. **Phytochemistry** 1976; 15: 1437–1439.

MI022   Saeed, A. R., K. A. Karamalla and A. H. Khattab. Polyphenolic compounds in the pulp of *Mangifera indica*. **J Food Sci** 1976; 41: 959.

MI023   Pharm, X. S. and G. K. Pharm. The extraction and determination of the flavanoid mangiferin in the bark and leaves of *Mangifera indica*. **Tap Chi Duoc Hoc** 1991; 5: 8–19.

MI024   Holdsworth, D. K. Traditional medicinal plants of Rarotonga, Cook Islands. Part II. **Int J Pharmacog** 1991; 29(1): 71–79.

MI025   Gorgue, C. M. P., M. M. J. Champ, Y. Lozano and J. Delort-Laval. Dietary fiber from mango by-products. Characterization and hypoglycemic effects determined by in vitro methods. **J Agr Food Chem** 1992; 40(10): 1864–1868.

MI026   Reddy, M. B., K. R. Reddy and M. N. Reddy. A survey of plant crude drugs of Anantapur District, Andhra Pradesh, India. **Int J Crude Drug Res** 1989; 27(3): 145–155.

MI027   Khan, M. A., S. S. Nizami, M. N. I. Khan and S. W. Azeem. Biflavone from *Mangifera indica*. **Pak J Pharm** Sci 1992; 5(2): 155–159.

MI028   Muanza, D. N., B. W. Kim, K. L. Euler and L. Williams. Antibacterial and antifungal activities of nine medicinal plants from Zaire. **Int J Pharmacog** 1994; 32(4): 337–345.

MI029   Schmeda-Hirschmann, G. and A. Rojas de Arias. A screening method for natural products on Triatomine bugs. **Phytother Res** 1992; 6(2): 68–73.

MI030   Diogenes, M. J. N., S. M. De Morias and F. F. Carvalho. Perioral contact dermatitis by cardol. **Int J Dermatol** 1995; 34(1): 72–73.

MI031   Khan, M. A. and M. N. I. Khan. Amino acid and sugar constituents of flowers of *Mangifera indica*. **Pak J Sci Ind Res** 1988; 31(12): 833–834.

MI032   Muanza, D. N., K. L. Euler, L. Williams and D. J. Newman. Screening for antitumor and anti-HIV activities of nine medicinal plants from Zaire. **Int J Pharmacog** 1995; 33(2): 98–106.

MI033   Lutete, T., K. Kambu, D. Ntondele, K. Cimanga and N. Luki. Antimicrobial activity of tannins. **Fitoterapia** 1994; 65(3): 276–278.

MI034   Singh, K. K. and J. K. Maheshwari. Traditional phytotherapy of some medicinal plants used by the Tharus of the Nainital District, Uttar Pradesh, India. **Int J Pharmacog** 1994; 32(1): 51–58.

MI035   Anis, M. and M. Iqbal. Medicinal plantlore of Aligarh, India. **Int J Pharmacog** 1994; 32(1): 59–64.

MI036   Gholap, A. S. and C. Bandyopadhvay. Characterization of green aroma of raw mango (*Mangifera indica*). **J Sci Food Agr** 1977; 28: 885.

MI037   Ghosal, S., K. Biswas and B. K. Chattopadhyay. Differences in the chemical constituents of *Mangifera indica* infected with *Aspergillus niger* and *Fusarium moniliformae*. **Phytochemistry** 1978; 17: 689–694.

MI038   Rukmini, C. and M. Vijayaraghavan. Nutritional and toxicological evaluation of mango kernel oil. **J Amer Oil Chem Soc** 1984; 61(4): 789–792.

MI039   Anjaneyulu, V., K. Harischandra, G. Prasad and R. Sambasiva. Triter-penoids of the root-bark of *Mangifera indica*. **Indian J Pharm Sci** 1982; 44(4): 85–87.

MI040   Bandyopadhyay, C., A. S. Gholap and V. R. Mamdapur. Characterization of alkenylresorcinol in mango (*Mangifera indica* L.) latex. **J Agr Food Chem** 1985; 33(3): 377–379.

MI041   Gaydou, E. M. and P. Bouchet. Sterols, methyl sterols, triterpene alcohols and fatty acids of the kernel fat of different Malagasy mango (*Mangifera indica*) varieties. **J Amer Oil Chem Soc** 1984; 61(10): 1589–1593.

MI042   Bandyopadhyay, C. Contribution of gas chromatography to food flavor research. **Pafai J** 1983; 5(3): 26–30.

MI043   Cojocaru, M., S. Droby, E. Glotter, A. Goldman, H. E. Gottlieb, B. Jacoby and D. Prusky. 5-(12-Heptadecenyl)-resorcinol, the major component of the antifungal activity in the peel of mango fruit. **Phytochemistry** 1986; 25(5): 1093–1095.

MI044   Hussain, M. G., M. E. Haque, M. A. Gafur, M. H. Ali and M. M. Ali. Studies on the kernel fat of mango of Rajshari region. **Bangladesh J Sci Ind Res** 1983; 18(1/4): 146–149.

MI045   Seetharam, K. A. and J. S. Pasricha. Condiments and contact dermatitis of the finger tips. **Indian J Dermatol Venereol Leprol** 1987; 53(6): 325–328.

MI046   Evans, D. A. and R. K. Raj. Extracts of Indian plants as mosquito larvicides. **Indian J Med Res** 1988; 88(1): 38–41.

MI047   Das, P. C., A. Das, S. Mandal, C. N. Islam, M. K. Dutta, B. B. Patra, S. Sikdar and P. K. Chakrabartty. Antiinflammatory and antimicrobial activities of the seed kernel of *Mangifera indica*. **Fitoterapia** 1989; 60(3): 235–240.

MI048   Patel, V. K. and H. Venkatakrishna-Bhatt. Folklore therapeutic indigenous plants in periodontal disorders in India (review, experimental and clinical approach). **Int J Clin Pharmacol Ther Toxicol** 1988; 26(4): 176–184.

MI049　Khan, M. A. and M. N. I. Khan. Alkyl gallates of flowers of *Mangifera indica*. **Fitoterapia** 1989; 60(3): 284.

MI050　Le Grand, A. Anti-infectious phytotherapy of the tree-savannah, Senegal (Western Africa) III: A review of the phytochemical substances and antimicrobial activity of 43 species. **J Ethnopharmacol** 1989; 25(3): 315–338.

MI051　Dennis, P. A. Herbal medicine among the Miskito of Eastern Nicaragua. **Econ Bot** 1988; 42(1): 16–28.

MI052　Alam, M. M., M. B. Siddiqui and W. Husain. Treatment of diabetes through herbal drugs in rural India. **Fitoterapia** 1990; 61(3): 240–242.

MI053　Anjaneyulu, V., K. Ravi, K. Harischanrda Prasad and J. D. Connolly. Triterpenoids from *Mangifera indica*. **Phyochemistry** 1989; 28(5): 1471–1477.

MI054　Miwa, M., Z. L. Kong, K. Shinohara and M. Watanabee. Macrophage stimulating activity of foods. **Agr Biol Chem** 1990; 54(7): 1863–1866.

MI055　Kambu, K., L. Tona, S. Kaba, K. Cimanga and N. Mukala. Antispasmodic activity of extracts proceeding of plant antidiarrheic traditional preparations used in Kinshasa, Zaire. **Ann Pharm Fr** 1990; 48(4): 200–208.

MI056　Miell, J., M. Papouchado and A. J. Marshall. Anaphylactic reaction after eating a mango. **Brit Med J** 1988; 297(6664): 1639–1640.

MI057　Chauhan, J. S., N. K. Singh and S. V. Singh. Screening of higher plants for specific herbicidal principle active against dodder, *Cuscuta reflexa* Roxb. **Indian J Exp Biol** 1989; 27(10): 877–884.

MI058　Caceres, A., E. Jauregu, D. Herrera and H. Logemann. Plants used in Guatemala for the treatment of dermatomucosal infections. 1: Screening of 38 plant extracts for anticandidal activity. **J Ethnopharmacol** 1991; 33(3): 277–283.

MI059　Craveiro, A. A., C. H. Andrade, F. J. Matos, J. W. Alencar and M. I. Machado. Volatile constituents of *Mangifera indica* Linn. **Rev Latinoamer Quim** 1980; 11: 129.

MI060　Kolhe, J. N., A. Bhaskar and N. V. Brongi. Occurrence of 3-oxo triterpenes in the unsaponifiable matter of some vegetable fats. **Lipids** 1982; 17: 166–168.

MI061　Yang, T. H. and A. Peng. Studies on the constituents of the peels of *Mangifera indica* L. **Tai-wan K'o Hsueh** 1981; 35(3): 69–73.

MI062　MacLeod, A. J. and N. G. De Troconis. Volatile flavour components of mango fruit. **Phytochemistry** 1982; 21: 2523–2526.

MI063　Joel, D. M., I. Harbach and A. M. Mayer. Laccase in Anacardiaceae. **Phytochemistry** 1978; 17: 796–797.

MI064　Gupta, M. P., T. D. Arias, M. Correa and S. S. Lamba. Ethnopharmacognostic observations on Panamanian medicinal plants. Part I. **Q J Crude Drug Res** 1979; 17(3/4): 115–130.

MI065　Billore, K. V. and K. C. Audichya. Some oral contraceptives-family planning tribal way. **J Res Indian Med Yoga Homeopathy** 1978; 13: 104–109.

MI066　Medina, F. R. and R. Woodbury. Terrestrial plants molluscicidal to Lymnaeid hosts of *Fasciliasis hepatica* in Puerto Rico. **J Agr Univ Puerto Rico** 1979; 63: 366–376.

MI067　Lu, Z. Y., H. D. Mao, M. R. He and S. Y. Lu. Studies on the chemical constituents of mangguo (*Mangifera indica*) leaf. **Chung Ts'ao Yao** 1982; 13: 3–6.

MI068　Anjaneyulu, V., K. Harischandra Prasad and G. Sambasiva Rao. Triterpenoids of the leaves of *Mangifera indica*. **Indian J Pharm Sci** 1982; 44: 58–59.

MI069　Van Den Berghe, D. A., M. Ieven, F. Mertens, A. J. Vlietinck and E. Lammens. Screening of higher plants for biological activities. II. Antiviral activity. **J Nat Prod** 1978; 41: 463–467.

MI070　Shaft, N. and M. Ikram. Quantitative survey of rutin-containing plants. Part 1. **Int J Crude Drug Res** 1982; 20(4): 183–186.

MI071　Vijayalakshimi, K., S. D. Mishra and S. K. Prasad. Nematicidal properties of some indigenous plant materials against second stage juveniles of *Meloidogyne incognita* (Koffoid and White) Chitwood. **Indian J Entomol** 1979; 41(4): 326–331.

MI072　Chen, W. S. Cytokinins of the developing mango fruit. Isolation, identification and changes in levels during maturation. **Plant Physiol** 1983; 71(2): 356–361.

MI073   Rouquayrol, M. Z., M. C. Fonteles, J. E. Alencar, F. Jose de Abreu and A. A. Craveiro. Molluscicidal activity of essential oils from Northeastern Brazilian plants. **Rev Brasil Pesq Med Biol** 1980; 13: 135–143.

MI074   Feroz, H., A. K. Khare and M. C. Srivastava. Review of scientific studies on anthelmintics from plants. **J Sci Res Pl Med** 1982; 3: 6–12.

MI075   John, D. One hundred useful raw drugs of the Kani Tribes of Trivandrum Forest Division, Kerala, India. **Int J Crude Drug Res** 1984; 22(1): 17–39.

MI076   Perera, P., D. Kanjanapoothi, F. Sandberg and R. Verpoorte. Screening for biological activity of different plant parts of *Tabernaemontana dichotoma*, known as divikaduru in Sri Lanka. **J Ethnopharmacol** 1984; 11(2): 233–241.

MI077   Singh, Y. N., T. Ikahihifo, M. Panuve and C. Slatter. Folk medicine in Tonga. A study of the use of herbal medicines for obstetric and gynaecological conditions and disorders. **J Ethnopharmacol** 1984; 12(3): 305–329.

MI078   Tripathi, R. K. R. and R. N. Tripathi. Reduction in bean common Mosaic Virus (BCMV) infectivity vis-a-vis crude leaf extract of some higher plants. **Experientia** 1982; 38(3): 349.

MI079   Tanaka, T., T. Sueyasu, G. I. Nonaka and I. Nishioka. Tannins and related compounds. XXI. Isolation and characterization of galloyl and P-hydroxybenzoyl esters of benzophenone and xanthone C-glucosides from *Mangifera indica* L. **Chem Pharm Bull** 1984; 32(7): 2676–2686.

MI080   Deka, L., R. Majumdar and A. M. Dutta. Some Ayurvedic important plants from District Kamrup (Assam). **Ancient Sci Life** 1983; 3(2): 108–115.

MI081   Aswal, B. S., D. S. Bhakuni, A. K. Goel, K. Kar, B. N. Mehrotra and K. C. Mukherjee. Screening of Indian plants for biological activity. Part X. **Indian J Exp Biol** 1984; 22(6): 312–332.

MI082   Tiwari, K. C., R. Majumder and S. Bhattacharjee. Folklore medicines from Assam and Arunachal Pradesh (District Tirap). **Int J Crude Res** 1979; 17(2): 61–67.

MI083   Singh, Y. N. Traditional medicine in Fiji. Some herbal folk cures used by Fiji Indians. **J Ethnopharmacol** 1986; 15(1): 57–88.

MI084   Polasa, K. and C. Rukmini. Mutagenicity tests of cashewnut shell liquid, rice-bran oil and other vegetable oils using the *Salmonella typhimurium*/microsome system. **Food Chem Toxicol** 1987; 25(10): 763–766.

MI085   Weniger, B., M. Rouzier, R. Daguilh, D. Henrys, J. H. Henrys and R. Anthon. Popular medicine of the Central Plateau of Haiti. 2. Ethnopharmacological inventory. **J Ethnopharmacol** 1986; 17(1): 13–30.

MI086   Kloss, H., F. W. Thiongo, J. H. Ouma and A. E. Butterworth. Preliminary evaluation of some wild and cultivated plants from snail control in Machakos District, Kenya. **J Trop Med Hyg** 1987; 90(4): 197–204.

MI087   Nisteswar, K. Review of certain indigenous antifertility agents. **Deerghayu International** 1988; 4(1): 4–7.

MI088   Koshimizu, K., H. Ohigashi, H. Tokuda, A. Kondo and K. Yamaguchi. Screening of edible plants against possible anti-tumor promoting activity. **Cancer Lett** 1988; 39(3): 247–257.

MI089   Ramirez, V. R., L. J. Mostacero, A. E. Garcia, C. F. Mejia, P. F. Pelaez, C. D. Medina and C. H. Miranda. Vegetales Empleados en Medicina Tradicional Norperuana. Banco Agrario Del Peru & NACL Univ, Trujillo, Peru, June 1988; 54pp.

MI090   Darias, V., L. Brando, R. Rabanal, C. Sanchez Mateo, R. M. Gonzalez Luis and A. M. Hernandez Perez. New contribution to the ethnopharmacological study of the Canary Islands. **J Ethnopharmacol** 1989; 25(1): 77–92.

MI091   Chabra, S. C., R. L. A. Mahunnah and E. N. Mshiu. Plants used in traditional medicine in Eastern Tanzania. I. Pteridophytes and angiosperms (Acanthaceae to Canellaceae). **J Ethnopharmacol** 1987; 21(3): 253–277.

MI092   Sharma, L. D., H. S. Bahga and P. S. Srivastava. In vitro anthelmintic screening of indigenous medicinal plants against *Haemonchus contortus* (Rudolphi, 1803) Cobbold, 1898 of sheep and goats. **Indian J Anim Res** 1971; 5(1): 33–38.

MI093   Malik, M. Y., A. A. Sheikh and W. H. Shah. Chemical composition of indigenous fodder tree leaves. **Pak J Sci** 1967; 19: 171.

MI094   Upadhya, G. S., G. Narayanaswamy and A. R. S. Kartha. Note on the comparative development of fatty acids in ripening seeds of 6 dicot species producing C16-C18 acid fats. **Indian J Agr Sci** 1974; 44: 620.

MI095   Malcolm, S. A. and E. A. Sofowora. Antimicrobial activity of selected Nigerian folk remedies and their constituent plants. **Lloydia** 1969; 32: 512–517.

MI096   Nigam, I. C. Studies of some Indian essential oils. **Agra Univ J Res Sci** 1962; 11: 147–152.

MI097   Chopra, R. N. Indigenous Drugs of India. Their Medical and Economic Aspects. The Art Press, Calcutta, India, 1933; 550pp.

MI098   Proctor, J. T. A. and L. L. Creasy. The anthocyanin of the mango fruit. **Phytochemistry** 1969; 8: 2108.

MI099   George, M. and K. M. Pandalai. Investigations on plant antibiotics. Part IV. Further search for antibiotic substances in Indian medicinal plants. **Indian J Med Res** 1949; 37: 169–181.

MI100   Makare, N., S. Bodhankar and V. Rangari. Immunomodulatory activity of alcoholic extract of *Mangifera indica* L. in mice. **J Ethnopharmacol** 2001; 78(2–3): 133–137.

MI101   Prashanth, D., A, Amrit, D. S. Samiulla, M. K. Asha and R. Padmaja. Alpha-Glucosidase inhibitory activity of *Mangifera indica* bark. **Fitoterapia** 2001; 72(6): 686–688.

MI102   Aderibigbe, A. O., T. S. Emudianughe and B. A. Lawal. Evaluation of the antidiabetic action of *Mangifera indica* in mice. **Phytother Res** 2001; 15(5): 456–458.

MI103   Prashanth, D., R. Padmaja and D. S. Samiulla. Effect of certain plant extracts on alpha-amylase activity. **Fitoterapia** 2001; 72(2): 179–181.

MI104   Garrida, G., D. Gonzalez, C. Delporte, N. Backhouse, G. Quintero, A. J. Nunez-Selles and M. A. Morales. Analgesic and anti-inflammatory effects of *Mangifera indica* L. extract (Vimang). **Phytother Res** 2001; 15(1): 18–21.

MI105   Sanchez, G. M., L. Re, A. Giuliani, A. J. Nunez-Selles, G. P. Davison and O. S. Leon-Fernandez. Protective effects of *Mangifera indica* L. extract, mangiferin and selected antioxidants against TPA-induced biomolecules oxidation and peritoneal macrophage activation in mice. **Pharmacol Res** 2000; 42(6): 565–573.

MI106   Martinez, G., R. Delgado, G. Perez, G. Garrido, A. J. Nunez-Selles and O. S. Leon. Evaluation of the in vitro antioxidant activity of *Mangifera indica* L. extract (Vimang). **Phytother Res** 2000; 14(6): 424–427.

MI107   Olle, D., A. Baron, Y. F. Lozano and J. M. Brillouet. Enzymatic degradation of cell wall polysaccharides from mango (*Mangifera indica* L.) puree. **J Agric Food Chem** 2000; 48(7): 2713–2716.

MI108   Tona, L., K. Kambu, N. Ngimbi, K. Mesia, O. Penge, M. Lusakibanza, K. Cimanga, T. De Bruyne, S. Apers, J. Totte, L. Pieters and A. J. Vlietinck. Antiamoebic and spasmolytic activities of extracts from some antidiarrhoeal traditional preparations used in Kinshasa, Congo. **Phytomedicine** 2000; 7(1): 31–8.

MI109   Yoosook, C., N. Bunyapraphatsara, Y. Boonyakiat and C. Kantasuk. Antiherpes simplex virus activities of crude water extracts of Thai medicinal plants. **Phytomedicine** 2000; 6(6): 411–419.

MI110   Aderibigbe, A. O., T. S. Emudianughe and B. A. Lawal. Antihyperglycaemic effect of *Mangifera indica* in rat. **Phytother Res** 1999; 13(6): 504–507.

18 | Manihot esculenta

Crantz.

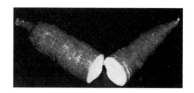

Common Names

Aikavitu	Nicaragua	Manioka	Samoa
Anaha	Nicaragua	Maniota	Venezuela
Belaselika	Nicaragua	Mannyok	Venezuela
Cassava	Brazil	Merelesita	Venezuela
Cassava	Guyana	Muhoko	Tanzania
Cassava	Nicaragua	Nao harnaka	Papua-New Guinea
Cassava	Nigeria	Noumea	Papua-New Guinea
Cassava	Tanzania	Sakarkanda	Papua-New Guinea
Cassava	Thailand	Sakarkanda	Fiji
Cassava	Venezuela	Sokobale	Fiji
Cassava	Zaire	Tapioka	Samoa
Coci	Zaire	Tapioka	Venezuela
Itk	Nicaragua	Tavioka	Venezuela
Kasaleka	Nicaragua	Vula'tolu	Venezuela
Kasera	Nicaragua	Yabia	Venezuela
Kasera	Fiji	Yabia damu	Venezuela
Katafaga	Fiji	Yauhra	Nicaragua
Manioc	Central Africa	Yuca	Guatemala
Manioc	Rodrigues Islands	Yuca	Nicaragua
Manioc	Sri Lanka	Yuca	Puerto Rico

BOTANICAL DESCRIPTION

A perennial shrub of the EUPHORBIACEAE family with slender, little-branched, erect nodose, glaborous stems, arising from a stock bearing thick, tuberous roots; usually growing to about 3 meters high. Leaves are spirally arranged, long-stalk to a blade deeply divided into 3 to 7 linear to elliptic-lanceolate lobes, exuding a milky sap when broken. Flowers are not often formed because plants are harvested before flowering takes place. Fruit is a small capsule; seeds are mottled and about 12 mm long.

ORIGIN AND DISTRIBUTION

Native probably to Brazil, it is now widespread in the tropics and subtropics. It is also cultivated and sometimes relict.

TRADITIONAL MEDICINAL USES

Central Africa. Leaf juice is taken orally as an abortifacient[ME003].

From: *Medicinal Plants of the World, vol. 1: Chemical Constituents, Traditional and Modern Medicinal Uses, 2nd ed.*
By: Ivan A. Ross © Humana Press Inc., Totowa, NJ

Colombia. Dried leaves, crushed together with leaves of *Tabernaemontana undulata*, are boiled to produce a tea that is considered an excellent vermifuge[ME014].

Fiji. Juice of grated tubers is taken orally for constipation and indigestion. Boiled tubers are eaten for diarrhea[ME038].

Haiti. Macerated dried leaves are put in a bath, or applied to the forehead for headache. For cutaneous infections, leaves are used in a bath[ME040].

Ivory Coast. Hot water extract of leaves is taken orally as an emmenagogue[ME002].

Samoa. The stem is inserted into the uterus and rotated as a means of inducing abortion[ME001]. Boiled tuber is taken orally for diarrhea[ME040].

Venezuela. Fresh pulverized tuber is eaten for diarrhea[ME015].

CHEMICAL CONSTITUENTS

(ppm unless otherwise indicated)

Amentoflavone: Lf[ME048]
Ascorbic acid: Rt[ME017]
Caffeic acid: Rt[ME017]
Ent-kaurene: Rt[ME006]
Ent-primara-8(14)-15-diene: Rt[ME006]
Glucose: Rt[ME017]
HCN: Lf 0.018–0.180%[ME030,ME035], St[ME007],
    Flour[ME009,ME010], Tuber[ME013,ME012],
    Rt Bk 1351[ME022]
Hydrogen sulfide: Lf 42–8573[ME018]
Iso-linamarin: Tb 0.79%[ME004]
Linamarin: Seedling[ME016],
    Tb 0.042–0.393%[ME004,ME005]
Linustatin: Seedling[ME016]
Lotaustralin: Seedling[ME016], Rt[ME020]
Malic Acid: Rt[ME017]
Methyl linamarin: Tb 80–113[ME005]
Neo linustatin: Seedling[ME016]
Oxalic acid: Lf 0.635%[ME011]
Podocarpusflavone A: Lf[ME048]
Quercetin: Rt[ME017]
Quercetin-3-0-a-L-rhamnosyl-glucoside:
    Lf[ME047]
Scopoletin: Rt[ME017]
Stachene(+): Rt[ME006]
Tyrosine: Rt[ME017]
Yucalexin A-16: Rt 0.1[ME006]

Yucalexin A-19: Rt 2.8[ME006]
Yucalexin B'-11: Rt 3[ME006]
Yucalexin B-14: Rt 1.1[ME006]
Yucalexin B-18: Rt 1.9[ME006]
Yucalexin B-20: Rt 1[ME006]
Yucalexin B-22: Rt 1.4[ME006]
Yucalexin B-5: Rt 0.6[ME006]
Yucalexin B-6: Rt 2.5[ME006]
Yucalexin B-7: Rt 1.3[ME006]
Yucalexin B-9: Rt 18.3[ME006]
Yucalexin P-10: Rt 2.1[ME006]
Yucalexin P-12: Rt 2.1[ME006]
Yucalexin P-13: Rt 0.3[ME006]
Yucalexin P-15: Rt 1.4[ME006]
Yucalexin P-17: Rt 0.3[ME006]
Yucalexin P-21: Rt 0.5[ME006]
Yucalexin P-4: Rt 0.4[ME006]
Yucalexin P-8: Rt 6.9[ME006]

PHARMACOLOGICAL ACTIVITIES AND CLINICAL TRIALS

Antibacterial activity. Ethyl acetate extract of dried aerial parts, at a concentration of 1.0 mg/ml on agar plate, was active on *Staphylococcus aureus*. Water and acetic acid extracts of the dried aerial parts, at concentrations of 1.0 mg/disk, were inactive on *Escherichia coli*, and the water extract was inactive on *Staphylococcus aureus*[ME045].

Anticrustacean activity. Ethyl acetate extract of dried aerial parts produced weak activity on *Artemia salina*, LC_{50} 2390 mcg/ml. The water extract was inactive, LC_{50} 4430 mcg/ml[ME045].

Antifertility effect. Fresh root as the diet of female rats was active. Significant reduction in frequency of pregnancy was observed. The average number of the litter and birth weights was significantly reduced[ME031].

Antifungal activity. Acetic acid extract of dried aerial parts, at a concentration of < 0.13 mg/ml on agar plate, was active on *Microsporum canis*, *Microsporum fulvum*, *Microsporum gypseum* and *Trichophytum gallinae*. The water extract was active on *Microsporum canis* and inactive on *Microsporum fulvum*, *Microsporum gypseum* and *Trichophytum gallinae*[ME045]. Water extract of fresh leaves, on agar plate, was inactive on Ustilago nuda, and strong activity was reported on Ustilago maydis[ME036].

Antihypercholesterolemic activity. Dried root in the ration of rats, at a dose of 68.0 gm/animal, was active. The animals were fed the ration daily for 3 months. There was an overall decrease in serum levels; however, high-density lipid cholesterol was increased, as compared to rats fed rice. Results significant at $P < 0.01$ level[ME019].

Antihyperlipemic activity. Dried root, in the ration of rats at a dose of 68.0 gm/animal, was active. Animals were fed the ration daily for 3 months. There were significant decreases in lipid and cholesterol levels over animals fed rice[ME019].

Antithyroid activity. Dried root ingested by human adults was active[ME033].

Antitumor activity. Ethanol (95%) extract of dried root, administered intraperitoneally to mice at a dose of 100.0 mcg/kg, was inactive on Sarcoma 180 (ASC); the water extract was active at the same dose[ME026].

Antiviral activity. Ethyl acetate extract of dried aerial parts, in cell culture, was active on Cytomegalovirus, LC_{50} 0.14 mcg/ml and Sindbis virus, LC_{50} 5.2 mg/ml when the viruses are exposed to the extract before infecting host cells, and LC_{50} 6.1 mg/ml when the infected host cells were exposed to the extract. The extract was inactive on Cytomegalovirus when hosts cells were exposed to the extract, LC_{50} > 100 mcg/ml. Water extract of dried aerial parts, in cell culture, was active on Cytomegalovirus, LC_{50} 0.18 mcg/ml and Sindbis virus, LC_{50} 26.0 mcg/ml when viruses were exposed to the extract before infecting hosts cells; Sindbis virus, LC_{50} 3.2 mcg/ml when infected host cells were exposed to the extract; inactive on Cytomegalovirus, LC_{50} > 100 when infected hosts cells were exposed to the extract[ME045].

Antiyeast activity. Ethyl acetate and water extracts of dried aerial parts, at con-centrations of 1.0 mg/disk, were inactive on Candida albicans and Saccharomyces cerevisiae[ME045].

Crown gall tumor inhibition. Water and acetic acid extracts of dried aerial parts, in cell culture, were active. LC_{50} 0.03 mcg/ml and 0.32 mcg/ml, respectively, were observed. Assay system is intended to predict for antitumor activity[ME045].

Diabetogenic activity. Dried tuber, in the ration of dogs, was active. Animals were fed diet in which cassava (rice, in controls) provided the carbohydrate. After 14 weeks, the plasma amino acid index of gluconeogenesis was 5.077 times greater in the cassava-fed compared to control animals. This value was 1.912 times greater than controls in a third group fed rice and HCN. Plasma lipase activity was significantly elevated in cassava-fed vs controls. Plasma thiocyanate levels were elevated in both cassava- and HCN-fed animals, but significantly more so in the latter. Pancreas showed hemorrhage, necrosis, fibrosis and atrophy of acinar tissue and fibrosis of islets. Hemorrhage was less prominent and fibrosis more so in HCN-fed animals[ME029]. Cassava fed to rats did not produce diabetes even after a year of feeding. There were transient changes in serum insulin and lipase levels, but the significance of these findings were not clear. There was no histopathological evidence of either acute or chronic pancreatitis, but there were changes of toxic hepatitis in the liver[ME102].

Embryotoxic effect. Dried root flour, in the ration of pregnant rats at a dose of 80.0% of the diet, was inactive. Dosing was on day 1–15 of gestation. Resorption occurred in 19%, and fetal malformation in 28%. Cassava starch from roots, in the ration of rabbits at concentrations of 15.0, 30, and 45% of the diet, was inactive[ME032].

Fish poison. Water extract of fresh root bark was active, LD_{50} 0.25%[ME042].

Glucose-6-phosphatase dehydrogenase stimulation. Dried root, in the ration of rats at a dose of 68.0 gm/animal, was active. Animals were fed the ration daily for 3 months. Liver enzyme levels were lower than animals fed on rice[ME019].

Goitrogenic activity. Dried tuber, in the ration of dogs, was inactive. Animals were fed diet in which cassava (rice, in controls) provided the carbohydrate. After 14 weeks T3 level had raised by roughly 40% in each group, whereas it had fallen by 36% in a third group fed rice and HCN. Thyroid weight after 14 weeks was not significantly different between control and cassava-fed groups, although it was significantly elevated above control in HCN treated group. Thiocyanate levels were elevated in cassava and HCN-fed groups, though only the latter demonstrated thyroid histopathology[ME028]. Fresh root, administered to mice by gastric intubation, was inactive[ME039].

Five hundred and eighty five households were selected in 3 areas with high prevalence of goiter. The relative impact of iodine deficiency (estimated by mean iodine excretion in the urine of family members) and cassava consumption (mean frequency of consumption by the household). Cassava consumption, even on a regular basis, neither caused nor increased goiter formation in that area. This was probably due to the local method of cassava root preparation, which reduces the amount of cyanogenic compounds consumed. Iodine deficiency was principally responsible for goiter formation[ME106].

Growth retardation effect. The effect of inadequately processed cassava was studied in 2 populations in The Democratic Republic of Congo. In the population (south) in which the cassava was not thoroughly processed, the mean urinary thiocyanate was much higher, whereas mean urinary sulphate excretion was equally low in the 2 populations. However, the mean urinary SCN/SO$_4$ molar ratio was higher in the south (0.20), indicating that 10–20% of sul-

phur amino acids were used for cyanide detoxication. No significant differences were found between the 2 populations in weight-for-height and weight-for-age indices but height-for-age index was significantly lower in children from the south, indicating more severe growth retardation in children exposed to dietary cyanide[ME103].

Hyperglycemic activity. Fresh root, ingested by human adults at variable dosage levels, was inactive. A study of 110 non-insulin dependent diabetics failed to find evidence that consumption of cassava flour induces diabetes[ME023]. Tuber, ingested by male human adult at a dose of 50.0 gm/person, was active[ME025].

Juvenile hormone activity. Acetone extract of stem was active[ME008].

Lipid metabolism effects. Dried roots, in the ration of rats at a dose of 68.0 gm/animal, were active. Animals were fed the ration daily for 3 months. Total serum cholesterol and triglyceride were lowered over rats fed rice. Glucose-6-phosphate dehydrogenase level in the liver was increased. Triglyceride lipase and lipoprotein lipase were decreased. Results were significant at $P < 0.01$ level[ME019].

Molluscicidal activity. Aqueous slurry (homogenate) of fresh entire plant was inactive on *Lymnaea columella* and *Lymnaea cubensis*, LD$_{100}$ > 1 ppm[ME034]. Water extract of oven–dried leaves was inactive on *Biomphalaria pfeifferi*[ME041]. Water extract of oven-dried stem showed weak activity on *Biomphalaria pfeifferi*[ME041].

Mutagenic activity. Fresh leaves, and acetone and methanol extracts of fresh leaves, at concentrations of 50 mg/plate on agar plate, were active on *Salmonella typhimurium* TA98. Mutagenicity was assayed after acid or enzymatic hydrolysis after leaves were boiled. Hexane extract of fresh leaves at a concentration of 500.0 mg/plate on agar plate was inactive on *Salmonella typhimurium* TA98. Chloroform extract of fresh leaves, at a concentration of 0.1 ml/plate on agar plate, was inactive on *Salmonella typhimurium* TA100, TA97 and TA98. The mutagenic effect was measured after boiling the leaves and metabolic activation had no effect on the results[ME024]. Chloroform extract of boiled root, at a concentration of 0.1 ml/plate on agar plate, was active on *Salmonella typhimurium* TA98, and inactive on TA97 and TA100. Metabolic activation had no effect on the results[ME024]. Chloroform extract of dried roots, at a concentration of 0.1 ml/plate on agar plate, was active on *Salmonella typhimurium* TA97 and TA98, and inactive on TA100. Mutagenic effect measured after boiling and metabolic activation had no effect on the results[ME024].

Neurological effects. Cassava, administered orally to albino rats for 30 days, alters the emotional status of the rats, with changes in the basal neurotransmitter levels in the hypothalamus[ME101]. A male agricultural worker in Brazil was suffering for 4 years from a predominantly crural spastic paraparesis. His main food was 'mandioca brava' or wild cassava that was insufficiently cooked. Study of the cerebrospinal fluid ruled out infection by HTLV and neurosyphilis. On magnetic resonance there was a slight thoracic atrophy[ME104]. Scopoletin was administered to 4-week old rats in rations of 3 groups of rats containing 0.07 microgram scopoletin/100 gm, 0.07 microgram scopoletin and 1.8 mg cyanide/100 gm, and 1.8 mg cyanide/100 gm, respectively. These levels of scopoletin and cyanide corresponded to levels found in a processed cassava diet. The first group was fed the same ration as the others but without scopoletin and cyanide. The rats were fed these rations for 12 months. Rats from each group were sacrificed at the third, sixth, ninth and twelfth months; the relative brain weight of the rats (% of body weight) and histology of their brains were also studied at twelfth month. The results indicated that the relative brain weight of the rats fed scopoletin and cyanide were significantly ($p < 0.05$) less than that of the control from the third month. There were no significant changes in the lipid peroxide levels of the rat brains in the various groups. Histological examination of the brains indicated that scopoletin is involved in the pathogenesis of the neuropathy seen in cassava consuming populations[ME105]. Cassava consumption reduced the motor coordination, but the changes in neurotransmitter levels due to cassava consumption (except for 5HT in corpus striatum) was identical with malnutrition-induced changes, indicating that the toxicity of chronic cassava consumption is mainly due to the associated protein calorie malnutrition[ME107].

Ovulation inhibition effect. Cassava starch from root, in the ration of rabbits at concentrations of 15%, 30% and 45% of the diet, was inactive[ME032].

Protein synthesis inhibition. Fresh leaves in buffer were active, IC_{50} 0.75 mg of protein per ml[ME027].

Respiration (cellular) inhibition. Dried tuber, in the ration of rats at a dose of 35.0% of the diet, was active. Effects were measured in the liver[ME021].

Teratogenic activity. Dried root flour, in the ration of pregnant rats at a dose of 80.0% of the diet, was active. Dosing was on days 1–15 of gestation. Resorption occurred in 19%, and fetal malformation occurred in 28%. Of the abnormal fetuses, all showed growth retardation, 19% had limb defects and 5.5% had microcephaly with open eye[ME037]. Fresh root, in the ration of female rats at a concentration of 50.0% of the diet, was inactive[ME031].

Thyroid stimulating hormone activity. Sun-dried root, ingested by human adults, was active[ME046].

Toxic effect (general). Hot water extract of fresh leaves, taken orally by human adults at variable dosage levels, was inactive. The leaves, which usually contain large quantities of cyanogenic glucosides, were processed into a traditional vegetable sauce "Mpondu" by simple methods that included blanching (10 minutes), mashing and boiling for 20–80 minutes. These methods enhanced the detoxification of the leaves, with blanching alone resulting in the loss of 57% of the bound (glycosidic) cyanide. It was presumed that losses of cyanide during these processes would be accounted for in volatile HCN, its derivatives and boiling water[ME030]. Entire plant, taken orally by human adult, was active[ME043,ME044]. Fresh root, as the entire diet of female rats, was active. There was an increased incidence of neonatal deaths among offspring, which had poor development, reduced brain weight and increased tendency toward biting littermates[ME031].

REFERENCES

ME001   McCuddin, C. R. Samoan Medicinal Plants and Their Usage. Office of Comprehensive Health Planning, Department of Medical Services. Government of American Samoa, 1974.

ME002   Bouquet, A. and M. Debray. Medicinal plants of the Ivory Coast. **Trav Doc Orstom** 1974; 32: 1.

ME003   Weeks, J. H. Among the Primitive Bakongo. Seeley, Service & Co., Ltd. England, 1914; 108.

ME004   Clapp, R. C., F. H. Bissett, R. A. Coburn and L. Long, Jr. Cyanogenesis in manioc: Linamarin and isolinamarin. **Phytochemistry** 1966; 5: 1323–1326.

ME005   Bissett, F. H., R. C. Clapp, R. A. Coburn, M. G. Ettlinger and L. Long, Jr. Cyanogenesis in manioc: Concerning lotaustralin. **Phytochemistry** 1969; 8: 2235–2247.

ME006   Sakai, T. and Y. Nakagawa. Diterpenic stress metabolites from cassava roots. **Phytochemistry** 1988; 27(12): 3769–3779.

ME007   Camarotti, A. J. Determination of hydrogen cyanide in *Manihot esculenta* using paper strips impregnated with isopurpurate. **Mem Inst Biocienc Univ Fed Pernambuco** 1974; 1: 107.

ME008   Prabhu, V. K. K. and M. John. Juvenomimetic activity in some plants. **Experientia** 1975; 31: 913.

ME009   Pieris, N., G. G. Premadasa and E. R. Jansz. A method for assay of total potential cyanide in manioc flour. **J Natl Sci Counc Sri Lanka** 1974; 1: 207.

ME010   Jansz, E. R., N. Pieris, E. E. Jeya Raj and D. J. Abeyratne. Cyanogenic glucoside content of manioc. II. Detoxification of manioc chips and flour. **J Natl Sci Counc Sri Lanka** 1975; 2: 129.

ME011   Valyasevi, A. and S. Dhanamitta. Bladder stone disease in Thailand. XVII. Effect of exogenous sources of oxalate on crystalluria. **Amer J Clin Nutr** 1974; 27: 877.

ME012   Pieris, N., E. R. Jansz and R. Kandage. Cyanogenic glucoside content of manioc. I. An enzymic method of determination applied to processed manioc. **J Natl Sci Counc Sri Lanka** 1974; 2: 67.

ME013   Pieris, N. and E. R. Jansz. Cyanogenic glucoside content of manioc. III. Fate of bound cyanide on processing and cooking. **J Natl Sci Counc Sri Lanka** 1975; 3: 41.

ME014   Schultes, R. E. De plantes toxicariie e Mundo Novo Tropicale commentationes. XIX. Biodynamic Apocynaceous plants of the Northwest Amazon. **J Ethnopharmacol** 1979; 1(2): 165–192.

ME015   Holdsworth, D. K. Traditional medicinal plants of Rarotonga, Cook Islands. Part II. Int **J Pharmacog** 1991; 29(1): 71–79.

ME016   Lykkesfeldt, J. and B. L. Moller. Cyanogenic glycosides in cassava, *Manihot esculenta* Crantz. **Acta Chem Scand** 1994; 48(2): 178–180.

ME017   Lalaguna, F. Purification of fresh cassava root polyphenols by solid-phase extraction with amberlite XAD-8 resin. **J Chromatogr** A 1993; 657(2): 445–449.

ME018   Ugochukwu, E. N. and I. U. W. Osisiogu. Hydrogen sulphide from leaves of *Manihot utilissima*. **Planta Med Suppl** 1977; 32: 105–109.

ME019   Premakumari, K. and P. A. Kurup. Lipid metabolism in rats fed rice and tapioca. **Indian J Med Res** 1982; 76: 488–493.

ME020   Brimer, L., S. B. Christensen, P. Molgaard and F. Nartey. Determination of cyanogenic compounds by thin-layer chromatography. 1. A densitometric method for quantification of cyanogenic glycosides, employing enzyme preparations (beta-glucuronidase) from Helix pomatia and picrate-impregnated ion-exchange sheet. **J Agr Food Chem** 1983; 31(4): 789–793.

ME021 Obidoa, O. and V. O. S. Ngodo. Effect of prolonged consumption of gari (cassava, *Manihot utilissima*) in rat hepatic energy metabolism. 1. Mitochondrial respiratory control. **Qual Plant Foods Hum Nutr** 1984; 34(3): 159–168.

ME022 Dufour, D. L. Cyanide content of cassava (*Manihot esculenta*, Euphorbiaceae) cultivars used by Tukanoan Indians in Northwest Amazonia. **Econ Bot** 1988; 42(2): 255–266.

ME023 Cooles, P. Diabetes and cassava in Dominica. **Trop Geograph Med** 1988; 40(3): 272–273.

ME024 De Messter, C., B. Rollmann, K. Mupenda and Y. Mary. The mutagenicity of cassava (*Manihot esculenta* Crantz) preparations. **Food Add Contam** 1990; 7(1): 125–136.

ME025 Akanji, A. O., I. Adeyefa, M. Charles-Davies and B. O. Osotimehin. Plasma glucose and thiocyanate responses to different mixed cassava meals in non-diabetic Nigerians. **Eur J Clin Nutr** 1990; 44(1): 71–77.

ME026 Itokawa, H., F. Hirayama, S. Tsuruoka, K. Mizuno, K. Takeya and A. Nitta. Screening test for antitumor activity of crude drugs (III). Studies on antitumor activity of Indonesian medicinal plants. **Shoyakugaku Zasshi** 1990; 44(1): 58–62.

ME027 Gasperi-Campani, A., L. Barbieri, M. G. Battelli and F. Stirpe. On the distribution of ribosome-inactivating proteins amongst plants. **J Anat Prod** 1985; 48(3): 446–454.

ME028 Kamalu, B. P. and J. C. Agharanya. The effect of a nutritionally-balanced cassava (*Manihot esculenta* Crantz) diet on endocrine function using the dog as a model. 2. Thyroid. **Brit J Nutr** 1991; 65(3): 373–379.

ME029 Kamalu, B. P. The effect of a nutritionally-balanced cassava (*Manihot esculenta* Crantz) diet on endocrine function using the dog as a model. 1. Pancreas. **Brit J Nutr** 1991; 65(3): 365–372.

ME030 Maduagwu, E. N. and I. B. Umoh. Detoxification of cassava leaves by simple traditional methods. **Toxicol Lett** 1982; 10: 245–248.

ME031 Olusi, S. O., O. L. Oke and A. Odusote. Effects of cyanogenic agents on reproduction and neonatal development in rats. **Biol Neonate** 1979; 36: 233–243.

ME032 Eshiett, N. O., A. A. Ademosun and T. A. Omole. Effect of feeding cassava root meal on reproduction and growth of rabbits. **J Nutr** 1980; 110: 697–702.

ME033 Bourdoux, P., F. Delange, M. Gerard, M. Mafuta, A. Hanson and A. M. Ermans. Antithyroid action of cassava in humans. **Int Dev Res Cent Rept IDRC** 1980; 61–8: 167–172.

ME034 Medina, F. R. and R. Woodbury. Terrestrial plants molluscicidal to Lymnaeid hosts of Fasciliasis hepatica in Puerto Rico. **J Agr Univ Puerto Rico** 1979; 63: 366–376.

ME035 Rosa de Battisti, C., F. F. F. Teles, D. T. Coelho, A. Jose da Silveira and C. M. Batista. Determination of hydrogen cyanide toxicity and total soluble carbohydrates in cassava (*Manihot esculenta*, Crantz). **Rev Ceres** 1981; 28: 521–525.

ME036 Singh, K. V. and R. K. Pathak. Effect of leaves extracts of some higher plants on spore germination of *Ustilago maydes* and *U. nuda*. **Fitoterapia** 1984; 55(5): 318–320.

ME037 Singh, J. D. The teratogenic effect of dietary cassava on the pregnant albino rat: A preliminary report. **Teratology** 1981; 24: 289–291.

ME038 Singh, Y. N. Traditional medicine in Fiji. Some herbal folk cures used by Fiji Indians. **J Ethnopharmacol** 1986; 15(1): 57–88.

ME039 Hershman, J. M., A. E. Pekary, M. Sugawara, M. Adler, L. Turner, J. A. Demetriou and J. D. Hershman. Cassava is not a goitrogen in mice. **Proc Soc Exp Biol Med** 1985; 180(1): 72–78.

ME040 Weniger, B., M. Rouzier, R. Daguilh, D. Henrys, J. H. Henrys and R. Anthon. Popular medicine of the Central Plateau of Haiti. 2. Ethnopharmacological inventory. **J Ethnopharmacol** 1986; 17(1): 13–30.

ME041 Kloss, H., F. W. Thiongo, J. H. Ouma and A. E. Butterworth. Preliminary evaluation of some wild and cultivated plants from snail control in Machakos District, Kenya. **J Trop Med Hyg** 1987; 90(4): 197–204.

ME042 Kulakkattolickal, A. Piscicidal plants of Nepal: Preliminary toxicity screening using grass carp (*Ctenopharyngodon idella*) fingerlings. **J Ethnopharmacol** 1987; 21(1): 1–9.

ME043 Wee, Y. C., P. Gopalakrishnakone and A. Chan. Poisonous plants in Singapore - A colour chart for identification with symptoms and signs of poisoning. **Toxicon** 1988; 26(1): 47.

ME044 Fernando, R. Plant poisoning in Sri Lanka. **Toxicon** 1988; 26(1): 20.

ME045 Macrae, W. D., J. B. Hudson and G. H. N. Towers. Studies on the pharmacological activity of Amazonian Euphorbiaceae. **J Ethnopharmacol** 1988; 22(2): 143–172.

ME046 Cliff, J., P. Lundquist, H. Rosling, B. Sorbo and L. Wide. Thyroid function in a cassava-eating population affected by epidemic spastic paraparesis. Acta Endocrinol 1986; 113(4): 523–528.

ME047 Subramanian, S. S., S. Nagarajan and N. Sulochana. Flavonoids of some Euphorbiaceous plants. Phytochemistry 1971; 10: 2548–2549.

ME048 Kamil, M., Ilyas, W. Rahman, M. Okigawa and N. Kawano. Biflavones from *Manihot utilissima*. Phytochemistry 1994; 13: 2619–2620.

ME049 Mathangi, D. C. and A. Namasivayam. Effect of cassava consumption on open-field behaviour and brain neurotransmitters in albino rats. Physiol Behav 2000; 70(1-2): 89–93.

ME050 Mathangi, D. C., R. Deepa, V. Mohan, M. Govindarajan and A. Namasivayam. Long-term ingestion of cassava (tapioca) does not produce diabetes or pancreatitis in the rat model. Int J Pancreatol 2000; 27(3): 203–208.

ME051 Banea-Mayambu, J. P., T. Tylleskar, K. Tylleskar, M. Gebre-Medhin and H. Roslin. Dietary cyanide from insufficiently processed cassava and growth retardation in children in Democratic Republic of Congo (formerly Zaire). Ann Trop Paediatr 2000; 20(1): 34–40.

ME052 Carod-Artal, F. J., A. P. Vargas and C. del Negro. Spastic paraparesis due to long term consumption of wild cassava (*Manihot esculenta*): a neurotic model of motor neuron disease. Rev Neurol 1999; 29(7): 610–613.

ME053 Ezeanyika, L. U., O. Obidoa and V. O. Shoyinka. Comparative effects of scopoletin and cyanide on rat brain, 1: histopathology. Plant Foods Hum Nutr 1999; 53(4): 351–358.

ME054 Dillon, J. C., D. Faivre, G. Ciornei, G. Sall. The consumption of cassava is not responsible for the etiology of endemic goiter in rural areas in Senegal. Sante 1999; 9(2): 93–99.

ME055 Mathangi, D. C., V. Mohan and A. Namasivayam. Effect of cassava on motor co-ordination and neurotransmitter level in albino rat. Food Chem Toxicol 1999; 37(1): 57–60.

19 | Momordica charantia

L.

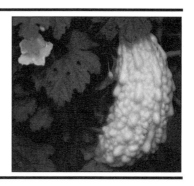

Common Names

African cucumber	USA	Cerasee	Trinidad
Amargoso	Philippines	Cerasee	West Indies
Ampalaya	Philippines	Concombre	West Indies
Ampalaya	USA-FL	Condiamor	Belize
Art pumpkin	West Indies	Condiamor	Guatemala
Asorosi	Haiti	Coraillie	West Indies
Assorossi	Haiti	Cun de amor	Puerto Rico
Balsam apple	West Indies	Cundeamor	Brazil
Balsam pear	Australia	Cundeamor	Cuba
Balsam pear	Bahamas	Cundeamor	Mexico
Balsam pear	Thailand	Cundeamor	Puerto Rico
Balsam pear	USA	Cundeamor	USA
Balsambirne	Bahamas	Embusabusu	Congo-Brazzaville
Balsamina	India	Eyezom	Guinea
Balsamina	Peru	Futoreishi	Japan
Balsamino	Panama	Kakara	India
Ban kareli	India	Kakayi	Nigeria
Baramasiya	India	Kakiral	India
Barbof	Senegal	Kakle	East Africa
Bitter cucumber	Thailand	Kakral	India
Bitter gourd	Fiji	Karala	India
Bitter gourd	India	Karawila	Sri Lanka
Bitter gourd	Thailand	Karela	Fiji
Bitter gourd	USA	Karela	India
Bitter melon	USA	Karela	Nepal
Bitter pear melon	Taiwan	Karela	USA
Bobobo	Ivory Coast	Karela	West Indies
Broomweed	Nicaragua	Kuguazi	West Indies
Caprika	West Indies	Lenzaa	Congo-Brazzaville
Carailla	Guyana	Lumba-lumba	East Africa
Carilla	USA	Lumbuzi	Thailand
Carilla	West Indies	Ma ra	Thailand
Cerasee	Bahamas	Machete	Puerto Rico
Cerasee	Bimini	Maiden apple	USA
Cerasee	Jamaica	Maiden apple	Virgin Islands

From: *Medicinal Plants of the World, vol. 1: Chemical Constituents, Traditional and Modern Medicinal Uses, 2nd ed.*
By: Ivan A. Ross © Humana Press Inc., Totowa, NJ

Maiden's blush	USA	Paprika	West Indies
Makalalaska	Nicaragua	Paroka	Guadeloupe
Manamat	East Africa	Pavakkachedi	India
Mange kuli	West Indies	Pepino montero	Nicaragua
Mara khee nok	Thailand	Periya laut	Malaysia
Mara	Thailand	Pom kouli	Guadeloupe
Margoze	Rodrigues Islands	Pomme nerveille	West Indies
Mbosa	Congo-Brazzaville	Pomme z'indiens	West Indies
Mbunbulu	Congo-Brazzaville	Pomme-coolie	Guadeloupe
Melao-de-sao caetano	Brazil	Qisaul-barri	India
Meleni	Brazil	Quisaul-barri	Saudi Arabia
Mexicaine	West Indies	Saga	Saudi Arabia
Miniklalasni	Nicaragua	Serimentok	India
Momotica	Curacao	Seripupa	India
Nagareishi	Japan	Sorosi	Nicaragua
Nania nania	Ivory Coast	Sorrow see	Belize
Nara cheen	Thailand	Sushavi	India
Nguene	Ivory Coast	Tasplira	Nicaragua
Nyanyra	Togo	Uchhe	India
Nyinya	East Africa	Ulhimar	India
Okookoo	Nigeria	Wild balsam pear	Bahamas
Panaminik	Nicaragua	Yesquin	Haiti
Papayilla	Peru	Zague zrou	Ivory coast

BOTANICAL DESCRIPTION

Slender-stemmed tendril climber of the CUCURBITACEAE family, the older stem is often flattened and fluted to 6 m or longer. Leaves alternate, cut into 5–7 narrow-based lobes. The lobes are mostly blunt, but have small marginal points, up to about 12 cm long, very thin-textured, and characteristically pungent and aromatic. Flowers are yellow on short (female) or long (male) peduncles that are short-lived. Fruit narrowed to both ends, ribbed with prominent tubercles on the ribs, 8 to 15 cm long, orange when ripe and then becoming softly fleshy and opening to reveal pendulous seeds covered with red pulp.

ORIGIN AND DISTRIBUTION

Originally found only in the tropics of the Old World, it has been spread by man throughout all the tropical regions of the world and is commonly found on fences and shrubs and in hedgerows.

TRADITIONAL MEDICINAL USES

Africa. Hot water extract of root is taken orally as an aphrodisiac[MC021].

Asia. Fresh fruit is consumed in large amounts for the treatment of diabetes[MC096].

Australia. Fresh fruit is cooked as a vegetable. After steeping in salt water, it is used as an anthelmintic and emetic. Hot water extract of root is taken orally as an abortifacient[MC026].

Bahamas. Hot water extract of dried vine is taken orally as an emmenagogue and for early abortion[MC142].

Belize. Hot water extract of dried leaves is taken frequently as a tea to treat diabetes[MC140].

Bimini. Fruit is eaten as a vegetable. Hot water extract of the vine is taken orally for diabetes, fevers, and as an abortifacient[MC122].

Brazil. Decoction of dried entire plant is taken orally as a vermifuge and febrifuge[MC188]. Decoction of dried stem is taken orally for fevers and malaria[MC051]. Diluted decoction (14.2%) of fresh leaves is taken orally to treat rheumatism. Cataplasm prepared from fresh leaves is applied externally to treat leprosy, especially to reduce the pain[MC009]. Dried fruit is used as insecticide. Unripe fruit is eaten to treat colds and as a purgative and abort-ifacient[MC071]. Ethanol (95%) extract of the entire plant is taken orally for colic and fevers. Hot water extract of the fruit is used externally to treat wounds. Fruit juice, mixed with Ricinus oil in equal parts, is taken orally as an anthelmintic. Hot water extract of root is taken orally as a purgative and to induce abortion; in large doses as an emetic, and the tincture is claimed to have an aphrodisiac effect[MC009]. Seeds are taken orally as an anthelmintic[MC196].

Congo. Extract of entire plant is taken orally for menstrual irregularities[MC020].

Costa Rica. Leaf extract is taken orally as an emmenagogue[MC127].

Cuba. Extract of the entire plant is taken by females to treat sterility[MC002]. Hot water extract of fruit and leaves is taken orally as an emmenagogue[MC202].

Curacao. Hot water extract of vine, decocted with sugar, is taken orally for high blood pressure[MC025].

East Africa. Hot water extract of root is taken orally as an abortifacient[MC193].

England. Hot water extract of dried fruit is taken orally for diabetes[MC091].

Fiji. Fresh fruit, toasted or fried in oil, is eaten for stomach worms, fever, phlegm, and diabetes. Fresh leaf juice is taken orally for hypertension, dysentery, and diabetes[MC169].

Ghana. Hot water extract of root is taken orally for malarial fever[MC190].

Guadeloupe. Water extract of fruit is taken orally for hyperglycemia[MC155].

Guam. Extract of the entire plant is used externally for malignant ulcers[MC193].

Guatemala. Hot water extract of fresh leaves is used externally for ringworm and fungal skin diseases[MC107].

Haiti. Decoction of dried aerial parts is taken orally for fever. Hot water extract of dried entire plant is taken orally for fever, to stimulate the appetite, for liver troubles, anemia and rage; ophthalmically, the decoction is used for eye infections and externally for cutaneous infections[MC180].

India. Butanol extract of dried leaves is taken orally as a galactagogue; the hot water extract is taken orally as an emmenagogue in dysmenorrhea and for leprosy, piles and jaundice. The leaf juice is taken orally as an anthelmintic. Fresh fruit is used as a common vegetable. Extract of the fruit is taken orally for jaundice, piles, leprosy, as an emmenagogue in dysmenorrhea, as a tonic for rheumatism and gout, and as a laxative[MC143]. Hot water extract of dried root is taken orally to induce abortion up to the fifth month of pregnancy[MC138,MC183,MC207]. Hot water extract of dried seeds is taken orally for diabetes, hepatic disorders, and pain relief in gout, pain relief in rheumatism and as an anthelmintic[MC103]. The extremely bitter effusion from boiled seeds, when taken orally, is said to produce instantaneous vomiting[MC131]. Hot water extract of flowers and leaves is taken orally each month to promote early abortion[MC023]. Hot water extract of fresh seeds is taken orally for diabetes[MC037]. Tender shoots, together with young leaves of *Leucas indica*, pepper, garlic and salt, are pulverized in equal quantities, made into pills and taken once a day for 9 consecutive days to treat pneumonia. Shoots, ground with pepper, camphor, young leaves of *Fluggea lencopyros* and young shoots and bark of mango are taken orally for 9 consecutive days to treat leukorrhagia[MC057]. Hot water extract of fruit is taken orally as an anthelmintic, antileprotic[MC193] and as a remedy for diabetes mellitus[MC046]. Fruits are eaten in large quantities as an abortifacient[MC002]. Hot water extract of dried fruit is taken orally for diabetes[MC035]. Fresh fruit is used as an ingredient in curries[MC091]. For hydrophobia, *Notonia grandiflora* juice is mixed with bitter gourd (*Momordica charantia* L.) powder and is taken orally[MC108]. Hot water extract of root is taken orally as an abortifacient[MC021, MC002,MC027,MC195]. Hot water extract of seeds is taken orally to produce instantaneous vomiting[MC126]. Seeds are taken orally as an anthelmintic[MC195]. Hot water extract of vine is taken orally as an emmenagogue[MC021]. Juice of the entire plant is taken orally as an abortifacient and an emmenagogue[MC019]. Leaves are eaten by children as a purgative[MC057] and anthelmintic[MC195]. Saponifiable fraction of unripe fruit is used as a vegetable. The juice is taken orally for diabetes mellitus[MC197]. Unripe, fresh fruit juice is taken orally for malarial fevers[MC098].

Iraq. Water extract of fruit is taken orally as an anthelmintic and for leprosy[MC193].

Ivory Coast. Leaves are crushed and the juice is taken orally with palm wine as an aphrodisiac[MC024].

Jamaica. Hot water extract of dried entire plant is used as a bush tea[MC208]. Hot water extract of dried fruit is taken orally for diabetes[MC154,MC072].

Malaysia. Hot water extract of the entire plant is taken orally as an abortifacient[MC018].

Mexico. Decoction of the entire plant is taken orally to treat diabetes and dysentery[MC064]. Extract of the root is used as an aphrodisiac[MC003]. Hot water extract of leaves is taken orally as an aphrodisiac[MC021].

Nepal. Leaf juice is taken orally as a purgative and emetic[MC001].

Nigeria. Fifteen to 20 dried leaves are crushed into 2–3 glasses of water; the filtrate is taken orally with salt to taste, as a treatment for diarrhea. Decoction of dried fruit and leaves is taken orally as a laxative and anthelmintic[MC054]. Fresh fruit and leaf juices are taken orally as an anthelmintic. Fresh entire plant is used externally for malignant ulcers[MC156]. Fresh fruit and leaves are eaten as a pot herb[MC149]. Leaf extract is used to treat breast cancer[MC156].

Panama. Hot water extract of leaf is taken orally as an antipyretic, choleretic and anti-

diabetic. Infusion of 10–12 leaves in 1 liter of water is taken 3–4 times daily[MC127].

Peru. Hot water extract of the dried fruit is taken orally as a purgative and for respiratory conditions, and externally on contusions and wounds. Hot water extract of the dried seed is taken orally as a vermifuge and for colic, and externally for suppurations[MC187].

Philippines. Decoction of dried entire plant is used as a bath for newborns. It is believed that it removes disease-causing elements from the skin. The petroleum benzene extract is taken orally for coughs in infants[MC167]. Hot water extract of root is taken orally to induce abortions. Hot water extract of vine is taken orally as a powerful emmenagogue[MC021].

Puerto Rico. Hot water extract of dried entire plant is taken orally for diabetes[MC032]. Hot water extract of the entire plant is taken orally as a treatment for diabetes mellitus[MC017]. Hot water extract of vine is taken orally for diabetes[MC012,MC021] and is rubbed on the skin to relieve itching[MC028].

Saudi Arabia. Hot water extract of dried fruit is taken orally for rheumatism, gout, liver and spleen disorders, pyrexia, colic, flatulence, menstrual suppression and diabetes[MC095,MC168].

Senegal. Hot water extract of dried entire plant is taken orally for intestinal pain and externally as a cicatrisant[MC172].

Sri Lanka. Extract of the fruit is taken orally as an anthelmintic[MC193]. Fresh fruit juice[MC067] and hot water extract[MC085] is taken orally for diabetes mellitus. Hot water extract of dried fruit is taken orally as a hypoglycemic agent[MC158].

Thailand. Decoction of dried fruit is taken orally as an anti-inflammatory[MC192]. The hot water extract is taken orally for diabetes[MC200]. Hot water extract of dried entire plant is taken orally as an antipyretic[MC209]. Hot water extract of dried leaf is taken orally as an antipyretic[MC206].

Togo. Decoction of dried leaf is taken orally for malaria[MC099].

Trinidad. Decoction of dried fruit, leaf and stem is taken orally for diabetes (noninsulin-dependent)[MC100].

Turkey. Dried fruit juice is taken orally as a treatment for peptic ulcers[MC059]. Fresh fruit is eaten as a treatment for ulcers[MC068].

USA. Hot water extract of fruit is administered rectally as a remedy for hemorrhoids. Externally, the fruit is used for snakebite, leprosy, itching, skin, burns and wounds. Unripe fruit is taken orally for bacillary dysentery; taken every 2 days, it relieves chronic colitis and in large doses it is an abortifacient. Unripe fruit juice is used externally to treat burns. Hot water extract is taken orally for thrush, as a substitute for quinine in intermittent fever, as a remedy for liver and spleen ailments, for gout and rheumatism, as a vermifuge and purgative and for menstrual difficulties[MC021].

Venezuela. Hot water extract of root is taken orally as an antimalarial[MC021].

Virgin Islands. Fruit is taken orally for a bad heart and diabetes[MC198].

West Africa. Extract of the root, together with the fruit and seeds, is taken orally as an abortifacient[MC002]. Fruit is taken orally as an abortifacient[MC193] and antidiabetic[MC130].

West Indies. Decoction (sweetened) of the hot water extract of leaves is taken orally as a powerful emmenagogue, for diabetes and hypertension and to treat worms and malarial fever. Fresh plant juice is taken orally for fever and to stimulate the appetite. The juice is applied ophthalmically for eye infection[MC180]. Fruit juice is taken orally for diabetes. Hot water extract of fresh or dried vine with salt is taken orally by women before and after childbirth. Seeds are taken orally as an anthelmintic. Hot water extract of the entire plant is taken orally as a laxative and abortifacient; infusion alone or with Bidens reptans is taken orally for menstrual troubles[MC125]. Hot water extract of vine is taken orally regularly each month by women to avoid childbirth by early abortion[MC021]. Infusion of dried leaves is used, as a tea to which are ascribed antidiabetic properties[MC096]

CHEMICAL CONSTITUENTS
(ppm unless otherwise indicated)

(-)-Menthol: Sd EO[MC081]
5-a stigmasta-7,22,25-trien-3-b-ol: Fr[MC011]
5-a stigmasta-7,22-dien-3-b-ol: Fr[MC011]
5-Hydroxytryptamine: Fr[MC007]
24-Methylene cycloartenol: Sd oil[MC082]
Alanine: Sd 0.0158%[MC151]
Alpha carotene epoxide: PC[MC050]
Alpha glucose: Sd[MC083]
Alpha momorcharin: Sd[MC173]
Alpha spinasterol: Fr[MC011]
Alpha-alpha trehalose: Sd[MC083]
Alpha-elaeostearic acid: Ke[MC008]
Arginine: Sd 0.0323%[MC151]
Asparagine: Sd[MC151]
Aspartic acid: Sd 0.009%[MC151]
Beta alanine: Fr[MC007]
Beta amyrin: Sd oil[MC082]
Beta carotene 5-6-epoxy: PC[MC050]
Beta carotene: PC[MC050]
Beta glucose: Sd[MC083]
Beta momorcharin: Sd 0.08%[MC166]
Beta sitosterol: Fr[MC117]
Calceolarioside E: Aer[MC113]
Capric acid: Sd oil[MC086]
Charantin: Fr 0.035–0.15%[MC197,MC005], Sd[MC159]
Charine: Fr[MC044]
Citrulline: Fr[MC010]
Cryptoxanthin: PC[MC050]
Cucurbita-5-24-dien-3-beta-ol,10-alpha: Sd oil[MC082]
Cucurbita-5-24-diene,3-beta-7-beta-23-trihydroxy-7-O-beta-D-glucoside: Lf[MC104]
Cucurbitacin B: Sd[MC075]
Cucurbitacin K: Sd[MC075]
Cycloartenol: Sd oil[MC082]
Delta carotene: PC[MC050]
Diosgenin: Fr[MC004], Sc[MC004]
Ethylene: Fr[MC124]
Galacturonic acid: Fr[MC006]
Gamma aminobutyric acid: Fr[MC007]
Gamma carotene: PC[MC050]
Gentisic acid: Lf[MC029]
Glutamic acid: Fr[MC007], Sd 0.0212%[MC151]
Glycine: Sd 38.2[MC151]
Goyaglycoside A: Fr[MC217]

Goyaglycoside B: Fr[MC217]
Goyaglycoside C: Fr[MC217]
Goyaglycoside D: Fr[MC217]
Goyaglycoside E: Fr[MC217]
Goyaglycoside F: Fr[MC217]
Goyaglycoside G: Fr[MC217]
Goyaglycoside H: Fr[MC217]
Goyasaponin I: Fr[MC217]
Goyasaponin II: Fr[MC217]
Goyasaponin III: Fr[MC217]
Hexadecan-1-ol: Sd EO[MC081]
Histidine: Sd[MC151]
Inhibitor BG-1-A: Sd[MC041]
Inulin: Cal Tiss[MC048], Fr[MC047]
Iso leucine: Sd[MC151]
Lauric acid: Fr[MC112], Sd oil[MC086]
Lectin inhibitor A: Sd[MC116]
Lectin: Sd[MC116]
Leucine: Sd[MC151]
Linoleic acid: Sd oil[MC086], Fr[MC112], Cot[MC152]
Linolenic acid: Sd oil[MC086], Fr[MC112], Cot[MC152]
Lutein: PC[MC050]
Lycopene: Sd[MC080], Fr[MC150], PC[MC050]
Lysine: Sd[MC151]
MAP-30: Sd[MC106]
Momorcharaside A: Sd[MC105]
Momorcharaside B: Sd[MC105]
Momorcharin I: Sd[MC056]
Momorcharin II: Sd[MC056]
Momordica agglutinin: Sd[MC078]
Momordica anti-HIV protein MAP-30:
    Sd[MC063]
Momordica charantia cytostatic factor or
    11,000 daltons: Fr[MC148]
Momordica charantia cytostatic factor or
    40,000 daltons: Fr[MC148]
Momordica charantia cytostatic factor:
    Fr[MC175]
Momordica charantia inhibitor protein:
    Sd[MC134]
Momordica charantia lectin: Sd[MC135]
Momordica charantia steroid glycoside:
    Fr[MC039]
Momordica charantia triterpene glycoside:
    Cot[MC160]
Momordica cucurbitane 3: Lf[MC104]
Momordica cucurbitane 6: Lf[MC104]
Momordica elastase inhibitor MEI-1:
    Sd[MC040]
Momordica protein MAP-30:
    Fr[MC053], Sd[MC053]
Momordica trypsin inhibitor MTI-I, Sd[MC040]

Momordica trypsin inhibitor MTI-II, Sd[MC040]
Momordicin 11: Lf[MC104]
Momordicin 8: Lf[MC104]
Momordicine I: Lf + St 0.07%[MC157]
Momordicine II: Lf + St 0.07%[MC157]
Momordicine III: Lf + St 0.12%[MC157]
Momordicine: Lf[MC009]
Momordicoside A: Fr[MC217],
    Sd 0.1287%[MC163]
Momordicoside B: Sd 0.0090%[MC163]
Momordicoside C: Fr[MC217],
    Sd 0.0114%[MC162]
Momordicoside D: Sd 0.00228%[MC162]
Momordicoside E: Fr 0.0037%[MC162]
Momordicoside E': Fr 0.00104%[MC147]
Momordicoside E-1: Fr 0.0756%[MC147]
Momordicoside EX: Fr 0.00126%[MC147]
Momordicoside F: Fr 0.0072%[MC147]
Momordicoside F': 0.0006%[MC147]
Momordicoside F-1: Fr 0.0434%[MC147]
Momordicoside F-2: Fr 0.004%[MC136]
Momordicoside G: Fr 0.01236%[MC136]
Momordicoside H: Fr 0.0074%[MC147]
Momordicoside I: Fr 0.0082%[MC147]
Momordicoside J: Fr 0.0008%[MC147]
Momordicoside K: Fr[MC146]
Momordicoside L: Fr 0.0036%[MC147]
Momordin 1c: Fr[MC226]
Momordin 2: Sd[MC043]
Momordin A: Sd[MC060]
Momordin B: Sd[MC042]
Momordin: Sd[MC078]
Multiflorenol: Sd oil[MC082]
Mutatochrome: PC[MC050]
Mycose: Sd[MC105]
Myristic acid: Sd oil[MC086]
Nerolidol: Sd EO[MC081]
Oleic acid: Fr[MC112], Cot 15.58%[MC152]
Ornithine: Sd 0.0063%[MC151]
P-insulin: Sd[MC087], Fr[MC087]
Palmitic acid: Fr[MC112], Sd oil[MC086],
    Cot 2.71–51.95%[MC152]
Palmitoleic acid: Fr[MC112]
Para cymene: Sd EO[MC081]
Pentadecan-1-ol: Sd EO[MC081]
Petroselinic acid: Sd[MC086]
Phytofluene: PC[MC050]
Proline: Fr[MC007]
Ribosome-inactivating protein 1: Sd[MC182]
Ribosome-inactivating protein 2: Sd[MC182]
Ribosome-inactivating protein 3: Sd[MC182]
Ribosome-inactivating protein 4: Sd[MC182]

Rosmarinic acid: Aer[MC113]
Rubixanthin: PC[MC050]
Serine: Sd 0.0040%[MC151]
Squalene: Sd EO[MC081]
Stearic acid: Sd oil[MC086], Fr[MC112], Cot[MC152]
Stigmast-5-ene-3-beta-25 diol: Fr[MC014]
Stigmasta-5-25-dien-3-beta-ol: Fr[MC117]
Stigmasta-5-25(27)-dien-3-beta-ol,3-0-(6'-0-palmitoyl-beta-D-glucosyl): Fr[MC101]
Stigmasta-5-25(27)-dien-3-beta-ol,3-0-(6'-0-stearoyl-beta-D-glucosyl): Fr[MC101]
Stigmasta-5-25-diene-3-beta-D-glucoside: Fr[MC013]
Stigmasta-7-22-25-trien-3-beta-ol: Fr[MC011]
Stigmasta-7-22-dien-3-beta-ol: Fr[MC011]
Stigmasterol: Fr[MC004]
Taraxerol: Sd oil[MC082]
Threonine: Sd 0.0017%[MC151]
Trehalose: Sd 0.3960%[MC151]
Trypsin inhibitor MCI-3: Sd[MC084]
Tyrosine: Sd 0.0517%[MC151]
V-insulin: Fr[MC110]
Verbascoside: Aer[MC113]
Vicine: Sd 0.0500-0.4000%[MC145,MC151]
Zeatin riboside: Sd[MC144]
Zeatin: Sd[MC144]
Zeaxanthin: PC[MC050]
Zeinoxanthin: PC[MC050]

PHARMACOLOGICAL ACTIVITIES AND CLINICAL TRIALS

Abortifacient effect. Ethanol/water (1:1) extract of dried aerial parts, administered orally to pregnant rats at a dose of 100.0 mg/kg, was inactive. Ethanol/water (1:1) extract of dried fruit, administered orally to rats at a dose of 100.0 mg/kg, was inactive[MC133]. Water extract of dried seed, administered intraperitoneally to pregnant rats at a dose of 8.0 mg/kg, was active. A fraction designated as AP–11 was tested[MC123]. Acetone extract of dried seed, administered intraperitoneally to pregnant mice at a dose of 4.0 mc/gm on day 12 of pregnancy, was active[MC166]. Water extract, administered intraperitoneally to pregnant mice at a dose of 0.04 mg/ml, was active[MC073]. Water extract of leaves, administered orally to female rats at a dose of 200.0 mg/kg, was inactive[MC199].

Adenyl cyclase inhibition. Dried fruit, in cell culture, was inactive[MC159].

Analgesic activity. Ethanol/water (1:1) extract of dried entire plant, administered intragastrically to mice, was inactive vs hot plate and tail clip methods. Ethanol/water (1:1) extract of dried fruit, administered intragastrically to mice, was inactive[MC055]. Methanol extract of dried seed, administered subcutaneously 30 minutes before challenge, was active in mice and equivocal in rats. Naloxone does not inhibit effect vs acetic acid-induced writhing[MC103].

Anthelmintic activity. Ethanol (95%) extract of fruit, at a concentration of 100.0 mg/ml, was active on *Ascaridia galli*. Ethanol (95%) extract of fruit juice, at a concentration of 0.1 ml, was active on *Ascaridia galli*[MC049]. Hot water extract of seed, at a concentration of 1:50, was active on *Haemonchus contortus*[MC195].

Antibacterial activity. Chloroform and ethanol (95%) extracts of dried fruit, at concentrations of 250.0 mg/ml on agar plate, were active on *Bacillus subtilis*, *Escherichia coli*, *Pseudomonas aeruginosa* and *Staphylococcus aureus*. Ethanol/water (1:1) extract, at a concentration of 1.0 mg/ml in broth culture, was inactive on *Pseudomonas aeruginosa*. Water extract, at a concentration of 250.0 mg/ml on agar plate, was active on *Bacillus subtilis*, *Escherichia coli* and *Pseudomonas aeruginosa*, and inactive on *Staphylococcus aureus*. Petroleum ether extract, at a concentration of 250.0 mg/ml on agar plate, was active on *Bacillus subtilis* and *Pseudomonas aeruginosa*, and inactive on *Staphylococcus aureus* and *Escherichia coli*[MC070]. Dried fruit, on agar plate, was active on *Sarcina lutea*. Chloroform, ether, water and methanol extracts of dried fruit, on agar plate, were active on *Escherichia coli*, *Pseudomonas aeruginosa*, *Salmonella typhosa*, *Sarcina lutea*, and *Shigella dysenteriae*, and produced strong activity on *Staphylococcus aureus*, MIC < 50.0 mg/disk. Water and methanol extracts also produced strong activity on *Bacillus subtilis*, MIC < 50.0 mg/disk. Petroleum ether extract was inactive on *Escherichia coli*, *Pseudomonas aeruginosa*, *Salmonella typhosa*, *Sarcina lutea*, *Shigella dysenteriae*, and *Staphylococcus aureus*[MC119]. Ethanol (95%) and hot water extracts of dried bark, on agar plate, were active on *Escherichia coli* and *Staphylococcus aureus*[MC205]. Ethanol (95%) and water extracts of dried seeds, at a concentration of 10.0 mg/ml on agar plate, were inactive on *Corynebacterium diphtheriae*, *Diplococcus pneumoniae*, *Staphylococcus aureus*, *Streptococcus pyogenes*, and *Streptococcus viridans*[MC115]. Ethanol (95%) extract of dried leaves, undiluted on agar plate, was inactive on *Staphylococcus aureus* and *Escherichia coli*; hot water extract was active[MC205]. Methanol extract of dried leaves, on agar plate at a concentration of 2.0 mg/ml, was active on *Corynebacterium diptheriae*, *Neisseria* species, *Pseudomonas aeruginosa*, *Salmonella* species, *Streptobacillus* species, and *Streptococcus* species, and inactive on *Staphylococcus aureus*[MC111]. Ethanol/water (1:1) extract of entire plant, at a concentration of 1.0 mg/ml in broth culture, was inactive on *Pseudomonas aeruginosa*[MC055]. Methanol extract of dried entire plant, at a concentration of 15.0 mg/ml on agar plate, was active on *Sarcina lutea*[MC165]. Methanol/water (1:1) extract of leaves, in broth culture, was active on *Staphylococcus aureus*, and inactive on *Bacillus subtilis*, *Escherichia coli*, *Proteus* species, *Pseudomonas aeruginosa* and *Staphylococcus albus*[MC045]. Unsaponifiable fraction of seed oil, on agar plate, was active on several Gram negative organisms[MC153].

Anticarcinogenic effect. Water extract of the fruit, administered orally to mice, produced an adverse effect on the general health and lifespan of the animals when used at a high concentration. But when the dose was reduced by half, the extract afforded protection from the development of skin tumor and increased life expectancy. Carcinogen-induced lipid peroxidation in liver and DNA damage in lymphocytes was reduced following treatment with the extract. The extract was also found to significantly activate the liver enzymes glutathione-S-transferase, glutathione peroxidase and catalase ($P < 0.001$), which showed a depression following exposure to the carcinogen[MC220].

Anticlastogenic activity. Fruit and leaf juice, administered intraperitoneally to mice at a dose of 50.0 ml/kg, was active on marrow cells vs mitomycin C-, tetracycline- and dimethylnitrosamine-induced micronuclei[MC065].

Anticonvulsant activity. Ethanol (70%) extract of fresh fruit, administered intraperitoneally to mice of both sexes at variable dosages, was inactive vs metrazole- and strychnine-induced convulsions. Ethanol (70%) extract of fresh leaves, administered intraperitoneally to mice of both sexes at variable dosage levels, was inactive vs metrazole- and strychnine-induced convulsions[MC149]. Ethanol/water (1:1) extract of dried entire plant, administered intraperitoneally to mice, was inactive vs supramaximal electroshock-induced convulsions. Ethanol/water (1:1) extract of dried fruit, administered intraperitoneally to mice, was inactive vs hot plate and tail clip methods[MC055].

Antifertility effect. Fresh leaf juice, administered orally to female mice, was active[MC201]. Unripe fruit juice, administered by gastric intubation to male rats at a dose of 5.0 ml/kg daily for 49 days, followed by mating, was active[MC141].

Antifungal activity. Ethanol (95%) extract of dried seeds, at a concentration of 10.0 mg/ml on agar plate, was inactive on *Microsporum canis*, *Microsporum gypseum*, *Phialophora jeanselmei*, *Piedraia hortae*, and *Trichophyton mentagrophytes*[MC115]. Ethanol/water (1:1) extract of dried entire plant, at a concentration of 1.0 mg/ml in broth culture, was inactive on *Aspergillus fumigatus* and *Trichophyton mentagrophytes*. Ethanol/water (1:1) extract of dried fruit, at a concentration of 1.0 mg/ml in broth culture, was inactive on *Aspergillus fumigatus* and *Trichophyton mentagrophytes*[MC055]. Hot water extract of fresh leaves, in broth culture at a concentration of 1.0 ml, was inactive on *Epidermophyton floccosum*, *Microsporum canis* and *Trichophyton mentagrophytes* var. algodonosa and granulare[MC107].

Anti-*Helicobacter pylori* activity. The fruit produced significant activity against the microorganism[MC225].

Antihepatotoxic activity. Hot water extract of dried aerial parts, at a concentration of 1.0 mg/plate in cell culture, was inactive on hepatocytes, measured by leakage of LDH and ASAT[MC074].

Antihistamine activity. Ethanol/water (1:1) extract of dried entire plant, at a concentration of 0.01 gm/ml, produced weak activity on guinea pig ileum[MC209].

Antihypercholesterolemic activity. Acetone extract of dried fruit, in the ration of rats at a dose of 250.0 mg/kg, was active vs alloxan-induce hyperglycemia[MC094]. Fruits, taken orally by male human adults at a dose of 2.0 gm/person, were active. Ten mildly diabetic patients (23–28 years of age) were used in the study. Fruit powder was given once daily for 11 days[MC109]. Freeze-dried fruit powder, administered orally to rats at concentrations of 0.5, 1 and 3% without and added dietary cholesterol (Exp 1) and those containing the powder at the level of 1% with or without 0.5% cholesterol and 0.15% bile acid (Exp II). No adverse effect of dietary powder on growth parameters and relative liver weight were noted. The powder resulted in a consistent decrease in serum glucose levels in rats fed cholesterol-free diets, but not in those fed cholesterol-enriched diets, although no dose-response was noted. Addition of cholesterol to the diets as compared to those without added cholesterol caused hypercholesterolemia and fatty liver. The powder had little effect on serum lipid parameters, except for high density lipoprotein cholesterol; high density lipoprotein cholesterol levels tended to decrease by dietary cholesterol, while they were consistently elevated by the dietary powder both in the presence and absence of dietary cholesterol, indicating an antiatherogenic activity. In addition, the powder exhibited a marked reduction in the hepatic total cholesterol and triglyceride levels both in the presence and absence of dietary cholesterol; the reduction of triglyceride levels in the absence of dietary cholesterol was in a dose-dependent manner[MC219].

Antihyperglycemic activity. Acetone extract of dried fruit, in the ration of rats at a dose of 250.0 mg/kg, was active. Blood sugar concentration decreased by 49% in 30 days. Blood sugar was maintained within normal limits for 2 weeks after treatment ceased vs alloxan-induced hyperglycemia[MC0940]. Benzene extract of dried fruit, administered intragastrically to rabbits at a dose of 1.0 gm/kg, was active. Alloxan-recovered rabbits were tested for glucose tolerance following sample treatment vs glucose-induced hyperglycemia[MC092]. Chloroform extract of dried fruit, administered intragastrically to female rats at a dose of 250.0 mg/kg, was inactive vs streptozotocin-induced hyperglycemia[MC070]. Decoction of dried fruit, taken orally by human adults at a dose of 500.0 mg/person, was active[MC036]. Ethanol (95%) extract of dried fruit, administered intragastrically to female rats at a dose of 250.0 mg/kg, was active vs streptozotocin-induced hyperglycemia; 75.0 mg/kg, administered intraperitoneally to rats, was inactive[MC174]. Dried powdered fruit, taken orally once daily for 11 days by 10 male patients with mild diabetes (23–28 years of age), at a dose of 2.0 gm/person, was active[MC109]. Water extract of dried fruit, administered intragastrically to female rats at a dose of 250.0 mg/kg, was active vs streptozotocin-induced hyperglycemia. The effect was potentiated when used with *Curcuma longa* and *Emblica offici-*

nalis[MC070]. The water extract, administered orally to rats at a dose of 4.0 gm/day for 2 months, was active vs alloxan-induced hyperglycemia. Onset of retinopathy was also retarded[MC184]. Acetone extract of dried fruit, at a dose of 250.0 mg/kg in the ration of rats, was inactive vs alloxan-induced hyperglycemia[MC094]. Decoction of dried fruit, leaves and stem, administered intraperitoneally to male mice at a dose of 0.5 ml/animal, was active vs streptozotocin-induced hyperglycemia. One ml of extract is equivalent to 10 gm of dried plant material. A single dose of the extract reduced plasma concentration by about 50% after 5 hours[MC100]. Decoction of fresh seeds, taken orally by human adults at variable dosage levels, was inactive. Three patients were studied; half of a seed was boiled in 5 cups of water until the volume was 2 cups. One cupful was given in the morning and 1 in the evening[MC037]. Methanol extract of shade-dried seeds, administered orally to rats at a dose of 10.0 mg/kg, was active vs adrenaline-induced hyperglycemia[MC185]. Dried fruit, administered intragastrically to rabbits at a dose of 1.0 gm/kg, was active vs alloxan-induced hyperglycemia[MC090]. Decoction of a 25% aqueous extract of dried fruit, administered intragastrically to mice at a dose of 0.5 ml/animal, was inactive vs alloxan-induced hyperglycemia; maximal change in blood sugar was 4.33%[MC095]. Hot water extract (25%) of dried fruit, administered by gastric intubation to mice at a dose of 0.5 ml, was inactive vs alloxan-induced hyperglycemia[MC168]. Dried fruit extract, together with a mixture of *Litchi chinensis* saponins and oleanolic acid, administered intraperitoneally to mice at a dose of 0.1 gm/kg, was active. Biological activity reported has been patented[MC114]. Dried fruit, taken orally by human adults, was active. A diabetic woman recovered from glycosuria after taking a kind of curry. Karela was an active ingredient[MC091]. Ethanol (95%) extract of dried aerial parts and fruits, administered

intragastrically to rats at a dose of 250.0 mg/kg, were inactive vs rats fasted for 18 hours, over fed rats, glucose-induced hyperglycemia and streptozotocin-induced hyperglycemia. With dosing for 21 days, the extract was also inactive vs glucose-induced hyperglycemia[MC093]. Ethanol (95%) extract of dried entire plant, administered intragastrically to rats at a dose of 250.0 mg/kg, was active vs rats fasted for 18 hours, overfed, glucose-induced hyperglycemic and streptozotocin-induced hyperglycemic rats, and when dosed for 21 days vs glucose-induced hyperglycemia[MC093]. Ethanol (95%) extract of fresh fruit, administered intra-gastrically to rats at a dose of 200.0 mg/kg, was active vs streptozo-tocin-induced-hyperglycemia. Blood sugar levels decreased 22%[MC058]. Fresh fruit, administered intra-gastrically to rats at a dose of 15.0 gm/animal, 5 gm each time, 3 times a day for 3 weeks, was active vs alloxan-induced hyperglycemia. Water extract of fresh fruit, administered intra-gastrically to rats at a dose of 1.0 gm/animal for a period of 3 weeks, was active vs alloxan-induced hyperglycemia. The reduction of the initial blood sugar level decreased from 220 mg% to 105 mg%. Water extract of fresh fruit, administered orally to male human adults at a dose of 1.0 gm/animal, was active vs alloxan-induced hyper-glycemia. Blood sugar was estimated after 2, 3, 4, and 7 weeks of treatment. The fall in blood sugar was highly significant at the termination of the treatment. The overall decrease in blood sugar was 54%[MC061]. Hot water extract of fresh fruit, administered intragastrically to rats of both sexes at a dose of 4.0 gm/animal, was active vs alloxan-induced hyperglycemia[MC097]. Fresh fruit juice, administered intragastrically to rabbit at a dose of 6.0 ml/kg, was active vs alloxan- and glucose-induced hyperglycemia[MC034]. Ethanol (95%) extract of fruit and fruit juice, administered orally to rabbits at doses of 3.0 ml/kg, were active vs alloxan-induced hyperglycemia[MC031]. Fresh fruit juice, taken orally by human adults at a dose of 50.0 ml/day for 8 to 11 weeks, was active. Improved glucose tolerance in diabetic patients was observed, results significant at $P < 0.01$ level[MC176]. When administered intragastrically to male rats at a dose of 5.0 ml/kg, the juice was active. A glucose tolerance test was used[MC038]. Fresh fruit juice, administered intragastrically to rats at a dose of 10.0 ml/kg daily for 30 days, was inactive vs streptozotocin-induced hyperglycemia[MC189]. Fresh fruit juice, taken by human adults at a dose of 100.0 ml 30 minutes before oral glucose load in the glucose tolerance test, was active. The results indicated improved glucose tolerance in 73% of the 18 patients with maturity onset diabetes[MC178]. Fried fruit, taken orally by human adults at a dose of 0.23 kg/day for 8 to 11 weeks, was active. Improved glucose tolerance in diabetic patients was observed, results significant at $P < 0.05$ level[MC176]. Fruit pulp juice, administered intragastrically to rats at a dose of 2.5 gm/kg, was inactive vs streptozotocin-induced hyperglycemia. The methanol extract was inactive[MC062]. Hot water extract of dried fruit, administered to diabetic rabbits at a dose of 10.20 mg/kg, was active[MC118]. Lyophilized extract of dried fruit, administered to rabbit at doses of 1.2 gm and 400 mg/kg, were inactive vs alloxan-induced hyperglycemia[MC120]. Hot water extract of fresh fruit juice, taken orally by human adults, was active on maturity onset diabetics vs glucose-induced hyperglycemia. A 73% improvement in glucose tolerance was observed[MC085]. Hot water extract of fruit juice, administered orally to rats at a dose of 5.0 ml/kg, was equivocal vs anterior pituitary extract-induced hyperglycemia[MC030]. Methanol extract of seed, administered intragastrically to rats at a dose of 2.5 gm/kg, was inactive vs streptozotocin-induced hyperglycemia[MC062]. Protein fraction (FM-1) of dried fruit was active on mice[MC089]. Seeds, administered by gastric intubation to rabbits, were active in streptozotocin-treated animals[MC143]. Water extract of fresh fruit, administered intragastrically to male mice at a dose of 0.5 gm/kg, was active. There was a significant decrease in non-fasting blood glucose levels of hyperglycemia-induced mice, results significant at $P < 0.01$ level[MC068]. Water extract of fresh fruit, administered intragastrically to mice at a dose of 16.0 gm/kg, was active vs streptozotocin-induced hyperglycemia[MC102]. Water extract of seed, administered orally to rabbits at a dose of 3.0 ml/kg, was inactive vs alloxan-induced hyperglycemia[MC031]. Diamed, a mixture composed of aqueous extracts of *Azadirachta indica*, *Cassia alata* and *Momordica charantia*, administered orally to rats at doses of 0.25, 0.30 and 0.35 gm/kg body weight for 30 days, produced a significant reduction in blood glucose, glycosylated hemoglobin, and an increase in plasma insulin and total hemoglobin. The effect was highly significant after administration of the 0.35 gm dose. The treatment also prevented a decrease in body weight. Oral glucose tolerance test in experimental diabetic rats indicated a significant improvement in glucose tolerance in the animals treated. The effect was comparable to 600 microgram/kg of gli benclamide[MC210]. The alcoholic and aqueous extracts of the fruit, administered orally to rats fed fructose for 15 days at doses of 100, 200 and 400 mg per day, increased serum glucose and insulin levels markedly and triglycerides levels marginally vs control. The 400 mg per day dose of the aqueous extract for 15 days substantially prevented hyperglycemia and hyperinsulinemia induced by a high diet in fructose (63.52 ± 2.9 vs 75.46 ± 2.4, respectively[MC212].

Anti-implantation effect. Ethanol/water (1:1) extract of dried aerial parts, administered orally to rats at a dose of 100.0 mg/kg, was inactive. Ethanol/water (1:1) extract of dried fruit, administered to rats at a dose of 100.0 mg/kg, was inactive[MC133]. Hot water extract of leaves, administered orally to rats at a dose of 500.0 mg/kg, was inactive[MC023].

Antilipolytic activity. Acetone extract of dried seed, at a concentration of 500.0 mcg/plate, was active on rat adipocytes vs ACTA- and epinephrine bitartrate-induced lipolysis. Acetone extract of unripe fresh fruit, at a concentration of 500.0 mcg/plate, was active on rat adipocytes vs ACTA-induced lipolysis, epinephrine bitartrate-induced lipolysis and glucagon-induced lipolysis[MC170]. Chromatographic fraction of decorticated seed, at a concentration of 300.0 mcg/ml, was active on hamster adipocytes. A concentration of 250.0 mg/ml was active on rat adipocytes, results significant at $P < 0.005$ level[MC079].

Antimalarial activity. Chloroform extract of aerial parts, administered subcutaneously to chicken at a dose of 42.0 mg/kg, was inactive on Plasmodium gallinaceum. A dose of 496.0 mg/kg, administered subcutaneously to ducklings, was inactive on Plasmodium cathemerium. Water extract at a dose of 3.44 gm/kg, administered orally to chicken, was inactive on Plasmodium gallinaceum; a dose of 2.37 gm/kg, administered orally to ducklings, was inactive on Plasmodium cathemerium and Plasmodium lophurae[MC016]. Ethanol (95%) extract of dried leaves produced weak activity on Plasmodium falciparum, IC_{50} 68.4 mg/ml[MC099]. Water extract of dried flowers, administered intragastrically to mice at a dose of 1.0 gm/kg, was inactive on Plasmodium berghei[MC052]. The aerial part was moderately active on Plasmodium falciparum chloroquine resistant strain[MC224].

Antimutagenic activity. Carbon tetrachloride and petroleum ether extracts of the unripe fruits, administered intragastrically to mice at doses of 5.0 mg/gm, given twice, were active. Methanol extract was inactive[MC101]. Methanol-insoluble fraction of dried leaves was active vs methylnitrosamine, methyl methane sulfonate and tetracycline-induced genotoxicity[MC066]. Ethanol (80%) extract of the fruit, administered orally to male F344 rats at concentrations of 0.1, 0.5 and 1.0 gm/kg body weight for 5 weeks during the initiation stage, and one week later given a subcutaneous dose of 15 mg/kg body weight of azoxymethane, once a week for 2 weeks, inhibited the mutagenicity of the heterocyclic amines 2-amino-3,4-dimethylimidazo-[4,5-f]quinoline and 2-amino-1-methyl-6-phenylimidazo[4,5-b]pyridine, and aflatoxin B1 in Salmonella mutation assay[MC213].

Antimycobacterial activity. Chloroform, water and methanol extracts of dried fruit, on agar plate, were active on Mycobacterium smegmatis. The ether extract produced strong activity, MIC 2.0 mg/disk. The petroleum ether extract was inactive[MC119].

Antiprotozoan activity. Ethanol/water (1:1) extract of dried entire plant, at a concentration of 125.0 mg/ml in broth culture, was active on Entamoeba histolytica[MC055]. Ethanol/water (1:1) extract of dried fruit, in broth culture, was active on Entamoeba histolytica, IC_{100} 25.0 mcg/ml[MC055].

Antipyretic activity. Ethanol/water (1:1) extract of dried entire plant, administered by gastric intubation to rabbits at variable dosages, was inactive vs yeast-induced pyrexia[MC209].

Antispermatogenic effect. Ethanol (95%) extract of fruit, administered orally to male dogs at a dose of 1.75 gm/animal, was active. Animals were dosed daily for 20 days, sacrificed and the organs examined. Seminiferous tubules lacked primary spermatocytes. 38.7% of the tubules contained normal spermatids. Spermatid abnormalities consisted of clear and vacuoled nuclei and formation of giant multinucleated cells. Interstitial cells did not show morphological evidence of lesions. After daily dosing for 40 days, tubule diameter decreased to 167 m (220 for controls). Testes exhibited variable degrees of spermatogenic arrest, mainly at spermatid stage disorganization, sloughing of immature cells and giant cell formation common in damaged tubules. Daily dosing for 60 days produced seminiferous tubules devoid of spermatozoa. Seventy-five percent completely lacked step 1–8 spermatid. Many tubules were devoid of cells except for sertoli cells and basal spermatogonia. Tubular diameters were minimal and lumen of epididymis and vas deferens devoid of spermatozoa. The extract, administered orally and subcutaneously to male gerbils at doses 200.0 mg/kg daily for 2 weeks, was active. Reduction in testicular weight and disruption of spermatogenesis without affecting seminal vesicles or prostate was observed[MC077].

Antitumor activity. Hot water extract of entire plant, administered intraperitoneally to rats at a dose of 0.4 mg/animal, produced weak activity on Sarcoma 180 (ASC). Slight increase in the life span was observed. When administered orally to human adults, at a dose of 15.0 ml/person 3 times daily for 62 days, it was active on cancer (human). The extract, when administered to 1 lymphatic leukemia patient, produced marked increase in hemoglobin content and a decrease in WBC[MC015]. Water extract of fresh fruit, administered intraperitoneally to mice at a dose of 100.0 mg/ml, was inactive on CBA/D1 cells. The drug was pre-incubated with tumor cells and then injected concomitantly. The extract was also active on LEUK–L1210; drug was pre-incubated with tumor cell line in vitro. Weak activity was produced on LEUK–P388, drug was also pre-incubated with tumor cell line in vitro[MC164]. Momordica protein of 30 kDa (MAP30) was tested on estrogen-independent and highly metastatic human breast tumor MDA-MB-231 both in vitro and in vivo. Treatment with MAP 30 resulted in inhibition of cancer cell proliferation as well as inhibition of the expression of HER2 gene in vitro. When MDA-MB-231 human breast cancer cells were transferred into SCID mice, the mice developed extensive metastases and all mice succumbed to tumor by day 46. Treatment of the human breast cancer bearing SCID mice with MAP30 at 10 microgram/injection EOD for 10 injections resulted in significant increases in survival, with 20–25% of the mice remaining tumor free for 96 days[MC222].

Antiulcer activity. Chloroform, ethanol (95%), and hexane extracts and essential oil, administered intragastrically to rats at doses of 500.0 mg/kg, were inactive[MC059]. Olive oil and ethanol extracts of the mature fruit, administered orally to rats with ethanol-induced ulcers, produced significant and dose-dependent anti-ulcerogenic activity. The dried-powdered fruit in filtered honey was also active[MC221].

Antiviral activity. Ethanol/water (1:1) extract of dried fruit, in cell culture at a concentration of 0.05 mg/ml, was inactive on Ranikhet and Vaccinia virus[MC055].

Antiyeast activity. Chloroform, ether and methanol extracts of dried fruit, on agar plate, were active on Candida albicans. Water extract produced strong activity, MIC 25 mg/disk. Petroleum ether extract was inactive[MC119]. Ethanol (95%) and water extracts of seeds, at a concentration of 10.0 mg/ml on agar plate, were inactive on Candida albicans and Candida tropicalis[MC115]. Ethanol/water (1:1) extract of dried entire plant, at a concentration of 1.0 mg/ml in broth culture, was inactive on Candida albicans, Cryptococcus neoformans and Sporotrichum schenckii. Ethanol/water (1:1) extract of dried fruit, at a concentration of 1.0 mg/ml in broth culture, was inactive on Candida albicans, Cryptococcus neoformans and Sporotrichum schenckii[MC055].

CNS depressant activity. Ethanol (70%) extract of fresh fruit, administered intraperitoneally to mice of both sexes at variable dosages, was active. Ethanol (70%) extract of fresh leaves, administered intraperitoneally to mice of both sexes at variable dosage levels, was active[MC149].

Cytotoxic activity. Dried fruit extract, in cell culture, was active on CA–755 and Leuk–CML (Human)[MC159]. Fresh fruit juice, in cell culture at a concentration of 0.14 mg/ml, was active on Melanoma-B cell-M9.

Viable cells decreased from 100% to 5% between 18 and 26 hours. The juice was also active on human lymphocytes and leukemic lymphocytes, ED$_{50}$ 0.35 and 0.16 mg/plate, respectively[MC139]. Hot water extract of entire plant, at a concentration of 4.0 mg/ml, was active on HEP 2 cells[MC015]. Water extract of dried fruit, in cell culture, was inactive on human lymphocytes[MC161]. Water extract of fresh fruit, in cell culture, was active on CBA/D1 cells, CD$_{10}$ 50.0 mcg/ml. The activity was highly dose-dependent[MC164]. Water extract of fresh fruit, in cell culture, was active on human lymphoblast and lymphocytes[MC128]. Water extract of seeds, in cell culture, was inactive on Sarcoma (Yoshida ASC), ED$_{50}$ > 1.0 mg/ml[MC022].

Diuretic activity. Ethanol/water (1:1) extract of dried entire plant, administered intragastrically to rats at a dose of 510.7 mg/kg, was inactive. Ethanol/water (1:1) extract of dried fruit, administered intragastrically to rats at a dose of 510.7 mg/kg, was inactive vs supramaximal electroshock-induced convulsions[MC055].

DNA Synthesis inhibition. Hot water extract of entire plant, at a concentration of 0.1 mg/ml, was active on sea urchin ova (antimitotic effect)[MC015]. Chromatographic fraction of dried fruit, in cell culture, was active on BKH-21 cells and vesicular stomatitis virus[MC161]. Ethanol (100%) extract of seed, in cell culture, was active on Sarcoma 180 (solid)[MC105].

Embryotoxic effect. Water[MC199] and hot water[MC023] extracts of leaves, administered orally to rats at 200.0 and 500.0 mg/kg, respectively, were inactive.

Estrogenic effect. Hot water extract of leaves, administered subcutaneously to rats at a dose of 20.0 mg/animal, was inactive[MC023].

Feeding deterrent (insect). Glycoside mixture of dried cotyledons, at a concentration of 2.0 mg/insect, was active on *Raphidopalpa foveicollis*[MC160]. Seed oil, at a concentration of 0.5%, was active on *Athalia promina*[MC132].

Fructose diphosphatase inhibition. Ethanol (95%) extract of fresh fruit, administered intragastrically to rats at a dose of 200.0 mg/kg, decreased the activity by 20%[MC058].

Gamma-glutamyltransferase induction. Unripe fruit juice, administered intragastrically to male rats at a dose of 10.0 ml/kg, was active, results significant at $P < 0.001$ level[MC085].

Gluconeogenesis inhibition. Hot water extract of fresh fruit juice was inactive on kidneys[MC085].

Glucose absorption inhibition. Acetone extract of oven-dried fruit, at a concentration of 125.0 mg/ml, was active on the rat small intestine. Ethanol (95%) extract was inactive on adipocytes. Aqueous high-speed supernatant of fresh fruit, at a concentration of 50.0 microliters, was active on the small intestine and inactive on adipocytes of rats[MC171]. Water extract of fresh fruit, administered intragastrically to mice at a dose of 16.0 gm/animal, was inactive vs streptozotocin-induced hyperglycemia[MC102].

Glucose oxidase inhibition. Aqueous high-speed supernatant of fresh fruit, at a concentration of 50.0 microliters, was active on rat adipocytes and liver homogenates[MC171]. Ethanol (95%) extract of oven-dried fruit, at a concentration of 125.0 mg/ml, was active on rat adipocytes and liver homogenates[MC171].

Glucose uptake induction. Fresh fruit juice, administered by gastric intubation to rats at a dose of 10.0 mg/kg, was active, results significant at $P < 0.001$ level[MC177]. Hot water extract of fresh fruit juice was active[MC085].

Glucose-6-phosphatase dehydrogenase stimulation. Ethanol (95%) extract of fresh fruit, administered intragastrically to rats at a dose of 200.0 mg/kg, was active vs streptozotocin-induced hyperglycemia[MC058].

Glucose–6–phosphatase inhibition. Ethanol (95%) extract of fresh fruit, administered intragastrically to rats at a dose of 200.0 mg/kg, was active vs streptozotocin-induced hyperglycemia. The activity decreased 23%[MC058].

Growth inhibitor activity. Hot water extract of the fruit, administered to rats at a dose of 2.0 mg/animal, was active on fetal development[MC015].

Guanylate cyclase inhibition. Water extract of fresh fruit, in cell culture, was active on human lymphoblasts, ED_{50} 0.3 mg/ml[MC128]. Dried fruit extract, in cell culture, was active[MC159]. Ethanol extract (defatted with petroleum ether) of fresh fruit was active, ED_{50} 170.0 mcg/ml[MC179]. Water extract of the fruit produced strong activity on rat colon, heart, kidney, liver, lung and stomach. Water extracts of seed and unripe fruit were inactive on rat liver[MC076]. Water extract of leaves produced strong activity on the rat liver[MC076].

Hematinic activity. Hot water extract of entire plant, taken orally by human adults at a dose of 15.0 ml/person 3 times daily for 62 days, was active. The extract, administered to 1 lymphatic leukemia patient, produced a marked increase in hemoglobin content of blood and decrease in WBC[MC015].

Hepatotoxic activity. Infusion of dried entire plant, taken orally by human children at variable dosage levels, was equivocal. It may be associated with the development of veno-occlusive disease of the liver in Jamaican children[MC208].

Hexokinase inhibition. Aqueous high-speed supernatant of fresh fruit, at a concentration of 50 ml, was active on rat liver homogenates. Ethanol (95%) extract of oven-dried fruit, at a concentration of 125.0 mg/ml, was active on rat liver homogenates[MC171].

HIV-1 reverse transcriptase inhibition. Protein MRK29, isolated for the ripe fruit and seed at a concentration of 18 micrograms/ml, inhibited the HIV-1 reverse transcriptase with 50% IR[MC211].

Hyperglycemic activity. Methanol extract of a commercial sample of entire plant, administered intragastrically to rats at a dose of 2.5 gm/kg, was active. The result was significant at 60 minutes[MC062]. Methanol extract of seeds, administered intragastrically to rats at a dose of 2.5 gm/kg, produced weak activity[MC062]. Protein fraction (FM-11) of dried fruit was active on mice[MC089].

Hyperlipidemic activity. Hot water extract of fresh fruit juice was active on adipose tissue vs triglyceride content of adipose tissue[MC085].

Hypoglycemic activity. Alkaloid fraction of vine, administered orally to rabbits, was inactive; the hot water extract was active[MC012]. Decoction of dried fruit, administered intragastrically to rabbits at a dose of 200.0 mg/kg, was active[MC036]. Ethanol (95%) extract of dried fruit, administered intragastrically to female rats at a dose of 250.0 mg/kg, was active[MC055]. Water extract of dried fruit, administered orally to female rats at a dose of 250.0 mg/kg, was active. The effect is potentiated if used with *Curcuma longa* and *Emblica officinalis*[MC070]. A dose of 10.0 mg/kg, administered orally to rabbits, produced a decrease in blood sugar of 15 mg relative to inert-treated control[MC035]. Decoction of dried fruit, leaves, and stem, in the drinking water of male mice at a concentration of 0.2%, was inactive. One ml of the extract is equivalent to 10 gm of dried plant material. Dosing was daily for 13 days. Plasma glucose and plasma insulin were measured. There was no significant alteration of body weight, food intake, fluid intake or plasma concentrations of glucose or insulin. Glucose tolerance, measured on day 13, was improved by treatment. Intraperitoneal administration of the decoction, at a dose of 0.3 ml/animal, was active, based on a glucose tolerance test. A single dose of extract was given and glucose and insulin levels were measured at 2, 4, 8, 8.5, and 9 hours. Following a single dose of the extract, basal plasma glucose concentrations were reduced after 4 and 8 hours. Glucose tolerance was also improved eight hours after dosing. Plasma insulin levels were unaffected by the extract[MC100]. Dried fruit, administered intragastrically to rabbits at a dose of 0.5 gm/kg, was active[MC090]. Dried plant juice, administered by gastric intubation and intravenously to rabbits, was active[MC159]. Dried unripe fruit juice, administered intragastrically to rabbits at a dose of 500.0 mg/animal, was inactive[MC033]. Ethanol/water (1:1) and saline extracts of shade dried seeds, administered orally to rats at doses of 20.0 mg/kg, and methanol extract at a dose of 10.0 mg/kg, were active[MC185]. Ethanol/water (1:1) and water extracts of fresh fruit, administered intragastrically to mice at doses of 0.5 gm/kg, were inactive[MC068]. Ethanol/water (1:1) extract of dried entire plant, administered intragastrically to rats at a dose of 250.0 mg/kg, was inactive[MC055]. Fresh fruit pulp juice, administered by gastric intubation to rats at a dose of 10.0 ml/kg, was active[MC158]. Fresh fruit, taken orally by human adults at a dose of 15.0 gm/day for 21 days, was equivocal. The fall in blood sugar was 25% of the initial level; however, statistically it is insignifi-cant[MC061]. Fresh fruit juice, administered intragastrically to rabbits at a dose of 6.0 ml/kg, was active[MC034]. Fruit juice, administered intragastrically to rabbits at doses of 200 and 500.0 mg/animal, was inactive[MC194]. Glycoside mixture of dried fruit, administered to rabbits at a dose of 10.0 mg/kg, was active. Lyophilized extract, administered to rabbits at doses of 1.2 gm and 400.0 mg/kg, were inactive[MC120]. Hot water extract, at doses of 5, 10 and 20 mg/kg, was inactive[MC118]. Hot water extract of 20 gm of air-dried fruit, administered by gastric intubation to dogs at a dose of 200.0 ml/animal, produced weak activity[MC154]. Fruit juice, administered intragastrically to rats at a dose of 2.5 gm/kg, was active, results significant at 60–120 minutes[MC062]. Ethanol/water (1:1) extract of dried entire plant, administered intravenously to dogs at variable dosages, was inactive[MC209]. Water extract of the fruit, tested on streptozotocin treated RIN cells and isolated islets in vitro, produced a reduction in streptozotocin-induced hyperglycemia in mice. It markedly reduced the streptozotocin-induced lipid peroxidation in pancreas of mice, RIN cells and islets. Further, it also reduced the streptozotocin-induced apoptosis in RIN cells indicating the mode of protection of the extract in RIN cells, islets and pancreatic beta-cells[MC218]. Aqueous homogenized suspension of the vegetable pulp, administered orally to 100 moderate non-insulin dependent diabetic subjects, produced a significant reduction ($P < 0.001$) of both fasting and post-prandial serum glucose levels. The hypoglycemic action was observed in 86% of the cases. Five percent of the cases showed lowering of fasting serum glucose only[MC223].

Hypotensive effect. Momordin, administered intravenously to normotensive rats, evoked mild hypotensive response, however, lacked dose dependence. It did not affect the blood pressure response to angiotensin I[MC216].

Hypothermic activity. Ethanol/water (1:1) extract of dried entire plant, administered intragastrically to rats, was inactive. Ethanol/water (1:1) extract of dried fruit, administered intragastrically to rats, was inactive[MC055].

Hypotriglyceridemic effect. Fruit extract, administered orally to streptozotocin-induced Type 1 diabetic rats for 10 weeks, indicated that the increased triglycerides and phospholipids returned to normal levels. In addition, the fruit juice exhibited an inhibitory effect on membrane lipoprotein under in vitro conditions[MC214].

Insecticide activity. Ethanol (95%) extract of dried meristem, at a concentration of 50.0 mcg, was inactive on *Rhodnius neglectus*[MC069]. Methanol and acetic acid extracts of dried fruit were inactive on *Spodoptera litura* larvae. Petroleum ether extract, at a concentration of 1.0 ppm, was active[MC117]. Water extract of dried leaves was inactive on *Oncopelatus fasciatus* and produced strong activity on

Blatella germanica; intravenous administration, at a dose of 40.0 ml/kg, produced strong activity on *Periplaneta americana*[MC204].

Insulin induction. Water extract of fresh unripe fruit, in cell culture at a concentration of 1.0 mg/ml, was active on pancreatic islets[MC088].

Leukopenic activity. Hot water extract of entire plant, taken orally by human adult at a dose of 15.0 ml/person 3 times daily for 62 days, was active. The extract, administered to 1 lymphatic leukemia patient, produced a marked increase in hemoglobin content of blood and a decrease in WBC[MC015].

Lipid metabolism effect. Acid/ethanol extract of unripe dried fruit and seeds, at variable concentrations, was active on adipocytes[MC181].

Lipid peroxide formation inhibition. Hot water extract of dried aerial parts, at a concentration of 1.0 mg/plate in cell culture, was inactive on hepatocytes and monitored by production of malonaldehyde[MC074].

Lipid synthesis stimulation. Chromatographic fraction of decorticated seed, at a concentration of 500.0 mcg/ml, was active on rat adipocytes, results significant at $P < 0.005$ level[MC079].

Lipolytic effect. Seeds, administered by gastric intubation to rabbits at a dose of 3.0 gm/animal, were active in streptozotocin-treated animals[MC115].

Liver glycogen increase. Fresh fruit juice, administered by gastric intubation to rats at a dose of 10.0 ml/kg, was active, results significant at $P < 0.01$ level[MC177]. Hot water extract of fresh fruit juice was active. Muscular glycogen level was also increased[MC085].

Metastasis inhibition. Chromatographic fraction of dried fruit, in cell culture, was active on vesicular stomatitis virus[MC161].

Molluscicidal activity. Aqueous slurry (homogenate) of fresh root was inactive on *Lymnaea columella* and *Lymnaea cubensis*, $LD_{100} > 1000$ ppm[MC137]. Ethanol (95%) and water extracts of dried fruit, at a concentra-

tion of 1000 ppm, produced weak activity on *Biomphalaria glabrata* and *Biomphalaria straminea*[MC203].

Oxygen radical inhibition. Fresh fruit juice at a concentration of 0.1 ml/units was active. The heat, acid and alkali-stable components of the extract acted as scavenger of both superoxide and hydroxyl radicals. At the given concentration, 90.16% scavenging of superoxide was seen. At a concentration of 0.33 ml/units, 87.70% scavenging of hydroxyl radical was seen[MC191].

Parasympatholytic activity. Ethanol/water (1:1) extract of the dried entire plant, at a concentration of 0.01 gm/ml, produced weak activity on guinea pig ileum[MC209].

Plant germination inhibition. Hot water extract of entire plant, at a concentration of 20.0 ppm, was active vs corn, cotton and broad beans[MC015].

Protein biosynthesis effect. Fruit extract, administered orally to Sprague-Dawley rats, produced an increase in muscle and liver protein levels, while there was a reduction in the levels of brain protein, muscle and liver glycogen. The activities of plasma L-alanine transaminase and alkaline phosphatase were reduced. The L-aspartate transaminase and adenosine triphosphatase activities were slightly elevated in whole plant extract treated rats while L-aspartate transaminase was unaffected by the ethanol extract but reduced the adenosine triphosphatase activity[MC215].

Protein synthesis inhibition. Chromatographic fraction of dried fruit, in cell culture, was active on BHK-21 cells and vesicular stomatitis virus[MC161]. Water extract of seed was active on rabbit reticulocyte lysate[MC129]. Water extract of dried seed, at a concentration of 10.0 mg/ml, produced strong activity (99% inhibition) on rabbit reticulocyte lysate[MC073].

Radical scavenging effect. Hot water extract of dried aerial parts, at a concentration of 250.0 mg/liter, was inactive. The activity was measured by discoloration of diphenylpicryl hydroxyl radical solution. Six-percent decoloration was observed[MC074].

Respiratory effect. Fresh fruit juice, administered by gastric intubation to rats at a dose of 10.0 ml/kg, was inactive[MC177].

RNA synthesis inhibition. Ethanol (100%) extract of seed, in cell culture, was active on Sarcoma 180 (solid)[MC105].

Spasmolytic activity. Ethanol/water (1:1) extract of dried entire plant was inactive on rat uterus[MC055]. Ethanol/water (1:1) extract of dried fruit was inactive on the uterus of rats[MC055].

Spermicidal effect. Unripe fruit juice was active on the rat sperm[MC141].

Toxic effect (general). Ethanol (95%) extract of fruit, administered orally to male gerbils at a dose of 1.10 gm/kg daily for 30 days, was inactive. At dose of 150.0 mg/kg, weak activity was produced. Twenty to 30% of the animals died within 30 days[MC077]. Ethanol/water (1:1) extract of dried entire plant, administered by gastric intubation and subcutaneously to mice at a dose of 10.0 gm/kg (dry weight of plant), was inactive[MC121]. Alkaloid fraction of vine, administered intraperitoneally to rats at a dose of 14.0 mg/kg, and to rabbits orally at a dose of 56.0 mg/animal, was inactive[MC012]. Decoction of dried fruit, taken orally by human adults at a dose of 500.0 mg/person, was inactive[MC036]. Fresh fruit juice, administered intragastrically to rabbits at a dose of 6.0 ml/kg, was active. Death occurred within 23 days when dosing continued. Two pregnant animals suffered from uterine hemorrhage and died. When administered intraperitoneally to rats at a dose of 15.0 ml/kg, death occurred within 18 hours[MC034].

Toxicity assessment (quantitative). Ethanol/water (1:1) extract of dried aerial parts, administered intraperitoneally to mice of both sexes, produced LD_{50} 681.0 mg/kg[MC133]. Ethanol/water (1:1) extract of dried entire plant, administered intraperitoneally to

mice, produced LD_{50} 681.0 mg/kg[MC055]. Water extract of fresh fruit, administered intraperitoneally and subcutaneously to mice, produced LD_{50} 16.0 and 27.0 mg/ml, respectively[MC164]. Water extract of the seed, administered intraperitoneally to rats, produced LD_{50} of 25.0 mg/kg[MC129]. Ethanol/water (1:1) extract of dried fruit, administered intraperitoneally to mice, produced a LD_{50} 681.0 mg/kg[MC055].

Trypsin inhibition. Chromatographic fraction of seed was active[MC040].

Tumor promotion inhibition. Methanol extract of fresh fruit, in cell culture at a concentration of 200.0 mcg, was inactive on Epstein–Barr virus vs 12-0-hexadecanoyl-phorbol-13-acetate-induced Epstein–Barr virus activation[MC186].

Uterine relaxation effect. Ethanol/water (1:1) extract of dried fruit, administered to nonpregnant rats, was inactive[MC133].

Uterine stimulant effect. Ethanol (95%) extract of dried root, administered intravenously to guinea pigs at a dose of 10.0 mg/ml, was active on the nonpregnant uterus[MC207]. Ethanol/water (1:1) extract of dried fruit, administered to nonpregnant rats, was inactive[MC133].

REFERENCES

MC001 Suwal, P. N. Medicinal Plants of Nepal. Ministry of Forests, Department of Medicinal Plants, Thapathali, Kathmandu, Nepal, 1970.

MC002 Quisumbing, E. Medicinal plants of the Philippines. **Tech Bull 16**, Rep Philippines, Dept Agr Nat Resources, Manilla 1951; 1.

MC003 Jiu, J. A survey of some medicinal plants of Mexico for selected biological activities. **Lloydia** 1966; 29: 250–259.

MC004 Khanna, P. and S. Mohan. Isolation and identification of diosgenin and sterols from fruits and in vitro cultures of *Momordica charantia*. **Indian J Exp Biol** 1973; 11: 58–60.

MC005 Lotlikar, M. M. and M. R. Rajarama. Note on hypoglycemic principle isolated from the fruits of *Momordica charantia.* **J Univ Bombay** 1960; 29: 223.

MC006 Vasistha, S. K., S. C. Vasistha and V. R. K. Rao. Chemical examination of *Momordica charantia.* III. Preparation of d-galacturonic acid and some new salts of it. **J Sci Res Banaras Hindu Univ** 1962; 12: 228.

MC007 Dhalla, N. S., K. C. Gupta, M. S. Sastry and C. L. Malhotra. Chemical composition of the fruit of *Momordica charantia.* **Indian J Pharmacy** 1961; 23: 128.

MC008 Kato, A. and T. Tsuchiya. Oils and fats in Japan. VIII. Alpha-eleostearic acid from the kernel fat of *Momordica charantia* seed. **Tokyo Kogyo Shikensho Hokoku** 1962; 57: 247.

MC009 Velez-Salas, F. Additional note on the antimalarial cundeamor. **Rev Farm** (Buenos Aires) 1944; 86: 512–516.

MC010 Inukai, F., Y. Suyama, I. Sato and H. Inatomi. Amino acids in plants. I. Isolation of citrulline from Cucurbitaceae. **Meiji Daigaku Nogakubu Kenkyu Hokoku** 1966; 20: 29.

MC011 Scrow, W. Constituents of *Momordica charantia.* II. Two new delta-7-sterols from *Momordica charantia.* **Chem Ber** 1966; 99: 3559.

MC012 Rivera, G. Preliminary chemical and pharmacological studies on "cundeamor", *Momordica charantia.* II. **Amer J Pharm** 1942; 114: 72.

MC013 Sucrow, W. Sterol glucoside and a new stigmastadienol from *Momordica charantia.* **Tetrahedron Lett** 1965; 1965: 2217.

MC014 Sucrow, W. Constituents of *Momordica charantia.* I. Delta 5,25-stigmastadien-3beta-ol and its beta-d-glucoside. **Chem Ber** 1966; 99: 2765.

MC015 West, M. E., G. H. Sidrak and S. P. W. Street. The anti-growth properties of extracts from *Momordica charantia.* **West Indian Med J** 1971; 20(1): 25–34.

MC016 Spencer, C. F., F. R. Koniuszy, E. F. Rogers et al. Survey of plants for antimalarial activity. **Lloydia** 1947; 10: 145–174.

MC017 Pons, J. A. and D. S. Stevenson. Effect of *Momordica charantia* (cundeamor) in diabetes mellitus. I. A test for hypoglycemic activity in an alcoholic extract.

Puerto Rico J Pub Health Trop Med 1943; 19: 196.

MC018 Gimlette, J. D. Malay Poisons and Charm Cures. J & A Churchill, London, 3rd Edition, 1929.

MC019 Saha, J. C., E. C. Savini and S. Kasinathan. Ecbolic properties of Indian medicinal plants. Part 1. **Indian J Med Res** 1961; 49: 130–151.

MC020 Bouquet, A. Feticheurs et Medecines Traditionelles du Congo (Brazzaville). Mem Orstom No. 36, 282 P. Paris, 1969.

MC021 Morton, J. F. The balsam pear - an edible, medicinal and toxic plant. **Econ Bot** 1967; 21: 57.

MC022 Tomita, M., T. Kurokawa, K. Onozaki, T. Osawa, Y. Sakurai and T. Ukita. The surface structure of murine ascites tumors. 11. Difference in cytotoxicity of various phytoagglutinins toward Yoshida Sarcoma cells in vitro. **Int J Cancer** 1972; 10: 602.

MC023 Saksena, S. K. Study of antifertility activity of the leaves of *Momordica* (Karela). **Indian J Physiol Pharmacol** 1971; 15: 79–80.

MC024 Kerharo, J. and A. Bouquet. Plantes Medicinales et Toxiques de la Cote-D'Ivoire - Haute-Volta. Vigot Freres, Paris, 1950; 297pp.

MC025 Morton, J. F. Folk-remedy plants and esophageal cancer in Coro, Venezuela. **Morris Arboretum Bull** 1974; 25: 24–34.

MC026 Webb, L. J. Guide to the Medicinal and Poisonous Plants of Queensland. CSIR Bull 232, Melbourne, 1948.

MC027 Watt, J. M. and M. G. Breyer-Brandwijk. The Medicinal and Poisonous Plants of Southern and Eastern Africa. 2nd Ed, E. S. Livingstone, Ltd., London, 1962.

MC028 Stimson, W. R. Ethnobotanical notes from Puerto Rico. **Lloydia** 1971; 34: 165.

MC029 Griffiths, L. A. On the distribution of gentisic acid in green plants. **J Exp Biol** 1959; 10: 437.

MC030 Gupta, S. S. Pituitary diabetes. III. Effect of indigenous antidiabetic-drugs against the acute hyperglycemic response of anterior pituitary extract in glucose fed albino rats. **Indian J Med Res** 1963; 51: 716.

MC031 Chatterjee, K. P. On the presence of an antidiabetic principle in *Momordica charantia*. **Indian J Physiol Pharmacol** 1964; 7: 240.

MC032 Rivera, G. Preliminary chemical and pharmacological studies on "cundeamor," *Momordica charantia* L. (Part 1). **Amer J Pharm** 1941; 113(7): 281–297.

MC033 Kulkarni, R. D. and B. B. Gaitonde. Potentiation of tolbutamide action by jasad bhasma and Karela (*Momordica charantia*). **Indian J Med Res** 1962; 50(5): 715–719.

MC034 Sharma, V. N., R. K. Sogani and R. B. Arora. Some observations on hypoglycemic activity of *Momordica charantia*. **Indian J Med Res** 1960; 48(4): 471–477.

MC035 Jain, S. R. and S. N. Sharma. Hypoglycaemic drugs of Indian indigenous origin. **Planta Med** 1967; 15(4): 439–442.

MC036 Khan, A. H. and A. Burney. A preliminary study of the hypoglycaemic properties of indigenous plants. **Pak J Med Res** 1962; 2: 100–116.

MC037 Ram, S. Karela and diabetes. **J Indian Med Assoc** 1956; 19: 181.

MC038 Gupta, S. S. and C. B. Seth. Effect of *Momordica charantia* Linn. (Karela) on glucose tolerance in albino rats. **J Indian Med Assoc** 1962; 39: 581–584.

MC039 Anansakunwatt, W., W. Thanakunrungsank and S. Larkrungsap. Chemical study in *Momordica charantia* L. Faculty of Pharmacy, Mahidol University, Bangkok, Thailand, **Undergraduate Special Project Report**, 1982; 1982: 32pp.

MC040 Hara, S., J. Makino and T. Ikenaka. Amino acid sequences and disulfide bridges of serine protinease inhibitors from bitter gourd (*Momordica charantia* Linn.) seeds. **J Biochem** (Tokyo) 1989; 105(1): 88–92.

MC041 Ogata, F., T. Miyata, N. Fujii, K. N. Yoshida, S. Makisumi and A. Ito. Purification and amino acid sequence of a bitter gourd inhibitor against an acidic amino acid-specific endopeptidase of *Streptomyces griseus*. **J Biol Chem** 1991; 266(25): 16,715–16,721.

MC042 Minami, Y., Y. Nakahara and G. Funatsu. Isolation and characterization of two momordins, ribosome-inactivating proteins from the seeds of bitter gourd

(*Momordica charantia*). **Biosci Biotech Biochem** 1992; 56(9): 1470–1471.

MC043 Wang, R. W., X. Chen, Y. Li and P. F. Shen. Immunotoxins composed of monoclonal antihuman T lymphocyte antibody and single chain ribosome-inactivating proteins: Antitumor effects in vitro and in vivo. **Zhongua Mazuixue Zazhi** 1992; 8(6): 356–360.

MC044 El-Gengaihi, S., M. S. Karawya, M. A. Selin, H. M. Motawe, N. Ibrahim and L. M. Faddah. A novel pyrmidine glycoside from *Momordica charantia* L. **Pharmazie** 1995; 50(5): 361–362.

MC045 Ogunlana, E. O. and E. Ramstad. Investigations into the antibacterial activities of local plants. **Planta Med** 1975; 27: 354.

MC046 Olaniyi, A. A. A neutral constituent of *Momordica foetida*. **Lloydia** 1975; 38: 361–362.

MC047 Khanna, P., T. N. Nag, S. C. Jain and S. Mohan. Recovering insulin from plant sources. **Patent-Ger Offen-** 2,432,334 1976; 17pp.

MC048 Khanna, P., T. N. Nag, S. C. Jain and S. Mohan. Improved process for isolation of insulin. **Patent-Brit-**1,435,664 1976.

MC049 Lal, J., S. Chandra, V. Raviprakash and M. Sabir. In vitro anthelmintic action of some indigenous medicinal plants on *Ascardia galli* worms. **Indian J Physiol Pharmacol** 1976; 20: 64.

MC050 Rodriquez, D. B., L. C. Raymundo, T. C. Lee, K. L. Simpson and C. O. Chichester. Carotenoid pigment changes in ripening *Momordica charantia* fruits. **Ann Bot (London)** 1976; 40: 615.

MC051 Brandao, M., M. Botelho and E. Krettli. Antimalarial experimental chemotherapy using natural products. **Cienc Cult** 1985; 37(7): 1152–1163.

MC052 Carvalho, L. H., M. G. L. Brandao, D. Santos-Filho, J. L. C. Lopes and A. U. Krettli. Antimalarial activity of crude extracts from Brazilian plants studies in vivo in *Plasmodium berghei*-infected mice and in vitro against *Plasmodium falciparum* in culture. **Braz J Med Biol Res** 1991; 24(11): 1113–1123.

MC053 Lee-Huang, S., P. L. Huang, P. L. Nara, H. C. Chen, H. F. Kung, P. Huang, H.

I. Huang and P. L. Huang. A plant protein useful for treating tumors and HIV infection. **Patent-Pct Int Appl-**92 06,106 1992; 58pp.

MC054 Bhat, R. B., E. O. Eterjere and V. T. Oladipo. Ethnobotanical studies from Central Nigeria. **Econ Bot** 1990; 44(3): 382–390.

MC055 Bhakuni, D. S., A. K. Goel, S. Jain, B. N. Mehrotra, G. K. Patnaik and V. Prakash. Screening of Indian plants for biological activity: Part XIII. **Indian J Exp Biol** 1988; 26(11): 883–904.

MC056 Zheng, S., G. Li and S. M. Yang. Purification and characterization of the analogs of momorcharin. **Shengwu Huaxue Zazhi** 1992; 8(4): 429–433.

MC057 Reddy, M. B., K. R. Reddy and M. N. Reddy. A survey of plant crude drugs of Anantapur District, Andhra Pradesh, India. **Int J Crude Drug Res** 1989; 27(3): 145–155.

MC058 Shibib, B. A., L. A. Khan and R. Rahman. Hypoglycemic activity of *Coccinia indica* and *Momordica charantia* in diabetic rats: Depression of the hepatic gluconeogenic enzymes glucose-6-phosphatase and fructose-1,6-bisphosphatase and elevation of both liver and red-cell shunt enzyme glucose-6-phosphatase. **Biochem J** 1993; 292(1): 267–270.

MC059 Yilkirim, O. F., B. S. Uydes, M. Ark, I. Kanzik and F. Akar. Investigation of the antiulcer effect of the fruits of *Momordica charantia* in rats. **Abstr 3rd Intern Symp Pharm Sci, Ankara Univ** 1993; Abstr-P85.

MC060 Minami, Y. J. and J. K. Funatsu. The complete amino acid sequence of momordin-A, a ribosome-inactivating protein from the seeds of bitter gourd (*Momordica charantia*). **Biosci Biotech Biochem** 1993; 57(7): 1141–1144.

MC061 Srivastava, Y., H. Venkatakrishna-Bhatt, Y. Verma and K. Venkaiah. Antidiabetic and adaptogenic properties of *Momordica charantia* extract: An experimental and clinical evaluation. **Phytother Res** 1993; 7(4): 285–289.

MC062 Ali, L., A. K. A. Khan, M. I. R. Mamun, M. Mosihuzzaman, N. Nahar, M. Nur-E-Alam and B. Rokeya. Studies on hypoglycemic effects of fruit pulp, seed, and whole plant of *Momordica charantia* on normal and diabetic model rats. **Planta Med** 1993; 59(5): 408–412.

MC063 Kee-Huang, S., H. C. Chen, H. F. Kung, P. L. Huang, P. L. Nara, L. B. Li, H. P. Qun, H. I. Huang and P. L. Huang. Plant proteins with antiviral activity against human immunodeficiency virus. Nat Prod Antiviral Agents, **Proc Am Chem Soc Agric Food Chem Div Symp** 1991; 1991: 153–170.

MC064 Zamora-Martinez, M. C. and C. N. P. Pola. Medicinal plants used in some rural populations of Oaxaca, Puebla and Veracruz, Mexico. **J Ethnopharmacol** 1992; 35(3) 229–257.

MC065 Lim-Sylianco, C. Y., J. A. Concha, A. P. Jocano and C. M. Lim. Antimutagenic effects of expressions from twelve medicinal plants. **Philippine J Sci** 1986; 115(1): 23–30.

MC066 Balboa, J. G. and C. Y. Lim-Sylianco. Antigenotoxic effects of drug preparations Akapulko and Ampalaya. **Philipp J Sci** 1992; 121(4): 399–411.

MC067 Tennekoon, K. H., S. Jeevathayaparan, P. Angunawala, E. H. Karunanayake and K. S. A. Jayasinghe. Effect of *Momordica charantia* on key hepatic enzymes. **J Ethnopharmacol** 1994; 44(2): 93–97.

MC068 Cakici, I., C. Hurmoglu, B. Tunctan, N. Abacioglu, I. Kanzik and B. Sener. Hypoglycaemic effect of *Momordica charantia* extracts on normoglycaemic or cyproheptadine-induced hyperglycaemic mice. **J Ethnopharmacol** 1994; 44(2): 117–121.

MC069 Schmeda-Hirschmann, G. and A. Rojas de Arias. A screening method for natural products on Triatomine bugs. **Phytother Res** 1992; 6(2): 68–73.

MC070 Sankaranarayanan, J. and C. I. Jolly. Phytochemical, antibacterial and pharmacological investigations on *Momordica charantia* Linn., *Emblica officinalis* Gaertn. and *Curcuma longa* Linn. **Indian J Pharm Sci** 1993; 55(1): 6–13.

MC071 Cunnick, J. and D. Takemoto. Bitter melon (*Momordica charantia*). **J Naturopathic Med** 1993; 4(1): 16–21.

MC072 Morrison, E. Local remedies... Yeh or Nay. **West Ind Med J Suppl** 1994; 2(43): 9.

MC073 Dong, T. X., T. B. Ng, R. N. S. Wong, H. W. Yeung and G. J. Xu. Ribosome inactivating protein-like activity in seeds of diverse Cucurbitaceae plants. **Int J Biochem** 1993; 25(3): 415–419.

MC074 Joyeux, M., F. Mortier and J. Fleurentin. Screening of antiradical, antilipoperoxidant and hepatoprotective effects of nine plant extracts used in Caribbean folk medicine. **Phytother Res** 1995; 9(3): 228–230.

MC075 Guha, J. and S. P. Sen. The cucurbitacins-A review. **Plant Biochem J** 1975; 2: 127.

MC076 Vesely, D. L., W. R. Graves, T. M. Lo, M. A. Fletcher and G. S. Levey. Isolation of a guanylate cyclase inhibition from the balsam pear (*Momordica charantia* Abreviata). **Biochem Biophys Res Commun** 1977; 77: 1294.

MC077 Dixit, V. P., P. Khanna and S. K. Bhargava. Effects of *Momordica charantia* fruit extract on the testicular function of dog. **Planta Med** 1978; 34: 280–286.

MC078 Lin, J. Y., M. J. Hou and Y. C. Chen. Isolation of toxic and non-toxic lectins from the bitter pear melon *Momordica charantia*. **Toxicon** 1978; 16: 653.

MC079 Ng, T. B., C. M. Wong, W. W. Li, H. W. Yeung. Insulin-like molecules in *Momordica charantia* seeds. **J Ethnopharmacol** 1986; 15(1): 107–117.

MC080 Yen, G. C. and L. S. Hwang. Lycopene from the seeds of ripe bitter melon (*Momordica charantia*) as a potential red food color. II. Storage stability, preparation of powdered lycopene and food applications. **Chung-kuo Nung Yeh Hua Hsueh Hi Chih** 1985; 23(1/2): 151–161.

MC081 Ishikawa, T., M. Kikuchi, T. Iida, S. Seto, T. Tamura and T. Matsumoto. Steam volatile constituents from seed Oils of *Momordica charantia* L. **Nihon Daigaku Kogakubu Kiyo Bunrui** 1985; 26: 165–173.

MC082 Kikuchi, M. T. Ishikawa, T. Iida, S. Seto, T. Tamura and T. Matsumoto. Triterpene alcohols in the seed Oils of *Momordica charantia* L. **Agr Biol Chem** 1986; 50(11): 2921–2922.

MC083 Ishikawa, T., M. Kikuchi, T. Iida, S. Seto, T. Tamura and T. Matsumoto. Carbohydrates in the seeds of *Momordica charantia* L. **Nihon Daigaku Kogakubu Kiyo, Bunrui A** 1987; 28: 165–170.

MC084 Zeng, F. Y., R. Q. Qian and Y. Wang. The amino acid sequence of a trypsin inhibitor from the seeds of *Momordica charantia* Linn. Cucurbitaceae. **Febs Lett** 1988; 234(1): 35–38.

MC085 Karunanayake, E. H. and J. Welihinda. Oral hypoglycaemic medicinal plants of Sri Lanka. **Abstr Princess Congress I**, Bangkok Thailand 1987; Abstr-BP-37.

MC086 Dave, G. R., R. M. Patel and R. J. Patel. Characteristics and composition of seeds and Oil of wild variety of *Momordica charantia* L., from Gujarat, India. **Fette Seifen Anstrichm** 1985; 87(8): 326–327.

MC087 Khanna, P., S. C. Jain, A. Panagariya and V. P. Dixit. Hypoglycemic activity of polypeptide-P from a plant source. **J Nat Prod** 1981; 44(6): 648–655.

MC088 Welihinda, J., G. Arvidson, E. Gylfe, B. Hellman and E. Karlsson. The insulin-releasing activity of the tropical plant *Momordica charantia*. **Acta Biol Med Germ** 1982; 41(12): 1229–1240.

MC089 Lei, Q. J., X. M. Jiang, A. C. Luo, Z. F. Liu, X. C. He, X. D. Wang, F. Y. Cui and P. I. Chen. Influence of balsam pear (the fruit of *Momordica charantia*) on blood sugar level. **Chung I Tsa Chih (Engl Ed)** 1985; 5(2): 99–106.

MC090 Akhtar, M. S., M. A. Athar and M. Yaqub. Effect of *Momordica charantia* on blood glucose level of normal and alloxan-diabetic rabbits. **Planta Med** 1981; 42(3): 205–212.

MC091 Aslam, M. and I. H. Stockley. Interaction between curry ingredient (karela) and drug (chlorpropamide). **Lancet** 1979; 607.

MC092 Venkanna Babu, B., R. Moorti, S. Pugazhenthi, K. M. Prabhu and P. Suryanarayana Murthy. Alloxan recovered rabbits and animal model for screening for hypoglycaemic activity of compounds. **Indian J Biochem Biophys** 1988; 25(6): 714–718.

MC093 Chandrasekar, B., B. Mukherjee and S. K. Mukherjee. Blood sugar lowering potentiality of selected Cucurbitaceae plants of Indian origin. **Indian J Med Res** 1989; 90(4): 300–305.

MC094 Singh, N., S. D. Tyagi and S. C. Agarwal. Effects of long term feeding of acetone extract of *Momordica charantia* (whole fruit powder) on alloxan diabetic albino rats. **Indian J Physiol Pharmacol** 1989; 33(2): 97–100.

MC095 Mossa, J. S. A study on the crude antidiabetic drugs used in Arabian folk medicine. **Int J Crude Drug Res** 1985; 23(3): 137–145.

MC096 Bailey, C. J., C. Day and B. A. Leatherdale. Traditional plant remedies for diabetes. **Diabetic Med** 1986; 3(2): 185–186.

MC097 Srivastava, Y., H. Venkatakrishna-Bhatt and Y. Verma. Effect of *Momordica charantia* Linn. pomous aqueous extract on cataractogenesis in murrin alloxan diabetics. **Pharmacol Res Commun** 1988; 20(3): 201–209.

MC098 Reddy, M. B., K. R. Reddy and M. N. Reddy. A survey of medicinal plants of Chenchu Tribes of Andhra Pradesh, India. **Int J Crude Drugs Res** 1988; 26(4): 189–196.

MC099 Greassor, M., A. Y. Kedjagni, K. Koumaglo, C. DeSouza, K. Agbo, K. Aklikokou and K. A. Amegbo. In vitro antimalarial activity of six medicinal plants. **Phytother Res** 1990; 4(3): 115–117.

MC100 Bailey, C. J., C. Day, S. L. Turner and B. A. Leatherdale. Cerasee, a traditional treatment for diabetes. Studies in normal and streptozotocin diabetic mice. **Diabetes Res** 1985; 2: 81–84.

MC101 Guevara, A. P., C. Lin-Sylianco, F. Dayrit and P. Finch. Antimutagens from *Momordica charantia*. **Mutat Res** 1990; 230(2): 121–126.

MC102 Day, C., T. Cartwright, J. Provost and C. J. Bailey. Hypoglycemic effect of *Momordica charantia* extracts. **Planta Med** 1990; 56(5): 426–429.

MC103 Biswas, A. R., S. Ramaswamy and J. S. Bapna. Analgesic effect of *Momordica charantia* seed extract in mice and rats. **J Ethnopharmacol** 1991; 31(1): 115–118.

MC104 Fatope, M. O., Y. Takeda, H. Yamashita, H. Okabe and T. Yamauchi.

New cucurbitane triterpenoids from *Momordica charantia*. **J Nat Prod** 1990; 53(6): 1491–1497.

MC105 Zhu, Z. L., Z. C. Zhong, Z. Y. Luo and Z. Y. Xiao. Studies on the active constituents of *Momordica charantia* L. **Yao Hsueh Hsueh Pao** 1990; 25(12): 898–903.

MC106 Lee-Huang, S., P. L. Huang, P. L. Nara, H. C. Chen, H. F. Kung, P. Huang, H. I. Huang and P. L. Huang. MAP-30: A new inhibitor of HIV-1 infection and replication. **Febs Lett** 1990; 272(1/2): 12–18.

MC107 Caceres, A., B. R. Lopez, M. A. Giron and H. Logemann. Plants used in Guatemala for the treatment of dermatophytic infections. I. Screeening for antimycotic activity of 44 plant extracts. **J Ethnopharmacol** 1991; 31(3): 263–276.

MC108 Nagaraju, N. and K. N. Rao. A survey of plant crude drugs of Rayalaseema, Andhra Pradesh, India. **J Ethnopharmacol** 1990; 29(2): 137–158.

MC109 Upadhyaya, G. L., A. Kumar and M. C. Pant. Effect of karela as hypoglycemic and cholesterolemic agent. **Jdai** 1983; 25(1): 12–15.

MC110 Baldwa, V. S., C. M. Bhandari, A. Pangaria and R. K. Goyal. Clinical trial in patients with diabetes mellitus of an insulin-like compound obtained from plant source. **Upsala J Med Sci** 1977; 82(1): 39–41.

MC111 Hussain, H. S. N. and Y. Y. Deeni. Plants in Kano ethnomedicine: Screening for antimicrobial activity and alkaloids. **Int J Pharmacog** 1991; 29(1): 51–56.

MC112 Yuwai, K. E., K. S. Rao, C. Kaluwin, G. P. Jones and D. E. Rivett. Chemical composition of *Momordica charantia* L. fruits. **J Agr Food Chem** 1991; 39(10): 1762–1763.

MC113 De Tommasi, N., F. De Simone, V. De Feo and C. Pizza. Phenylpropanoid glycosides and rosmarinic acid from *Momordica balsamina*. **Pianta Med** 1991; 57(2): 201.

MC114 Liu, Y. Pharmaceutical composition containing extracts of fruits and vegetables for treating and preventing diabetes. **Patent-US-**4,985-248 1991; 6pp.

MC115 Naovi, S. A. H., M. S. Y. Khan and S. B. Vohora. Anti-bacterial, anti-fungal and anthelmintic investigations on Indian medicinal plants. **Fitoterapia** 1991; 62(3): 221–228.

MC116 Barbieri, L., M. Zamboni, E. Lorenzoni, L. Montanaro, S. Sperti and F. Stirpe. Inhibitor of protein synthesis in vitro by proteins from the seeds of Momordica charantia (bitter pear melon). **Biochem J** 1980; 186: 443–452.

MC117 Tuntivanich, U., S. Tiwakornpunnarai and C. Dejsupa. Studies of insecticidal activity of organic compounds in Momordica charantia Linn. **Sci Thailand** 1981; 38(3): 750–754.

MC118 Praphapraditchote, K., C. Nookhwan and R. Mekmanee. Hypoglycemic effect of Momordica charantia in rabbits. **Abstr 6ᵗʰ Congress of the Pharmacological and Therapeutic Society of Thailand** 1984; 75pp.

MC119 Maneelrt, S. and A. Satthampongsa. Antimicrobial activity of Momordica charantia. **Undergraduate Special Project Report** 1978; 18pp.

MC120 Praphaditchote, K. Hypoglycemic effect of Momordica charantia Linn. in rabbits. **Master Thesis** 1984; 59pp.

MC121 Mokkhasmit, M., K. Swatdimongkol and P. Satrawana. Study on toxicity of Thai medicinal plants. **Bull Dept Med Sci** 1971; 12(2/4): 36–65.

MC122 Halberstein, R. A. and A. B. Saunders. Traditional medical practices and medicinal plant usage on a Bahamian Island. **Cul Med Psychiat** 1978; 2: 177–203.

MC123 Shum, L. K. W., V. E. C. Coi and H. W. Yeung. Effects of Momordica charantia seed extract on the rat mid-term placenta. (Abstract). **Abstr International Symposium on Chinese Medicinal Materials Research, Hong Kong** 1984; Abstr-78.

MC124 Kays, S. J. and M. J. Hayes. Induction of ripening in the fruits of Momordica charantia by ethylene. **Trop Agr (Trinidad)** 1978; 55: 167.

MC125 Ayensu, E. S. Medicinal Plants of the West Indies. **Unpublished Manuscript** 1978; 110pp.

MC126 Koelz, W. N. Notes on the ethnobotany of Lahul, a province of the Punjab. **Q J Crude Res** 1979; 17: 1–56.

MC127 Gupta, M. P., T. D. Arias, M. Correa and S. S. Lamba. Ethnopharmacognostic observations on Panamanian medicinal plants. Part 1. **Q J Crude Drug Res** 1979; 17(3/4): 115–130.

MC128 Takemoto, D. J., R. Kresie and D. Vaughn. Partial purification and characterization of a guanylate cyclase inhibition with cytotoxic properties from the bitter melon (Momordica charantia). **Biochem Biophys Res Commun** 1980; 94: 332–339.

MC129 Gasperi-Campani, A., L. Barbieri, P. Morelli and F. Stirpe. Seed extracts inhibiting protein synthesis in vitro. **Biochem J** 1980; 186: 439–441.

MC130 Oliver-Bever, B. Oral hypoglycaemic plants in West Africa. **J Ethnopharmacol** 1980; 2(2): 119–127.

MC131 Koelz, W. N. Notes on the ethnobotany of Lahul, a province of the Punjab. **Q J Crude Drug Res** 1979; 17: 1–56.

MC132 Kumar, A., G. D. Tiwari and N. D. Pandey. Studies on the antifeeding and insecticidal properties of bitter gourd (Momordica charantia L.) against mustard sawfly Athalia proxima Klug. **Pestology** 1979; 3(5): 23–25.

MC133 Dhawan, B. N., M. P. Dubey, B. N. Mehrotra, R. P. Rastogi and J. S. Tandon. Screening of Indian plants for biological activity. Part IX. **Indian J Exp Biol** 1980; 18: 594–606.

MC134 Licastro, F., C. Franceschi, L. Barbieri and F. Stirpe. Toxicity of Momordica charantia lectin and inhibitor for normal and leukemic lympocytes. **Virchows Arch B** 1980; 33: 257–265.

MC135 Horejsi, V., M. Ticha, J. Novotny and J. Kocourek. Studies on lectins. XLVII. Some properties of d-galactoside binding lectins isolate from the seeds of Butea frondosa, Erythrina indica and Momordica charantia. **Biochim Biophys Acta** 1980; 623: 439–448.

MC136 Okabe, H., Y. Miyahara and T. Yamauchi. Bitter principles and their related compounds in the fruits of Momordica charantia L. **Symposium on the Chemistry of Natural Products, Osaka** 1981; 24: 95–102.

MC137 Medina, F. R. and R. Woodbury. Terrestrial plants molluscicidal to Lymnaeid hosts of Fasciliasis hepatica in

Puerto Rico. **J Agr Univ Puerto Rico** 1979; 63: 366–376.

MC138   Commachan, M. and S. S. Khan. Plants in aid of family planning programme. **Sci Life** 1981; 1: 64–66.

MC139   Takemoto, D. J., C. Dunford and M. M. McMurray. The cytotoxic and cytostatic effects of the bitter melon (*Momordica charantia*) on human lymphocytes. **Toxicon** 1982; 20: 593–599.

MC140   Arnason, T., F. Uck, J. Lambert and R. Hebda. Maya medicinal plants of San Jose Succotz, Belize. **J Ethnopharmacol** 1980; 2(4): 345–364.

MC141   Koentjoro-Soehadi, T. and I. G. P. Santa. Perspectives of male contraception with regards to Indonesian traditional drugs. **Proc Second Congress of Indonesian Society of Andrology**, Bali, Indonesia 1982; 12pp.

MC142   Morton, J. F. Caribbean and Latin American folk medicine and its influence in the United States. **Q J Crude Drug Res** 1980; 18(2): 57–75.

MC143   Kedar, P. and C. H. Chakrabarti. Effects of bitter gourd (*Momordica charantia*) seed & glibenclamide in streptozotocin induced diabetes mellitus. **Indian J Exp Biol** 1982; 20: 232–235.

MC144   Iyer, R. I., P. K. Nagar and P. K. Sircar. Endogenous cytokinins in seeds of bittergourd *Momordica charantia* L. **Indian J Exp Biol** 1981; 19: 766–767.

MC145   Dutta, P. K., A. K. Chakravarty, U. S. Chowdhury and S. C. Pakrashi. Studies on Indian medicinal plants. Part 64. Vicine, a favism-inducing toxin from *Momordica charantia* Linn. seeds. **Indian J Chem Ser B** 1981; 20: 669–671.

MC146   Okabe, H., Y. Miyahara and T. Yamauchi. Studies on the constituents of *Momordica charantia* L. 4. Characterization of the new cucurbitacin glycosides of the immature fruits. (2). Structures of the bitter glycosides, momordicosides K and L. **Chem Pharm Bull** 1982; 30: 4334–4340.

MC147   Okabe, H., Y. Miyahara and T. Yamauchi. Studies in the constituents of *Momordica charantia*. 3. Characterization of new cucurbitacin glycosides of the immature fruits. (1). Structures of momordicosides G, F1, F2 and I. **Chem Pharm Bull** 1982; 30: 3977–3986.

MC148   Takemoto, D. J., C. Jilka and R. Kresie. Purification and characterization of a cytostatic factor from the bitter melon *Momordica charantia*. **Prep Biochem** 1982; 12: 355–375.

MC149   Adesina, S. K. Studies on some plants used as anticonvulsants in Amerindian and African traditional medicine. **Fitoterapia** 1982; 53: 147–162.

MC150   Yen, G. C., L. S. Hwang and T. C. Lee. Lycopene from the seeds of ripe bitter melon (*Momordica charantia*) as a potential red food colorant. 1. Identification, survey of lycopene content and ripening test. **Chung-kuo Nung Yeh Hus Hsueh Hui Chih** 1981; 19: 227–235.

MC151   Barron, D., M. Kaouadji and A. M. Mariotte. Comparative study of two medicinal Cucurbitaceae. 1. Seeds metabolism and amino acid composition. **Planta Med** 1982; 46: 184–186.

MC152   Halder, T. and V. N. Gadgil. Fatty acids of callus tissues of six species of Cucurbitaceae. **Phytochemistry** 1983; 22(9): 1965–1967.

MC153   Sharma, A. K. Bacterial growth inhibition of unsaponifiable matter of fixed Oil from *Momordica charantia*. **Indian Drugs Pharm Ind** 1981; 16: 29–30.

MC154   Morrison, E. Y. S. A. and M. West. A preliminary study of the effects of some West Indian medicinal plants on blood sugar levels in the dog. **West Indian Med J** 1982; 31: 194–197.

MC155   Vitalyos, D. Phytotherapy in domestic traditional medicine in Matouba-Papaye (Guadeloupe). **Dissertation-Ph.D.-Univ Paris** 1979; 110pp.

MC156   Okoli, B. E. Wild and cultivated cucurbits in Nigeria. **Econ Bot** 1984; 38(3): 350–357.

MC157   Yasuda, M., M. Iwamoto, H. Okabe and T. Yamauchi. Structures of momordicines I, II and III. The bitter principles in the leaves and vines of *Momordica charantia* L. **Chem Pharm Bull** 1984; 32(5): 2044–2047.

MC158   Karunanayake, E. H., J. Welihinda, S. R. Sirimanne and G. Sinnadorai. Oral hypoglycaemic activity of some medicinal plants of Sri Lanka. **J Ethnopharmacol** 1984; 11(2): 223–231.

MC159   Ng, T. B. and H. W. Yeung. Bioactive constituents of Cucurbitaceae plants with special emphasis on *Momordica charantia* and *Trichosanthes kirilowii*. **Proc 5th Asian Symposium on Medicinal Plants and Spices Seoul Korea** 1984; 5: 183–196pp.

MC160   Chandravadana, M. V. and A. B. Pal. Triterpenoid feeding deterrent of *Raphidopalpa foveicollis* L. (red pumpkin beetles) from *Momordica charantia* L. **Curr Sci** 1983; 52(2): 87–89.

MC161   Takemoto, D. J., C. Jilka, S. Rockenbach and J. V. Hughes. Purification and characterization of a cystostatic factor with anti-viral activity from the bitter melon. **Prep Biochem** 1983; 13(5): 397–421.

MC162   Miyahara, Y., H. Okabe and T. Yamauchi. Studies on the constituents of *Momordica charantia* L. II. Isolation and characterization of minor seed glycosides, momordicosides C, D and E. **Chem Pharm Bull** 1981; 29: 1561–1566.

MC163   Okabe, H., Y. Miyahara, T. Yamauchi, K. Miyahara and T. Kawasaki. Studies on the constituents of *Momordica charantia* L. I. Isolation and characterization of momordicosides A and B, glycosides of a pentahydroxy-cucurbitane triterpene. **Chem Pharm Bull** 1980; 28(9): 2753–2762.

MC164   Jilka, C., B. Strifler, G. W. Fortner, E. F. Hays and D. J. Takemoto. In vivo antitumor activity of the bitter melon (*Momordica charantia*). **Cancer Res** 1983; 43(11): 5151–5155.

MC165   Laurens, A., S. Mboup, M. Tignokpa, O. Sylla and J. Masquelier. Antimicrobial activity of some medicinal species of Dakar markets. **Pharmazie** 1985; 40(7): 482–485.

MC166   Yeung, H. W., W. W. Li, L. K. Law and W. Y Chan. Purification and partial characterization of momorcharins, abortifacient proteins from the Chinese drug, Kuguazi (*Momordica charantia*) seeds. Advances in Chinese Medicinal Materials Research, World Scientific Press, Philadelphia, Pa 1984; 311–318pp.

MC167   Velazco, E. A. Herbal and traditional practices related to material and child health care. Rural **Reconstruction Review** 1980; 35–39.

MC168   Mossa, J. S. A study on the crude antidiabetic drugs used in Arabian folk medicine. **Int J Crude Drug Res** 1985; 23(3): 137–145.

MC169   Singh, Y. N. Traditional medicine in Fiji: Some herbal folk cures used by Fiji Indians. **J Ethnopharmacol** 1986; 15(1): 57–88.

MC170   Wong, C. M., T. B. Ng and H. W. Yeung. Screening of *Trichosanthes kirilowii*, *Momordica charantia* and *Cucurbitas maxima* (Family Cucurbitaceae) for compounds with antilipolytic activity. **J Ethnopharmacol** 1985; 13(3): 313–321.

MC171   Meir, P. and Z. Yaniv. An in vitro study on the effect of *Momordica charantia* glucose uptake and glucose metabolism in rats. **Planta Med** 1985; 1: 12–16.

MC172   Tignokpa, M., A. Laurens, S. Mboup and O. Sylla. Popular medicinal plants of the markets of Dakar (Senegal). **Int J Crude Drug Res** 1986; 24(2): 75–80.

MC173   Chan, W. Y., P. P. L. Tam, H. L. Choi, T. B. Ng and H. W. Yeung. Effects of momorcharins on the mouse embryo at the early organogenesis stage. **Contraception** 1986; 34(5): 537–544.

MC174   Chakraborty, T. and G. Poddar. Herbal drugs in diabetes - Part 1. Hypoglycaemic activity of indigenous plants in streptozotocin (STZ) induced diabetic rats. **J Inst Chem (India)** 1984; 56(1): 20–22.

MC175   Takemoto, D. J., C. Jilka, S. Rockenbach and J. V. Hughes. Purification and characterization of a cytostatic factor with anti-viral activity from the bitter melon. **Prep Biochem** 1983; 13(4): 371–393.

MC176   Leatherdale, B. A., R. K. Panesar, G. Singh, T. W. Atkins, C. J. Bailey and A. H. C. Bignell. Improvement in glucose tolerance due to *Momordica charantia* (Karela). **Brit Med J** 1981; 282(6279): 1823–1824.

MC177   Welihinda, J. and E. H. Karunanayake. Extra-pancreatic effects of *Momordica charantia* in rats. **J Ethnopharmacol** 1986; 17(3): 247–255.

MC178   Welihinda, J., E. H. Karunanayake, M. H. R. Sheriff and K. S. A. Jayasinghe. Effect of *Momordica charantia* on the glucose tolerance in maturity onset diabetes. **J Ethnopharmacol** 1986; 17(3): 277–282.

MC179 Takemoto, D. J., C. Dunford, D. Vaughn, K. J. Kramer, A. Smith and R. G. Powell. Guanylate cyclase activity in human leukemic and normal lymphocytes. **Enzyme** 1982; 27: 179–188.

MC180 Weniger, B., M. Rouzier, R. Daguilh, D. Henrys, J. H. Henrys and R. Anthon. Popular medicine of the Central Plateau of Haiti. 2. Ethnopharmacological inventory. **J Ethnopharmacol** 1986; 17(1): 13–30.

MC181 Ng, T. B., C. M. Wong, W. W. Li and H. W. Yeung. Acid-ethanol extractable compounds from fruits and seeds of the bitter gourd *Momordica charantia*: Effects on lipid metabolism in isolated rat adipocytes. **Amer J Chin Med** 1987; 15(1/2): 31–42.

MC182 Yeung, H. W., W. W. Li, Z. Feng, L. Barbieri and F. Stirpe. Trichosanthin, alpha-momorcharin and beta-momorcharin: Identity of abortifacient and ribosome-inactivating proteins. **Int J Peptide Protein Res** 1988; 31(3): 265–268.

MC183 Kamboj, V. P. A review of Indian medicinal plants with interceptive activity. **Indian J Med Res** 1988; 4: 336–355.

MC184 Srivastava, Y., H. Venkatakrishna-Bhatt, Y. Verma and A. S. Perm. Retardation of retinopathy by *Momordica charantia* L. (bitter gourd) fruit extract in alloxan diabetic rats. **Indian J Exp Biol** 1987; 25(8): 571–572.

MC185 Dubey, D. K., A. R. Biswas, J. S. Bapna and S. C. Pradhan. Hypoglycaemia and antihyperglycaemic effects of *Momordica charantia* seed extracts in albino rats. **Fitoterapia** 1987; 58(6): 387–394.

MC186 Koshimizu, K., H. Ohigashi, H. Tokuda, A. Kondo and K. Yamaguchi. Screening of edible plants against possible anti-tumor promoting activity. **Cancer Lett** 1988; 39(3): 247–257.

MC187 Ramirez, V. R., L. J. Mostacero, A. E. Garcia, C. F. Mejia, P. F. Pelaez, C. D. Medina and C. H. Miranda. Vegetales empleados en medicina tradicional Norperuana. Banco Agrario Del Peru & NACL Univ, Trujillo, Peru, June 1988; 54pp.

MC188 Hirschmann, G. S. and A. Rojas De Arias. A survey of medicinal plants of Minas Gerais, Brazil. **J Ethnopharmacol** 1990; 29(2): 159–172.

MC189 Karunanayake, E. H., S. Jeevathayaparan and K. H. Tennekoon. Effect of *Momordica charantia* fruit juice on streptozotocin-induced diabetes in rats. **J Ethnopharmacol** 1990; 30(2): 199–204.

MC190 Boye, G. L. Studies on antimalarial action of *Cryptolepis sanguinolenta* extract. **Proc Int Symp on East-West Med**, Seoul, Korea 1989; 243–251pp.

MC191 Sreejayan and M. N. A. Rao. Oxygen free radical scavenging activity of the juice of *Momordica charantia* fruits. **Fitoterapia** 1991; 62(4): 344–346.

MC192 Panthong, A., D. Kanjanapothi and W. C. Taylor. Ethnobotanical review of medicinal plants from Thai traditional books, Part 1. Plants with antiinflammatory, anti-asthmatic and antihypertensive properties. **J Ethnopharmacol** 1986; 18(3): 213–228.

MC193 Ayensu, E. S. Medicinal Plants of West Africa. Reference Publications, Inc, 1978.

MC194 Kulkarni, R. D. and B. B. Gaitonde. Potentiation of tolbutamide action by jasad bhasma and karela (*Momordica charantia*). **Indian J Med Res** 1962; 50: 715–719.

MC195 Sharma, L. D., H. S. Bahga and P. S. Srivastava. In vitro anthelmintic screening of indigenous medicinal plants against *Haemonchus contortus* (Rudolphi, 1803) Cobbold, 1898 of sheep and goats. **Indian J Anim Res** 1971; 5(1): 33–38.

MC196 Friese, F. W. Certain little-known anthelmintics from Brazil. **Apoth ZTG** 1929; 44: 180.

MC197 Lotlikar, M. M. and M. R. Rajarama Rao. Pharmacology of a hypoglycaemic principle isolated from the fruits of *Momordica charantia*. **Indian J Pharmacy** 1966; 28: 129.

MC198 Oakes, A. J. and M. P. Morris. The West Indian weedwoman of the United States Virgin Islands. **Bull Hist Med** 1958; 32: 164.

MC199 Prakash, A. O. and R. Mathur. Screening of Indian plants for antifertility activity. **Indian J Exp Biol** 1976; 14: 623–626.

MC200   Mueller-Oerlinghausen, B., W. Ngamwathana and P. Kanchanapee. Investigation into Thai medicinal plants said to cure diabetes. **J Med Assoc Thailand** 1971; 54: 105–111.

MC201   Stepka, W., K. E. Wilson and G. E. Madge. Antifertility investigation on Momordica. **Lloydia** 1974; 37: 645C.

MC202   Roig y Mesa, J. T. Plantas Medicinales, Aromaticas o Venemosas de Cuba. Ministerio de Agricultura, Republica de Cuba, Havana 1945; 872pp.

MC203   Pinheiro de Sousa, M. and M. Z. Rouquayrol. Molluscicidal activity of plants from Northeast Brazil. **Rev Bras Fpesq Med Biol** 1974; 7(4): 389–394.

MC204   Heal, R. E., E. F. Rogers, R. T. Wallace and O. Starnes. A survey of plants for insecticidal activity. **Lloydia** 1950; 13: 89–162.

MC205   George, M. and K. M. Pandalai. Investigations on plant antibiotics. Part IV. Further search for antibiotic substances in Indian medicinal plants. **Indian J Med Res** 1949; 37: 169–181.

MC206   Wasuwat, S. A list of Thai medicinal plants, ASRCT, Bangkok, Report No. 1 on Res. Project. 17. **ASRCT** Bangkok Thailand 1967; 17: 22pp.

MC207   Jamwal, K. S. and K. K. Anand. Preliminary screening of some reputed abortifacient indigenous plants. **Indian J Pharm** 1962; 24: 218–220.

MC208   Jelliffe, D. B., G. Bras and K. L. Stuart. The clinical picture of veno-occlusive disease of the liver in Jamaican children. **Ann Trop Med Parasitol** 1954; 48: 386–396.

MC209   Mokkhasmit, M., K. Swasdimongkol, W. Ngarmwathana and U. Permphiphat. Pharmacological evaluation of Thai medicinal plants. (Continued). **J Med Assoc Thailand** 1971; 54(7): 490–504.

MC210   Pari, L., R. Ramakrishnan and S. Venkateswaran. Antihyperglycaemic effect of Diamed, a herbal formulation, in experimental diabetes in rats. **J Pharm Pharmacol** 2001; 53(8): 1139–1143.

MC211   Jiratchariyakul, W., C. Wiwat, M. Vongsakul, A. Somanabandhu, W. Leelamanit, I. Fugii, N. Suwannaroj and Y. Ebizuka. HIV inhibitor from Thai bitter gourd. **Planta Med** 2001; 67(4): 350–353.

MC212   Vikrant, V., J. K. Grover, N. Tandon, S. S. Rathi and N. Gupta. Treatment with extracts of Momordica charantia and Eugenia jambolana prevents hyperglycemia and hyperinsulinemia in fructose fed rats. **J Ethnopharmacol** 2001; 76(2): 139–143.

MC213   Chiampanichayakul, S., K. Kataoka, H. Arimochi, S. Thumvijit, T. Kuwahara, H. Nakayama, U. Vinitketkumnuen and Y. Ohnishi. Inhibitory effects of bitter melon (Momordica charantia Linn.) on bacterial mutagenesis and aberrant crypt focus formation in the rat colon. **J Med Invest** 2001; 48(1–2): 88–96.

MC214   Ahmed, I., M. S. Lakhani, M. Gillett, A. John and H. Raza. Hypotriglyceridemic and hypocholesterolemic effects of antidiabetic Momordica charantia (karela) fruit extract in streptozotocin-induced diabetic rats. **Diabetes Res Clin Pract** 2001; 51(3): 155–161.

MC215   Araba, B. G. Stimulation of protein biosynthesis in rat hepatocytes by extracts of Momordica charantia. **Phytother Res** 2001; 15(2): 95–98.

MC216   Wang, H. X and T. B. Ng. Studies on the anti-mitogenic, anti-phage and hypotensive effects of several ribosome inactivating proteins. **Comp Biochem Physiol C Toxicol Pharmacol** 2001; 128(3): 359–366.

MC217   Murakami, T., A. Emoto, H. Matsuda and M. Yoshikawa. Medicinal foodstuffs. XXI. Structures of new cucurbitane-type triperpene glycosides, goyaglycosides- a, -b, -c, -d, -e, -f, -g, and -h, and new oleanane-type triterpene saponins, goyasaponins I, II, and II, from the fresh fruit of Japanese Momordica charantia L. **Chem Pharm Bull (Tokyo)** 2001; 49(1): 54–63.

MC218   Sitasawad, S. L., Y. Shewade and R. Bhonde. Role of bittergourd fruit juice in stz-induced diabetic state in vivo and in vitro. **J Ethnopharmacol** 2000; 73 (1–2): 71–79.

MC219   Jayasooriya, A. P., M. Sakono, C. Yukizaki, M. Kawano, K. Yamamoto, N. Fukuda. Effects of Momordica charantia powder on serum glucose levels and various lipid parametes in rats fed with cholesterol-free and cholesterol-enriched diets. **J Ethnopharmacol** 2000; 72(1–2): 331–336.

MC220 Ganguly, C., S. De and S. Das. Prevention of carcinogen-induced mouse skin papilloma by whole fruit aqueous extract of *Momordica charantia*. **Eur J Cancer Prev** 2000; 9(4): 283–288.

MC221 Gurbuz, I., C. Akyuz, E. Yesilada and B. Sener. Anti-ulcerogenic effect of *Momordica charantia* L. fruits on various ulcer models in rats. **J Ethnopharmacol** 2000; 71(1–2): 77–82.

MC222 Lee-Huang, S., P. L. Huang, Y. Sun, H. C. Chen, H. F. Kung, P. L. Huang and W. J. Murphy. Inhibition of MDA-MB-231 human breast tumor xenografts and HER2 expression by anti-tumor agents GAP31 and MAP30. **Anticancer Res** 2000; 20(2A): 653–659.

MC223 Ahmad, N., M. R. Hassan, H. Halder and K. S. Bennoor. Effect of *Momordica*

charantia (Karolla) extracts on fasting and postprandial serum glucose levels in NIDDM patients. **Bangladesh Med Res Counc Bull** 1999; 25(1): 11–13.

MC224 Munoz, V., M. Sauvain, G. Bourdy, J. Callapa, I. Rojas, L. Vargas, A. Tae and E. Deharo. The search for natural bioactive compounds through a multidisciplinary approach in Bolivia. Part II. Antimalarial activity of some plants used by Mosetene Indians. **J Ethnopharmacol** 2000; 69(2): 139–155.

MC225 Yesilada, E., I. Gurbuz and H. Shibata. Screening of Turkish anti-ulcerogenic folk remedies for anti-*Helicobacter pylori* activity. **J Ethnopharmacol** 1999; 66(3): 289–293.

MC226 Matsuda, H., Y. Li, J. Yamahara and M. Yoshikawa. Inhibition of gastric emptying by triterpene saponin, momordin Ic, in mice: roles of blood glucose, capsaicin-sensitive sensory nerves, and central nervous system. **J Ethnopharmacol Exp Ther** 1999; 289(2): 729–734.

20 | Moringa pterygosperma

Gaertn.

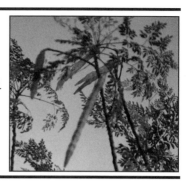

Common Names

Ba da dai	Indonesia	Malunggay	Philippines
Ben aile	New Caledonia	Mangai	India
Ben aile	Senegal	Maranga	Mauritius
Ben nut tree	Mauritius	Marum	Malaysia
Ben nut tree	West Indies	Marum	Thailand
Brede mourounge	Rodrigues Islands	Ma-rum	Thailand
Chum ngay	Indonesia	Mbum	Senegal
Daintha	India	Meetho sirgavo	India
Dandalonbin	India	Meethosaragavo	India
Danthalons	India	Merunggai	Malaysia
Da-tha-lwon	India	Moringa tree	West Indies
Dhak I houm	Indonesia	Moringa	India
Diaboy	Senegal	Moringa	West Indies
Drum stick tree	Fiji	Moringue	Angola
Drum stick tree	India	Munaga	India
Drum stick	India	Munga	India
Drum stick	Nepal	Mungay	India
Drum stick	Sri Lanka	Munigha	India
Getha	Saudi Arabia	Muringa	India
Horse radish tree	India	Murunga	Sri Lanka
Horse radish tree	Malaysia	Murungai	India
Horse radish tree	Nepal	Musing	India
Horseradish tree	Fiji	Nebeday	Senegal
Horseradish tree	Guam	Neboday	Senegal
Horseradish tree	Indonesia	Nebreday	Senegal
Horseradish tree	Mauritius	Neveday	Senegal
Horseradish tree	Nigeria	Nevorday	Senegal
Horseradish tree	USA	Nevredie	Senegal
Horseradish tree	West Indies	Noboday	Senegal
Horseradish	India	Nobody	Senegal
Kelor pea	Malaysia	Radish tree	India
Kelor	Indonesia	Ramunggai	Malaysia
Kelor	Malaysia	Ravinta	India
Malungai	Guam	Sahajan	India
Malungal	Philippines	Sahajana	India

From: *Medicinal Plants of the World, vol. 1: Chemical Constituents, Traditional and Modern Medicinal Uses, 2nd ed.*
By: Ivan A. Ross © Humana Press Inc., Totowa, NJ

Sahanjana	India	Shajmah	India
Sahjan	India	Shajna	India
Sahjna	India	Shejan	India
Sahjna	Pakistan	Shigru	India
Saijan	Fiji	Shobanjan	Nepal
Saijan	Guyana	Shobhanjana	India
Sainjan	India	Sigru	India
Sainjna	India	Soanjna	Fiji
Sajana	India	Sobhanja	India
Sajina	India	Sobhanjan	India
Sajna	Bangladesh	Sobhanjana	India
Sajna	Fiji	Sobhanjanavriksha	India
Sajna	India	Sohawjana	Nepal
Salijan	India	Sojna	India
Sanjna	India	Sonth	India
Sapsap	Senegal	Sunara	India
Saragavo	India	Sundan	India
Segat	India	Sunja	India
Segra	India	West Indian ben	India
Sehjan	India	Wolof	Senegal
Shahjnah	India	Yovoviti	Togo
Shajiwan	Nepal	Zoliv	Haiti

BOTANICAL DESCRIPTION

A tree of the MORINGACEAE family that grows 10 to 15 meters high. It is a rapidly growing tree that resembles a legume, has tripinnate leaves, a gummy bark and fragrant flowers with white petals. The brown, 3-angled fruits are up to 45 cm long and have winged seeds. The flowers are 1.5 to 2 cm long. Fertile filaments are villous at the base; ovary hairy; pods 15 to 30 cm long and pendulous.

ORIGIN AND DISTRIBUTION

A native of India now found in East and Southeast Asia, Polynesia and the West Indies.

TRADITIONAL MEDICINAL USES

Andaman Islands. Fruits and leaves are eaten as a vegetable[MP053].

Colombia. Hot water extract of the plant is taken orally as an abortive[MP094].

East Africa. Hot water extract of the root bark is taken orally as an abortifacient[MP033].

East Indies. Hot water extract of the root bark is taken orally as a menstrual promoter, a diuretic and a stimulant[MP109].

Fiji. Dried leaves ground with garlic, salt, black pepper and turmeric are used as a treatment for dog bites. Dried leaves, ground with black pepper are applied externally for headache. Fresh leaf juice, mixed with honey, is used as an ointment for sore eyes. The fresh leaf juice is taken orally to induce vomiting (useful in poisoning)[MP090].

Guam. Hot water extract of seeds is taken orally to treat fevers, and as a tonic[MP017].

Haiti. Decoction of dried leaves is taken orally for nervous shock[MP091].

India. Fifteen grams of root bark, mixed with 20 corns of black pepper, is taken orally to produce abortion[MP098]. Decoction of dried leaves is taken orally for abortion[MP049], and externally for rheumatism[MP059] and wound healing[MP076]. Leaves, made into a paste with salt are used to treat edema[MP085]. Dried fruit is taken orally for 20 days to produce sterility. A mixture of the fruits of *Clerodendrum* *indicum, Sesamum orientale, Moringa pterygosperma* and *Piper nigrum* is mixed with sugar[MP070]. The mixture is also taken as a tonic[MP081]. Hot water extract of the dried fruit is taken orally for headache and for giddiness[MP087]. Dried gum is applied externally for headache[MP057]. Dried seeds, after frying, are eaten[MP076]. Dried stem bark of *Moringa pterygosperma*, together with *Cuminum cyminum, Trigonella foenumgraecum* and *Murraya koenigii*, is taken orally for backache[MP059]. Flowers are taken orally as a stimulant and aphrodisiac. Hot water extract is taken orally as a tonic and cholagogue[MP099]. Fresh flowers are used as a vegetable[MP076]. Fresh seedpods are used as a vegetable[MP076]. Gum is administered intravaginally to produce abortion[MP098]. Hot water extract of dried flower is taken orally in Ayurvedic and Unani medicine as an aphrodisiac and stimulant[MP079]. Hot water extract of dried fruit and leaves is taken orally for dysentery and diarrhea[MP087]. Hot water extract of dried root and stem bark is taken orally as an abortifacient and emmenagogue[MP093]. Hot water extract of dried root bark is taken orally for fertility control[MP075]. Hot water extract of stem bark is taken orally in Ayurvedic medicine as an abortive, antipyretic and a tonic[MP016]. In Ayurvedic and Unani medicine, hot water extracts of the dried bark and dried root are taken orally by pregnant women as abortifacients[MP079]. Juice of fresh bark is taken orally to relieve acute stomachaches. Juices of *Erythrina variegata* and *Moringa oleifera* barks are mixed. Also, for stomachache, juice of bark is mixed with *Ferula asafoetida* and salt, and taken orally. Externally, the juice is used as a treatment for mange in horses[MP112]. Leaf juice, mixed with honey, is used as an eye ointment for conjunctivitis[MP052]. Leaves are taken orally as an aphrodiasic[MP030] and to treat wounds. For wound treatment, the leaves are pounded with turmeric and buttermilk and then applied[MP048]. Powdered dried root and stem is used externally for rheumatism pains.

For asthma and cough, 50 mg of the powder dissolved in water is taken orally. Stem bark is taken orally to produce permanent sterility. Five gram of stem bark from an old tree together with 2 seeds of *Piper nigrum*, 1 gram of *Cuminum cyminum* seeds and a few pieces of *Allium sativum* are ground into a paste, the paste is swallowed after the third day of delivery and a bland diet is followed. This is repeated 3 times. After 2 to 3 months, the woman should not participate in coitus[MP096]. Fresh stem bark is used to produce abortion. The gum from the stem bark is rubbed with milk, made into a paste, and applied to the vagina and up into the cervix. The gum is very tough, swells rapidly when moistened, and produces abortion by dilating the cervix[MP096].

Indonesia. Hot water extract of the plant is taken orally to provoke the menses, and as an abortive[MP008,MP029].

Malaysia. Hot water extract of the bark is taken orally to stimulate the menses[MP035]. Hot water extract of the root is taken orally for amenorrhea[MP028]. It may also produce abortion[MP035].

Mauritius. Hot water extract of the bark is taken orally as a purgative, vermifuge and antispasmodic[MP107].

Nepal. Hot water extract of flowers is taken orally as an aphrodisiac. Hot water extract of the dried bark is taken orally by pregnant women as an abortifacient. Hot water extract of the root is taken orally as a stimulant, for intermittent fever and epilepsy and as an abortifacient[MP001].

New Caledonia. Gum is taken orally as an abortifacient[MP026]. Leaves are rubbed over the breast to reduce milk flow[MP114].

Nigeria. Hot water extract of fresh root is taken orally as an analgesic, hypotensive and sedative[MP082]. Hot water extract of the dried root and stem is taken orally to treat arthritis[MP077].

Philippines. Decoction of dried leaves is taken orally as a galactagogue. A decoction of *Solanum nigrum, Moringa pterygosperma* and beach pebbles is used[MP088]. Extract of leaves is used as a galactagogue[MP002].

Saudi Arabia. Hot water extract of the dried fruit is taken orally for diabetes, ascites, edema, spleen enlargement, inflammatory swellings, abdominal tumors, colic, dyspepsia, fever, ulcers, paralysis, lumbago and skin diseases[MP058,MP089].

Senegal. Extract of the entire dried plant is used for sprains in adult, headache and neuralgia in children and adults, rheumatism and arthritis in adults, rickets in children and adults, bronchitis in children and adults and as an antipyretic in children and adults. Dried exudate is used as an astringent for various medicinal purposes. Juice of fresh inflorescence is placed in the eyes for eye problems[MP114].

Thailand. Hot water extract of dried root is taken orally as a cardiotonic, stimulant for fainting[MP066], and antipyretic[MP115].

Togo. Decoction of dried leaves and twigs is taken orally for malaria[MP060].

USA. Fresh leaves are taken orally as a diuretic[MP031].

West Indies. Flowers are boiled and the decoction taken orally as a cough remedy[MP055]. Hot water extract of root bark is used as a diuretic, stimulant, menstrual promoter and abortive[MP109]. Seeds are taken orally as a purgative[MP067]. Warmed leaves are used as a dressing for syphilitic ulcers[MP067].

CHEMICAL CONSTITUENTS

(ppm unless otherwise indicated)

3-Methoxy quercetin: Lf[MP062]
3-O-(6-O-oleoyl-beta-D-glucopyranosyl)-beta-sitosterol: Sd[MP122]
4- Hydroxy phenylacetonitrile: Sd[MP063]
4-(Alpha-L-rhamnosyloxy)-benzyl isothiocyanate): Sd[MP122]
4-Hydroxy phenylacetamide: Sd[MP063]
4-Hydroxy phenylacetic acid: Sd[MP063]
Alanine: Sd[MP003]
Alpha-tocopherol: Lf 9.0%[MP116]
Amylase: Lf[MP068]
Arachidic acid: Sd oil[MP022]

Arginine: Sd[MP003]
Ascorbic acid oxidase: Fr[MP006]
Ascorbic acid: Fr Ju[MP004], Lf[MP076]
Athomin: Rt Bk[MP101]
Baurenol: Bk[MP010]
Behenic acid: Sd oil[MP076]
Benzyl glucosinolate: Sd[MP046]
Beta carotene: Lf[MP117], Fr[MP102]
Beta sitosterol: Sd oil[MP121], St Bk[MP016]
Beta-sitosterol-3-O-beta-D-glucopyranoside: Sd[MP122]
Calcium: Fl[MP099], Fr 0.4%[MP038]
Campesterol: Sd oil[MP121]
Choline: Lf 0.42%[MP076], Fr 0.42%[MP076]
Delta-tocopherol: Sd oil 7.76%[MP121]
Essential oil: Bk 50[MP011]
Gamma-tocopherol: Sd oil 1.5%[MP121]
Glycerol-1-(9-octadecanoate): Sd[MP122]
Gossypitin: Lf[MP062]
Gum: Fl[MP080]
Histidine: Sd[MP003]
Hydroxy proline: Sd[MP003]
Iso-butyl thiocynate: Pl[MP110]
Iso-thiocynate: Pl[MP110]
Kaempferol: Fl[MP014,MP039]
Lauric acid: Sd oil[MP023]
Leucine: Sd[MP003]
Lignoceric acid: Sd oil[MP023,MP022]
Linoleic acid: Sd oil[MP054,MP022]
Moringine: Bk[MP012,MP011], Rt Bk[MP030]
Moringinine: Bk[MP011], Rt Bk[MP030]
Moringyne: Sd[MP040]
Myristic acid: Sd oil[MP022]
Niazicin B: Lf 1.06[MP044]
Niazimicin: Lf 18.2–2.5[MP042,MP043]
Niaziminin A: Lf 2.8–10.3[MP043,MP042]
Niaziminin B: Lf 0.7[MP043]
Niazinin A: Lf 2.3–13.7[MP043,MP042]
Niazinin B: Lf 2.6–14.5[MP043,MP042]
Niazirin: Lf 4.5[MP043]
Niazirinin: Lf 2.7[MP043]
Nicotinic acid: Fr 2[MP076], Lf 8[MP076]
O-ethyl-4-(alpha-L-rhamnosyloxy)benzyl carbamate: Sd[MP122]
Oleic acid: Sd oil 67.48%[MP054]
Oxalic acid: Fr 0.042–0.101%[MP038,MP076], Lf 0.101%[MP076]
Palmitic acid: Sd oil 3.4–9.3%[MP054,MP076]
Pentadecanoic acid: Sd oil[MP023]
Phosphorus: Fr 0.45%[MP038]
Potassium: Fl[MP099]
Proline: Sd[MP003]

Protein: Fr 2.5–19.5%[MP076,MP038,MP005],
  Sd 46.5%[MP103], Lf 6.7–29%[MP076,MP105]
Pterygospermin: Rt[MP007,MP037], St Bk[MP009],
  Sd[MP013], Bk[MP100]
Quercetagetin: Lf[MP062]
Quercetin: Fl[MP039]
Quercetin-3-glycoside: Fl[MP014]
Rhamnetin: Fl[MP014]
Rhamnetin-3-glycoside: Fl[MP014]
Rutin: Lf 2.6%[MP084]
Serine: Sd[MP003]
Spirochin: Rt[MP104]
Spirochine: Rt[MP009]
Starch: Lf[MP068]
Stearic acid:
  Sd oil 7.4–10.5%[MP076,MP054,MP022]
Stigmasterol: Sd oil[MP121]
Sulfur: Rt[MP037]
Threonine: Sd[MP003]
Valine: Sd[MP003]
Vitamin A: Lf 113 IU/gm[MP076],
  Fr 1.8 IU/gm[MP076]
Vitamin B-1: Lf 0.6[MP076], Fr 0.5[MP076]
Vitamin B-2: Lf 0.5[MP076], Fr 0.7[MP076]
Zeatin Ribose: Fr[MP078]
Zeatin: Fr[MP078]

PHARMACOLOGICAL ACTIVITIES AND CLINICAL TRIALS

Abortifacient activity. Ethanol/water (1:1) extract of root, administered orally to rats at a dose of 200.0 mg/kg, was inactive[MP108]. Ethanol/water (50%) extract of leaves and twigs, administered by gastric intubation to pregnant rats at a dose of 100.0 mg/kg, was inactive[MP097]. Ethanol/water (1:1) extract of dried aerial parts, administered orally to pregnant rats, was inactive[MP073]. Ethanol/water (1:1) extract of the entire plant, administered by gastric intubation to pregnant rats at a dose of 100.0 mg/kg, was inactive[MP097].

Adrenolytic activity. Ethanol (95%) and water extracts of leaves, administered intravenously to dogs, were inactive[MP024].

Analgesic activity. Ethanol/water (1:1) extract of dried leaves and dried stem, administered intraperitoneally to mice at a dose of 500.0 mg/kg, was inactive vs tail pressure method[MP020]. Ethanol/water (1:1) extract of flowers, administered by gastric intubation to mice, was inactive vs hot plate and tail clip methods[MP097].

Anthelmintic activity. Dried bark powder, fresh leaf juice, dried root powder and dried leaf powder, at a concentration of 1.0 ml, were active on *Ascaris lumbricoides*[MP064]. Dried plant, taken orally by human adults of both sexes, was active, IC_{100} 2.0 gm. Equal parts of a mixture containing *Butea frondosa*, *Moringa pterygosperma*, *Piper nigrum*, *Azadirachta indica*, and *Embelia ribes* was used. Dosing was 3 times daily for 4–8 weeks. Eleven cases of Ascariasis, 9 cases of ancylostomiasis and 9 cases of *Hymenolepsis nana* were treated. Stool specimens were found negative at end of treatment period[MP071]. Powdered dried seeds, at a concentration of 1.0 ml, were inactive on *Ascaris lumbricoids*[MP064].

Antibacterial activity. Powdered dried bark, at a concentration of 100.0 microliters on agar plate, was inactive on *Escherichia coli*, *Pseudomonas aeruginosa*, *Shigella flexneri*, *Staphylococcus aureus*, and *Streptococcus pyogenes*[MP064]. Ethanol (95%) extract of dried flowers, undiluted on agar plate, was active on *Escherichia coli* and *Staphylococcus aureus*[MP113]. Powdered dried root, at a concentration of 100.0 microliters on agar plate, was inactive on *Escherichia coli*, *Pseudomonas aeruginosa*, *Shigella flexneri*, *Staphylococcus aureus* and *Streptococcus pyogenes*[MP064]. Ethanol (95%) extract of dried fruit, undiluted on agar plate, was active on *Escherichia coli* and *Staphylococcus aureus*[MP113]. Saline extract of leaves, at a concentration of 1:20 on agar plate, was active on *Staphylococcus aureus* and inactive on *Pasteurella pestis*[MP106]. Powdered dried leaves, at a concentration of 100.0 microliters on agar plate, were inactive on *Shigella flexneri*, *Staphylococcus aureus*, *Streptococcus pyogenes*, *Escherichia coli*, and *Pseudomonas aeruginosa*[MP064]. Ethanol (95%) extract of dried leaves, undiluted on agar plate, was active on *Escherichia coli* and *Staphylococcus aureus*[MP113]. Fresh leaf juice, at a concentration of 100.0 microliters on agar plate, was active on *Pseudomonas aeruginosa* and inactive on *Escherichia coli*, *Shigella flexneri*, *Staphylococcus aureus*, and *Streptococcus pyogenes*[MP064]. Ethanol (95%) extract of dried root, undiluted on agar plate, was active on *Escherichia coli* and *Staphylococcus aureus*[MP113]. Water and hexane extracts of dried seeds, applied externally to mice at a dose of 10.0%, were active on *Staphylococcus aureus*[MP065]. Powdered dried seeds, at a concentration of 100.0 microliters on agar plate, were active on *Staphylococcus aureus*[MP064], and inactive on *Escherichia coli*, *Pseudomonas aeruginosa*, *Shigella flexneri*, and *Streptococcus pyogenes*[MP064]. Water extract of dried seeds, at a concentration of 1:10 on agar plate, was active on *Bacillus cereus*, *Bacillus megaterium*, *Bacillus subtilis*, *Sarcina lutea*, and *Staphylococcus aureus*. The extract was equivocal on *Escherichia coli*, *Salmonella edinburgi* and *Serratia marcesens*; inactive on *Klebsiella aerogenes* and produced weak activity on *Proteus mirabilis* and *Streptococcus faecalis*[MP074].

Anticonvulsant activity. Ethanol/water (1:1) extracts of dried leaves and dried stem, administered intraperitoneally to mice at a dose of 500.0 mg/kg, were inactive vs electroshock-induced convulsions[MP020]. Ethanol (70%) extract of the fresh root, administered intraperitoneally to mice of both sexes at variable dosage levels, was active vs metrazole and strychnine-induced convulsions[MP082].

Antifertility effect. Ethanol (95%), water and petroleum ether extracts of bark, administered to female mice, were inactive[MP018].

Antifungal activity. Powdered dried bark, powdered dried root, powdered dried seeds, fresh leaves and powdered dried leaves, at a concentration of 1.0 ml on agar plate, were inactive on *Epidermophyton floccosum*, *Microsporum canis*, *Microsporum gypseum*, *Trichophyton mentagrophytes*, and *Trichophyton rubrum*[MP064] (plant pathogens). Water extract of dried seeds, at a concentration of 1:10 on agar plate, was active on *Botrytis allii*,

Coniophora cerebella, *Penicillium expansum*, *Phytophthora cactorum*, and *Polyporus versicolor*. The extract was equivocal on *Fusarium oxysporum* F. sp. Lycopersici, and inactive on *Aspergillus oryza*[MP074].

Antihemolytic activity. The dried entire plant, at a concentration of 0.2 ml, was active on red blood cells[MP095].

Antihepatotoxic activity. Ethanol (95%) extract of dried leaves, administered by gastric intubation to mice at a dose of 300.0 mg/kg, was inactive vs CCl_4-induced hepatotoxicity[MP086].

Antihistamine activity. Ethanol/water (1:1) extract of dried root, at a concentration of 0.001 gm/ml, was active on guinea pig ileum[MP115].

Anti-implantation effect. Ethanol (95%), water and petroleum ether extracts of bark, administered orally to female rats, were inactive[MP018]. Ethanol/water (1:1) extract of dried aerial parts, administered orally to hamsters, was active, and inactive when administered to rats[MP073]. Ethanol/water (50%) extract of entire plant, administered by gastric intubation to pregnant hamsters at a dose of 100.0 mg/ kg, was inactive[MP097]. Water extract of dried leaves, administered by intravenous infusion to rats at a dose of 750.0 mg/kg, was active vs carrageenin-induced pedal edema[MP045].

Anti-inflammatory activity. Hot water extract of bark, administered orally to rats, was inactive vs formalin-induced pedal edema[MP027]. Water extracts of dried flowers and dried stem, administered by intravenous infusion to rats at a dose of 1.0 gm/kg, were inactive vs carrageenin-induced pedal edema. Water extract of dried root and dried seeds, administered by intravenous infusion to rats at a dose of 750.0 mg/kg, was active vs carrageenin-induced pedal edema[MP045].

Antimalarial activity. Ethanol (95%) extract of dried leaves and twigs produced weak activity on *Plasmodium falciparum*, IC_{50} 60.0 mcg/ml[MP060]. Water extract of the bark, administered orally to chicken at a dose of 1.82 gm/kg, was inactive on *Plasmodium gallinaceum*[MP015].

Antimycobacterial activity. An extract of the entire plant, on agar plate, was active on *Mycobacterium tuberculosis*[MP032]. Water extract of dried seeds, at a concentration of 1:10 on agar plate, was active on *Mycobacterium phlei*[MP074].

Antispasmodic activity (unspecified type). Water extract of dried flowers, at a concentration of 1.0 gm, was inactive on rat duodenum vs ACh-induced contractions[MP045]. Ethanol/water (1:1) extract of fruits was active on guinea pig ileum vs ACh- and histamine-induced spasms[MP021]. Ethanol (95%) and water extracts of leaves were active on guinea pig ileum vs ACh- and histamine-induced spasms. Water extract of dried leaves, at a concentration of 1000 mg, was inactive on rat duodenum vs ACh-induced contractions[MP045]. Ethanol/water (1:1) extract of dried leaves and dried stem were inactive on guinea pig ileum vs ACh- and histamine-induced spasms[MP020]. Water extract of dried root and dried stem, at a concentration of 1.0 gm, were inactive on rat duodenum vs ACh-induced contrac-tions[MP045]. Ethanol/water (1:1) extract of dried root, at a concentration of 0.001 gm/ml, was active on guinea pig ileum[MP115]. Ethanol/water (1:1) extract of rootbark was active on guinea pig ileum vs ACh- and histamine-induced spasms[MP020]. Ethanol/water (1:1) extract of rootwood was active on guinea pig ileum vs ACh- and histamine-induced spasms[MP020]. Water extract of dried seeds, at a concentration of 1 gm, was active on rat duodenum. Contractions were inhibited 32.6% vs ACh-induced contractions[MP045].

Antitumor activity. Ethanol/water (1:1) extract of dried aerial parts, administered intraperitoneally to mice, was active on LEUK-P388[MP073]. Ethanol/water (1:1) extract of dried leaves, administered intrap-

eritoneally to mice, was inactive on LEUK-P388 and LEUK-L1210[MP020]. Ethanol (95%) extract of dried leaves, administered intraperitoneally to mice at a dose of 100.0 mg/kg, was inactive on Sarcoma 180(ASC)[MP061]. The seeds, tested for antitumor promoting activity using an in vitro assay which tested their inhibitory effects on Epstein-Barr virus antigen (EBV-EA) activation in Raji cells induced by the tumor promoter, 12-O-tetradecanoyl-phorbol-13-acetate (TPA), produced inhibitory activity against EBV-EA activation. Compounds 4(alpha-L-rhamno-syloxy)-benzyl isothiocyanate, niazimicin, and beta-sitosterol-3-O-beta-D-glucopyra-noside showed significant activities. Niazimicin was further subjected to in vivo tests and found to have potent antitumor promoting activity in the two-stage carcinogenesis in mouse skin using 7,12-dimethylbenz(a)anthracene as a initiator and TPA as a tumor promoter[MP122].

Antiulcer activity. Methanol extract of dried flower buds, administered by gastric intubation to rats at a dose of 4.0 gm/kg, was active[MP050]. Methanol extract of dried leaves, administered by gastric intubation to mice at a dose of 2.0 gm/kg, was inactive vs stress-induced ulcers (water-immersion)[MP056].

Antiviral activity. Ethanol/water (50%) extract of flowers, at a concentration of 0.05 mg/ml in cell culture, was inactive on Vaccinia virus[MP097]. Ethanol/water (50%) extract of leaves and twigs, at a concentration of 0.05 mg/ml in cell culture, was inactive on Vaccinia virus[MP097]. Ethanol/water (1:1) extract of rootbark, at a concentration of 50.0 mcg/ml in cell culture, produced weak activity on Vaccinia virus[MP021].

Antiyeast activity. Powdered dried leaves, powdered dried root, powdered dried bark and powdered dried seeds, at a concentration of 100.0 microliters on agar plate, were inactive on *Candida albicans*[MP064]. Fresh leaf juice, at a concentration of 100.0 microliters on agar plate, was inactive on

Candida albicans[MP064]. Water extract of dried seeds, at a concentration of 1:10 on agar plate, was active on *Candida pseudotropicalis*, *Candida reukaufii* and *Pyricularia oryza*, and equivocal on *Saccharomyces carlsbergenesis*[MP074].

Barbiturate sleeping time decrease. Ethanol (95%) extract of dried leaves, administered by gastric intubation to mice at a dose of 300.0 mg/kg, was inactive vs CCl_4-induced hepatotoxicity[MP086].

Carcinogenesis inhibition. Water extract of dried leaves, in the ration of mice at a dose of 600.0 mg/per gm diet, was active vs benzo(A)pyrene-induced carcinogenesis and 3-methyl-4-dimethylaminoazobenzene-induced carcinogenesis[MP047].

CNS depressant activity. Water and ethanol (95%) extracts of leaves, administered intraperitoneally to dogs and mice were active[MP024]. Ethanol (70%) extract of fresh root, administered intraperitoneally to mice of both sexes at variable dosage levels, produced strong activity[MP082].

Cytotoxic activity. Ethanol/water (1:1) extract of dried leaves, in cell culture, was inactive on CA-9KB, $ED_{50} > 20.0$ mcg/ml[MP020]. Ethanol/water (1:1) extract of fruits was inactive on CA-9KB in cell culture, $ED_{50} > 20$ mcg/ml[MP021]. Ethanol/water (1:1) extract of the aerial parts, in cell culture, was active on CA-9KB, $ED_{50} < 20.0$ mcg/ml[MP073]. Ethanol/water (1:1) extract of root bark, in cell culture, was inactive on CA-9KB, $ED_{50} > 20.0$ mcg/ml. Ethanol/water (1:1) extract of rootwood, in cell culture, was inactive on CA-9KB, $ED_{50} > 20.0$ mcg/ml[MP021].

Diuretic activity. Ethanol/water (1:1) extracts of dried leaves and dried stem, administered intraperitoneally to saline loaded male rats at doses of 250.0 mg/kg, were inactive. Urine was collected for 4 hours post-drug[MP020]. Water extracts of dried leaves, dried stem, dried root and dried seeds, administered to rats by intravenous infusion at doses of 25.0 mg/kg, were active[MP045].

Embryotoxic effect. Ethanol (70%) extract of bark administered orally to female rats at dosages of 200, 400 and 800 mg/kg, were inactive[MP069]. Ethanol/water (1:1) extract of root, administered orally to rats at a dose of 200.0 mg/kg, was ina-tive[MP108]. Water extract of shade-dried bark, administered orally to rats on days 1–7 at a dose of 400 mg/kg, was active[MP092]. Water extract of dried leaves, administered intragastrically to pregnant rats at a dose of 175.0 mg/kg, was active[MP049]. Water extract of shade-dried root, administered orally to rats on days 1–7 at a dose of 200.0 mg/kg, was active[MP092].

Estrogenic effect. Leaves, in the ration of mice, were inactive[MP034].

Hepatorenal activity. Methanol extract root, administered intraperitoneally at dose of 3.5, 4.6, and 7.0 mg/kg daily and 35, 46, and 70 mg/kg weekly, produced no alteration in hematological and biochemical parameters at love and moderate dose levels. However, the moderate dose levels in weekly treatment changed serum aminotransferase and plasma cholesterol levels significantly. High dose, in addition to the above parameters, changed total bilirubin, non-protein nitrogen, and blood urea and plasma protein. The high dose, at daily treatment, moderate, and high dose of the weekly treatment, increased WBC count and decreased clotting time significantly[MP120].

Hyperglycemic activity. Hot water extract of dried fruits, administered by gastric intubation to rats at a dose of 0.5 ml/animal, produced a maximal change in blood sugar of 15.3% (increase) vs alloxan-induced hyperglycemia[MP058]. Ethanol/water (1:1) extract of dried leaves, administered orally to rats at a dose of 250.0 mg/kg, produced more than 30% drop in blood sugar level[MP020]. Ethanol/water (1:1) extract of the entire plant, administered by gastric intubation to rats at a dose of 250.0 mg/kg, was active[MP097].

Hypocholesterolemic effect. Crude extract of the leaves with a high-fat diet decreased the high-fat-diet-induced increases in serum, liver, and kidney cholesterol levels by 14.35% (115–103.2 mg/100 ml of serum), 6.40% (9.4–8.8 mg/gm wet weight) and 11.09% (1.09–0.97 mg/gm wet weight), respectively. The effect on the serum cholesterol was statistically significant and there was no significant effect on serum total protein, However, the crude extract increased serum albumin by 15.22% (46–53 gm/l)[MP119].

Hypoglycemic activity. Ethanol/water (1:1) extract of flowers, administered by gastric intubation to rats at a dose of 250.0 mg/kg, was active[MP097].

Hypoproteinemia activity. Ethanol (95%) extract of fresh leaves, administered intravenously to rats at a dose of 10.0 mg/kg, was active[MP043].

Hypotensive activity. Ethanol (95%) and water extracts of leaves, administered intravenously to dogs, were active[MP024]. Ethanol/water (1:1) extracts of dried leaves and dried stem, administered intravenously to dogs at doses of 50.0 mg/kg, were inactive[MP020]. Ethanol/water (1:1) extract of dried root, administered intravenously to dogs at variable dosage levels, produced weak activity[MP115]. Rootbark, administered intravenously to cats at a dose of 0.01 mg/animal, was active. Duration of activity was 20–30 minutes[MP021]. Water extract of dried stem bark, at a dose of 20.0 mg/kg, administered intravenously to dogs, was active[MP051].

Hypothermic activity. Methanol extract dried leaves, administered intragastrically to mice at a dose of 2.0 gm/kg, was inactive[MP056]. Ethanol/water (1:1) extract of dried stem, administered intraperitoneally to mice at a dose of 500.0 mg/kg, was inactive[MP020].

Immunostimulant activity. Powdered root, administered intravenously to female mice at a dose of 100.0 mg/kg, was inactive vs rate of clearance of colloidal carbon[MP072].

Inotropic effect. Water extract of dried stem bark, at concentrations of 1.0 mcg/ml

and 10 ng/ml, produced negative and positive effects, respectively, on frog hearts. The reported biological activity is highly dose-dependent[MP051].

Interferon induction stimulation. Ethanol/water (1:1) extract of dried aerial parts, at a concentration of 0.012 mg/ml in cell culture, was active on Ranikhet virus, and inactive on Vaccinia virus[MP083].

Mutagenic activity. Chloroform extract of roasted seeds, administered intraperitoneally to mice at a dose of 0.15 mg/gm, was inactive. Ethyl acetate extract, administered intraperitoneally to mice at a dose of 0.33 mg/kg, was active. The effects were determined by the micronucleus test[MP041].

Myocardial depressant activity. Water and 95% ethanol extracts of leaves were active on the rabbit heart[MP024].

Polygalacturonase inhibition. Hot water extract of bark was active[MP036].

Protopectinase inhibition. Hot water extract of bark was active[MP036].

Semen coagulation effect. Ethanol/water (1:1) extract of the dried aerial parts was inactive on rat semen[MP073].

Skeletal muscle relaxant activity. Ethanol (95%) and water extracts of the plant were active on the rectus abdominus muscle of frogs[MP024]. Water extract of dried stem bark, at a concentration of 10.0 mg/ml, was inactive on the rectus abdominus muscle of frogs[MP051].

Smooth muscle relaxant activity. Water extract of dried stem bark, at a concentration of 10.0 mg/ml, was inactive on guinea pig ileum and rat stomach[MP051].

Spermicidal effect. Ethanol/water (1:1) extract of the dried aerial parts was inactive on the rat sperm[MP073].

Toxic effect. Leaves, in the ration of rats on a 60-day feeding, produced no toxicity[MP111]. Ethanol/water (1:1) extract of dried root, administered to mice by gastric intubation and subcutaneously at a dose of 10.0 gm/kg (dose expressed as dry weight of plant), was inactive[MP066].

Toxicity assessment (Quantitative). Ethanol/water (1:1) extract of dried aerial parts, administered intraperitoneally to mice of both sexes, produced LD_{50} 8.0 mg/kg[MP073]. Ethanol/water (1:1) extract of flowers, administered to mice intraperitoneally, produced $LD_{50} > 1000$ mg/kg[MP097]. Dried leaves, fed to mice, produced LD_{50} 1850 mg/kg[MP086]. Ethanol/water (1:1) extract of the leaves, administered intraperitoneally to mice, produced a maximum tolerated dose of 1.0 gm/kg[MP021]. Ethanol/water (1:1) extract of leaves and roasted seeds, administered intraperitoneally to mice, both produced $LD_{50} > 1.0$ gm/kg[MP020].

Thyroid hormone effect. Leaf extract, administered orally to adult Swiss rats at a dose of 175 mg/kg daily for 10 days, increased serum triiodothyronine concentration and hepatic lipid peroxidation decreased with a concomitant increase in the serum thyroxine concentration, in female rats, while in males no significant changes were observed. At a dose of 350 mg/kg daily for the same duration, almost similar reduction in the serum triiodothyronine concentration increased by approximately 30% and an increase in thyroxine concentration was also observed. The result suggested the inhibiting nature of the extract in the peripheral conversion of thyroxine to triiodothyronine, the principal source of the generation of the latter hormone[MP118].

Uterine stimulant effect. Ethanol/water (1:1) extract of dried aerial parts was active on the nonpregnant rat uterus[MP073]. Water extract of bark was inactive on the nonpregnant rat uterus[MP019]. Water and ethanol (95%) extracts of leaves were inactive on the rat uterus[MP024]. Water extract, at a concentration of 225.0 gm/liter, was active on guinea pig uterus[MP025].

Wound healing acceleration. Hexane extract of dried seeds, applied externally on mice at a dose of 10.0%, was active on *Sta-phylococcus aureus* vs pyoderma induced by *Staphylococcus aureus*[MP055].

REFERENCES

MP001   Suwal, P. N. Medicinal Plants of Nepal. Ministry of Forests, Department of Medicinal Plants, Thapathali, Kathmandu, Nepal, 1970.

MP002   Quisumbing, E. Medicinal plants of the Philippines. **Tech Bull 16**, Rep Philippines, Dept Agr Nat Resources, Manilla 1951; 1.

MP003   Tandon, S. P., K. P. Tiwari and A. P. Gupta. Amino acid content of the seed of *Moringa concanensis*. **Proc Nat Acad Sci India Sert A** 1967; 37: 121–123.

MP004   Srinivasan, M. Ascorbic acid from drumstick *Moringa pterygosperma*. **Curr Sci** 1935; 4: 407.

MP005   Rau, Y. V. S. and V. Ranganathan. Protein of Indian vegetables drumstick (*Moringa pterygosperma* or guilandina or hyperanthera). **J Indian Inst Sci Ser A** 1937; 20(7): 49.

MP006   Spruyt, J. P. (Non) specific properties of type vitamin C oxidases of the juices of the kelor pea *Moringa oleifera*. **Z Vitaminforsch** 1940; 10: 185.

MP007   Raghunandana Rao, R. and G. Mariam. Investigations on plant antibiotics. III. Studies on pterygospermin, the antibacterial principle of the roots of *Moringa pterygosperma*. **Indian J Med Res** 1949; 37: 159.

MP008   Couvee. Compilation of herbs, plants, crops supposed to be effective in various complaints and illnesses. **J Sci Res** 1952; 1s: 1.

MP009   Kerharo, J. Nebreda (*Moringa oleifera*), a popular Senegalese remedy. Therapeutic use in African chemistry and pharmacology. **Plant Med Phytother** 1969; 3: 214.

MP010   Anjaneyulu, B., V. B. Rao, A. K. Ganguly, T. R. Govindachari, B. S. Joshi, V. N. Kamat, A. H. Manmade, P. A. Mohamed, A. D. Rahimtula, A. K. Saksena, D. S. Varde and N. Viswanathan. Chemical investigation of some Indian plants. **Indian J Chem** 1965; 3: 237.

MP011   Ghosh, S., R. N. Chopra and A. Dutta. Chemical examination of the bark of

Moringa pterygosperma. **Indian J Med Res**. 1935; 22: 785.

MP012 Chakravarti, R. N. Chemical identity of moringine. **Bull Calcutta Sch Trop Med** 1955; 3: 162.

MP013 Badgett, B. L. The mustard oil glucoside from *Moringa oleifera* seed ascorbic acid analogs with deoxy side chains. **Diss Abstr** 1964; 25: 1556.

MP014 Nair, A. G. R. and S. Sankara Subramanian. Pigments of the flowers of *Moringa pterygosperma*. **Curr Sci** 1962; 31: 155.

MP015 Spencer, C. F., F. R. Koniuszy, E. F. Rogers et al. Survey of plants for antimalarial activity. **Lloydia** 1947; 10: 145–174.

MP016 Kinel, F. A. and J. Gedeon. Products from *Moringa pterygosperma*. **Arch Pharm(Weinheim)** 1957; 290: 302.

MP017 Haddock, R. L. Some medicinal plants of Guam including English and Guamanian common names. Report Regional Tech Mtg Med Plants, Papeete, Tahiti, Nov, 1973, South Pacific Commissioner, Noumea, New Caledonia 1974; 79pp.

MP018 Bhaduri, B., C. R. Ghose, A. N. Bose, B. K. Moza and U. P. Basu. Antifertility activity of some medicinal plants. **Indian J Exp Biol**. 1968; 6: 252–253.

MP019 Dhawan, B. N. and P. N. Saxena. Evaluation of some indigenous drugs for stimulant effect on the rat uterus. A preliminary report. **Indian J Med Res** 1958; 46(6): 808–811.

MP020 Dhar, M. L., M. M. Dhar, B. N. Dhawan, B. N. Mehrotra, R. C. Srimal and J. S. Tandon. Screening of Indian plants for biological activity. Part IV. **Indian J Exp Biol** 1973; 11: 43–54.

MP021 Dhar, M. L., M. M. Dhar, B. N. Dhawan, B. N. Mehrotra and C. Ray. Screening of Indian plants for biological activity: Part I. **Indian J Exp Biol** 1968; 6: 232–247.

MP022 Sengupta, A. and M. P. Gupta. Seed fat composition of *Moringaceae* family. **Fette Seifen Anstrichm** 1970; 72: 6.

MP023 Ferrao, A. M. B. C. and J. E. M. Ferrao. Fatty acids in oil of moringue (*Moringa oleifera*). **Agron Angolana** 1970; 30: 3.

MP024 Siddiqu, S. and M. I. Khan. Pharmacological study of *Moringa pterygosperma*. **Pak J Sci Ind Res** 1968; 11: 268–272.

MP025 Saha, J. C., E. C. Savini and S. Kasinathan. Ecbolic properties of Indian medicinal plants. Part I. **Indian J Med Res** 1961; 49: 130–151.

MP026 Rageau, J. Les Plantes Medicinales de la Nouvelle-Cal Edonie. Trav & Doc De Lorstom No. 23. Paris, 1973.

MP027 Chaturvedi, G. N. and R. H. Singh. Experimental studies on the antiarthritic effect of certain indigenous drugs. **Indian J Med Res** 1965; 53: 71.

MP028 Gimlette, J. D. A Dictionary of Malayan Medicine, Oxford Univ. Press., New York, USA, 1939.

MP029 Petelot, A. Les Plantes Medicinales du Cambodge, du Laos et du Vietnam, Volume 1–4. Archives des Recherches Agronomiques et Pastorales au Vietnam No. 23, 1954.

MP030 Chorpa, R. N., P. De and N. N. De. *Moringa pterygosperma*. **Indian J Med Res** 1932; 20: 533.

MP031 Morton, J. F. Ornamental plants with toxic and/or irritant properties. II. **Proc Fla State Hort Soc** 1962; 75: 484.

MP032 Schramm, G. Plant and animal drugs of the old Chinese Materia Medica in the therapy of pulmonary tuberculosis. **Planta Med** 1956; 4(4): 97–104.

MP033 Watt, J. M. and M. G. Breyer-Brandwijk. The Medicinal and Poisonous Plants of Southern and Eastern Africa. 2nd Ed. E. S. Livingstone, Ltd., London 1962.

MP034 Agliout, F. B. and L. S. Castillo. Estrogen content of legumes in the Philippines. **Philippine Agr** 1963; 46: 673.

MP035 Burkhill, I. H. Dictionary of the Economic Products of the Malay Peninsula. Ministry of Agriculture and Cooperatives, Kuala Lumpur, Malaysia. Volume II, 1966.

MP036 Prasad, V. and S. C. Gupta. Inhibitory effect of bark and leaf decoctions on the activity of pectic enzymes of *Alternaria tennis*. **Indian J Exp Biol** 1967; 5: 192.

MP037 Kurup, P. A. and P. L. Narasima Rao. Antibiotic principle from *Moringa pterygosperma*. I. Purification. **J Indian Inst Sci** 1952; 34: 219.

MP038   Basu, K. P. and D. Ghosh. Availability of CA in lady's finger (*Hibiscus esculentus*), cabbage (*Brassica oleracea capitata*), drumstick (*Moringa oleifera*) and amaranth tender (*Amaranthus gangeticus*). I. Experiments. **Indian J Med Res** 1943; 31: 29.

MP039   Pankadamani, K. S. and T. R. Seshadri. Survey of anthoxanthins. **Proc Indian Acad Sci Ser A** 1952; 36: 157.

MP040   Memon, G. M., S. A. Memon and A. R. Memon. Isolation and structure elucidation of moringyne – A new glycoside from seeds of *Moringa oleifera* Lam. **Pak J Sci Ind Res** 1985; 28(1): 7–9.

MP041   Villasenor, I. M., P. Finch, C. Y. Lim-Sylianco and F. Dayrit. Structure of a mutagen from roasted seeds of *Moringa oleifera*. **Carcinogenesis** 1989; 10(6): 1085–1087.

MP042   Faizi, S., B. S. Siddiqui, R. Saleem, S. Siddiqui, K. Aftab and A. U. H. Gilani. Isolation and structure elucidation of novel hypotensive agents, niazinin A, niazinin B, niazimicin and niaziminin A + B from *Moringa oleifera*: The first naturally occurring thiocar-bamates. **J Chem Soc Perkin Trans I** 1992; 23: 3237–3241.

MP043   Faizi, S., B. S. Siddiqui, Saleemr, S. Siddiqui, K. Aftab and A. H. Gilani. Isolation and structure elucidation of new nitrile and mustard oil glycosides from *Moringa oleifera* and their effect on blood pressure. **J Nat Prod** 1994; 57(9): 1256–1261.

MP044   Faizi, S., B. S. Siddiqui, R. Saleem, S. Siddiqui, K. Aftab and A. U. H. Gilani. Fully acetylated carbamate and hypotensive thiocarbamate glycosides from *Moringa oleifera*. **Phytochemistry** 1995; 38(4): 957–963.

MP045   Caceres, A., A. Saravia, S. Rizzio, L. Zabala, E. DeLeon, and F. Nave. Pharmacologic properties of *Moringa oleifera*. 2. Screening for antispasmodic, antiinflammatory and diuretic activity. **J Ethnopharmacol** 1992; 36(3): 233–237.

MP046   Villasenor, I. M., F. M. Dayrit and C. Y. Lim-Sylianco. Studies on *Moringa oleifera* seeds. II. Thermal degradation of roasted seeds. **Philippine J Sci** 1990; 119(1): 33–39.

MP047   Aruna, K. and V. M. Sivarama-krishnan. Anticarcinogenic effects of some Indian plant products. **Food Chem Toxicol** 1992; 30(11): 953–956.

MP048   Reddy, M. B., K. R. Reddy and M. N. Reddy. A survey of plant crude drugs of Anantapur District, Andhra Pradesh, India. **Int J Crude Drug Res** 1989; 27(3): 145–155.

MP049   Nath, D., N. Sethi, R. K. Singh and A. K. Jain. Commonly used Indian abortifacient plants with special reference to their teratologic effects in rats. **J Ethnopharmacol** 1992; 36(2): 147–154.

MP050   Akhtar, A. H. and K. U. Ahmad. Antiulcerogenic evaluation of the methanolic extracts of some indigenous medicinal plants of Pakistan in aspirin-ulcerated rats. **J Ethnopharma-col** 1995; 46(1): 1–6.

MP051   Limaye, D. A., A. Y. Nimbkay, R. Jain and M. Ahmad. Cardiovascular effects of the aqueous extract of *Moringa pterygosperma*. **Phytother Res** 1995; 9(1): 37–90.

MP052   Girach, R. D., Aminuddin, P. A. Siddioui and S. A. Khan. Traditional plant remedies among the Kondh of District Dhenkanal (Orissa). **Int J Pharmacog** 1994; 32(3): 274–283.

MP053   Awasthi, A. K. Ethnobotanical studies on the Negrito Islanders of Andaman Islands, India - The Great Andamanese. **Econ Bot** 1991; 45(2): 274–280.

MP054   Khan, F. W., P. Gul and M. N. Malik. Chemical composition of oil from *Moringa oleifera*. **Pak J For** 1975; 25: 100.

MP055   Morton, J. F. Medicinal and other plants used by people on North Caicos (Turks and Caicos Islands, West Indies). **J Crude Drug Res** 1977; 15: 1–24.

MP056   Yamazaki, M., Y. Maebayashi, N. Iwase and T. Kaneko. Studies on pharmacologically active principles from Indonesian crude drugs. I. Principle prolonging pentobarbital-induced sleeping time from *Curcuma xanthorrhiza* Roxb. **Chem Pharm Bull** 1988; 36(6): 2070–2074.

MP057   Shah, G. L. and G. V. Gopal. Ethnomedical notes from the tribal inhabitants of the North Gujarat (India). **J Econ Taxon Botany** 1985; 6(1): 193–201.

MP058 Mossa, J. S. A study on the crude antidiabetic drugs used in Arabian folk medicine. **Int J Crude Drug Res** 1985; 23(3): 137–145.

MP059 Reddy, M. B., K. R. Reddy and M. N. Reddy. A survey of medicinal plants of Chenchu Tribes of Andhra Pradesh, India. **Int J Crude Drugs Res** 1988; 26(4): 189–196.

MP060 Greassor, M., A. Y. Kedjagni, K. Koumaglo, C. DeSouza, K. Agbo, K. Aklikokou and K. A. Amegbo. In vitro antimalarial activity of six medicinal plants. **Phytother Res** 1990; 4(3): 115–117.

MP061 Itokawa, H., F. Hirayama, S. Tsuruoka, K. Mizuno, K. Takeya and A. Nitta. Screening test for antitumor activity of crude drugs (III). Studies on antitumor activity of Indonesian medicinal plants. **Shoyakugaku Zasshi** 1990; 44(1): 58–62.

MP062 Daniel, M. Polyphenols of some Indian vegetables. **Curr Sci** 1989; 58(23): 1332–1334.

MP063 Villasenor, I. M., C. Y. Lim-Sylianco and F. Dayrit. Mutagens from roasted seeds of Moringa oleifera. **Mutat Res** 1989; 224(2): 209–212.

MP064 Caceres, A., O. Cabrera, O. Morales, P. Mollinedo and P. Mendia. Pharmacological properties of Moringa oleifera. 1. Preliminary screening for antimicrobial activity. Pyodermia. **J Ethnopharmacol** 1991; 33(3): 213–216.

MP065 Caceres, A. and S. Lopez. Pharmacological properties of Moringa oleifera. 3. Effect of seed extracts in the treatment of experimental Pyodermia. **Fitoterapia** 1991; 62(5): 449–450.

MP066 Mokkhasmit, M., K. Swasdimongkol and P. Satrawaha. Study on toxicity of Thai medicinal plants. **Bull Dept Med Sci** 1971; 12(2/4): 36–65.

MP067 Ayensu, E. S. Medicinal plants of the West Indies. **Unpublished Manuscript** 1978; 110pp.

MP068 Rao., J. V. S., G. R. Rao, C. M. Krishna and G. G. Rao. Diurnal rhythmicity of ascorbic acid, carbohydrate fractions and activity in Moringa pterygosperma leaves. **Comp Physiol Ecol** 1979; 4: 243–245.

MP069 Rao, V. S. N., P. Dasaradhan and K. S. Krishnaiah. Antifertility effect of some indigenous plants. **Indian J Med Res** 1979; 70: 517–520.

MP070 Lal, S. D. and K. Lata. Plants used by the Bhat community for regulating fertility. **Econ Bot** 1980; 34: 273–275.

MP071 Tyagi, R. K., M. K. Tyagi, H. R. Goyal and K. Sharma. A clinical study of Krimi Roga. **J Res Indian Med Yoga Homeopathy** 1978; 13: 130–132.

MP072 Anon. Antifertility agents. **Annu Rept Central Drug Res Inst**, Lucknow India 1978; 1–10pp.

MP073 Dhawan, B. N., M. P. Dubey, B. N. Mehrotra, R. P. Rastogi and J. S. Tandon. Screening of Indian plants for biological activity. Part IX. **Indian J Exp Biol** 1980; 18: 594–606.

MP074 Eilert, U., S. B. Wolter and A. Nahrstedt. The antibiotic principle of seeds of Moringa oleifera and Moringa stenopetala. **Planta Med** 1981; 42: 55–61.

MP075 Commachan, M. and S. S. Khan. Plants in aid of family planning programme. **Sci Life** 1981; 1: 64–66.

MP076 Ramachandran, C., K. V. Peter and P. K. Gopalakrishnan. Drumstick (Moringa oleifera). A multipurpose Indian vegetable. **Econ Bot** 1980; 34: 276–283.

MP077 Iwu, M. M. and B. N. Anyanwu. Phytotherapeutic profile of Nigerian herbs. 1. Antiinflammatory and antiarthritic agents. **J Ethnopharmacol** 1982; 6(3): 263–274.

MP078 Nagar, P. K., R. I. Iyer and P. K. Sircar. Cytokinins in developing fruits of Moringa pterygosperma Gaertn. **Physiol Plant** 1982; 55: 45–50.

MP079 Kapoor, S. L. and L. D. Kapoor. Medicinal plant wealth of the Karimnagar District of Andhra Pradesh. **Bull Med Ethnobot Res** 1980; 1: 120–144.

MP080 Bhattacharya, S. B., A. K. Das and N. Banerji. Chemical investigations on the gum exudate from sajna (Moringa oleifera). **Carbohydr Res** 1982; 102: 253–262.

MP081 Shah, N. C. Herbal folk medicine in Northern India. **J Ethnopharmacol** 1982; 6(3): 293–301.

MP082 Adesina, S. K. Studies on some plants used as anticonvulsants in Amerindian and African traditional medicine. **Fitoterapia** 1982; 53: 147–162.

MP083 Babbar, O. P., M. N. Joshi and A. R. Madan. Evaluation of plants for antiviral activity. **Indian J Med Res Suppl** 1982; 76: 54–65.

MP084 Shaft, N. and M. Ikram. Quantitative survey of rutin-containing plants. Part 1. **Int J Crude Drug Res** 1982; 20(4): 183–186.

MP085 John, D. One hundred useful raw drugs of the Kani Tribes of Trivandrum Forest Division, Kerala, India. **Int J Crude Drug Res** 1984; 22(1): 17–39.

MP086 Singh, N., R. Nath, D. R. Singh, M. L. Gupta and R. P. Kohli. An experimental evaluation of the protective effects of some indigenous drugs on carbon tetrachloride-induced hepatotoxicity in mice and rats. **Q J Crude Drug Res** 1978; 16(1): 8–16.

MP087 Jain, S. P. and D. M. Verma. Medicinal plants in the Folk-lore of North-East Haryana. **Nat Acad Sci Lett (India)** 1981; 4(7): 269–271.

MP088 Velazco, E. A. Herbal and traditional practices related to material and child health care. **Rural Reconstruction Review** 1980; 35–39.

MP089 Mossa, J. S. A study on the crude anti-diabetic drugs used in Arabian folk medicine. **Int J Crude Drug Res** 1985; 23(3): 137–145.

MP090 Singh, Y. N. Traditional medicine in Fiji. Some herbal folk cures used by Fiji Indians. **J Ethnopharmacol** 1986; 15(1): 57–88.

MP091 Weniger, B., M. Rouzier, R. Daguilh, D. Henrys, J. H. Henrys and R. Anthon. Popular medicine of the Central Plateau of Haiti. 2. Ethnopharmacological inventory. **J Ethnopharmacol** 1986; 17(1): 13–30.

MP092 Shukla, S., R. Mathur and A. O. Prakash. Anti-implantation efficacy of *Moringa oleifera* Lam. and *Moringa concanensis* Nimmo in rats. **Int J Crude Drug Res** 1988; 26(1): 29–32.

MP093 Kamboj, V. P. A review of Indian medicinal plants with interceptive activity. **Indian J Med Res** 1988; 4: 336–355.

MP094 Gonzalez, F and M. Silva. A survey of plants with antifertility properties described in the South American folk

medicine. **Abstr Princess Congress 1, Thailand,** Dec. 1987; 20pp.

MP095 Kausalya, S., L. Padmanabhan and S. Durairajan. Effect of certain plant extracts on chlorpromazine induced haemolysis of human normal erythrocytes in vitro - A preliminary report. **Clinician** 1984; 48(12): 460–464.

MP096 Vedavathy, S., K. N. Rao, M. Rajaiah and N. Nagaraju. Folklore information from Rayalaseema region, Andhra Pradesh for family planning and birth control. **Int J Pharmacog** 1991; 29(2): 113–116.

MP097 Abraham, Z., S. D. Bhakuni, H. S. Garg, A. K. Goel, B. N. Mehrotra and G. K. Patnaik. Screening of Indian plants for biological activity. Part XII. **Indian J Exp Biol** 1986; 24: 48–68.

MP098 Chopra, R. N., R. L. Badhwar and S. Ghosh. Poisonous Plants of India. Manager of Publications, Government of India Press, Calcutta. Volume 1, 1949.

MP099 Rangaswami, S. and S. Sankarasubramanian. Chemical components of the flowers of *Moringa pterygosperma*. **Curr Sci** 1946; 15: 316–317.

MP100 Kurup, P. A. and P. L. Narasimha Rao. Antibiotic principle from *Moringa pterygosperma*. II. Chemical nature of pterygospermin. **Indian J Med Res** 1954; 42: 85.

MP101 Sen Gupta, K. P., N. C. Ganguli and B. Battacharjee. Bacteriological and pharmacological studies of a vibriocidal drug derived from an indigenous source. **Antiseptic** 1956; 53: 287.

MP102 Orataliza, I. C., I. F. Del Rosario, M. Minda Caedo and A. P. Alcaraz. The availability of carotene in some Philippine vegetables. **Philippine J Sci** 1969; 98: 123.

MP103 Padilla, S. P. and F. A. Soliven. Chemical analysis for possible sources of oils of forty-five species of oil-bearing seeds. **Philippine Agr** 1933; 22: 408.

MP104 Chatterjee, G. S. and S. R. Maitra. A note on physiological and clinical findings of the active principle (spirochin) on the *Moringa pterygosperma*. **Sci Cult** 1951; 17: 43–44.

MP105 Malik, M. Y., A. A. Sheikh and W. H. Shah. Chemical composition of indigenous fodder tree leaves. **Pak J Sci** 1967; 19: 171.

MP106 Collier, W. A. and L. Van De Piji. The antibiotic action of plants, especially the higher plants, with results with Indonesian plants. **Chron Nat** 1949; 105: 8.

MP107 Asprey, G. F. and P. Thornton. Medicinal Plants of Jamaica. IV. **West Indian Med J** 1955; 4: 145–165.

MP108 Prakash, A. O. and R. Mathur. Screening of Indian plants for antifertility activity. **Indian J Exp Biol** 1976; 14: 623–626.

MP109 Dragendorff, G. Die Heilpflanzen der Verschiedenen Volker und Zeiten, F. Enke, Stuttgart, Book 1898; 885pp.

MP110 Das, B. R. and P. L. Rao. Antibiotic principles from *Moringa pterygosperma.* IX. Inhibition of transaminase by isothiocyanates. **Ijar** 1958; 46: 75–76.

MP111 Devadatta, S. C. and R. C. Appanna. Availability of calcium in some of the leafy vegetables. **Proc Indian Acad Sci Ser B** 1954; 39: 236–242.

MP112 Singh, A. and J. D. Kohli. A plea for research into indigenous drug employed in veterinary practice. **Indian Vet J** 1956; 32: 271–280.

MP113 George, M. and K. M. Pandalai. Investigations on plant antibiotics. Part IV. Further search for antibiotic substances in Indian medicinal plants. **Indian J Med Res** 1949; 37: 169–181.

MP114 Kerhado, J. Nebreday (*Moringa oleifera*), a popular Senegalese remedy. Therapeutic use on African chemistry and pharmacology. **Plant Med Phytother** 1969; 3: 214–219.

MP115 Mokkhasmit, M., K. Swasdimongkol, W. Ngarmwathana and U. Perm-phiphat. Pharmacological evaluation of Thai medicinal plants. (Continued). **J Med Assoc Thailand** 1971; 54(7): 490–504.

MP116 Ching, L. S. and S. Mohamed. Alpha-tocopherol content in 62 edible tropical plants. **J Agric Food Chem** 2001; 49(6): 3101–3105.

MP117 Nambiar, V. S. and S. Seshadri. Bioavailability trials of beta-carotene from fresh and dehydrated drumstick leaves (*Moringa oleifera*) in rat model. **Plant Foods Hum Nutr** 2001; 56(1): 83–95.

MP118 Tahiliani, P. and A. Kar. Role of *Moringa oleifera* leaf extract in the regulation of thyroid hormone status in adult male and female rats. **Pharmacol Res** 2000, 41(3): 319–323.

MP119 Ghasi, S., E. Nwobodo and J. O. Ofili. Hypocholesterolemic effects of crude extract of leaf of *Moringa oleifera* Lam. in high-fat diet fed Wistar rats. **J Ethnopharmacol** 2000; 69(1): 21–25.

MP120 Mazumder, U. K., M. Gupta, S. Chakrabarti and D. Pal. Evaluation of hematological and hepatorenal functions of methanolic extract of *Moriniga oleifera* Lam. root treated mice. **Indian J Exp Biol** 1999; 37(6): 612–614.

MP121 Tsaknis, J., S. Lalas, V. Gergis, V. Dourtoglou and V. Spiliotis. Characterization of *Moringa oleifera* variety Mbololo seed oil of Kenya. **J Agri Food Chem** 1999; 47(11): 4495–4499.

MP122 Guevara, A. P., C. Vargas, H. Sakurai, Y. Fujiwara, K. Hashimoto, T. Maoka, M. Kozuka, Y. Ito, H. Tokuda and H. Nishino. An antitumor promoter from *Moringa oleifera* Lam. **Mutat Res** 1999; 440(2): 181–188.

21 | Persea americana

P. mill

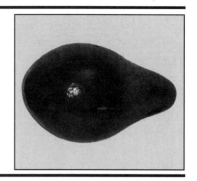

Common Names

A'aboca	West Indies	Avocado	Mexico
Abacateiro	Brazil	Avocado	Nicaragua
Abacateiro	Cuba	Avocado	Sri Lanka
Afia	Guinea	Avocado	Trinidad
Aguacate	Argentina	Avocado	Turkey
Aguacate	Belize	Avocado	West Indies
Aguacate	Brazil	Avocado pear	Indonesia
Aguacate	Colombia	Avocado pear	Israel
Aguacate	Cuba	Avocado pear	Jamaica
Aguacate	Guatemala	Avocado pear	South Africa
Aguacate	Honduras	Avocat	Mauritius
Aguacate	Mexico	Avocat	Rodrigues Islands
Aguacate	Nicaragua	Buite	Colombia
Aguacate	Panama	Butter pear	Nicaragua
Aguacate	Paraguay	Cura	Cuba
Aguacate	Puerto Rico	Curo	Colombia
Aguacatero	Canary Islands	Hoja de palto	Easter Island
Aguacatillo	Mexico	Kukataj	Mexico
Aguate	Peru	Kuulup	Nicaragua
Agucatillo	Cuba	On	Belize
Ahuacaquahuitl	Mexico	Palta	Argentina
Alligator pear	West Indies	Palta	Cuba
Aquacate	Guatemala	Palta	Peru
Aquacate	Mexico	Palto	Peru
Auacatl	Mexico	Pear	Belize
Avocado	Argentina	Pear	Guyana
Avocado	Australia	Pear	Nicaragua
Avocado	Cuba	Sarin	Nicaragua
Avocado	Indonesia	Sikya	Nicaragua
Avocado	Israel	Wagadi	Nicaragua
Avocado	Jamaica	Zaboka	Haiti
Avocado	Japan	Zaboka	West Indies

From: *Medicinal Plants of the World, vol. 1: Chemical Constituents, Traditional and Modern Medicinal Uses, 2nd ed.*
By: Ivan A. Ross © Humana Press Inc., Totowa, NJ

BOTANICAL DESCRIPTION

Tree of the LAURACEAE family with straggling-ascending branches, usually up to about 15 meters high, sometimes much taller. Leaves spirally arranged, often clustered near the branch ends, narrowly to broadly elliptical or obovate, usually pointed at the tip, up to 20 cm long and over 15 cm broad, with well-developed petioles, glaucous beneath. Flowers in a much-branched compact panicle shorter than the leaves, greenish-yellow. Fruits variable in size and shape according to the variety, usually shiny and green or brownish when ripe, often pear-shaped, up to about 15 cm long; flesh soft, greenish or yellow, oily, surrounding one large loose round seed.

ORIGIN AND DISTRIBUTION

Native of Mexico, now widespread in the tropics and subtropics. Avocado is cultivated commercially in Florida, California and Hawaii in the USA, as well as in several South American countries, South Africa, Australia and tropical Asia.

TRADITIONAL MEDICINAL USES

Belize. Hot water extract of dried leaves is taken orally for cough[PA056].

Bolivia. Hot water extract of dried fruits is taken orally for amenorrhea. Hot water extract of dried leaves is taken orally as for amenorrhea[PA068].

Brazil. Hot water extract of buds is taken orally as an emmenagogue and antisyphiletic. Hot water extract of fresh leaves is taken orally to treat hypertension or induce diuresis[PA064]. Hot water extract of leaves is taken orally as a diuretic. Hot water extract of the fruit is taken orally as an aphrodisiac by males[PA076].

Canary Islands. Dried bark is used as a food. Hot water extract of dried seeds is taken orally as a diuretic[PA069].

Colombia. Extract of the mesocarp is administered orally to cows as an abortifa-cient[PA002]. Hot water extract of dried leaves is taken orally as an emmenagogue and treatment for sterility. Hot water extracts of dried seeds and fruit are taken orally for sterility in women, and as an emmenagogue[PA068]. Hot water extract of leaves is used as an emmenagogue[PA002]. Hot water extract of the seeds is claimed to have antifertility properties[PA054].

Costa Rica. Infusion of young leaves is taken orally as an emmenagogue and abortifacient[PA034].

Cuba. Hot water extract of shoots is taken orally as an abortifacient[PA077].

Ecuador. Hot water extract of the plant is taken orally as a contraceptive[PA068].

Guatemala. Roasted seeds are eaten as a remedy for diarrhea[PA072].

Haiti. Decoction of dried bark is taken orally for amenorrhea. Dried fruit is eaten for liver troubles. Fresh seeds are eaten for hepatitis, liver troubles and amenorrhea. Juice from fresh seeds is applied to eye for eye problems[PA065].

Honduras. Hot water extract of the fruit is taken orally by male adults as a sexual stimulant[PA006].

Indonesia. Hot water extract of dried leaves is taken orally as an antihypertensive[PA053].

Jamaica. Fruits are considered "great provocatives," hence the Spaniards did not like their wives to indulge too much. Hot water extract of leaves is taken orally as a cure for high blood pressure[PA074].

Mauritius. Hot water extract of dried leaves is taken orally as an emmenagogue[PA051].

Mexico. Extract of the bark and leaves is taken orally as an emmenagogue[PA001]. Decoction of fresh branches is taken orally to treat infertility in adult females[PA063]. Decoction of Corymbosa stem, plants of *Satureja brownei* or *Satureja xalapensis* and 1 seed of *Persea americana* are boiled or extracted in alcohol. The decoction is taken in the morning after breakfast for anemia[PA061]. Decoction of dried leaves is taken orally as a remedy for coughs and colds. Half a leaf of *Persea americana* is boiled with leaves of *Lippia dulcis* and one half cup is taken[PA061]. To relax the body before childbirth, avocado pit, avocado leaves and salt are used in a bath[PA062]. For premature contractions, avocado leaves and salt are used in a bath. The patients also take boiled water with 10 drops of "Esencia maravaillosa" (commercial preparation)[PA062]. Decoction of fresh leaves and seeds is taken orally for contraception and dysmenorrhea, to enhance childbirth and as an emmenagogue. Leaves and seeds prepared with pine smoke and fat is used externally as a poultice for wounds and bruises[PA063]. Decoction of leaves is taken orally to treat diarrhea[PA026]. Hot water extract of the leaf is taken orally as an emmenagogue[PA077] and diuretic[PA076]. Decoction of the fresh bark is used externally for skin blemishes; orally to prevent miscarriage and speed up postpartum recovery, to treat hemorrhage between menstrual periods and menorrhagia[PA063]. Fruit pulp is used as an aphrodisiac[PA077]. Hot water extract of bark, at a dose of 2 full soupspoons every 2 hours, is taken as an emmenagogue[PA034]. Hot water extract of buds is taken orally as an emmenagogue and an antisyphiletic[PA076]. Hot water extract of seeds, mixed with moneyworth, wood sorrel and spurge, is taken orally by women suffering from excessive bleeding after abortion[PA032]. Hot water extract of the fruit is taken orally as an aphrodisiac[PA076] and emmenagogue[PA001]. Hot water extract of trunk bark is taken orally as an emmenagogue[PA077]. Seed oil is used externally as an astringent, to treat sores and to remove scars[PA014].

Panama. Hot water extract of leaves is taken orally to treat hypertension and as an emmenagogue[PA049].

Paraguay. Extract of the plant is taken orally as an abortifacient and emmenagogue[PA015]. Hot water extract of leaves, together with *Aristolochia triangularis* and *Jacaranda mimosifolia*, is taken orally for fertility regulation in females[PA004,PA033].

Peru. Hot water extract of dried seeds is taken orally for amoebic dysentery and as an antidiarrheal, antidiabetic and astringent. Externally, the extract is used to wash wounds and for baldness[PA067]. Hot water extract of leaves is taken orally as an abortifacient by the Kichos Indians[PA005].

South Africa. Fruit pulp is eaten as an aphrodisiac and emmenagogue[PA007].

Trinidad. Water extract of grated seeds is taken orally every other day as a remedy for diabetes[PA073].

West Africa. Hot water extract of leaves is taken orally as a diuretic[PA008].

West Indies. Hot water extract of leaves is taken orally as an antidiarrheal[PA046].

CHEMICAL CONSTITUENTS
(ppm unless otherwise indicated)

(5E,12Z,15Z)-2-hydroxy-4-oxoheneicosa-5,12,15-trienyl: Fr[PA083]

(2E,12Z,15Z)-2-hydroxy-4-oxoheneicosa-12,15-dienyl: Fr[PA083]

(5E,12Z)-2-hydroxy-4-oxoheneicosa-5,12-dienyl: Fr[PA082]

(2R,4R)-2,4-dihydroxyheptadec-16-enyl: Fr[PA082]

(2R,4R)-2,4-dihydroxyheptadec-16-ynyl: Fr[PA082]

5-Dehydro-avenasterol: Sd oil 1.6–6.8%[PA057]

5-Hydroxy-tryptamine: Fr[PA011,PA050]

7-Dehydro-avenasterol: Sd oil 0.9–1.7%[PA057]

1,2,4-Triacetoxyheptadeca-16-ene: Sd[PA071]

Abscisic acid: Fr[PA017], Sd[PA079]

Alpha cubebene: Lf EO[PA022]

Alpha phellandrene: Lf EO[PA022]

Alpha pinene: Lf EO[PA022]

Alpha terpinene: Lf EO[PA022]

Alpha tocopherol: Sd oil[PA047]

Apigenin: Lf[PA023]

Astragalin: Lf[PA023]

Beta myrcene: Lf EO[PA022]

Beta ocimene: Lf EO[PA022]

Beta pinene: Lf EO[PA022]

Beta sitosterol: Lf[PA008]

Campesterol: Sd oil 4.9–6.3%[PA057]

Camphene: Lf EO[PA022]

Carvone: Lf EO[PA022]

Catechin: Sd[PA009], Lf[PA080]

Catechin, epi: Sd[PA009], Lf[PA080], Fr Pe[PA080]
Chaviccol methyl ester: Lf EO 90.03%[PA043]
Cholesterol: Sd oil 1.1–2.3%[PA057,PA047]
Cineol: Lf EO[PA022]
Cyanidin: Lf[PA060]
Cynaroside: Lf[PA023]
D-Limonene: Lf EO[PA022]
Decan-1-ol acetate: Lf EO[PA022]
Dihydro-phaseic acid: Fr[PA058]
Dimethyl-sciadinonate: Lf[PA018]
Dopamine: Fr[PA050]
Estragole: Fr Pe 60–90%[PA019],
   Lf EO 90.03%[PA021]
Eugenol methyl ether: Lf EO[PA022]
Fructose: Fr[PA048]
Gamma terpinene: Lf EO[PA022]
Glucose: Fr[PA048]
Heptadecane-1-2-4-triol: Sd[PA071]
Hex-cis-3-en-1-oil: Lf EO[PA022]
Hexan-1-al: Lf EO[PA022]
Luteolin: Lf[PA023]
Mannoheptulose: Fr 0.6–3.1%[PA048]
Methyl ether chavicol: Lf EO 90.03%[PA043]
N-Hexadecane: Lf EO[PA022]
N-Octane: Lf EO[PA022]
Nerol acetate: Lf EO[PA022]
Octan-1-ol: Lf EO[PA022]
Oleic acid: Fr[PA016]
Palmitic acid: Fr[PA016]
Pentan-1-ol: Lf EO[PA022]
Persea proanthocyanidin: Sd[PA010]
Perseitol: Fr 0.4–3.8%[PA048]
Persenone A: Fr[PA085]
Persenone B: Fr[PA087]
Procyanidins: Lf[PA060], Fr Pe[PA080]
Quercetin: Lf[PA008]
Quercetin-3-diglucoside: Lf[PA023]
Sabinene: Lf EO[PA022]
Sciadinonic acid dimethyl ester: Lf[PA045]
Scopoletin: Lf[PA023]
Stearic acid: Fr[PA016]
Stigmast-7-en-3-beta-ol: Sd oil[PA057]
Stigmasterol: Sd oil[PA057]
Vitamin A: Sd oil[PA047]
Vitamin D: Sd oil[PA047]

PHARMACOLOGICAL ACTIVITIES AND CLINICAL TRIALS

Allergenic activity. Fresh fruit, eaten by human adults of both sexes, was active. The effect was investigated by an immunoblot-ting technique in sera of allergenic patients[PA031]. Fruit, taken by human adults, was active. Skin prick tests produced positive IgE-mediated reactions with varying symptoms from rhinoconjunctivitis to anaphylactic shock[PA029].

Analgesic activity. Flavonoid fraction of dried seeds, administered intraperitoneally to mice at a dose of 80.0 mg/kg, was active vs hot plate method[PA052].

Antibacterial activity. Methanol/water (1:1) extract of leaves, in broth culture, was inactive on *Bacillus subtilis*, *Escherichia coli*, *Proteus vulgaris*, *Pseudomonas aeruginosa*, *Staphylococcus albus*, and *Staphylococcus aureus*[PA013]. Petroleum ether extract of seeds, on agar plate, was active on *Sarcina lutea* and *Staphylococcus aureus*, and inactive on *Bacillus subtilis*, *Escherichia coli* and *Salmonella typhosa*[PA075].

Anticlastogenic activity. Fruit juice, at a dose of 50.0 ml/kg, administered intraperitoneally to mice, was active on marrow cells vs mitomycin C- and dimethylnitrosamine-induced micronuclei[PA027].

Antiedema activity. Methanol extract of fruit, applied externally to mice at a dose of 2.0 mg/ear, was active. The inhibition ratio was 8 vs 12-0-tetradecanoylphorbol-13-acetate (TPA)-induced ear inflammation[PA024].

Antifungal activity. Chloroform extract of freeze-dried fruit peel, on agar plate, was active on *Cladosporium cladosporiodes*[PA012]. (E,Z,Z)-1-Acetoxy-2-hydroxy-4-oxoheneicosa-5,12,15-triene, isolated for the fruit idioblast cells, inhibited spore germination of the fungal pathogen *Colletotrichum gloeosporioides*[PA086].

Antigiardiasis activity. Decoction of leaves and stem, at a concentration of 4.0 mg/ml, produced weak activity on *Giardia intestinalis*[PA028].

Antihepatotoxic activity. Fruits, administered orally to rats with liver damage caused by D-galactosamine, produced extraordinarily potent liver injury suppressing activity as measured by changes in the levels of plasma alanine aminotransferase and aspartate amiotransferase[PA083].

Antihypertensive activity. Water extract of dried leaves, administered intravenously to rats at a concentration of 0.1 ml/animal, was active vs nicotine- and norepinephrine-induced hypertension[PA053]. Methanol:dichloromethane extract of the leaves inhibited the [3H]-AT II binding (angiotensin II ATI receptor) more than 50%[PA084].

Antimalarial activity. Ethanol (95%) and hexane extracts of dried leaves and stem, administered by gastric intubation to mice at a dose of 100.0 mg/kg (daily for 4 days), were inactive on *Plasmodium berghei*[PA020].

Antiyeast activity. Ethanol (60%) extract of dried leaves, on agar plate, was inactive on *Candida albicans*[PA042].

Barbiturate potentiation. Flavonoid fraction of dried seeds, administered intraperitoneally to mice at a dose of 80.0 mg/kg, was active[PA052].

Cell proliferation inhibition. Water extract of dried leaves, at a concentration of 200.0 mcg/ml, was inactive on lymphocytes vs phytohemagglutinin-induced proliferation. The effect is reversible[PA030].

Chronotropic effect (positive). Ethanol/water (1:1) extract of fresh leaves, administered by gastric intubation to rats at a dose of 40.0 ml/kg, was inactive[PA064].

Collagen synthesis inhibition. Seed oil, administered to rats by gastric intubation at a dose of 10%, was active. Weanling animals were fed a diet supplemented with the oil for 8 weeks, after which dorsal skin was assayed for moisture, protein total collagen and soluble collagen. Only the latter had increased by 36% vs control[PA040].

Comutagenic activity. Fruit juice, administered intraperitoneally to mice at a dose of 50.0 ml/kg, was active on marrow cells vs tetracycline-induced micronuclei[PA027].

Death. Dried fruit, administered orally to canary, was active. One canary and 3 cock-

atiels died after eating avocado. Necropsy of the canary revealed enlarged spleen, subcutaneous edema and phlebitis (judged unrelated to avocado ingestion). The cockatiels showed hydropericardium, possibly due to avocado. Deaths of all birds were attributed to avocado intoxication. Fruit pulp, administered by gastric intubation to budgerigars and canaries at doses of 1.0 and 0.7 ml/animal, was active. The birds were given doses of a mixture of 8.7 gm avocado pulp mixed with 2.0 ml water. Two of 4 budgerigars given 2 doses died, all budgerigars given 4 doses died and 1 canary given 4 doses died. Necropsy showed excessive epicardial fluid, generalized lung congestion and nonsuppurative inflammation. Death was attributed to lung congestion caused by avocado[PA037].

Diuretic activity. Ethanol/water (1:1) extract of fresh leaves, administered to rats by gastric intubation at a dose of 40.0 ml/kg, was active. The extract consists of five parts fresh plant material in 100 parts water/ethanol[PA036].

Hypertensive activity. Fresh fruit eaten by human adults was active. There was an induction of a hypertensive crisis in a patient on monoamine-oxidase inhibitor therapy[PA044]. Ethanol (95%) and water extracts of dried leaves and stem, administered intravenously to dogs and by gastric intubation to rats at a dose of 0.1 ml/kg, were active[PA003]. Ethanol/water (1:1) extract of fresh leaves, at a dose of 40.0 ml/kg, produced weak activity[PA064]. Flavonoid fraction of dried seeds, administered intravenously to male rats at a dose of 2.0 mg/kg, produced weak activity[PA052].

Larvicidal activity. Leaves (undiluted), in the ration of *Bombyx mori* larvae, were active[PA045].

Lysyl oxidase inhibition. Seed oil, administered by gastric intubation to rats at a dose of 10.0%, was active. Weanling animals were fed a diet supplemented with the oil for 8 weeks, after which dorsal skin was assayed. A

56% decrease in activity was observed[PA040]. Unsaponifiable fraction, at a concentration of 0.5%, was active on rat skin. Enzyme activity was decreased by 30%[PA038].

Molluscicidal activity. Ethanol (95%) extract of dried leaves, at a concentration of 100.0 ppm, was inactive on *Biomphalaria glabrata* eggs and adults. The hexane-ethyl acetate extract was inactive on eggs and adults[PA039]. Ethanol (95%) and hot water extracts of seeds, at a concentration of 10,000 ppm, were active on *Biomphalaria straminea*[PA070]. Ethanol (95%) and water extracts of dried seeds, at concentrations of 10,000 ppm, were inactive on *Biomphalaria glabrata* and *Biomphalaria straminea*[PA078]. Homogenate of fresh entire plant was inactive on *Lymnaea columella* and *Lymnaea cubensis*. Fruits, leaves and roots were tested[PA055].

Nitric oxide synthase suppression. Persenone A, at a concentration of 20 microM, almost completely suppressed both inducible nitric oxide synthase and cyclo-oxygenase protein expression induced by lipopolysaccharide and interferon in a mouse machrophage cell line RAW 264.7[PA085].

Phagocytosis stimulation. Unsaponifiable fraction of dried fruit, administered intraperitoneally to male mice at a dose of 0.5 ml/animal, was active[PA059].

Pharmacokinetic study. Seed oil applied to the skin is rapidly absorbed[PA035].

Smooth muscle relaxant activity. Ethanol (95%) extract of dried leaves and stem, at a concentration of 33 ml/liter, was active on rabbit duodenum[PA003].

Smooth muscle stimulant activity. Flavonoid fraction of dried seeds produced weak activity on guinea pig ileum[PA052].

Spasmogenic activity. Ethanol (95%) extract of the leaves, at a concentration of 3.3 ml/liter and water extract at a concentration of 0.33 ml/liter administered intraperitoneally to guinea pigs, were active on the ileum[PA003].

Superoxide generation inhibitors. (2R)0(12Z,15Z)-2-hydroxy-4-oxoheneicosa-12,15-dien⁺⁺⁺-1-yl acetate, and two compounds, persenone A and B, isolated from the fruit, inhibited superoxide and nitric oxide generation in cell culture systems[PA087].

Toxic effect. Powdered freeze-dried fruit, administered to budgerigar by gastric intubation at a concentration of 1.0 ml, was active[PA025]. Seed oil, at variable concentrations, was inactive. Various tests involving creams and other beauty care products with avocado oil concentrations as high as 10% showed little or no irritation. Undiluted seed oil applied by patches was inactive. Patches remained on subject for 48 hours and test was repeated in 14 days. No sensitization occurred. Seed oil, administered subcutaneously to rats at a dose of 0.25 ml/animal, was inactive. Daily dosing for 30 days produced no gross pathological effects. Seed coat, taken orally by human adults at a dose of 625.0 mg/kg, was inactive[PA035].

Toxicity assessment (quantitative). The minimum toxic dose for ethanol (95%) extract of dried leaves and stem was 1.0 ml/animal when administered intraperitoneally to mice. The water extract was 0.5 ml/animal[PA003]. Flavonoid fraction of dried seeds, administered intraperitoneally to mice, LD_{50} 340.0 mg/kg[PA052].

Tumor promotion inhibition. Methanol extract of fresh fruits, at a concentration of 200.0 mcg in cell culture, was active on Epstein-Barr virus vs 12-0-hexadecanoyl-phorbol-13-acetate-induced Epstein-Barr virus activation[PA066].

Uterine stimulant effect. Ethanol (95%) extract of leaves and stem, at a concentration of 0.33 ml/liter, was active on rat uterus. The water extract, at a concentration of 0.033 ml/liter, produced strong activity[PA003].

WBC-macrophage stimulant. Water extract of freeze-dried fruit at a concentration of 2.0 mg/ml was inactive. Nitrite formation was used as an index of the macrophage stimulating activity to screen effective foods[PA041].

REFERENCES

PA001 Quisumbing, E. Medicinal plants of the Philippines. **Tech Bull 16**, Rep Philippines, Dept Agr Nat Resources, Manilla 1951; 1.

PA002 Garcia-Barriga, H. Flora Medicinal de Colombia. Volume 1. Universidad Nacional, Bogota, 1974.

PA003 Feng, P. C., L. J. Haynes, K. E. Magnus, J. R. Plimmer and H. S. A. Sherrat. Pharmacological screening of some West Indian Medicinal Plants. **J Pharm Pharmacol** 1962; 14: 556–561.

PA004 Hnatyszyn, O., P. Arenas, A. R. Moreno, R. V. D. Rondina and J. D. Coussio. Preliminary phytochemical study of Paraguayan medicinal plants. 1. Plants regulating fertility from medicinal folklore. **Rev Soc Cient** 1974; 14: 23.

PA005 Tessman, G. Die Indianer Nordost-Perus, Grundlegende Forschunger Fur Eine Systematischen, De Gruyter Co., Hamburg, Germany, 1930.

PA006 Girard, R. The medicine chest of the Chorti Indians. **Bol Indigenista** 1947; 7(4): 347.

PA007 Watt, J. M. and M. G. Breyer-Brandwijk. The Medicinal and Poisonous Plants of Southern and Eastern Africa. 2nd Ed, E. S. Livingstone, Ltd., London, 1962.

PA008 Nogueira Prista, L. and A. Correia Alves. Phytochemical study of the leaves of *Persea americana*. **Garcia Orta** 1961; 9: 501.

PA009 De Oliveira, M. M., M. R. P. Sampaio, F. Simon, B. Gilbert and W. B. Mors. Antitumor activity of condensed flavonols. **An Acad Brasil Cienc** 1972; 44: 41.

PA010 Geissman, T. A. and H. F. K. Dittmar. A proanthocyanidin from avocado seed. **Phytochemistry** 1965; 4: 359–368.

PA011 Willaman, J. J. and H. L. Li. Alkaloid-bearing plants and their contained alkaloids, 1957–1968. **Lloydia** 1970; 33S; 1–286.

PA012 Adikaram, N. K. B., D. R. Ewing, A. M. Karunaratne and E. M. K Wijeratne. Antifungal compounds from immature avocado fruit peel. **Phytochemistry** 1992; 31(1): 93–96.

PA013 Ogunlana, E. O. and E. Ramstad. Investigation into the antibacterial actvities of local plants. **Planta Med** 1975; 27: 354.

PA014 Ortiz De Montellano, B. Empirical Aztec medicine. **Science** 1975; 188: 215–220.

PA015 Moreno, A. R. Two Hundred Sixty-Eight Medicinal Plants Used to Regulate Fertility in Some Countries of South America, Unpublished (Stenciled) Review in Spanish, 1975.

PA016 Harwood, J. L. Fatty acid biosynthesis by avocado pear. **Lipids** 1974; 9: 850–.

PA017 Milborrow, B. V. The origin of the methyl groups of abscisic acid. **Phytochemistry** 1975; 14: 2403.

PA018 Murakoshi, S., A. Isogai, C. F. Chang, T. Kamikado, A. Sakurai and S. Tamura. The effects of two components from avocado leaves (*Persea americana*) and related compounds on the growth of silkworm larvae, Bombyx mori. **Nippon Oyo Dobutsu Konchu Gakkaishi** 1976; 20: 87.

PA019 Opdyke, D. L. J. Monographs on fragrance raw materials. Methyl chavicol. **Food Cosmet Toxicol** 1976; 14: 601–603.

PA020 Brandao, M., M. Botelho and E. Krettli. Antimalarial experimental chemotherapy using natural products. **Cienc Cult** 1985; 37(7): 1152–1163.

PA021 Sarer, E. and G. Kokdl. Investigation on avocado leaf oil. **Ankara Univ Eczacilik Fak Derg** 1990; 20(1/2): 18–24.

PA022 King, J. R. and R. J. Knight. Volatile components of the leaves of various avocado cultivars. **J Agr Food Chem** 1992; 40(7): 1182–1185.

PA023 Merici, F., A. H. Merici, F. Yilmaz, G. Yunculer and O. Yunculer. Flavonoids of avocado (*Persea americana*) leaves. **Acta Pharm Turc** 1992; 34(2): 61–63.

PA024 Yasukawa, K., A. Yamaguchi, J. Arita, S. Sakurai, A. Ikeda and M. Takido. Inhibitory effect of edible plant extracts on 12-0-tetradecanoylphorbol-

13-acetate-induced ear oedema in mice. **Phytother Res** 1993; 7(2): 185–189.

PA025   Shopshire, C. M., E. Stauber and M. Arai. Evaluation of selected plants for acute toxicosis in budgerigars. **J Amer Vet Assn** 1992; 200(7): 936–939.

PA026   Zamora-Martinez, M. C. and C. N. P. Pola. Medicinal plants used in some rural populations of Oaxaca, Puebla and Veracruz, Mexico. **J Ethnopharmacol** 1992; 35(3) 229–257.

PA027   Lim-Sylianco, C. Y., J. A. Concha, A. P. Jocano and C. M. Lim. Antimutagenic effects of expressions from twelve medicinal plants. **Philippine J Sci** 1986; 115(1): 23–30.

PA028   Ponce-Macotela, M., I. Navarro-Alegria, M. N. Martinez-Gordillo and R. Alvarez-Chacon. In vitro antigiardiasic activity of plant extracts. **Rev Invest Clin** 1994; 46(5): 343–347.

PA029   Blanco, C., T. Carrillo, R. Castillo, J. Quiralte and M. Cuevas. Avocado hypersensitivity. **Allergy** 1994; 49(6): 454–459.

PA030   Moraes, V. L. G., L. F. M. Santos, S. B. Castro, L. H. Loureiro, O. A. Lima et al. Inhibition of lymphocyte activation by extracts and fractions of *Kalanchoe*, *Alternathera*, *Paullinia* and *Mikania* species. **Phytomedicine** 1994; 1(3): 199–204.

PA031   Lavaud, F., A. Prevost, C. Cossart, L. Guerin, J. Bernard and S. Kochman. Allergy to latex, avocado pear, and 0banana. Evidence for a 30 KD antigen in immunoblotting. **J Allergy Clin Immunol** 1995; 95(2): 557–564.

PA032   Latorre, D. L. and F. A. Latorre. Plants used by the Mexican Kickapoo Indians. **Econ Bot** 1977; 31: 340–357.

PA033   Arenas, P. and R. Moreno Azorero. Plants of common use in Paraguayan folk medicine for regulating fertility. **Econ Bot** 1977; 31: 298–301.

PA034   Morton, J. F. Some folk medicine plants of Central American markets. **Q J Crude Drug Res** 1977; 15: 165.

PA035   Anon. Final report of the safety assessment for avocado oil. **J Environ Pathol Toxicol** 1980; 4: 93–103.

PA036   De A Ribeiro, R., F. Barros, M. Margarida, R. F. Melo, C. Muniz, S. Chieia, M. G. Wanderley, C. Gomes

and G. Trolin. Acute diuretic effects in conscious rats produced by some medicinal plants used in the state of Sao Paulo, Brasil. **J Ethnopharmacol** 1988; 24(1): 19–29.

PA037   Hargis, A. M., E. Stauber, S. Casteel and D. Eitner. Avocado (*Persea americana*) intoxication in caged birds. **J Amer Vet Med Assoc** 1989; 194(1): 64–66.

PA038   Werman, M. J., S. Mokady and I. Neeman. Partial isolation and characterization of a new natural inhibitor of lysyl oxidase from avocado seed oil. **J Agr Food Chem** 1990; 38(12): 2164–2168.

PA039   De Souza, C. P., M. L. Lima De Azevedo, J. L. C. Lopes, J. Sarti, D. D. Santos Filho et al. Chemoprophylaxis of schistosomiasis. Molluscicidal activity of natural products. **An Acad Brasil Cienc** 1984; 56(3): 333–338.

PA040   Werman, M. J., S. Mokady, M. E. Nimni and I. Neeman. The effect of various avocado oils on skin collagen metabolism. **Conn Tiss Res** 1991; 26(1/2): 1–10.

PA041   Miwa, M., Z. L. Kong, K. Shinohara and M. Watanabee. Macrophage stimulating activity of foods. **Agr Biol Chem** 1990; 54(7): 1863–1866.

PA042   Caceres, A., E. Jauregu, D. Herrera and H. Logemann. Plants used in Guatemala for the treatment of dermatomucosal infections. 1. Screening of 38 plant extracts for anticandidal activity. **J Ethnopharmacol** 1991; 33(3): 277–283.

PA043   Sarer, E. and G. Kokdil. Investigations on avocado leaf oil. **Ankara Univ Eczacilik Fak Derg** 1990; 20(1/2): 18–24.

PA044   Anon. Avocado pear-MAO inhibitor interaction. **Pharm Int** 1982; 3(4): 122.

PA045   Chang, C. F., A. Isogai, T. Kamikado, S. Murakoshi, A. Sakurai and S. Tamura. Isolation and structure elucidation of growth inhibitors for silkworm larvae from avocado leaves. **Agr Biol Chem** 1975; 39: 1167–1168.

PA046   Ayensu, E. S. Medicinal plants of the West Indies. **Unpublished Manuscript** 1978; 110pp.

PA047   Sardi, J. C. and O. A. Torres. Study on avocado (*Persea americana*) oil. **Arch Bioquim Quim Farm** 1978; 20: 45–49.

PA048 Wilson III, C. W., P. E. Saw and S. Nagy. Analysis of monosacchardies in avocado by HPLC. **Liq Chromatogr Anal Food Beverages** 1979; 1: 225–236.

PA049 Gupta, M. P., T. D. Arias, M. Correa and S. S. Lamba. Ethnopharmacognostic observations on Panamanian medicinal plants. Part 1. **Q J Crude Drug Res** 1979; 17(3/4): 115–130.

PA050 Bick, R. C. and W. Sinchai. Alkaloids of the Lauraceae. **Heterocycles** 1978; 9: 903–945.

PA051 Sussman, L. K. Herbal medicine on Mauritius. **J Ethnopharmacol** 1980; 2(3): 259–278.

PA052 De Oliviera, M. M., M. Santos, and A. C. Coni. Analgesic activity of dimeric proanthocyanidins -preliminary experiments. **ARQ Inst Biol Sao Paulo** 1975; 42: 145–150.

PA053 Padmawinata, K. and E. Hoyaranda. The effect of juice of *Averrhoa carambola* fruits and the aqueous extract of *Persea americana* leaves on rat blood pressure. **Abstr 4th Asian Symp Med Plants Spices**, Bangkok, Thailand. Sept. 15–19, 1980.

PA054 Gonzalez, J. Medicinal plants in Colombia. **J Ethnopharmacol** 1980; 2(1): 43–47.

PA055 Medina, F. R. and R. Woodbury. Terrestrial plants molluscicidal to Lymnaeid hosts of *Fasciliasis hepatica* in Puerto Rico. **J Agr Univ Puerto Rico** 1979; 63: 366–376.

PA056 Arnason, T., F. Uck, J. Lambert and R. Hebda. Maya medicinal plants of San Jose Succotz, Belize. **J Ethnopharmacol** 1980; 2(4): 345–364.

PA057 Sciancalepore, V. and W. Dorbessan. Sterol composition of oil of avocado (*Persea americana* Mill.). **Grasas Aceites (Seville)** 1982; 33: 273–275.

PA058 Hirai, N. and K. Koshimizu. A new conjugate of dihydrophaesic acid from avocado fruit. **Agr Biol Chem** 1983; 47(2): 365–371.

PA059 Delaveau, P., P. Lallouette and A. M. Tessier. Stimulation of the phagocytic activity of reticuloendothelial system by plant drugs. **Planta Med** 1980; 40: 49–54.

PA060 Bate-Smith, E. C. Phytochemistry of proanthocyanidins. **Phytochemistry** 1975; 14(4): 1107–1113.

PA061 Martinez, M. A. Medicinal plants used in a Totonac community of the Sierra Norte de Puebla. Tuzamapan de Galeana, Puebla, Mexico. **J Ethnopharmacol** 1984; 11(2): 203–221.

PA062 Cosminsky, S. Knowledge of body concepts of Guatemala wives. Chapter 12. Anthropology of Human Birth, 1982; 233–252pp.

PA063 Browner, C. H. Plants used for reproductive health in Oaxaca, Mexico. **Econ Bot** 1985; 39(4): 482–504.

PA064 De Ribeiro, R., M. M. R. Fiuza De Melo, F. De Barros, C. Gomes and G. Trolin. Acute antihypertensive effect in conscious rats produced by some medicinal plants used in the state of Sao Paulo. **J Ethnopharmacol** 1986; 15(3): 261–269.

PA065 Weniger, B., M. Rouzier, R. Daguilh, D. Henrys, J. H. Henrys and R. Anthon. Popular medicine of the Central Plateau of Haiti. 2. Ethnopharmacological inventory. **J Ethnopharmacol** 1986; 17(1): 13–30.

PA066 Koshimizu, K., H. Ohigashi, H. Tokuda, A. Kondo and K. Yamaguchi. Screening of edible plants against possible anti-tumor promoting activity. **Cancer Lett** 1988; 39(3): 247–257.

PA067 Ramirez, V. R., L. J. Mostacero, A. E. Garcia, C. F. Mejia, P. F. Pelaez, C. D. Medina and C. H. Miranda. Vegetales empleados en medicina tradicional Norperuana. **Banco Agrario Del Peru & NACL Univ Trujillo**, Peru, June 1988; 54pp.

PA068 Gonzalez, F and M. Silva. A survey of plants with antifertility properties described in the South American folk medicine. **Abstr Princess Congress 1** Thailand, Dec. 1987; 20pp.

PA069 Darias, V., L. Brando, R. Rabanal, C. Sanchez Mateo, R. M. Gonzalez Luis and A. M. Hernandez Perez. New contribution to the ethnopharmacological study of the Canary Islands. **J Ethnopharmacol** 1989; 25(1): 77–92.

PA070 Silva, M. J. M., M. Pinheiro de Sousa and M. Z. Rouquayrol. Molluscicidal activity of plants from Northeastern Brazil. **Rev Brasil Farm** 1971; 52: 117–123.

PA071 Neeman, I., A. Lifshitz and Y. Kashman. New antibacterial agent isolated from the avocado pear. **Appl Microbiol** 1970; 19: 470–473.

PA072   Logan, M. H. Digestive disorders and plant medicine in Highland Guatemala. **Anthropos** 1973; 68: 537–543.

PA073   Simpson, G. E. Folk medicine in Trinidad. **J Amer Folklore** 1962; 75: 326–340.

PA074   Asprey, G. F. and P. Thornton. Medicinal plants of Jamaica. III. **West Indian Med J** 1955; 4: 69–82.

PA075   Gallo, P. and H. Valeri. The antibiotic activity of the seed of avocado pear (*Persea americana*). **Rev Med Vet Parasitol** 1953; 12: 125–129.

PA076   Dragendorff, G. Die Heilpflanzen der Verschiedenen Volker und Zeiten, F. Enke, Stuttgart, Book 1898; 885pp.

PA077   Roig Y Mesa, J. T. Plantas Medicinales, Aromaticas o Venenosas de Cuba. Ministerio De Agricultura, Republica De Cuba, Havana, 1945; 872pp.

PA078   Pinheiro de Sousa, M. and M. Z. Rouquayrol. Molluscicidal activity of plants from Northeast Brazil. **Rev Bras Fpesq Med Biol** 1974; 7(4): 389–394.

PA079   Gazit, S. and A. Blumenfeld. Inhibitor and auxin activity in the avocado fruit. **Physiol Plant** 1972; 27: 77–82.

PA080   Thompson, R. S., D. Jacques, E. Haslam and R. J. N. Tanner. Plant proanthocyanidins. Part 1. Introduction: The isolation, structure and distribution in nature of plant procyanidins. **J Chem Soc Perkin Trans I** 1972; 1387–1399.

PA081   Appelboom, T., J. Schuermans, G. Verbruggen, Y. Henrotin and J. Y. Reginster. Symptoms modifying effect of avocado.soybean unsaponifiables (ASU) in knee osteoarthritis. A double blind, prospective, placebo-controlled study. **Scand J Rheumatol** 2001; 30(4): 242–247.

PA082   Hashimura, H., C. Ueda, J. Kawabata and T. Kasai. Acetyl-CoA carboxylase inhibitors from avocado (*Persea ameri-cana* Mill) fruits. **Biosci Biotechnol Biochem** 2001; 65(7): 1656–1658.

PA083   Kawagish, H., Y. Fukumoto, M. Hatakeyama, P. He, H. Arimoto, T. Matsuzawa, Y, Arimoto, H. Suganuma, T. Inakuma and K. Sugiyama. Liver injury suppressing compounds from avocado (*Persea americana*). **J Agri Food Chem** 2001; 49(5): 2215–2221.

PA084   Caballero-George, C., P. M. Vanderheyden, P. N. Solis, L. Pieters, A. A. Shahat, M. P. Gupta, G. Vauquelin and A. J. Vlietinck. Biological screening of selected medicinal Panamanian plants by radioligand-binding techniques. **Phytomedicine** 2001; 8(1): 59–70.

PA085   Kim, O. K., A. Murakami, D. Takahashi, Y. Nakamura, K. Torikai, H. W. Kim and H. Ohigashi. An avocado constituent, persenone A, suppressed expression of inducible forms of nitric oxide synthase and cyclooxygenase in macrophages, and hydrogen peroxide generation in mouse skin. **Biosci Biotechnol Biochem** 2000; 64(11): 2504–2507.

PA086   Domergue, F., G. L. Helms, D. Prusky and J. Browse. Antifungal compounds from idioblast cells isolated from avocado fruits. **Phytochemistry** 2000; 54(2): 183–189.

PA087   Kim, O. K., A. Murakami, Y. Nakamura, N. Takeda, H. Yoshizumi and H. Ohigashi. Novel nitric oxide and superoxide generation inhibitors, persenone A and B, from avocado fruit. **J Agric Food Chem** 2000; 48(5): 1557–1563.

22 | Phyllanthus niruri

L.

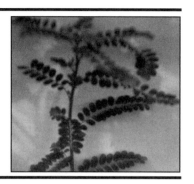

Common Names

Bhoomi amalaki	India	Gale-wind grass	West Indies
Bhui amla	Bangladesh	Graine en bas fievre	French Guiana
Bhui-amla	India	Hurricane weed	West Indies
Bhuianvalah	India	Jar amla	Fiji
Bhuimy-amli	East Indies	Jar-amla	India
Bhuin-amla	Pakistan	Kizha nelli	India
Bhumyamalaki	India	Mapatan	Papua-New Guinea
Cane peas senna	West Indies	Mimosa	West Indies
Carry-me seed	Fiji	Niruri	Pakistan
Carry-me seed	West Indies	Para-parai mi	Paraguay
Chamber bitters	West Indies	Pei	Admiralty Islands
Chancapiedra	Peru	Phyllanto	Brazil
Chickweed	West Indies	Pombinha	East Indies
Creole senna	Virgin Islands	Querba pedra	Brazil
Daun marisan	East Indies	Quinine weed	West Indies
Derriere-dos	Haiti	Sampa-sampalukan	Philippines
Deye do	Haiti	Sasi	Papua-NewGuinea
Elrageig	Sudan	Se	Papua-New Guinea
En bas	West Indies	Shka-nin-du	Mexico
Eruption plant	Papua-New Guinea	Viernes santo	Puerto Rico
Gale-o-wind	Bimini	Ya-tai-bai	Thailand
Gale wind grass	Fiji	Yerba de san pablo	Philippines

BOTANICAL DESCRIPTION

A herb of the EUPHORBIACEAE family that grows up to 60 cm. The plant is bitter in taste, the leaves are small, green, and short-petioled with a thin and glaucous under surface. The flowers are unisexual, monoecious, minute, greenish and inconspicuous, short-stalked and borne in pairs in the axils of the leaves. The fruit is a capsule, globose, slightly depressed at the top with 6 enervations. In the roots, the secondary growth starts very early and is well pronounced. There is a distinct cambium. No starch grains, mineral crystals or latex vessels are seen in either the root or stem.

ORIGIN AND DISTRIBUTION

The plant originated in India, usually occurring as a winter weed throughout the hotter parts; now widespread throughout the

From: *Medicinal Plants of the World, vol. 1: Chemical Constituents, Traditional and Modern Medicinal Uses, 2nd ed.*
By: Ivan A. Ross © Humana Press Inc., Totowa, NJ

tropics and subtropics in sandy regions during rainy seasons.

TRADITIONAL MEDICINAL USES

Admiralty Islands. Hot water extract of dried bark and leaves is taken orally for acute venereal disease. The extract (500 ml) is taken twice daily for up to 6 months[PN061].

Argentina. The plant is used as an emmenagogue by the rural populace[PN016].

Bimini. Hot water extract of the entire plant is taken orally to reduce fevers and as a laxative[PN052].

Brazil. Decoction of dried root is taken orally for jaundice. Decoction of dried seeds is taken orally for diabetes. Hot water extract of dried fruit is taken orally for diabetes. Infusion of dried leaves and stems is taken orally to treat kidney and bladder calculi. Infusion of the dried entire plant administered orally, is used to dissolve kidney and bladder stones, and for renal diseases[PN080].

Dominican Republic. Hot water extract of leaves is taken orally as a popular fever remedy[PN084].

East Africa. Hot water extract of the aerial parts is taken orally as a diuretic[PN089].

East Indies. Hot water extract of the entire plant is taken orally for menstrual troubles/complaints and diabetes, as a purgative and tonic[PN090].

Fiji. Decoction of dried leaves and roots is taken orally for fever and for good health. Dried entire plant, ground in buttermilk is taken orally for jaundice. Fresh leaf juice is used externally for cuts and bruises. For eye diseases, the juice is mixed with castor oil and applied to the eye. Infusion of dried leaves is taken orally for dysentery and diarrhea. Infusion of the green root is taken orally to treat heavy menstrual flow[PN072].

French Guiana. Hot water extract of leaves is taken orally as a cholagogue[PN017].

Haiti. Decoction of dried leaves is taken orally or used in bath for fever, and orally for indigestion[PN077]. Hot water extract of dried entire plant is taken orally as a spasmolytic and for fever[PN058].

India. Decoction of the dried aerial parts is taken orally for diarrhea[PN025] and jaundice[PN065]. Fresh plant juice is taken orally for genitourinary disorders[PN070]. The fruit is used externally for tubercular ulcers, scabies and ringworm[PN030]. Hot water extract of dried entire plant is taken orally, as a diuretic[PN021], for gonorrhea, urogenital tract infections[PN042], diabetes[PN010], jaundice[PN094,PN064], leucorrhea[PN045] and asthma, in Ayurvedic medicine[PN068]. Hot water extract of dried leaves is taken orally for diabetes. Hot water extract of fresh shoots is taken orally for dysentery and jaundice[PN042]. Hot water extract of leaves is taken orally as a stomachic[PN030], for menorrhagia[PN007] and intermittent fever[PN087]. Water extract of roots is taken orally as a galactagogue[PN006].

Malaysia. Hot water extract of leaves is taken orally after a miscarriage and as an emmenagogue[PN007].

Mexico. Hot water extract of dried leaves is an emetic when taken as a strong tea[PN091].

Papau-New Guinea. Fresh leaf and root juices are taken orally for venereal diseases. Decoction of dried entire plant is taken orally to treat venereal diseases[PN043]. For malaria, the decoction is taken orally and used to bathe the patient. For tuberculosis, a single dose of the decoction is taken orally[PN067]. Decoction of dried leaf is taken orally as a treatment for diarrhea. A cupful of the decoction is taken daily[PN027].

Peru. Hot water extract of dried entire plant is taken orally as a diuretic, for gallstones and renal calculi[PN079].

Philippines. Decoction of dried entire plant is used as a bath for newborns. It is believed to remove disease-causing elements from the skin. Orally, the decoction is used for coughs in infants[PN069]. Hot water extract of the entire plant is taken orally as an emmenagogue[PN001,PN005].

Puerto Rico. Hot water extract of leaf and stem is taken orally for fevers[PN004].

Sudan. Hot water extract of dried leaves is taken orally as an analgesic[PN060].

Tanzania. Hot water extract of fresh entire plant is taken orally for gonorrhea[PN071].

Thailand. Hot water extract of the entire plant is taken orally as an antipyretic[PN093]. Hot water extract of the dried aerial parts is taken orally as a diuretic and antipyretic, and for malaria[PN037]. Hot water extract of dried entire plant is taken orally as an anti-inflammatory agent[PN092].

Virgin Islands. Hot water extract of the plant is taken orally to increase the appetite[PN085].

West Indies. Hot water extract of roots, together with hot water extract of *Citrus aurantifolia* roots, is taken orally to increase appetite. Hot water extract of the entire plant is taken orally, for malaria and malarial fever. Water extract of the leaves and roots is taken orally for diabetes, and as a diuretic[PN053,PN088].

CHEMICAL CONSTITUENTS

(ppm unless otherwise indicated)

(–)-Epi-catechin: Rt Cult[PN020]
(–)-Epi-catechin-3-gallate: Rt Cult[PN020]
(–)-Epi-gallocatechin: Rt Cult[PN020]
(–)-Epi-gallocatechin-3-O-gallate: Rt Cult[PN020]
(–)-Limonene: Lf EO 4.5%[PN083]
(–)-Nor-serurinine: Pl[PN082]
(+)-Catechin: Rt Cult[PN020]
(+)-Gallocatechin: Rt Cult[PN020]
4-Hydroxy-lintetralin: Lf 200[PN013,PN011]
4-Hydroxy-sesamin: Pl[PN029]
4-Methoxy-nor-securinine: Aer, Lf, Rt, St[PN065]
2,3-dimethoxy-iso-lintetralin: Lf 2[PN013]
24-Isopropyl cholesterol: Aer 18[PN033]
Ascorbic acid: Lf 0.41%[PN032]
Astragalin: Lf[PN031,PN041]
Beta sitosterol: Lf[PN002]
Corilagin: Pl 7[PN040]
Cymene: Lf EO 11%[PN083]
Demethylenedioxy niranthin: Lf 2[PN013]
Dotriacontanoic acid: Aer 65[PN033]
Ellagic acid: Pl 108-972[PN038,PN040,PN021]
Eriodictyol-7-O-alpha-L-rhamnoside: Rt[PN030]
Estradiol: Pl 3[PN050]
Fisetin-41-O-beta-D-glucoside: Pl 400[PN063]
Gallic acid: Rt Cult[PN020],
    Pl 2.7-27[PN040,PN038]

Geranin: Pl 0.23%[PN038]
Hinokinin: Pl[PN014]
Hydroxy niranthin: Lf 4[PN011]
Hypophyllanthin: Pl[PN008],
    Lf 0.05-0.17%[PN087,PN013,PN002], Aer[PN089]
Iso-lintetralin: Pl 3.4[PN014]
Iso-quercitrin: Lf[PN031,PN041]
Kaempferol-4-O-alpha-L-rhamnoside:
    Rt[PN030]
Linnanthin: Lf 2[PN013]
Linoleic acid: Sd oil 21%[PN057]
Linolenic acid: Sd oil 51.4%[PN057]
Lintetralin: Lf 5-15[PN014,PN013], Aer[PN033]
Lupeol acetate: Rt[PN009,PN054]
Lupeol: Rt[PN009,PN054]
Niranthin: Lf 9-430[PN013,PN002], Aer[PN033]
Nirphyllin: Aer 7[PN012]
Nirtetralin: Pl[PN014,PN056], Lf 9-930[PN013,PN002]
Nirurin: Pl 400[PN066]
Nirurine: Aer 39.8[PN076]
Nirurinetin: Pl[PN066]
Nor-securinine: Rt[PN030]
Phyllanthenol: Aer 20[PN015]
Phyllanthenone: Aer 8[PN015]
Phyllantheol; Aer 15[PN015]
Phyllanthin: Aer 400[PN074],
    Lf 1100-3250[PN081,PN087]
Phyllanthine: Rt, Lf, St[PN065]
Phyllanthus: Pl[PN042]
Phyllester: Aer 12[PN033]
Phyllnirurin: Aer 6[PN012]
Phyllochrysine: Lf, St[PN055]
Phylltetrin: Aer[PN033]
Phyltetralin: Pl[PN056], Lf 0.14%[PN013]
Quercetin: Lf[PN031,PN041], Pl[PN063]
Quercitrin: Lf[PN031,PN041], Pl[PN063]
Repandusinic acid A: Pl[PN021]
Repandusinic acid: Pl 0.12%[PN019]
Ricinoleic acid: Sd oil 1.2%[PN039]
Rutin: Pl[PN063], Lf[PN031,PN041]
Salicylic acid methyl ester: Lf EO[PN083]
Seco-4-hydroxy-lintetralin: Lf 20[PN011]
Trans-phytol: Pl[PN049]
Triacontan-1-al: Aer 60[PN074]
Triancontan-1-ol: Aer 560[PN074]

PHRMACOLOGICAL ACTIVITIES AND CLINICAL TRIALS

Aldose reductase inhibition. Ethanol (70%) extract of dried entire plant was active, IC_{50} 1.0 mcg/ml[PN040].

Analgesic activity. Methanol extract of dried callus tissue, administered intraperitoneally to mice at a concentration of 10.0 mg/kg, was active vs acetic acid-induced writhing and formalin-induced pedal edema. At 50.0 mg/kg, the extract was inactive vs tail flick response to radiant heat[PN026]. Ethanol/water (1:1) extract of dried entire plant, administered intragastrically to male mice at a dose of 50 mg/kg, was active. The extract, administered intraperitoneally to male mice at a dose of 0.3 mg/kg, was also active. In both cases, antinociceptive effects were demonstrated using 5 different models of nociception[PN028].

Angiotensin-converting enzyme inhibition. Chromatographic fraction of dried entire plant, at a concentration of 100.0 mcg/ml, was active[PN038].

Antibacterial activity. Water extract of fresh entire plant, at a concentration of 1.0% on agar plate, was inactive on *Neisseria gonorrhea*[PN071]. Saline extract of leaves, at a concentration of 10% on agar plate, was active on *Pasteurella pestis* and *Staphylococcus aureus*, and inactive on *Escherichia coli*[PN086]. Chloroform extract of dried leaves, at a concentration of 1.0 gm/ml on agar plate, was inactive on *Bacillus subtilis*, *Escherichia coli*, *Pseudomonas aeruginosa*, and *Staphylococcus aureus*. The methanol extract was active on *Staphylococcus aureus*, and inactive on *Bacillus subtilis*, *Escherichia coli*, and *Pseudomonas aeruginosa*[PN060].

Antidiarrheal activity. Ethanol/water (1:1) extract of the dried aerial parts, at a concentration of 300 mg, was inactive for antidiarrheal activity on both guinea pig and rabbit ileums vs *Escherichia coli*-Inte Rotoxin-induced diarrhea[PN025].

Antifungal activity. Petroleum ether extract of whole plant produced antifungal activity on *Helminthosporium sativa*. The leaf extract produced antifungal activity on *Alternaria alternata*, and had no activity on *Curvalaria lunata*[PN051].

Antihepatotoxic activity. Hexane extract of dried aerial parts, at a concentration of 1.0 mg/ml in cell culture, was active on rat hepatocytes, results significant at $P < 0.01$ level vs CCl_4-induced hepatotoxicity. The extract was inactive vs galactosamine-induced toxicity[PN074]. Dried entire plant, administered by gastric intubation to sheep at a dose of 1.0 gm/kg, was active. The animals were dosed daily for 10 days after receiving the hepatotoxic paracetamol. A mixture of *Andrographis paniculata*, *Phyllanthus niruri*, and *Solanum nigrum* was used. Changes induced by toxin were ameliorated by treatment. Changes included anemia, leukocytosis with neutrophilia and lymphopenia, increased coagulation, decreased glucose, cholesterolemia, hypotriglyceridemia jaundice and elevation of AST and ALT[PN024]. Powdered dried entire plant, administered by gastric intubation to rats at a dose of 200.0 mg/kg, was active on liver homogenate vs ethanol-treated rats dosed for 45 days. Triglyceride, cholesterol and phospholipid contents in fatty liver were reduced to normal levels[PN036]. Water extract of dried leaves, administered by gastric intubation to rats at a concentration of 2.0 ml/kg, was active. The activity was as effective as pretreatment vs CCl_4-induced hepatotoxicity[PN075].

Antihypercholesterolemic activity. Dried entire plant, in the ration of rats, was active. Fatty liver was induced with alcohol. The plant material reduced the increased deposition of triglycerides, cholesterol and phospholipids in the liver, heart and kidney that resulted from alcohol treatment[PN078].

Antihyperglycemic activity. Water extract of dried entire plant, administered by gastric intubation to rats, was active vs alloxan-induced hyperglycemia[PN042].

Antihyperlipemic activity. Water extract of dried entire plant, in the ration of rats, was active. Fatty liver was induced with alcohol. The plant material reduced the increased deposition of triglycerides, cholesterol and phospholipids in the liver, heart, and kidney that resulted from the alcohol treatment[PN078].

Antimalarial activity. Ethanol extract of the entire plant produced more than 60% inhibition of *Plasmodium falciparum* growth, in vitro, at a test concentration of 6 microgram/ml[PN096]. The ethanolic, dichloromethane and lyophilized aqueous extracts of the whole plant were evaluated for its antimalarial activity in vivo, in 4-day, suppressive assays against *Plasmodium berghei* ANKA in mice. No toxic effect of mortality was observed in the mice treated, orally, as a single dose of 500 mg/kg body weight, or as the same dose given twice weekly for 4 weeks. No significant lesions were observed, by eye or during histopathological examinations, in the hearts, lungs, spleens, kidneys, livers, large intestines or brains of any mouse. At a dose of 200 mg/kg, the ethanolic and dichloro-methane extracts produced significant chemosuppressions of parasitaemia, when administered orally[PN097].

Antimutagenic activity. Water extract of dried leaves, administered by gastric intubation to mice at a dose of 10.0 ml/kg, was active vs nickle-induced clastogenicity[PN018].

Antipyretic activity. Ethanol/water (1:1) extract of the entire plant, administered by gastric intubation to rabbits at variable dosage levels, was inactive vs yeast-induced pyrexia[PN093].

Antispasmodic activity. Ethanol/water (1:1) extract of the entire plant was active on guinea pig ileum vs ACh- and histamine-induced spasms[PN003].

Antitumor activity. Ethanol/water (1:1) extract, administered intraperitoneally to mice, was active on LEUK (Friend Virus-Solid)[PN003]. Ethanol (95%) and water extracts of dried aerial parts, at doses of 100.0 mg/kg, were inactive on Sarcoma 180(ASC)[PN044].

Anti-urolithiasis effect. The aqueous extract of the plant, in vitro, exhibited a potent and effective non-concentration-dependent inhibitory effect on a model of CaOx crystal endocytosis by Madin-Darby canine kidney cells. The response was present even at very high (pathologic) CaOx concentrations and no toxic effect was detected[PN095].

Antiviral activity. Ethanol (95%) extract of dried aerial parts was active on hepatitis B virus. Antiviral activity was measured in serum of patients who were positive for the hepatitis B virus[PN046]. Water extract of the dried entire plant, administered to woodchucks at a dose of 9.0 mg/animal, was active vs hepatitis in long-term chronic carriers of woodchuck hepatitis. No effect was seen in either experimental or control animals. When experimental animals were later switched to intraperitoneal administration, two of them showed a drop in antigen titer (two others died of unrelated causes). No control animals showed any effects[PN094]. Water extract of the dried entire plant, administered by gastric intubation to woodchucks, was active on woodchuck hepatitis virus. Biological activity reported has been patented[PN035]. Water extract of the dried entire plant, administered intraperitoneally to woodchucks at a concentration of 9.0 mg/animal, was active vs hepatitis in recently infected woodchucks. Three out of 4 experimental animals showed elimination of woodchuck hepatitis surface antigen and woodchuck hepatitis DNA polymerize after 72 days. They remained negative for 300 days. Control animal did not show any change. Water extract of the dried entire plant, administered intraperitoneally to woodchucks at a concentration of 9.0 mg/animal, was active vs hepatitis in long-term chronic carriers of woodchuck hepatitis. Titer of woodchuck hepatitis surface antigen was lowered relative to untreated controls. Half of a ml of the extract was given once a week[PN094]. Water extract of dried entire plant (plants cultivated in USA), tested on hepatitis virus in cell culture, was inactive vs hepadnavirus DNA polymerase, IC_{50} 381.0 and 410.0 mcg/ml[PN038]. Ethanol (95%) extract of fresh entire plant, tested on Tobacco Mosaic virus in cell culture, was equivocal. The viral inhibitory activity was 7%[PN022]. Fresh leaf and fresh root extracts, at a concentration of 4.0%, were active on Peanut Mosaic virus, Tobacco Mosaic virus and Tobacco Ring Spot virus[PN073].

Cardiotoxic activity. Ethanol/water (1:1) extract of the entire plant, administered intravenously to dogs at variable concentrations, was inactive[PN093].

Chromosome aberration inhibition. Water extract of dried fruit and leaf, administered by gastric intubation to mice at a dose of 685.0 mg/kg, was active vs chromosome damage induced by lead nitrate and aluminum sulphate in bone marrow chromosomes. Dosing was for 7 days[PN047].

Chronotropic effect (positive). Ethanol/water (1:1) extract of the entire plant, administered to dogs intravenously at variable dosages, was inactive[PN093].

Cytotoxic activity. Ethanol/water (1:1) extract of entire plant, in cell culture, was inactive on CA-9KB, ED_{50} > 20.0 mcg/ml[PN003].

DNA polymerase inhibition. Water extract of dried entire plant, at a concentration of 50.0 mg/ml, was active vs activity of woodchuck hepatitis virus DNA polymerase; 50.0 mg/ml produced 25% inhibition. Methanol and water extracts, at variable dosages, were also active. The biological activity reported in these studies has been patented[PN035].

Hepatitis B surface antigen inactivation. Water extract of dried entire plant, at a concentration of 0.2 mg/ml, was active on hepatitis virus vs reaction of woodchuck hepatitis surface antigen with hepatitis B (Human) antibody. A concentration of 0.63 mg/ml was active on hepatitis B virus vs reaction of hepatitis B surface antigen with hepatitis B antibody[PN094]. Water and methanol extracts of the dried entire plant, at vari-

able concentrations, were active. The biological activity reported has been patented[PN035]. Water extract of dried leaves, was active. Hepatitis B surface antigen inactivation was assayed, IC_{50} 650 ng/ml. The methanol extract was also active, IC_{50} 1.2 mcg/ml. Water extract of dried leaves was active. Hepatitis B surface antigen inactivation was assayed, IC_{50} 3.30 mcg/ml[PN023]. Chloroform extract[PN059] and water extract[PN034] of dried leaves, stem and dried roots, at a concentration of 2.0%, were active.

Hypoglycemic activity. Water extract of the dried entire plant, administered orally to rabbits at a dose of 10.0 mg/kg, was inactive. A drop in blood sugar of 15 mg relative to inert-treated control indicated positive results[PN010].

Hypotensive activity. Ethanol/water (1:1) extract of the entire plant, administered intravenously to dogs at variable dosage levels, was inactive[PN093].

Molluscicidal activity. Ethanol (95%) extract of dried stem, at a concentration of 250.0 ppm, was inactive on *Biomphalaria pfeifferi* and *Bulinus truncatus*. Petroleum ether extract, at a concentration of 25.0 ppm, was active on *Biomphalaria pfeifferi* and *Bulinus truncatus*[PN062].

Nematocidal activity. Decoction of bark, at a concentration of 1.0 mg/ml, was active on *Toxacara canis*[PN048].

Reverse transcriptase inhibition. Water extract of the dried entire plant was active on HIV-1 virus, ID_{50} 50.0 mcg/ml[PN021].

Spasmolytic activity. Methanol extract of dried callus tissue, at a concentration of 320.0 mcg/ml, was inactive on guinea pig ileum vs ACh-induced contractions[PN026].

Toxicity assessment (quantitative). Ethanol/water (1:1) extract of the entire plant, administered orally to mice, tolerated a maximum dose of 1.0 gm/kg[PN003]. Water extract of the dried entire plant, at a dose of 0.1 mcg/animal, was inactive. No weight loss was found 7 days after treatment with the extract[PN094].

REFERENCES

PN001 Quisumbing, E. Medicinal plants of the Philippines. **Tech Bull 16**, Rep Philippines, Dept Agr Nat Resources, Manilla 1951; 1.

PN002 Anjaneyulu, A. S. R., K. J. Rao and C. Subrahmanyam. Crystalline constituents of Euphorbiaceae. XII. Isolation and structural elucidation of three new lignans from the leaves of *Phyllanthus niruri*. **Tetrahedron** 1973; 29: 1291.

PN003 Dhar, M. L., M. M. Dhar, B. N. Mehrotra and C. Ray. Screening of Indian plants for biological activity. Part 1. **Indian J Exp Biol** 1968; 6: 232–247.

PN004 Loustalot, A. J. and C. Pagan. Local "fever" plants tested for presence of alkaloids. **El Crisol (Puerto Rico)** 1949; 3(5): 3.

PN005 Anon. Description of the Philippines. Part I., Bureau of Public Printing, Manila, 1903.

PN006 Petelot, A. Les Plantes Medicinales du Cambodge, du Laos et du Vietnam, Volume 1–4. Archives Des Recherches Agronomiques et Pastorales au Vietnam No. 23, 1954.

PN007 Burkhill, I. H. Dictionary of the Economic Products of the Malay Peninsula. Ministry of Agriculture and Cooperatives, Kuala Lumpur, Malaysia. Volume II, 1966.

PN008 Ramachandra Row, L., P. Satyanarayana and C. Srinivasulu. Crystalline constituents of Euphor-biaceae – XI. Revised structure of hypophyllanthin from *Phyllanthus niruri*. **Tetrahedron** 1970; 26: 3051.

PN009 Chauhan, J. S., M. Sultan and S. K. Srivastava. Chemical investigation of the roots of *Phyllanthus niruri*. **J Indian Chem Soc** 1979; 56: 326.

PN010 Jain, S. R. and S. N. Sharma. Hypoglycaemic drugs of Indian indigenous origin. **Planta Med** 1967; 15(4): 439–442.

PN011 Satyanarayana, P., P. Subrahmanyam, K. N. Viswanatham and R. S. Ward. New seco- and hydroxy-lignans from *Phyllanthus niruri*. **J Nat Prod** 1988; 51(1): 44–49.

PN012 Singh, B., P. K. Agrawal and R. S. Thakur. A new lignan and a new neolignan from *Phyllanthus niruri*. **J Nat Prod** 1989; 52(1): 48–51.

PN013 Satyanarayana, P. and S. Venkateswarlu. Isolation, structure and synthesis of new diarylbutane lignans from *Phyllanthus niruri* – 1: Synthesis of 5'desmethoxy niranthin and an antitumor extractive. **Tetrahedron** 1991; 47(42): 8931–8940.

PN014 Huang, Y. L., C. C. Chen and J. C. Ou. Isolintetralin: A new lignan from *Phyllanthus niruri*. **Planta Med** 1992; 58(5): 473–474.

PN015 Singh, B., P. K. Agrawal and R. S. Thakur. Euphane triterpenoids from *Phyllanthus niruri*. **Indian J Chem Ser B** 1989; 28(4): 319–321.

PN016 Moreno, A. R. Two Hundred Sixty-Eight Medicinal Plants Used to Regulate Fertility in Some Countries of South America. Unpublished (Stenciled) Review in Spanish, 1975.

PN017 Luu, C. Notes on the traditional pharmacopoeia of French Guyana. **Plant Med Phytother** 1975; 9: 125–135.

PN018 Agarwa, K., H. Dhir, A. Sharma and G. Taluker. The efficacy of two species of Phyllanthus in counteracting nickel clastogenicity. **Fitoterapia** 1992; 63(1): 49–54.

PN019 Niguchi, H., T. Ogata and H. Matsumoto. Anti-retrovirus pharmaceuticals containing repandusinic acid A or its salts. **Patent-Japan Kokai Tokkyo Koho-**03 206,044 1991; 5pp.

PN020 Ishimaru, K., K. Yoshimatsu, T. Yamakawa, H. Kamada and K. Shimomura. Phenolic constituents in tissue cultures of *Phyllanthus niruri*. **Phytochemistry** 1992; 31(6): 2015–2018.

PN021 Ogata, T., H. Higuchi, S. Mochida, H. Matsumoto, A. Kato, T. Endo, A. Kaji and H. Kaji. HIV-1 reverse transcriptase inhibitor from *Phyllanthus niruri*. **AIDS Res Human Retroviruses** 1992; 8: 1937–1944.

PN022 Khan, M., D. C. Jain, R. S. Bhakuni, M. Zaim and R. S. Thakur. Occurrence of some antiviral sterols in *Artemisa annua*. **Plant Sci** 1991; 75: 161–165.

PN023 Pousset, J. L., J. P. Levesque, P. Coursaget and F. X. Galen. Hepatitis B surface antigen (HBSAg) inactivation and antiotension-converting enzyme

(ACE) inhibition in vitro by *Combretum glutinosum* Perr. (Combretaceae) extract. **Phytother Res** 1993; 7(1): 101–102.

PN024   Bhaumik, A. and M. C. Sharma. Therapeutic efficacy of two herbal preparations in induced hepatopathy in sheep. **J Res Indian Med** 1993; 12(1): 33–42.

PN025   Gupta, S., J. N. S. Yadava and J. S. Tandon. Antisecretory (antidiarrheal) activity of Indian medicinal plants against *Escherichia coli* enterotoxin-induced secretion in rabbit and guinea pig ileal loop models. **Int J Pharmacog** 1993; 31(3): 198–204.

PN026   Santo, A. R. S., V. C. Filho, R. Niero, A. M. Viana, F. N. Moreno, M. M. Campos, R. A. Yunes, J. B. Calixto. Analgesic effects of callus culture extracts from selected species of Phyllanthus in mice. **J Pharm Pharmacol** 1994; 46(9): 755–759.

PN027   Holdsworth, D and L. Balun. Medicinal plants of the East and West Sepik Provinces, Papau New Guinea. **Int J Pharmacog** 1992; 30(3): 218–222.

PN028   Santos, A. R. S., V. C. Filho, R. A. Yunes and J. B. Calixto. Further studies on the antinociceptive action of the hydroalcoholic extracts from plants on the genus Phyllanthus. **J Pharm Pharmacol** 1995; 47(1): 66–71.

PN029   Quader, M. A., M. Khatun and M. Mosihuzzaman. Isolation of 4-hydroxysesamin and ent-norsecurinine from *Phyllanthus niruri* and their chemotaxonomic significance. **J Bangladesh Acad Sci** 1994; 18(2): 229–234.

PN030   Chauhan, J. S., M. Sultan and S. K. Srivastava. Two new glycoflavones from the roots of the *Phyllanthus niruri*. **Planta Med Suppl** 1977; 32: 217–222.

PN031   Tea Keth Nara, J. Gleye, E. Lavergne de Cerval and E. Stanislas. Flavonoids of *Phyllanthus niruri*, *Phyllanthus urinaria*, and *Phyllanthus orbiculatus*. **Plant Med Phytother** 1977; 11: 82.

PN032   Sinha, S. K. P. and J. V. V. Dogra. Variation in the level of vitamin C, total phenolics and protein in *Phyllanthus niruri* Linn. during leaf maturation. **Natl Acad Sci Lett (India)** 1981; 4(12): 467–469.

PN033   Singh, B., P. K. Agrawal and R. S. Thakur. Chemical constituents of *Phyllanthus niruri* Linn. **Indian J Chem Ser B** 1986; 25: 600–602.

PN034   Thyagarajan, S. P., K. Thiruneelakantan, S. Subramanian and T. Sundaravelu. In vitro inactivation of HBSAg by *Eclipta alba* Hassk. and *Phyllanthus niruri* Linn. **Indian J Med Res Suppl** 1982; 76S: 124–130.

PN035   Venkateswaran, P. S., I. Millman and B. S. Blumberg. Composition, pharmaceutical preparation and method for treating viral hepatitis. **Patent-US-4,673,575** 1987; 10pp.

PN036   Umarani, D., T. Devaki, P. Govindaraju and K. R. Shanmugasundaram. Ethanol induced metabolic alterations and the effect of *Phyllanthus niruri* in their reversal. **Ancient Sci Life** 1985; 4(3): 174–180.

PN037   Kitisin, T. Pharmacological studies. 3. *Phyllanthus niruri*. **Siriraj Hospital Gaz** 1952; 4: 641–649.

PN038   Ueno, H., S. Horie, Y. Nishi, H. Shogawa, M. Kawasaki, S. Suzuki et al. Chemical and pharmaceutical studies on medicinal plants in Paraguay. Geraniin, an angiotensin-converting enzyme inhibitor from "paraparai mi," *Phyllanthus niruri*. **J Nat Prod** 1988; 51(2): 357–359.

PN039   Ahmad, M. U., S. K. Husain and S. M. Osman. Ricinoleic acid in *Phyllanthus niruri* seed oil. **J Amer Oil Chem Soc** 1981; 58(6): 673–674.

PN040   Shimizu, M., S. Horie, S. Terashima, H. Ueno, T. Hayashi, M. Arisawa, S. Suzuki, M. Yoshizaki and N. Morita. Studies on aldose reductase inhibitors from natural products. II. Active components of a Paraguayan crude drug "para-parai mi", *Phyllanthus niruri*. **Chem Pharm Bull** 1989; 37(9): 2531–2532.

PN041   Nara, T. K., J. Gleye, E. L. de Cerval and E. Stanislas. Flavonoides de *Phyllanthus niruri* L., *Phyllanthus urinaria* L., *Phyllanthus orbiculatus* L. C. Rich. **Plant Med Phytother** 1977; 11(2): 82–86.

PN042   Hukeri, V. I., G. A. Kalyani and H. K. Kakrani. Hypoglycemic activity of flavonoids of *Phyllanthus fraternus* in rats. **Fitoterapia** 1988; 59(1): 68–70.

PN043   Holdsworth, D., O. Gideon and B. Pilokos. Traditional medicine of New Ireland, Papau New Guinea Part III Konos, Central New Ireland. **Int J Crude Drug Res** 1989; 27(1): 55–61.

PN044   Itokawa, H., F. Hirayama, S. Tsuruoka, K. Mizuno, K. Takeya and A. Nitta. Screening test for antitumor activity of crude drugs (III). Studies on antitumor activity of Indonesian medicinal plants. **Shoyakugaku Zasshi** 1990; 44(1): 58–62.

PN045   Jain, S. P. Tribal remedies from Saranda Forest, Bihar, India. 1. **Int J Crude Drug Res** 1989; 27(1): 29–32.

PN046   Mehrotra, R., S. Rawat, D. K. Kulshreshtha, G. K. Patnaik and B. N. Dhawan. In vitro studies on the effect of certain natural products against hepatitis B virus. **Indian J Med Res B** 1990; 92(2): 133–138.

PN047   Dhir, H., A. K. Roy, A. Shama and G. Talukder. Protection afforded by aqueous extracts of Phyllanthus species against cytotoxicity induced by lead and aluminum salts. **Phytother Res** 1990: 4(5): 172–176.

PN048   Kiuchi, F., M. Hioki, N. Nakamura, N. Miyashita, Y. Tsuda and K. Kondo. Screening of crude drugs used in Sri Lanka for nematocidal activity on the larva of *Toxacaria canis*. **Shoyakugaku Zasshi** 1989; 43(4): 288–293.

PN049   Singh, B., P. K. Agrawal and S. Thakur. Isolation of trans-phytol from *Phyllanthus niruri*. **Planta Med** 1991; 57(1): 98.

PN050   Mannan, A. and K. Ahmad. A short note on the occurrence of sex hormones in Bangladesh plants. **Bangladesh J Biol Sci** 1976; 5: 45.

PN051   Bhatnagar, S. S., H. Santapau, J. D. H. Desa et al. Biological activity of Indian Medicinal Plants. Part 1. Antibacterial, antitubercular, and anti-fungal action. **Indian J Med Res** 1961; 49: 799.

PN052   Halberstein, R. A. and A. B. Saunders. Traditional medical practices and medicinal plant usage on a Bahamian Island. **Cul Med Psychiat** 1978; 2: 177–203.

PN053   Ayensu, E. S. Medicinal plants of the West Indies. **Unpublished Manuscript** 1978; 110pp.

PN054   Chauhan, J. S., M. sultan and S. K. Srivastava. Chemical investigation of the roots of *Phyllanthus niruri*. **J Indian Chem Soc** 1979; 56: 326A.

PN055   Cuellar Cuellar, A. and P. F. Estevez. A preliminary phytochemical study of Cuban plants. V. *Phyllanthus niruri* Euforbiaceae. **Rev Cubana Farm** 1980; 14: 63–68.

PN056   Ganeshpure, P. A., G. E. Schneiders and R. Stevenson. Structure and synthesis of hypophyllanthin, nirtetralin, phytetralin and lintetralin. **Tetrahedron** 1981; 22: 393–396.

PN057   Ahmad, M. U., S. K. Husain and S. M. Osman. Ricinoleic acid in *Phyllanthus niruri* seed oil. **J Amer Oil Chem Soc** 1981; 58: 673–674.

PN058   Weninger, B., M. Haag-Berrurier and R. Anton. Plants of Haiti used as anti-fertility agents. **J Ethnopharmacol** 1982; 6(1): 67–84.

PN059   Thyagarajan, S. P., K. Thiruneelakantan, S. Subramanian and T. Sundaravelu. In vitro inactivation of HBSAg by *Eclipta alba* Hassk. and *Phyllanthus niruri* Linn. **Indian J Med Res Suppl** 1982; 76: 124–130.

PN060   Farouk, A., A. K. Bashir and A. K. M. Salih. Antimicrobial activity of certain Sudanese plants used in folkloric medicine. Screening for antibacterial activity (I). **Fitoterapia** 1983; 54(1): 3–7.

PN061   Holdsworth, D. and B. Wamoi. Medicinal plants of the Admiralty Islands, Papau, New Guinea. Part I. **Int J Crude Drug Res** 1982; 20(4): 169–181.

PN062   Ahmed, E. M., A. K. Bashir and Y. M. El Kheir. Investigations of molluscicidal activity of certain Sudanese plants used in folk-medicine. Part IV. **Planta Med** 1984; 1: 74–77.

PN063   Gupta, D. R. and B. Ahmed. A new flavone glycoside from *Phyllanthus niruri* Linn. **Shoyakugaku Zasshi** 1984; 38(3): 213–215.

PN064   John, D. One hundred useful raw drugs of the Kani Tribes of Trivandrum Forest Division, Kerala, India. **Int J Crude Drug Res** 1984; 22(1): 17–39.

PN065   Mulchandani, N. B. and S. A. Hassarajani. 4-Methoxy-nor-securinine, a new alkaloid from *Phyllanthus niruri*. **Planta Med** 1984; 1: 104,105.

PN066   Gupta, D. R. and B. Ahmed. Nirurin: A new prenylated flavanone glycoside from *Phyllanthus niruri*. **J Nat Prod** 1984; 47(6): 958–963.

PN067   Holdsworth, D. Phytomedicine of the Madang Province, Papua, New Guinea Part I. Karkar Island. **Int J Crude Drug Res** 1984; 22(3): 111–119.

PN068   Sircar, N. N. Pharmaco-therapeutics of Dasemani drugs. **Ancient Sci Life** 1984; 3(3): 132–135.

PN069   Velazco, E. A. Herbal and traditional practices related to maternal and child health care. **Rural Reconstruction Review** 1980; 35–39.

PN070   Sahu, T. R. Less known uses of weeds as medicinal plants. **Ancient Sci Life** 1984; 3(4): 245–249.

PN071   Khan, M. R., G. Ndaalio, M. H. H. Nkunya, H. Wevers. Studies on the rationale of African traditional medicine. Part II. Preliminary screening of medicinal plants for anti-gonoccoci activity. **Pak J Sci Ind Res** 1978; 27(5/6): 189–192.

PN072   Singh, Y. N. Traditional medicine in Fiji. Some herbal folk cures used by Fiji Indians. **J Ethnopharmacol.** 1986; 15(1): 57–88.

PN073   Saigopal, D. V. R., V. S. Prasad and P. Sreenivasulu. Antiviral activity in extracts of *Phyllanthus fraternus* Webst. (*P. niruri*). **Curr Sci** 1986; 55(5): 264–265.

PN074   Syamasundar, K. V., B. Singh, R. S. Thakur, A. Husain, Y. Kiso and H. Hikino. Antihepatotoxic principles of *Phyllanthus niruri* herbs. **J Ethnopharmacol** 1985; 14(1): 41–44.

PN075   Rao, Y. S. Experimental production of liver damage and its protection with *Phyllanthus niruri* and *Capparis spinosa* (both ingredients of LIV.52) in white albino rats. **Probe** 1985; 117–119.

PN076   Petchnaree, P., N. Bunyapraphatsara, G. A. Cordell, H. J. Cowe, P. J. Cox, R. A. Howie and S. L. Patt. X-ray crystal and molecular structure of nirurine, a novel alkaloid related to the securinega alkaloid skeleton, from *Phyllanthus niruri* (Euphorbiaceae). **J Chem Soc Perkin Trans I** 1986; 1551–1556.

PN077   Weniger, B., M. Rouzier, R. Daguilh, D. Henrys, J. H. Henrys and R. Anthon. Popular medicine of the Central Plateau of Haiti. 2. Ethnopharmacological inventory. **J Ethnopharmacol** 1986; 17(1): 13–30.

PN078   Umarani, D., T. Devaki, P. Govindaraju and K. R. Shanmugasundaram. Ethanol induced metabolic alterations and the effect of *Phyllanthus niruri* in their reversal. **Ancient Sci Life** 1985; 4(3): 174–180.

PN079   Ramirez, V. R., L. J. Mostacero, A. E. Garcia, C. F. Mejia, P. F. Pelaez, C. D. Medina and C. H. Miranda. Vegetales empleados en medicina tradicional Norperuana. **Banco Agrario Del Peru & NACL Univ Trujillo**, Peru, June 1988; 54pp.

PN080   Hirschmann, G. S. and A. Rojas de Arias. A survey of medicinal plants of Minas Gerais, Brazil. **J Ethnopharmacol** 1990; 29(2): 159–172.

PN081   Ramachandra, Row, L., C. Srinivasulu, M. Smith and G. S. R. Subba Rao. Crystalline constituents of Euphorbiaceae. V. New lignans from *Phyllanthus niruri*. The constitution of phyllanthin. **Tetrahedron** 1966; 22: 2899.

PN082   Rouffiac, R. and J. Parello. Chemical study of the alkaloids of *Phyllanthus niruri* L. (Euphobiaceae). Presence of the optical antipode of norsecurinine. **Plant Med Phytother** 1969; 3: 220–223.

PN083   Freise, F. W. Essential oils from Brazilian Euphorbiaceae. **Perfum Essent Oil Rec** 1935; 26: 219.

PN084   Ricardo, M. S. Investigation of quinine in *Phyllanthus niruri*. **Anales Univ Santo Domingo** 1944; 8: 295.

PN085   Oakes, A. J. and M. P. Morris. The West Indian weedwoman of the United States Virgin Islands. **Bull Hist Med** 1958; 32: 164.

PN086   Collier, W. A. and L. Van De Piji. The antibiotic action of plants, especially the higher plants, with results with Indonesian plants. **Chron Nat** 1949; 105: 8.

PN087   Krishnamurti, G. V. and T. R. Seshadri. The bitter principle of *Phyllanthus niruri*. **Proc Indian Acad Sci Ser A** 1946; 24: 357–364.

PN088   Asprey, G. F. and P. Thornton. Medicinal plants of Jamaica. III. **West Indian Med J** 1955; 4: 69–82.

PN089 Stanislas, E., R. Rouffiac and J. J. Foyard. *Phyllanthus niruri* alkaloids, flavonoids, and lignans. **Plant Med Phytother** 1967; 1: 136–141.

PN090 Dragendorff, G. Die Heilpflanzen der Verschiedenen Volker und Zeiten, F. Enke, Stuttgart, Book 1898; 885pp.

PN091 Schultes, R. E. De plantis toxicariis a mundo novo tropicale commentationes. IV. **Bot Mus Leafl Harv Univ** 1969; 22(4): 133–164.

PN092 Wasuwat, S. A list of Thai medicinal plants, ASRCT, Bangkok, Report No. 1 on Res. Project. 17. ASRCT Bangkok Thailand 1967; 17: 22pp.

PN093 Mokkhasmit, M., K. Swasdimongkol, W. Ngarmwathana and U. Permphiphat. Pharmacological evaluation of Thai medicinal plants. (Continued). **J Med Assoc Thailand** 1971; 54(7): 490–504.

PN094 Venkateswaran, P. S., I. Millman and B. S. Blumberg. Effects of an extract from *Phyllanthus niruri* on hepatitis B and woodchuck hepatitis viruses: In vitro and in vivo studies. **Proc Nat Acad Sci (USA)** 1987; 84(1): 274–278.

PN095 Campos, A. H. and N. Schor. *Phyllanthus niruri* inhibits calcium oxalate endocytosis by renal tubular cells: its role in urolithiasis. **Nephron** 1999; 81(4): 393–397.

PN096 Tona, L., N. P. Ngimbi, M. Tsakala, K. Mesia, K. Cimaga, S. Apers, T. De Bruyne, L. Pieters, J. Totte and A. S. J. Vlietinck. Antimalarial activity of 20 crude extracts from nine African medicinal plants used in Kinshasa, Congo. **J Ethnopharmacol** 1999; 68(1-3): 193–203.

PN097 Tona, L., K. Mesia, N. P. Ngimbi, B. Chrimwami, Okond'ahoka, K. Cimanga, T. de Bruyne, S. Apers, N. Hermans, J. Totte, L. Pieters and A. J, Vlietinck. In-vivo antimalarial activity of *Cassia occidentalis, Morinda morindoides* and *Phyllanthus niruru*. **Ann Trop Med Parasitol** 2001; 95(1): 47–57.

23 | Portulaca oleracea

L.

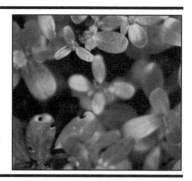

Common Names

Amloniya	Fiji	Makabling	West Indies
Baldroegas	Madeira	Mutunu	Tanzania
Baraloniya	Fiji	Olasiman	West Indies
Barbin	Qatar	Pappukura	India
Barbir	Qatar	Pigweed	Fiji
Beldroega	Brazil	Portulaca	Italy
Beldroegas	Madeira	Posely	Nicaragua
Bredo de porco	Brazil	Pourpier	Dominica
Buklut-ul-hakima	India	Pourpier	West Indies
Burra-lonia	India	Purchiacchella	Italy
Common purslane	Madeira	Purslane	Dominica
Common purslane	USA	Purslane	Europe
Coupie	Dominica	Purslane	Jamaica
Coupie	West Indies	Purslane	Netherlands
Croupier	French Guiana	Purslane	USA
Demze	Guinea	Purslane	West Indies
Dorcellana	Italy	Pusley	Europe
Erba vasciulella	Italy	Pusley	Guyana
Farfena	Oman	Pusley	Virgin Islands
Goni	India	Pussley	West Indies
Khurfa	India	Pussly	Jamaica
Khursa	Fiji	Pussly	West Indies
Khutura	India	Rigia	Qatar
Koolfa	India	Rigla	Egypt
Koupye	Haiti	Shoi-bee-reum	Egypt
Kulfa	India	Small purslain	India
Kupye	West Indies	Suvandacheera	India
Kurfa	India	Tarbari	India
Langiruh	Brunei	Tokmakan	Turkey
Lonika	India	Tukhm khurfa	Pakistan
Loonia	India	Verdolaga	Brazil
Lulimilwasenga	Tanzania	Verdolaga	Canary Islands
Machixian	China	Verdolaga	Cuba

From: *Medicinal Plants of the World, vol. 1: Chemical Constituents, Traditional and Modern Medicinal Uses, 2nd ed.*
By: Ivan A. Ross © Humana Press Inc., Totowa, NJ

Verdolaga	Nicaragua	Verdolaga	Spain
Verdolaga	Peru	Verdulaga	Spain
Verdolaga	Puerto Rico		

BOTANICAL DESCRIPTION

An annual, prostrate or spreading, succulent, branched herb of the PORTULACAEAE family; quite glabrous; 10–50 cm long. The stems are often purplish. Leaves are fleshy and flat, obtuse, oblong-obovate, base cuneate, 1 to 2.5 cm long. Flowers are sessile, axillary and terminal with few-flowered heads. The heads are solitary or cymose, the buds compressed. Petals: five, yellow and about as long as the sepals. Stamens: 8–12.

ORIGIN AND DISTRIBUTION

A very common weed of cultivated and undisturbed land. Native to the Old World tropics. Now found in both temperate and tropical zones, from South Europe where it is cultivated as a vegetable, to China.

TRADITIONAL MEDICINAL USES

Brazil. Seeds are taken orally as an emmenagogue[PO072]. The wilted entire plant is said to cause death in cattle when ingested[PO008].

Canary Islands. Hot water extract of dried aerial parts is taken orally as a diuretic, calculolithic and for migraine[PO062].

China. Hot water extract of leaves is taken orally for arthritis. Hot water extract of stem is taken orally for arthritis[PO077].

Dominica. Leaves are employed as a plaster to ease pain of menstruation[PO067].

Europe. Aerial parts have been eaten as a vegetable since early Roman times[PO070].

Fiji. Dried leaf and stem are taken orally for stomachache and paralysis[PO049].

French Guiana. Hot water extract of leaves is taken orally as a cholagogue[PO018]..

Haiti. Decoction of the dried leaves is taken orally for asthenia[PO052].

Hawaii. Water extract of plant is taken orally for asthma[PO028]..

India. Hot water extract of dried leaves is taken orally as a diuretic and for liver diseases[PO042]. Leaves and shoot are cooked as a vegetable[PO029,PO036]. Seeds are taken orally as a vermifuge[PO042]. Seeds steeped in wine are taken orally as an emmenagogue. In Ayurvedic and Unani medicine, the seeds are taken orally as a vermifuge[PO040], and the shoots are used as food[PO086].

Indo-China. Seeds are taken orally to provoke menses[PO001].

Italy. Decoction of dried leaves is taken orally as a diuretic and for gastronomic purposes[PO064].

Jamaica. Hot water extract of entire plant is taken orally as a vermifuge[PO068].

Malaysia. Hot water extract of dried entire plant is taken orally for chest pain[PO045].

New Caledonia. Seeds are taken orally as an emmenagogue[PO006].

Nigeria. Hot water extract of fresh entire plant is taken orally as a sedative and heart tonic[PO041]. Hot water extract of fresh leaves and stem is taken orally for muscular aches and pains[PO053].

Peru. Hot water extracts of dried seeds and of dried stems are taken orally as an antiscorbutic, antidysenteric, emmenagogue and vermifuge, and for jaundice[PO057].

Sierra Leone. Infusion of dried leaves is taken orally with palm oil as an abortifacient[PO046].

Tanzania. Decoction of hot water extract of the entire plant is washed over the breasts as a galactagogue[PO010].

Virgin Islands. Hot water extract of aerial parts is taken orally for intestinal worms[PO065].

West Indies. Hot water extract of aerial parts is taken orally to provoke menses[PO007]. Hot water extract of leaves is taken orally for painful menstruation[PO038]. Seeds are taken orally to provoke menses[PO001].

CHEMICAL CONSTITUENTS

(ppm unless otherwise indicated)

Alanine: Pl[PO017]
Alpha tocopherol: Lf[PO020]
Ascorbic acid: Aer[PO044,PO071,PO047], Lf[PO020]
Aspartic acid: Pl[PO039]
Behenic acid: Sd oil[PO031]
Beta amyrin: Aer[PO019]
Beta carotene: Lf 220–300[PO080,PO020]
Beta sitosterol: Aer[PO019]
Caffeic acid: Pl[PO025]
Campesterol: Aer[PO019]
Capric acid: Aer[PO019]
Cinnamic acid: Lf, St[PO025]
Citric acid: Lf, St[PO025]
Digalactosyldiacyl glycerol: Lf[PO020]
DNA: Pl[PO030], Sd[PO037]
Fatty acids: Lf[PO020]
Ferulic acid: Pl[PO015]
Iso-palmitic acid: Aer[PO019]
Kaempferol: Aer[PO021]
KCL: Pl[PO009]
Lauric acid: Aer[PO019], Sd oil[PO031]
Linoleic acid: Aer[PO019], Sd oil[PO031]
Linolenic acid: Sd oil[PO031]
Linolenic acid (Omega-3): Aer[PO032]
Malic acid: Pl 0.5%[PO039,PO025]
Monogalactosyl-diactyl glycerol: Lf[PO020]
Myristic acid: Aer[PO019], Sd oil[PO031]
Norepinephrine: Aer[PO013]
Oleic acid: Aer[PO019], Sd oil[PO031]
Oleracin-I: Pl[PO015], St[PO076]
Oleracin-II: Pl[PO015], St[PO076]
Oxalic acid: Aer[PO075], Pl[PO009]
Palmitic acid: Aer[PO019], Sd oil[PO031]
Palmitoleic acid: Aer[PO019], Sd oil[PO031]
Phorbic acid: Lf[PO074]
Phosphatidyl choline: Lf[PO020]
Phosphatidyl glycerol: Lf[PO020]
Phosphatidyl inositol: Lf[PO020]
Phosphatidyl serine: Lf[PO020]
Phosphatidyl ethanolamine: Pl[PO020]
Portulaca polysaccharide: Lf, St[PO034]
Potassium oxalate: Lf, St[PO025]
Protein: Seedling[PO037]
Quercetin: Aer[PO021], Lf, St[PO025]
RNA: Seedling[PO037]
Stearic acid: Aer[PO019]
Stigmasterol: Aer[PO019]
Vitamin A: Aer[PO047]

PHARMACOLOGICAL ACTIVITIES AND CLINICAL TRIALS

Aldose reductase inhibition. Hot water extract of dried aerial parts, at a concentration of 0.01 mg/ml, was inactive. The effect was tested on bovine lens aldase reductase[PO022].

Analgesic activity. Ethanol (95%) extract of fresh leaves, administered intragastrically to mice at a dose of 1.0 gm/kg, was active vs benzoyl peroxide-induced writhing and inactive vs tail-flick response to hot water[PO061]. Ethanol (10%) extract of the aerial parts (dried leaves and stem), administered intraperitoneally and topically, produced significant activity when compared with the synthetic drug, diclofenac sodium as the positive control[PO081].

Antiandrogenic effect. Ethanol (95%) extract of dried seeds, administered subcutaneously to mice at a dose of 50.0 mg/animal, was active[PO043].

Antibacterial activity. Acetone extract of dried leaves, undiluted on agar plate, was active on *Pseudomonas aeruginosa* and *Salmonella* B, and inactive on *Salmonella newport*, *Escherichia coli*, *Salmonella typhi*, *Sarcina lutea*, *Serratia marcescens*, *Shigella flexneri*, *Staphylococcus albus*, and *Staphylococcus aureus*. Ethanol (95%) extract was active on *Escherichia coli*, *Pseudomonas aeruginosa*, *Salmonella typhi*, *Sarcina lutea*, *Serratia marcescens*, *Shigella flexneri*, *Staphylococcus albus*, and *Staphylococcus aureus*; and inactive on *Salmonella* B and *Salmonella newport*. Water extract was active on *Escherichia coli*, *Pseudomonas aeruginosa*, *Serratia marcescens* and *Shigella flexneri*; inactive on *Salmonella* B, *Salmonella newport*, *Salmonella typhi*, *Sarcina lutea*, *Staphylococcus albus*, and *Staphylococcus aureus*. Acetone extract of dried stem, undiluted on agar plate, was active on *Salmonella* B, *Salmonella typhi*, *Serratia marcescens* and *Staphylococcus albus*; inactive on *Escherichia coli*, *Pseudomonas aeruginosa*, *Salmonella newport*, *Sarcina lutea*, *Shigella* *flexneri*, and *Staphylococcus aureus*. Ethanol (95%) extract was active on *Escherichia coli*, *Pseudomonas aeruginosa*, *Salmonella* B, *Salmonella typhi*, *Sarcina lutea*, *Serratia marcescens*, *Shigella flexneri*, *Staphylococcus albus* and *Staphylococcus aureus*; inactive on *Salmonella newport*. Water extract was active on *Escherichia coli*, *Salmonella newport*, *Salmonella typhi*, *Serratia marcescens*, *Shigella flexneri*, and *Staphylococcus aureus*; inactive on *Pseudomonas aeruginosa*, *Salmonella* B, *Sarcina lutea* and *Staphylococcus albus*[PO063]. Hot water and methanol extracts of the aerial parts, at a concentration of 1.2 mg/disc on agar plate, were inactive on *Streptococcus mutans* strains MT5091 and OMZ176[PO055]. Hot water extract of entire plant, on agar plate, was inactive on *Alcaligenes calcoaceticus*, *Escherichia coli*, *Klebsiella pneumonia*, *Proteus vulgaris*, *Pseudomonas aeruginosa*, *Salmonella typhimurium*, *Staphylococcus aureus* and *Streptococcus faecalis*, MIC > 1600 mcg/ml[PO050].

Anticonvulsant activity. Ethanol (70%) extract of fresh entire plant, administered intraperitoneally to mice of both sexes at variable dosage levels, was inactive vs metrazole- and strychnine-induced convulsions[PO041].

Antifertility effect. Hot water extract of entire plant, administered subcutaneously to female mice, was inactive[PO004].

Antifungal activity. Acetone, ether, ethanol (95%) and chloroform extracts of the dried aerial parts, on agar plate, were inactive on *Trichophyton rubrum*[PO073]. Water extract of fresh shoots, undiluted on agar plate, was equivocal on *Helminthosporium turcicum*[PO066]. Ethyl acetate extract of the plant produced a specific activity against dermatophytes of the genera Trichophyton[PO079].

Antihyperglycemic activity. Dried entire plant, administered intragastrically to rabbits at a dose of 2.0 gm/kg, was inactive vs alloxan-induced hyperglycemia[PO035].

Antiinflammatory activity. Ethanol (10%) extract of the aerial parts (dried leaves and stem), administered intraperitoneally and topically, produced significant activity when compared with the synthetic drug, diclofenac sodium as the positive control[PO081].

Antimycobacterial activity. Hot water extract of entire plant, on agar plate, was inactive on *Mycobacterium smegmatis*[PO050]. Leaf juice, on agar plate, produced weak activity on *Mycobacterium tuberculosis*, MIC < 1:40[PO005].

Antinematodal activity. Ethanol (95%) extract of entire plant was active on *Meloidogyne incognita*[PO012].

Antispermatogenic effect. Ethanol (95%) extract of dried seeds, administered subcutaneously to mice at a dose of 50.0 mg/animal, was active[PO043].

Antitumor activity. Ethanol/chloroform extract of fresh entire plant, administered intraperitoneally to mice at a dose of 360.0 mg/kg, was inactive on CA-755 and Leuk-L1210. A dose of 450.0 mg/kg was inactive on Sarcoma 180(ASC)[PO069]. Water extract of dried entire plant, administered intraperitoneally to mice at a dose of 150.0 mg/kg on days 5, 6 and 7, was active on CA-Ehrlich-ascites. The methanol extract produced weak activity[PO014].

Antiulcer activity. Methanol extract of dried aerial parts, administered intragastrically to mice at a dose of 2.0 gm/kg, was inactive vs stress-induced ulcers (water-immersions)[PO033].

Antiviral activity. Hot water extract of dried aerial parts, at a concentration of 0.5 mg/ml in VERO cell cultures, was inactive on Herpes simplex 1 virus, measles virus and poliovirus[PO024].

Antiyeast activity. Hot water extract of entire plant, on agar plate, was inactive on *Candida albicans*[PO050].

Chronotropic effect (negative). Water extract of fresh leaves and stem, at a concentration of 0.55 mg/ml, was active on rabbit atrium. The effect was not inhibited by atropine. It affected both spontaneously beating and electrically paced atria. The effect was reversed by the addition of calcium[PO056].

CNS Depressant activity. Ethanol (defatted with petroleum ether) extract of entire plant, administered intraperitoneally to mice at a dose of 1.0 gm/kg, produced weak activity[PO002].

Cytotoxic activity. Methanol extract of dried leaves, at a concentration of 100.0 mcg/ml in cell culture, was inactive on Chinese hamster V79 cells[PO027].

Hypertensive activity. Water extract of fresh leaves and stem, administered intravenously to rats at a dose of 1.4 mg/kg, was active. Effect abolished by phentolamine, reduced by propranolol and unaffected by atropine[PO056].

Hypoglycemic activity. Dried entire plant, administered intragastrically to rabbits at doses of 0.5 and 1.0 gm/kg, produced no effect after 4, 8 and 25 hours. At doses of 1.5 and 2.0 gm/kg, significant effect was observed after 8 and 12 hours[PO035]. Seeds, in a mixture with 7 other plants, administered orally to male rats at a dose of 4.0 gm/animal, were active[PO016].

Hypotensive activity. Ethanol (95%) and water extracts of leaves and stem, administered intravenously to dogs at doses of 0.1 ml/kg, were active[PO003].

Hypothermic activity. Methanol extract of dried aerial parts, administered intragastrically to mice at a dose of 2.0 gm/kg, was inactive[PO033].

Inotropic effect (negative). Water extract of fresh leaves and stem, at a concentration of 0.55 mg/ml, was active on the rabbit atrium. The effect was not inhibited by atropine and affected both spontaneously beating and electrically paced atria. The effect was reversed by the addition of calcium[PO056].

Molluscicidal activity. Aqueous slurry (homogenate) of fresh fruit, fresh leaves and fresh roots were inactive on *Lymnaea columella* and *Lymnaea cubensis*, LD_{100} > 1000 ppm[PO078].

Neuropharmacological effect. Ethanol (10%) extract of the plant, administered intraperitoneally to rats and mice, produced significant reduction in the locomotor activity in mice; anti-nociceptive activity in rats using Tail Flick Method, and increase in the onset of pentylenetetrazole-induced convulsions in mice and muscle relaxant activity in in vitro and in vivo experiments. The anti-nociceptive activity of the extract in rats was attenuated by naloxone pre-treatment indicating the involvement of opioid receptors in its anti-nociceptive effects[PO082].

Paralyzing activity. Ethanol (95%) extract of frozen leaves, at a concentration of 2.0 mg/ml, was active on chicken nerve-muscle preparation. Augmentation was followed by blockade. The effect was simulated by K^+, which appears to be the active species[PO026].

Plaque formation suppressant. Water and methanol/water (1:1) extracts of dried aerial parts, at a concentration of 0.1 mg/ml, produced weak activity on *Streptococcus mutans*. The methanol extract was active[PO048].

Platelet activating factor binding inhibition. Methanol extract of dried entire plant, at a dose of 400.0 mcg/ml, produced weak activity on rabbit platelets[PO023].

Skeletal muscle relaxing activity. Aqueous (dialyzed) fresh leaf and stem, at concentrations of 2.0 and 1.81 mg/ml, were active on rat phrenic nerve (diaphragm) vs K^+- and electrically-induced contractions, respectively. A dose of 30.0 mg/animal, administered intravenously to chicks, was active vs electrically-induced contractions. Ether extract, at concentration of 5.0 mg/ml, was active vs K^+, caffeine and electrically-induced contractions[PO059]. Water extract, at a concentration of 3.0 mg/ml, was active on frog sciatic nerve, sartorius muscle, rat rectus abdominus and phrenic nerve (diaphragm)[PO053]. Methanol extract, at a dose of 3.0 mg/ml, was active on rat phrenic nerve (diaphragm) vs caffeine- and electrically-induced contractions, IC_{50} 2.16

mg/ml[PO059]. Water extract, administered intraperitoneally to rat at a dose of 200 mg/kg, was active. A dose of 5.0 gm/kg, administered orally to rat, produced weak activity[PO051]. A dose of 70.0 mg/person, used externally on human adults, was active vs resting and partially contracted muscles, and maximally contracted muscle in healthy subjects[PO060]. Hot water extract of fresh leaves, at a concentration 3.0 mg/ml, was active on frog rectus abdominus and rat phrenic nerve (diaphragm). Methanol extract, at a concentration of 2.2 mg/ml, was active on frog rectus abdominus and rat phrenic nerve (diaphragm)[PO054].

Skeletal muscle stimulant activity. Aqueous (dialyzed) fresh leaf and stem, at a concentration of 0.82 mg/ml, was active on rat phrenic nerve (diaphragm). A concentration of 1.2 mg/ml was active on rat rectus abdominus. Ether extract, at a concentration of 1.66 mg/ml, was active on rat phrenic nerve (diaphragm), and a concentration of 8.2 mg/ml was active on rat rectus abdominus. Water extract, at a concentration of 2.5 mg/ml and methanol extract at a concentration of 1.03 mg/ml, were active on rat phrenic nerve (diaphragm). The methanol extract, at a concentration of 5.8 mg/ml, was active on rat rectus abdominus. Twitch tension occurred before relaxation in each case vs electrically induced contractions[PO058].

Smooth muscle relaxant activity. Ethanol (95%) and water extracts of leaves and stem, at a concentration of 0.33 ml/liter, were active on rabbit duodenum[PO003]. Water extract of fresh leaves and stem, at a concentration of 0.03 mg/m, was active on guinea pig taenia coli. A concentration of 0.05 mg/ml was active on guinea pig fundus (stomach). The activities were reduced by phentolamine, and further reduced with the addition of propranolol. A concentration of 0.025 mg/ml was active on rabbit jejunum. The activity was reduced by phentolamine,

further reduced with the addition of propranolol, and unaffected by guanethidine or tetrodoxin[PO060]. A concentration of 0.02 mg/ml was active on rabbit aorta, attenuated or inhibited by phentolamine and unaffected by guanethidine or tetrodoxin[PO056]. When applied externally at a dose of 70.0 mg/person, the extract was active vs maximally contracted muscle in patients with spasticity[PO060].

Spasmogenic activity. Ethanol (95%) and water extracts of leaves and stem, administered intraperitoneally to guinea pigs at a concentration of 33.0 ml/liter, were active on the ileum[PO003].

Spasmolytic activity. Water extract of fresh leaves and stem, at a concentration of 2.0 mg/ml, was active on rat diaphragm vs electrically induced contractions[PO025].

Toxic effect (general). Fresh leaves, administered orally to cows at a dose of 48.0 gm/kg, were inactive[PO008].

Toxicity assessment (quantitative). Water extract of leaves and stem, administered intraperitoneally to mice, produced a minimum toxic dose of 1.0 ml/animal[PO003]. Water extract of fresh leaves and stem, administered intraperitoneally to mice, produced LD_{50} 1040 mg/kg[PO051].

Uterine stimulant effect. Ethanol (95%) and water extracts of leaves and stem, at a concentration of 0.33 ml/liter, were active on rat uterus[PO003]. Water extract of leaves was active on the uterus of pregnant and nonpregnant rats and mice[PO011].

Vasoconstrictor activity. Ethanol (95%) extract of leaves and stem, at a concentration of 0.33 ml/liter, was active on rat hind quarters (isolated)[PO003].

REFERENCES

PO001   Quisumbing, E. Medicinal plants of the Philippines. **Tech Bull 16**, Rep Philippines, Dept Agr Nat Resources, Manilla 1951; 1.

PO002   Fong, H. H. S., N. R. Farnsworth, L. K. Henry, G. H. Svoboda and M. J. Yates.

Biological and phytochemical evaluation of plants. X. Test results from a third two-hundred accessions. **Lloydia** 1972; 35(1): 35–48.

PO003 Feng, P. C., L. J. Haynes, K. E. Magnus, J. R. Plimmer and H. S. A. Sherrat. Pharmacological screening of some West Indian medicinal plants. **J Pharm Pharmacol** 1962; 14: 556–561.

PO004 Matsui, A. D. S., J. Rogers, Y. K. Woo, W. C. Cutting. Effects of some natural products on fertility in mice. **Med Pharmacol Exp** 1967; 16: 414.

PO005 Fitzpatrick, F. K. Plant substances active against *Mycobacterium tuberculosis*. **Antibiot Chemother** 1954; 4: 528.

PO006 Rageau, J. Les Plantes Medicinales de la Nouvelle-Cal Edonie. Trav & Doc De Lorstom No. 23. Paris, 1973.

PO007 Murray, J. A. Plants and Drugs of Sind. Richardson and Co., London, 1881.

PO008 Canella, C. F. C., C. H. Tokarnia and J. Dobereiner. Experiments with plants supposedly toxic to cattle in Northeastern Brazil, with negative results. **Pesqui Agropecu Brasil Ser Vet** 1966; 1: 345–352.

PO009 Schermerhorn, J. W. and M. W. Quimby. Order Centrospermae. **Lynn Index** 1957; 1.

PO010 Haerdi, F. Native medicinal plants of Ulanga District of Tanganyika (East Africa). Dissertation, Verlag Fur Recht Und Gesellschaft Ag, Basel. **Dissertation-Ph.D.-Univ Basel** 1964.

PO011 Sharaf, A. Food plants as a possible factor in fertility control. **Qual Plant Mater Veg** 1969; 17: 153.

PO012 Abivardi, C. Studies on the effects of nine Iranian anthelmintic plant extracts on the root-knot nematode *Meloidogyne incognita*. **Phytopathol** 1971; 71: 300–308.

PO013 Willaman, J. J. and H. L. Li. Alkaloid-bearing plants and their contained alkaloids, 1957-1968. **Lloydia** 1970; 33S: 1–286.

PO014 Kosuge, T., M. Yokota, K. Sugiyama, T. Yamamoto, M. Y. Ni and S. C. Yan. Studies on antitumor activities and antitumor principles of Chinese herbs. 1. Antitumor activities of Chinese herbs. **Yakugaku Zasshi** 1985; 105(8): 791–795.

PO015 Imperato, F. Acylate betacyanins of *Portulaca oleracea*. **Phytochemistry** 1975; 14: 2091–1092.

PO016 Kazmi, H., M. Aslan, Z. U. Khan and M. I. Bureny. A report on the trial of a Unani prescription for diabetes. **Rawal Med** 1974; 3(2): 67.

PO017 Kennedy, R. A. and W. M. Laetsch. Formation of carbon-14-labeled alanine from pyruvate during short term photosynthesis in a C-4 plant. **Plant Physiol** 1974; 54: 608.

PO018 Luu C. Notes on the traditional pharmacopoeia of French Guyana. **Plant Med Phytother** 1975; 9: 125–135.

PO019 Sayed, H. M. and M. A. Abdel-Hafiz. Pharmacognostical study of *Portulaca oleracea* L. growing in Egypt. Part I. Botanical study of the stems, leaves and investigation of the lipid content. **Bull Pharm Sci Assiut Univ** 1985; 8(1): 41–60.

PO020 Simopoulos, A. P., H. A. Norman, J. E. Gillaspy and J. A. Duke. Common purslane: A source of Omega-3 fatty acids and antioxidants. **J Amer Coll Nutr** 1992; 11(4): 374–382.

PO021 Hertog, M. G. L., P. C. H. Hollman and M. B. Katani. Content of potentially anticarcinogenic flavonoids of 28 vegetables and 9 fruits commonly consumed in The Netherlands. **J Agr Food Chem** 1992; 40(12): 2379–2383.

PO022 Shin, K. H., M. S. Chung, Y. I. Chae, K. Y. Yoon and T. S. Cho. A survey for aldose reductase inhibition of herbal medicines. **Fitoterapia** 1993; 64(2): 130–133.

PO023 Son, K. H., S. H. Kim, K. Y. Jung and H. W. Chang. Screening of platelet activating factor (PAF) antagonists from medicinal plants. **Korean J Pharmacog** 1994; 25(2): 167–170.

PO024 Kurokawa, M., H, Ochiai, K. Nagasaka, M. Neki, H. X. Xu, S. Kadota, S. Sutardio, T. Matsumoto, T. Namba and K. Shiraki. Antiviral traditional medicines against Herpes Simplex Virus (HSV-1), Poliovirus, and Measles virus In Vitro and their therapeutic efficacies for HSV-1 infection in mice. **Antiviral Res** 1993; 22(2/3): 175–188.

PO025 Parry, O., J. A. Marks and F. K. Okwuasaba. The skeletal muscle relaxant action of *Portulaca oleracea*: Role of potassium ions. **J Ethnopharmacol** 1993; 40(3): 187–194.

PO026   Habtemariam, S., A. L. Harvey and P. G. Waterman. The muscle relaxant properties of *Portulaca oleracea* are associated with high concentration of potassium ions. **J Ethnopharmacol** 1993; 40(3): 195–200.

PO027   Hirobe, C., D. Palevitch, K. Takeya and H. Itokawa. Screening test for antitumor activity of crude drugs (IV). Studies on cytotoxic activity of Israeli medicinal plants. **Nat Med** 1994; 48(2): 168–170.

PO028   Hope, B. E., D. G. Massey and G. Fournier-Massey. Hawaiian materia medica for asthma. **Hawaii Med J** 1993; 52(6): 160–166.

PO029   Maikhuri, R. K. and A. K. Gangwar. Ethnobiological notes on the Khasi and Garo tribes of Meghalaya, Northeast India. **Econ Bot** 1993; 47(4): 345–357.

PO030   Adachi, T. and S. Shiotsuki. Studies of biochemical genetics on flower color and its application to flower breeding. VII. Some problems on the extraction of DNA from Portulaca plant and tissue culture. **Miyazaki Daigaku Nogakubu Kenkyu Hokoku** 1976; 23(1): 65.

PO031   Afaque, S., I. Ahmad, M. S. Siddiqui and S. M. Osman. Studies on minor seed oils – VIII. **J Oil Technol Ass India** 1984; 15(2): 63–64.

PO032   Simopoulos, A. P. and N. Salem, Jr. Purslane: A terrestrial source of Omega-3 fatty acids. **N Engl J Med** 1987; 315(13): 833.

PO033   Yamazaki, M., Y. Maebayashi, N. Iwase and T. Kaneko. Studies on pharmacologically active principles from Indonesian crude drugs. I. Principle prolonging pentobarbital-induced sleeping time from *Curcuma xanthorrhiza* Roxb. **Chem Pharm Bull** 1988; 36(6): 2070–2074.

PO034   Barbakadze, V. V., R. A. Gakhokidze, Z. S. Shengeliya and A. I. Usov. Preliminary investigation of water-soluble polysaccharides from Georgian plants. **Chem Nat Comp** 1989; 25(3): 281–286.

PO035   Akhtar, M. S., Q. M. Khan and T. Khaliq. Effects of *Portulaca oleracae* (Kulfa) and *Taraxacum officinale* (Dhudhal) in normoglycaemic and alloxan-

treated hyperglycaemic rabbits. **J Pak Med Assoc** 1985; 35: 207–210.

PO036   Saklani, A. and S. K. Jain. Ethnobotanical observations on plants used in Northeastern India. **Int J Crude Drug Res** 1989; 27(2): 65–73.

PO037   Reger, B. J. and I. E. Yates. Protein and nucleic acid syntheses in dark dormant common purslane (*Portulaca oleracea*) seed. **Weed Sci** 1978; 26: 669.

PO038   Ayensu, E. S. Medicinal plants of the West Indies. **Unpublished Manuscript** 1978; 110pp.

PO039   Karadge, B. A. and G. V. Joshi. Carbon assimilation and Crassulacean acid metabolism in *Portulaca oleracea* Linn. **Indian J Exp Biol** 1980; 18: 631–634.

PO040   Kapoor, S. L. and L. D. Kapoor. Medicinal plant wealth of the Karimnagar District of Andhra Pradesh. **Bull Med Ethnobot Res** 1980; 1: 120–144.

PO041   Adesina, S. K. Studies on some plants used as anticonvulsants in Amerindian and African traditional medicine. **Fitoterapia** 1982; 53: 147–162.

PO042   Ikram, M. A review on the medicinal plants. **Hamdard** 1981; 24(1/2): 102–129.

PO043   Verma, O. P., S. Kumar and S. N. Chatterjee. Antifertility effects of common edible *Portulaca oleracea* on the reproductive organs of male albino mice. **Indian J Med Res** 1982; 75: 301–310.

PO044   Bruno, S., A. Amico and L. Stefanizzi. Vitamin C content of edible and medicinal plants of the Apulian Region. **Boll Soc Ital Biol Sper** 1980; 56(20): 2067–2070.

PO045   Goh, S. H., E. Soepadmo, P. Chang, U. Barnerjee, et al. Studies on Malaysian medicinal plants. Preliminary results. **Proc 5th Asian Symposium on Medicinal Plants and Spices South Korea** 1984; August 20–24. 5: 473–483.

PO046   Macfoy, C. A. and A. M. Sama. Medicinal plants in Pujehun District of Sierra Leone. **J Ethnopharmacol** 1983; 8(2): 215–223.

PO047   Zennie, T. M. and C. D. Ogzewalla. Ascorbic acid and vitamin A content of edible wild plants of Ohio and Kentucky. **Econ Bot** 1977; 31: 76–79.

PO048   Namba, T., M. Tsunezaku, Y. Takehana, S. Nunome, et al. Studies on dental caries prevention by traditional

Chinese medicines. IV. Screening of crude drugs for anti-plaque action and effects on *Artemisia capillaris* spikes on adherence of *Streptococcus mutans* to smooth surfaces and synthesis of glucan. **Shoyakugaku Zasshi** 1984; 38(3): 253–263.

PO049 Singh, Y. N. Traditional medicine in Fiji. Some herbal folk cures used by Fiji Indians. **J Ethnopharmacol**. 1986; 15(1): 57–88.

PO050 Franzblau, S. G. and C. Cross. Comparative in vitro antimicrobial activity of Chinese medicinal herbs. **J Ethnopharmacol** 1986; 15(3): 279–288.

PO051 Parry, O., F. K. Okwuasaba and C. Ejike. Skeletal muscle relaxant action of an aqueous extract of *Portulaca oleracea* in the rat. **J Ethnopharmacol** 1987; 19(3): 247–253.

PO052 Weniger, B., M. Rouzier, R. Daguilh, D. Henrys, J. H. Henrys and R. Anthon. Popular medicine of the Central Plateau of Haiti. 2. Ethnopharmacological inventory. **J Ethnopharmacol** 1986; 17(1): 13–30.

PO053 Okwuasaba, F., C. Ejike and O. Parry. Skeletal muscle relaxant properties of the aqueous extract of *Portulaca oleracea*. **J Ethnopharmacol** 1986; 17(2): 139–160.

PO054 Okwuasaba, F., C. Ejike and O. Parry. Comparison of the skeletal muscle relaxant properties of *Portulaca oleracea* extracts with dantrolene sodium and methoxyverapamil. **J Ethnopharmacol** 1987; 20(2): 85–100.

PO055 Namba, T., M. Tsunezuka, K. H. Bae and M. Hattori. Studies on dental caries prevention by traditional Chinese medicines. Part 1. Screening of crude drugs for antibacterial action against *Streptococcus mutans*. **Shoyakugaku Zasshi** 1981; 35(4): 295–302.

PO056 Parry, O., F. Okuasaba and C. Ejike. Effect of an aqueous extract of *Portulaca oleracea* leaves on smooth muscle and rat blood pressure. **J Ethnopharmacol** 1988; 22(1): 33–44.

PO057 Ramirez, V. R., L. J. Mostacero, A. E. Garcia, C. F. Mejia, P. F. Pelaez, C. D. Medina and C. H. Miranda. Vegetales empleados en medicina tradicional Norperuana. **Banco Agrario Del Peru & NACL Univ Trujillo**, Peru, June 1988; 54pp.

PO058 Okwuasaba, F., O. Parry and C. Ejike. Investigation into the mechanism of action of extracts of *Portulaca oleracea*. **J Ethnopharmacol** 1987; 21(1): 91–97.

PO059 Okwuasaba, F., O. Parry and C. Ejike. Effects of extracts of *Portulaca oleracea* on skeletal muscle in vitro. **J Ethnopharmacol** 1987; 21(1): 55–63.

PO060 Okwuasaba, F., O. Parry and C. Ejike. Preliminary clinical investigation into the muscle relaxant actions of an aqueous extract of *Portulaca oleracea* applied topically. **J Ethnopharmacol** 1987; 21(1): 99–106.

PO061 Costa, M., L. C. Di Stasi, M. Kirizawa, S. L. J. Mendacolli, C. Gomes and G. Trolin. Screening in mice of some medicinal plants used for analgesic purposes in the state of Sao Paulo. **J Ethnopharmacol** 1989; 27(1/2): 25–33.

PO062 Darias, V., L. Brando, R. Rabanal, C. Sanchez Mateo, R. M. Gonzalez Luis and A. M. Hernandez Perez. New contribution to the ethnopharmacological study of the Canary Islands. **J Ethnopharmacol** 1989; 25(1): 77–92.

PO063 Misas, C. A. J., N. I. M. R. Hernandez and A. M. L. Abraham. Contribution to the biological evaluation of Cuban plants. V. Rev Cub Med Trop 1979; 31: 37–43.

PO064 Lokar, L. C. and L. Poldini. Herbal remedies in the traditional medicine of the Venezia Guilia Region (Northeast Italy). **J Ethnopharmacol** 1988; 22(3): 231–239.

PO065 Oakes, A. J. and M. P. Morris. The West Indian weedwoman of the United States Virgin Islands. **Bull Hist Med** 1958; 32: 164.

PO066 Nene, Y. L., P. N. Thapliyal and K. Kumar. Screening of some plant extracts for antifungal properties. **Labdev J Sci Tech** 1968; 6B(4): 226–228.

PO067 Hodge, W. H. and D. Taylor. The ethnobotany of the Island Caribes of Dominica. **WEBBIA** 1956; 12: 513–644.

PO068 Asprey, G. F. and P. Thornton. Medicinal plants of Jamaica. IV. **West Indian Med J** 1955; 4: 145–165.

PO069 Abbott, B. J., J. Leiter, J. L. Hartwell, M. E. Caldwell, J. L. Beal, R. E. Perdue

Jr. and S. A. Schepartz. Screening data from the cancer chemotherapy national service center screening laboratories. XXXIV. Plant extracts. **Cancer Res** 1966; 26: 761–935.

PO070   Roca-Garcia, H. Weeds: A link with the past. **Arnoldia (Boston)** 1970; 30(3): 114–115.

PO071   Cross, F. B. The effect of certain cultural practices on the ascorbic acid content of some horticultural plants. **Dissertation-Ph.D.-Univ Missouri** 1939; 123pp.

PO072   Roig Y Mesa, J. T. Plantas Medicinales, Aromaticas o Venenosas de Cuba. Ministerio de Agricultura, Republica de Cuba, Havana, 1945; 872pp.

PO073   Lee, H. K. and Y. S. Chung. Antifungal activities of medicinal plants in Korea. **Kisul Yon'guso Pogo** 1963; 2: 76–78.

PO074   Nordal, A., A. Krogh and G. Ogner. The occurrence of phorbic acid in plants. **Acta Chem Scand** 1965; 19(7): 1705–1708.

PO075   Mathams, R. H. and A. K. Sutherland. The oxalate content of some Queensland pasture plants. **Queensl J Agr Sci** 1952; 9: 317–334.

PO076   Piatelli, M. and L. Minale. Pigments of Centrospermae-II. Distribution of betacyanins. **Phytochemistry** 1964; 3(5): 547–557.

PO077   Kong, Y. C. Plants used for rheumatism, arthritis and related conditions in Chinese traditional medicine. **Personal Communication** 1977.

PO078   Medina, F. R. and R. Wodbury. Terrestrial plants molluscicidal to lymnaid hosts of *Fasciliasis hepatica* in Puerto Rico. **J Agr Univ Puerto Rico** 1979; 63: 366–376.

PO079   Oh, K. B., I. M. Chang, K. J. Hwang and W. Mar. Detection of antifungal activity in *Portulaca oleracea* by a single-cell bioassay system. **Phytother Res** 2000; 14(5): 329–332.

PO080   Liu, L., P. Howe, Y. F. Zhou, Z. Q. Xu, C. Hocart and R. Zhan. Fatty acids and beta-carotene in Australian purslane (*Portulaca oleracea*) varieties. **J Chromatogr** A 2000; 893(1): 207–213.

PO081   Chan, K., M. W. Islam, M. Kamil, R. Radhakrishnan, M. N. Zakaria, M. Habibullah and A. Attas. The analgesic and anti-inflammatory effects of *Portulaca oleracea* L. subsp. Sativa (Haw.) Celak. **J Ethnopharmacol** 2000; 73(3): 445–451.

PO082   Radhakrishnan, R., M. N. Zakaria, M. W. Islam, H. B. Chen, M. Kamil, K. Chan and A. Al-Attas. Neuropharmacological actions of *Portulaca oleraceae* L. v. sativa (Hawk). **J Ethnopharmacol** 2001; 76(2): 171–176.

24 | Psidium guajava

L.

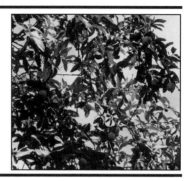

Common Names

Abas	Guam	Guayaba	Paraguay
Amba	Nepal	Guayaba	Puerto Rico
Amrood	India	Guayabe	Guatemala
Amrud	Fiji	Guayabero	Canary Islands
Amrut	Fiji	Guayabo	Canary Islands
Arasa	Paraguay	Guayabo	Mexico
Banjiro	Brazil	Guayabo	Peru
Banziro	Brazil	Guayava	Guatemala
Bilauti	Nepal	Guega	Papua-New Guinea
Borimak	Nicaragua	Gwawa	Papua
Bugoyab	Senegal	Ipera	Rwanda
Djambu bidji	Indonesia	Jaama	India
Djambu klutuk	Indonesia	Jambu biji	Indonesia
Fa-rang	Thailand	Kautonga	Indonesia
Goavy	Madagascar	Kiswahili	Tanzania
Goejaba	Suriname	Krue	Nicaragua
Goiabeira	Brazil	Ku'ava	Nicaragua
Goyav	Haiti	Kuabas	Nicaragua
Guava	Fiji	Kuava	Nicaragua
Guava	Ghana	Kuawa	Nicaragua
Guava	Guam	Kuiaba	Papua-New Guinea
Guava	Guyana	Kuliabs	Malaysia
Guava	Indonesia	Mabera	Tanzania
Guava	Mexico	Maduriam	India
Guava	Nepal	Mansala	India
Guava	Nicaragua	Motiram	India
Guava	Papua-New Guinea	Mpera	Tanzania
Guava	Sierra Leone	Mugwavha	Venda
Guava	Sri Lanka	Ngoaba	Guinea
Guava	Tanzania	Psidiium	Taiwan
Guava	USA	Quwawa	Taiwan
Guyaba	Cuba	Sigra	Nicaragua
Guayaba	Guatemala	Sikra	Nicaragua
Guayaba	Nicaragua	Tuava	Cook Islands

From: *Medicinal Plants of the World, vol. 1: Chemical Constituents, Traditional and Modern Medicinal Uses, 2nd ed.*
By: Ivan A. Ross © Humana Press Inc., Totowa, NJ

Tuava	Easter Island	Xalxocotyl	Mexico
Tuava	Rarotonga	Xalxoctl	Mexico
Wariafa	Nicaragua		

BOTANICAL DESCRIPTION

A spreading tree of the MYRTACEAE family which may grow as high as 15 meters, with bark peeling in large thin flakes. Leaves are simple, opposite, oblong, elliptic or ovate, in pairs on 4-angled twigs, elliptical or oblong, 7–14 cm long and 4–6 cm wide; consisting of obtuse or micronulate apex; margin entire or slightly curved; with broadly cuneate or obtuse base. Blades are more or less hairy beneath; the veins parallel and conspicuously raised below; petiole 5–10 mm long. Flowers are white, axillary, solitary or 2 to 3 together on slender peduncles, about 3 cm in diameter; consisting of calyx-tube campanulate, deeply divided into 4–5 lobes above the ovary; petals are large and broad, spreading; stamens are numerous, about length of petals, free, inserted on disk. Fruit globose or pear-shaped, tipped with remnants of the calyx lobes, the pulp is white or pink, juicy, containing many small, hard, seeds. The plant can be propagated by seeds, grafting or cutting.

ORIGIN AND DISTRIBUTION

A native of Central America, sometimes cultivated but also very common as an adventive in pastures and wayside thickets throughout the tropics and subtropics.

TRADITIONAL MEDICINAL USES

Andaman Islands. The ripe fruit is used as a food[PG034].

Bolivia. A few drops of liquid from boiled leaves of *Psidium guajava* is mixed with a tablespoon of *Orbignya martiana* fruit oil and taken orally 4 times a day for coughs[PG068].

Brazil. Dried fruit is taken orally to treat diarrhea, stomachache and diabetes[PG016].

Canary Islands. Hot water extract of dried fruit is used as an antihemorrhoidal[PG089].

China. Extract of roots is taken orally by monks in south China to suppress libido[PG099].

Cook Islands. Dried leaves of *Psidium guajava* and *Citrus aurantium* are crushed and taken orally for pain around the navel. Infusion of dried leaves is taken orally to relieve postpartum pain and rid the body of residual stale blood. For sores, dried leaves are chewed with or without coconut oil and then applied to the sores[PG075].

Fiji. Dried fruit is taken orally for constipation. Infusion of dried leaves and root is taken orally for diarrhea and indigestion. Fresh leaf juice is taken orally for dysentery and upset stomach[PG080].

Ghana. Peeled twig is used as a chewing stick[PG061].

Guam. Hot water extract of leaves is administered intravaginally to treat vaginitis and to promote conception[PG002].

Guatemala. Decoction of dried bark and leaves is taken orally to treat fevers, respiratory ailments and skin infections[PG030]. Dried fruit is powdered and eaten for stomach cramps[PG095]. Infusion of dried leaves is taken orally to treat infections[PG025]. The hot water extract is applied externally for dermatomucosal lesions and ringworm[PG049].

Haiti. Decoction of dried leaves is taken orally for diarrhea. Fresh fruit juice is taken orally for diarrhea[PG082].

India. Crushed fresh flowers, together with the juice from buds squeezed through muslin cloth, are taken orally as an anthelmintic. Decoction of dried leaves is taken orally for diarrhea and as an antiemetic[PG046]. Hot water extract of dried leaves is used in bath for high fever and headache[PG065]. Dried fruit is used for jaundice. One dose consists of the juice of 1 fruit of *Psidium guajava*, 0.25 liter goat's milk and the root of an unidentified herb, possibly Sida. One dose is taken on alternate days.

Three doses give significant relief[PG078]. Hot water extract of dried bark is taken orally as a remedy for stomachache[PG065].

Indonesia. Hot water extract of leaves is taken orally as an emmenagogue[PG004].

Ivory Coast. Dried stem is used as a chewing stick[PG043].

Japan. Extract of roots is taken orally by Japanese monks as a suppressant of libido[PG099].

Madagascar. Hot water extract of young leaves is taken orally for diarrhea[PG045].

Malaysia. Hot water extracts of bark and leaf are taken orally to expel the placenta and as an emmenagogue[PG008]. Water extract of dried bark and leaves is taken orally for after-birth disorders[PG072].

Mexico. Hot water extract of bark is taken orally for dysentery. Hot water extract of fruit is taken orally as a digestive. Hot water extract of leaves is used externally as a treatment for mange[PG017]. The extract is also taken orally for diarrhea[PG026]. Infusion of dried leaves is taken orally for diarrhea[PG031].

Nigeria. Water extract of dried root is taken orally for diarrhea[PG023].

Panama. Hot water extract of flowers and fruits is taken orally as an emmenagogue. Hot water extract of fresh bark is taken orally for diarrhea. The decoction is taken as 1 dose. Hot water extract of fruit is taken orally for diarrhea. For this purpose, decoction of fruits is taken in water as 1 dose[PG060].

Papua-New Guinea. Fresh leaf juice is taken orally for diarrhea. Young top leaves are squeezed and the juice taken with water[PG074].

Peru. Hot water extract of dried bark is taken orally as an astringent, antihemorrhagic and antidiarrheal, and for stomach pain. Hot water extract of dried leaves is taken orally for stomach pain, and as an astringent, antihemorrhagic and antidiarrheal. Hot water extract of dried roots is taken orally as an astringent, antihemorrhagic and antidiarrheal, and for stomach pain[PG087].

Philippines. Hot water extract of dried bark is used in steam baths postpartum. *Psidium guajava*, *Commiphora myrrha* and incense are added to the bath[PG077].

Rarotonga. Fresh leaf juice is taken orally for dysentery[PG019].

Rwanda. Hot water extract of dried leaves is taken orally for dysentery[PG088].

Senegal. Dried stem is used as toothbrush. Hot water extract of dried leaves is taken orally for diarrhea. Hot water extract of the green fruit is taken orally for dysentery. Hot water extract of young shoots is taken orally for diarrhea[PG043].

Sierra Leone. Decoction of dried leaves is taken orally for diarrhea during pregnancy[PG071].

Taiwan. Fresh fruit juice is taken orally to treat diabetes mellitus[PG018]. Hot water extract of dried branches is taken orally for liver diseases[PG086].

Tanzania. Decoction of dried leaves is taken orally to treat malaria[PG024]. Hot water extract of fresh leaves is taken orally for skin diseases[PG079].

Thailand. Hot water extract of dried leaves is taken orally for diabetes[PG097].

Venda. Decoction of dried roots is taken orally for venereal diseases. The decoction of *Opuntia vulgaris* and *Psidium guajava* is taken twice a daily[PG070].

CHEMICAL CONSTITUENTS
(ppm unless otherwise indicated)

1-8-Cineol: Fr[PG056], EO[PG037], Lf EO[PG051]

13-Hydroperoxide lyase: Fr[PG104]

2-3-4-6-Tetra-0-galloyl glucose: Rt[PG076]

2-Alpha-hydroxy ursolic acid: Lf EO[PG059], Fr[PG084]

2-Ethyl thiophene: Fr[PG029]

2-Methyl propan-2-ol; Fr 1.0%[PG091]

2-Methyl propane-1-thiol; Fr[PG029]

2-Methyl propyl acetate: Fr 0.5%[PG091]

2-Phenethyl acetate: Fr 0.2%[PG091]

2-Furfural: Fr[PG091]

2-Methyl furfural: Fr[PG091]

3-O-Methyl ellagic acid: Bk[PG012]

3-3-Di-O-methyl ellagic acid: Bk[PG012]

3-Methyl butan-1-ol: Fr 0.3%[PG091]

3-Methyl thiophene: Fr[PG029]
5-Ethoxy thiazole: Fr[PG029]
6-Mercapto hexan-1-ol: Fr[PG029]
Acetaldehyde: Fr 0.2%[PG091]
Acetone: Fr 0.8%[PG091,PG001]
Acetyl furan: Fr[PG091]
Acutissimin A: Bk 0.086%[PG016]
Acutissimin B: Bk 3.7[PG016]
Alpha amyrin: Fr[PG084]
Alpha copaene: Fr Pe EO[PG056], Fr 0.1%[PG091]
Alpha humulene: Fr Pe EO[PG056],
    Fr 0.6%[PG091,PG054]
Alpha pinene: Fr[PG056], Lf EO[PG051,PG059]
Alpha terpineol: Fr[PG056]
Alpha selinene: Fr[PG054,PG091]
Amritoside: St Bk 40[PG011], Lf 850[PG010],
    Wd[PG055]
Arabinose: Fr (unripe)[PG009]
Arabinose hexahydroxydiphenyl acid ester:
    Fr (unripe) 0.1%[PG009]
Arjunolic acid: Rt 0.01%[PG096], Fr[PG084]
Aromadendrene: Fr Pe EO[PG056]
Ascorbic acid: Fr[PG013,PG084]
Asiatic acid: Fr[PG084]
Benzaldehyde: Fr 0.1%[PG091]
Benzothiazole: Fr[PG029]
Beta amyrin: Fr[PG084]
Beta bisabolene: Fr Pe EO[PG056],
    Fr 0.2%[PG091,PG054]
Beta caryophyllene: Fr 0.45%[PG091,PG054]
Beta copaene: Fr[PG054]
Beta humulene: Fr[PG054]
Beta pinene: Fr[PG054], Lf EO[PG059]
Beta selinene: Fr[PG054]
Beta sitosterol: Fr[PG084,PG003], Lf EO[PG059],
    Rt[PG076,PG036], Wd[PG055]
Brahmic acid: Fr[PG084]
Butanedione: Fr 2.0%[PG091]
Butanoic acid ethyl ester: Fr 8.7%[PG091]
Butanone: Fr 2.2%[PG091]
Butyl acetate, 3-methyl: Fr 0.1%[PG091]
Butyl acetate: Fr 0.1%[PG091,PG001]
Butyraldehyde: Fr[PG001]
Calamenene: Fr[PG056]
Calcium oxalate: Fr (unripe)[PG009]
Camphene: Fr[PG056]
Carophyllene oxide: EO[PG037], Fr[PG056]
Caryophyllene: EO[PG037], Fr[PG056]
Castalagin: Bk 0.17%[PG016]
Casuarinin: Lf 0.021%[PG063],
    Bk 0.004%[PG016]
Catechin (+): Bk 0.029%[PG016]

Cineol: EO[PG006]
Cis-beta ocimene: Fl [PG056]
Curcumene: Fr[PG054]
Daucosterol: Fr[PG084]
Decanoic acid ethyl ester: Fr 0.1%[PG091]
Delta elemene: EO[PG037]
Delta cadinene: Fr Pe EO[PG056], Fr[PG054]
Diisopropyl disulfide: Fr[PG029]
Dimethyl disulfide: Fr[PG029]
Dimethyl sulfone: Fr[PG029]
Dimethyl trisulfide: Fr[PG029]
Dodecanoic acid ethyl ester: Fr[PG091]
Ellagic acid: Bk[PG012], Fl[PG044],
    Fr (unripe)[PG009], Lf 150[PG010],
    St Bk 40[PG011]
Ethanol: Fr 25.8%[PG091]
Ethyl acetate: Fr 26.2%[PG091,PG001]
Ethyl butyrate: Fr[PG001]
Eugenigrandin A: Bk 0.08%[PG016]
Eugenol: EO[PG037]
Farnesene: Fr[PG054]
Foeniculin: Lf[PG042]
Gallic acid ethyl ester: Rt[PG036,PG076]
Gallic acid: Fr (unripe)[PG009], Rt[PG036,PG076],
    Wd[PG055]
Gallocatechin (+): Lf[PG027], Bk 0.057%[PG016]
Gamma muurolene: Fr[PG056]
Gentisic acid: Lf[PG007]
Glucose: Fr (unripe)[PG009]
Glucuronic acid: Fr[PG084]
Grandinin: Bk 0.037%[PG016]
Guaijavarin: Lf[PG031]
Guaijaverin: Lf 0.035%[PG010], Fl[PG009,PG044],
    Fr[PG009]
Guajavin B: Bk 211[PG016]
Guajavin: Bk 24.5[PG016]
Guavin A: Lf[PG015]
Guavin B: Lf[PG067]
Guavin C: Lf[PG015]
Guavin D: Lf[PG015]
Heptan-1-al: Fr[PG001]
Hex-3-en-1-ol acetate: Fr Pe EO[PG056]
Hex-cis-3-en-1-ol acetate: Fr 0.5%[PG091]
Hex-cis-3-en-1-ol: Fr1.0%[PG091]
Hex-cis-3-enoic acid: Fr Pu 0.2[PG038]
Hexadecanoic acid ethyl ester: Fr[PG091]
Hexagalloyl glucose: Rt[PG076]
Hexan-1-al: Fr 3.2%[PG091,PG001]
Hexan-1-ol acetate: Fr Pe EO[PG056]
Hexanoic acid ethyl ester: Fr 15.5%[PG091]
Hexanoic acid methyl ester: Fr 0.3%[PG091]
Hexyl acetate: Fr 0.3%[PG091]

Hyperoside: Lf[PG031]
Iso-quercetin: Lf[PG031]
Iso-strictinin: Lf 30[PG063]
Leucocyanidins: Fl[PG009], Fr .02%[PG009], Lf[PG010], Rt[PG036], St Bk 0.4%[PG011]
Leucocyanin: Rt[PG076]
Limonene: Fr Pe EO[PG056], Fr[PG054,PG091], Lf EO[PG059]
Linalool: EO[PG037]
Lupeol: Fr[PG084]
Mannose: Lf EO[PG059]
Maslinic acid: Fr[PG084], Lf[PG093], Lf EO[PG059]
Menthol: Lf EO[PG059]
Methanol: Fr[PG001]
Methyl ethyl ketone: Fr[PG001]
Mongolicain A: Bk[PG016]
Myrcene: EO[PG037], Fr[PG091]
N-Octane: Fr[PG091]
Nonan-1-al: Fr[PG001]
Octan-1-al: Fr[PG001]
Octan-1-ol: Fr[PG091]
Octanoic acid ethyl ester: Fr[PG091]
Octyl acetate: Fr[PG091]
Oleanolic acid: Fl[PG044], Lf[PG093], Wd[PG055]
Para cymene: Fr[PG056]
Para-methyl styrene: Fr 0.3%[PG091]
Pedunculagin: Lf 0.06%[PG091], Bk 27[PG016]
Pendunculagin: Lf[PG014]
Pentane-2-thiol: Fr[PG029]
Procyanidin B-1: Lf[PG067], Bk 4.5[PG016]
Procyanidin B-2: Lf[PG067]
Procyanidin B-3: Lf[PG067]
Prodelphinidin B-1: Bk[PG016]
Psidinin A: Bk 0.016%[PG016]
Psidinin B: Bk 24.5[PG016]
Psidinin C: Bk 23.4[PG016]
Psiguavin: Bk 38.2[PG016]
Quercetin: Lf[PG010,PG042], Fl[PG009,PG044], Rt[PG036,PG076], Wd[PG055]
Quercetin-3-0-gentiobioside: Lf[PG031]
Stachyurin: Lf 15[PG063]
Strictinin: Lf 62.5[PG063]
Sucrose: Lf EO[PG059]
Tannin: Rt[PG036]
Tellimagrandin 1: Lf 237.5[PG063]
Tetradecanoic acid ethyl ester: Fr 0.2%[PG091]
Toluene: Fr 0.2%[PG091]
Trans-cinnamic acid: Fr Pu 0.4[PG038]
Ursolic acid: Lf[PG093]
Valeraldehyde: Fr[PG001]
Valolaginic acid: Bk 114[PG016]
Vescalagin carboxylic acid: Bk 20.5[PG016]

Zeatin nucleotide: Fr[PG057]
Zeatin riboside: Fr[PG057]
Zeatin: Fr[PG057]

PHARMACOLOGICAL ACTIVITIES AND CLINICAL TRIALS

ACh release inhibition. Methanol extract of dried leaves, at a concentration of 800.0 mcg/ml, was active on guinea pig ileum[PG042]. Quercetin, extracted from the plant, induced a reduction of the acetylcholine-evoked release[PG100].

Analgesic activity. Dried fruit, administered intraperitoneally to male rats at a dose of 50.0 mg/kg, was active vs acetic acid-induced writhing[PG032]. Ethanol/water (1:1) extract of the aerial parts, administered intraperitoneally to mice at a dose of 0.094 mg/kg, was inactive vs tail pressure method[PG092].

Anti-HCG activity. Ethanol (60%) extract of roots, administered subcutaneously to immature female rats, was active[PG005].

Anti-PMS activity. Ethanol (60%) extract of roots, administered subcutaneously to immature female rats, was active[PG005].

Antibacterial activity. Acetone extract of dried bark and leaves, at a concentration of 50.0 mg/disc, was active on *Staphylococcus aureus*, and produced weak activity on *Streptococcus pneumonia*. The extract was active on *Streptococcus pyogenes*, MIC 10.0 mg/disc. Hexane extract, at a concentration of 50.0 mg/disc on agar plate, produced weak activity on *Staphylococcus aureus*, *Streptococcus pneumonia* and *Streptococcus pyogenes*. Methanol extract, at a concentration of 50.0 mg/disc on agar plate, was active on *Streptococcus pneumonia* and *Streptococcus pyogenesi*, and inactive on *Staphylococcus aureus*, MIC 5.0 mg/disc[PG030]. Acetone extract of dried leaves, undiluted on agar plate, was active on *Escherichia coli*, *Pseudomonas aeruginosa*, *Salmonella B*, *Salmonella newport*, *Salmonella typhi*, *Sarcina lutea*, *Serratia marcescens*, *Shigella flexneri*, *Staphylococcus albus* and *Staphylococcus aureus*. The ethanol (95%) extract was active on *E. coli*, *P. aeruginosa*, *Salmonella*

B, S. newport, S. typhi, S. flexneri and S. albus, and inactive on S. lutea, Serratia marcescens and S. aureus. Water extract was active on P. aeruginosa, S. lutea, S. marcescens, S. flexneri, S. albus and S. aureus, and inactive on Salmonella B, S. newport and S. typhi[PG090]. Acetone extract of dried stem, undiluted on agar plate, was inactive on Escherichia coli, Pseudomonas aeruginosa, Salmonella B, Salmonella newport, Salmonella typhi, Sarcina lutea, Serratia marcescens, Shigella flexneri, Staphylococcus albus and Staphylococcus aureus. The ethanol (95%) extract was active on E. coli, P. aeruginosa, S. newport, S. typhi, Sarcina lutea, Serratia marcescens, Shigella flexneri and S. albus, and inactive on Salmonella B and S. aureus. The water extract was active on Escherichia coli, P. aeruginosa, S. marcescens, S. flexneri, S. albus and S. aureus, and inactive on Salmonella B, S. newport, S. typhi and Sarcina lutea[PG090]. Ethanol (95%) extract of dried bark, at a concentration of 5.0 mg/ml on agar plate, was active on Staphylococcus aureus and Bacillus subtilis, and inactive on Escherichia coli and Pseudomonas aeruginosa. From extract of 10 ml/gm plant material, 0.1 ml of extract was placed in the well on the plate[PG085]. Ethanol (95%) extract of dried leaves, at a concentration of 1000 mcg/ml on agar plate, was active on Salmonella D, Shigella dysenteriae 1, Shigella flexneri 2A and 4A. The extract was inactive on Salmonella B, Salmonella typhi Type 2, Shigella boydii, Shigella boydii 5, Shigella dysenteriae 2, Shigella flexneri 3A and Shigella sonnei[PG088]. Ethanol/water (1:1) extract of the aerial parts, at a concentration greater than 25.0 mcg/ml on agar plate, was inactive on Bacillus subtilis, Escherichia coli, Salmonella typhosa, Staphylococcus aureus and Agrobacterium tumefaciens[PG092]. Hot water extract of dried leaves, undiluted on agar plate, was active on Staphylococcus aureus and Sarcina lutea[PG098]. Saline extract of leaves, at a concentration of 1–40 on agar plate, was active on Staphylococcus aureus and inactive on Escherichia coli[PG094]. Tannin frac-

tion of dried leaves, at a concentration of 100.0 mcg/ml on agar plate, was active on Escherichia piracoli. A concentration of 110 mcg/ml was active on Escherichia coli; 60.0 mcg/ml active on Citrobacter diversus; 85.0 mcg/ml active on Klebsiella pneumonia and Shigella flexneri; 95.0 mcg/ml active on Salmonella enteritidis and Staphylococcus aureus[PG033]. Water extract of fresh leaves, at a concentration of 1.0% on agar plate, was active on Neisseria gonorrhea[PG079]. Aqueous extract of the leaf, investigated by plate count, disk inhibition zone and turbidity techniques, indicated that a concentration of 6.5 mg/ml produced complete inhibition of 9 strains of Staphylococcus aureus[PG102]. Ethanol, water, and acetone-diluted extracts of the sprout displayed halos exceeding 13 mm for both Escherichia coli and Staphylococcus aureus. The ethanol (50%) extract most effectively inhibited E. coli, while those in 50% acetone were less effective[PG105].

Anticholinergic activity. Water extract of dried fruits was active on rat ileum vs ACh-induced contractions[PG058].

Anticonvulsant activity. Ethanol/water (1:1) extract of aerial parts, administered to mice at a dose of 0.094 mg/kg, was inactive vs electroshock-induced convulsions[PG092].

Anticough activity. Water extract of the leaf, administered orally to rats and guinea pigs at doses of 2 and 5 gm/kg, decreased the frequency of cough induced by capsaicin aerosol by 35 and 54%, respectively, as compared to control, within 10 min after injection of the extract. The activity was less potent than 3 mg/kg dextromethorphan, which decreased frequency of cough by 78%. An experiment of isolated rat tracheal muscle indicated that the extract directly stimulated muscle contraction and also synergized with the stimulatory effect of pilocarpine. This effect was antagonized by an atropine[PG101].

Antidiarrheal activity. Decoction of dried leaves, administered to rats by gastric intubation at a dose of 10.0 ml/kg, was active vs microlax-induced diarrhea[PG020]. Ethanol (95%) extract of dried leaves, administered by gastric intubation to mice at a dose of 750.0 mg/kg, produced weak activity. A dose of 0.5 ml of castor oil per 20 kg of body weight was given to induce diarrhea[PG088].

Antiedema activity. Dried fruit, administered intraperitoneally to male rats at a dose of 100.0 mg/kg, was active vs acetic acid-induced peritoneal proteinexudation[PG032].

Antifungal activity. Acetone, ethanol (95%) and water extracts of dried stem, at a concentration of 50% on agar plate, was inactive on *Neurospora crassa*. Acetone, water and ethanol (95%) extracts of dried leaves, at a concentration of 50% on agar plate, were inactive on *Neurospora crassa*[PG069]. Hot water extract of dried leaves, at a concentration of 1.0 ml in broth culture, was active on *Epidermophyton floccosum*, and inactive on *Microsporum canis*, *Microsporum gypseum*, *Trichophyton mentagrophytes* var. algodonosa and *Trichophyton rubrum*. Ethanol (95%) extract of dried bark, at a concentration of 50.0 mg/ml on agar plate, was inactive on *Aspergillus niger*. From the extract of 10 ml/gm plant material, 0.1 ml was placed in the well of the plate[PG085]. Ethanol/water (1:1) extract of the aerial parts, at a concentration greater than 25.0 mcg/ml on agar plate, was inactive on *Microsporum canis*, *Trichophyton mentagrophytes* and *Aspergillus niger*[PG092]. Hot water extract of dried leaves, undiluted on agar plate, was inactive on *Aspergillus niger*[PG098]. Water extract of fresh leaves, at a concentration of 1:1 on agar plate, was active on *Fusarium oxysporum* F. sp. Lentis. The extract represented 1 gm dried leaves in 1.0 ml of water[PG028].

Antigonadotrophin effect. Ethanol/water (1:1) extract of roots, at a dose of 600.0 mg/animal in the ration of male rats, was inactive. The water and ethanol/water (1:1) extracts, administered subcutaneously to male rats at a dose of 15.0 mg/animal, induced sex organ atrophy[PG099].

Antihyperglycemic activity. Ethanol/water (50%) extract dried leaves, administered by gastric intubation to rats at a dose of 200.0 mg/kg, was active vs alloxan-induced hyperglycemia[PG081]. Water extract of fresh fruit, administered by gastric intubation to rats at doses of 5.0 and 8.0 gm/kg, was active vs streptozotocin-induced hyperglycemia[PG018]. Fresh fruit juice, administered intraperitoneally to mice at a dose of 1.0 gm/kg, was active vs alloxan-induced hyperglycemia. The juice, taken orally by human adults at a dose of 1.0 gm/kg, was active, results significant at $P < 0.05$ level[PG064].

Anti-inflammatory activity. Dried fruit, administered intraperitoneally to male rats at a dose of 100.0 mg/kg, was active vs formaldehyde-induced arthritis, and at a dose of 25.0 mg/kg vs carrageenin-induced pedal edema[PG032]. Ethanol/water (1:1) extract of the aerial parts, administered orally to rats at a dose of 0.094 mg/kg, was inactive vs carrageenin-induced pedal edema. The animals were dosed 1 hour before carrageenin injections[PG092].

Antilipolytic activity. Ethanol/water (50%) extract of dried leaves, at a concentration of 100.0 mcg/ml, was active on the adipocytes-epidermal fat pad of rats. The N-butanol soluble portion of 50% ethanol extract was active vs epinephrine-induced lipolysis. A concentration of 200.0 mcg/ml of the aqueous soluble portion of ethanol extract was active vs epinephrine-induced lipolysis, results significant at $P < 0.01$ level. A concentration of 500.0 mcg/ml of the extract was active on the adipocytes-epididimal fat pad of rats vs epinephrine-induced lipolysis, results significant at $P < 0.01$ level[PG081].

Antimalarial activity. Acetic acid, ethanol (95%) and water extracts of dried leaves were active on *Plasmodium falciparum*, ED_{50} 10.0 mcg/ml, 36.0 mcg/ml, and 80.0 mcg/ml, respectively[PG024]. Chloroform extract of dried leaves was inactive on *Plasmodium falciparum* vs hypoxanthine uptake by plasmodia, IC_{50} 499.0 mcg/ml. Petroleum ether extract of dried leaves was weakly active on *Plasmodium falciparum* vs hypoxanthine uptake by plasmodia, IC_{50} 49.0 mcg/ml[PG047].

Antimutagenic activity. Chloroform extract of fresh fruit, at a concentration of 100.0% on agar plate, was active on *Salmonella typhimurium* TA97 vs 2-aminofluorene- and 4-nitro-o-phenylenediamine-induced mutagenesis. The extract was inactive on *Salmonella typhimurium* TA100 and TA1535 vs sodium azide-induced mutagenesis; *Salmonella typhimurium* TA98 vs 2-aminofluorene- and 4-nitro-o-phenylene-diamine-induced mutagenesis. The water extract, at a concentration of 100.0% on agar plate, was active on *Salmonella typhimurium* TA100 vs 2-aminofluorene- and sodium azide-induced mutagenesis and on *Salmonella typhimurium* TA97 and TA98 vs 2-aminofluorene- and 4-nitro-o-phenylene-diamine-induced mutagenesis[PG021]. Chromatographic fraction of fresh leaves, at a concentration of 1.0 mg/plate on agar plate, was active on *Escherichia coli* vs UV-induced mutation[PG027]. Methanol extract of dried fruit, at a concentration of 50.0 microliters/disc on agar plate, was inactive on *Bacillus subtilis* NIG-1125 HIS MET and *Escherichia coli* B/R-WP2-TRP. Methanol extract of dried leaves, at a concentration of 50.0 microliters/disc on agar plate, was inactive on *Bacillus subtilis* NIG-1125 HIS MET and produced weak activity on *Escherichia coli* B/R-WP2-TRP[PG073]. Methanol extract of freeze-dried leaves, at a concentration of 5.0 mg/plate on agar plate, was active on *Escherichia coli* WP-2 vs MNNG-induced mutation and UV-induced mutagenicity[PG039].

Antimycobacterial activity. Hot water extract of dried leaves, undiluted on agar plate, was active on *Mycobacterium phlei*[PG098].

Antioxidant effect. Pulp and peel contained 2.62–7.79% extractable polyphenols. Using the free radical scavenging (DPPH),

ferric reducing antioxidant power assay (FRAP), and inhibition of copper-catalyzed in vitro human low-density lipoprotein (LDL) oxidation, all fractions indicated a remarkable antioxidant capacity, and this activity was correlated with the corresponding total phenolic content. A 1 gm portion of peel (dry weight) contained DPPH activity, FRAP activity, and inhibition of copper-induced in vitro LDL oxidation, equivalent to 43 mg, 116 mg, and 176 mg of Trolox, respectively[PG106].

Antipyretic activity. Dried fruit, administered intraperitoneally to male rats at a dose of 50.0 mg/kg, was active vs yeast-induced pyrexia[PG032].

Antispasmodic activity. Ethanol/water (1:1) extract of the aerial parts was inactive on guinea pig ileum vs ACh- and histamine-induced spasms[PG092]. Water extract of dried fruits was active on rat ileum vs ACh-induced contractions[PG058].

Antiviral activity. Ethanol/water (1:1) extract of the aerial parts, at a concentration of 50.0 mcg/ml in cell culture, was inactive on Vaccinia virus[PG092].

Antiyeast activity. Ethanol (60%) extract of dried leaves, on agar plate, was active on *Candida albicans*[PG053]. Ethanol (95%) extract of dried bark, at a concentration of 50.0 mg/ml, was inactive on *Candida albicans*. From the extract of 10 ml/gm plant material, 0.1 ml was placed in the well of the plate[PG085]. Ethanol/water (1:1) extract of the aerial parts, at a concentration of 25.0 mg/ml, was inactive on *Candida albicans* and *Cryptococcus neoformans*[PG092]. Hot water extract of dried leaves, undiluted on agar plate, was inactive on *Saccharomyces cerevisiae*[PG098].

Carcinogenic activity. Water extract of unripe fruits, administered subcutaneously to female mice at a dose of 35.0 gm/animal weekly for 77 weeks, was inactive. Of 15 rats, none developed tumors. When administered to male rats, 2 of 15 developed tumors[PG035].

Central nervous system effect. Hexane, ethyl acetate, and methanol extracts of the leaves at concentrations of 20, 100, 500, and 1250 mg/kg, produced mostly dose-dependent antinociceptive effects in chemical and thermal tests of analgesia. The extracts also produced dose-dependent prolongation of pentobarbitone-induced sleeping time. However, they had variable and mostly non-significant effects on locomotor coordination, locomotor activity or exploration. In the pharmacological tests used, the ethyl acetate extract appeared to be the most active, followed by the hexane and then the methanol extracts[PG103].

Cytotoxic activity. Chloroform extract of dried leaves, in cell culture, was active on CA-9KB, ED_{50} 7.9 mcg/ml. The ethanol (95%) extract was active on LEUK-P388, ED_{50} 7.6 mcg/ml, and inactive on CA-9KB-V1 (vinblastine resistant), ED_{50} > 20.0 mcg/ml[PG022].

Diuretic activity. Ethanol/water (1:1) extract of the aerial parts, administered intraperitoneally to rats at a dose of 0.047 mg/kg, was inactive vs saline-loaded animals. Urine was collected for 4 hours post-drug administration[PG092].

Estrous cycle disruption effect. Ethanol (95%) and hot water extracts of roots, administered subcutaneously to rats at a dose of 20.0 mg/animal, and ethanol/water (1:1) extract, administered orally at a dose of 300.0 mg/animal daily, were active[PG099].

Gastric emptying time increase. Water and methanol extracts of dried roots, administered intraperitoneally to rats at a dose of 250.0 mg/kg, were active[PG023].

Glutamate-pyruvate-transaminase inhibition. Ethanol/water (1:1) extract of dried branches, at a concentration of 1.0 mg/ml in cell culture, was active on rat liver cells vs CCl_4-induced hepatotoxicity and PGE-1-induced pedal edema[PG086].

Granuloma formation inhibition. Dried fruit, administered intraperitoneally to male rats at a dose of 25.0 mg/kg, was active vs cotton pellet granuloma[PG032].

Hyperglycemic activity. Hot water extract of dried leaves, administered orally to mice at a dose of 5.0 gm/kg, was active. A 16% rise in blood sugar was observed[PG097].

Hypoglycemic activity. Ethanol/water (1:1) extract of dried leaves, administered orally to mice and rabbits at a dose of 5.0 gm/kg, was inactive[PG097]. Ethanol/water (1:1) extract of the aerial parts, administered orally to rats at a dose of 250 mg/kg, was inactive. Less than 30% drop in blood sugar level was observed[PG092].

Hypothermic activity. Ethanol/water (1:1) extract of the aerial parts, administered intraperitoneally to mice at a dose of 0.094 mg/kg, was inactive[PG092].

Insulin biosynthesis stimulation. Ethanol/water (50%) extract of dried leaves, administered to rats by gastric intubation at a dose of 200.0 mg/kg, was inactive vs alloxan-induced hyperglycemia[PG081].

Intestinal motility inhibition. Water extract of dried roots, administered intraperitoneally to rats at a dose of 250.0 mg/kg, was active[PG023].

Locomotor activity decrease. Decoction of dried leaves, administered by gastric intubation to rats at a dose of 10.0 ml/kg, was active[PG020].

Molluscicidal activity. Aqueous slurry (homogenate) of fresh entire plant (fruits, roots, and leaves), was inactive on *Lymnaea columella* and *Lymnaea cubensis*, LD_{100} > 1M ppm[PG062]. Water extract of oven-dried leaves was active on *Biomphalaria pfeifferi*[PG083]. Water saturated with fresh leaf essential oil, at a concentration of 1:10, was inactive on *Biomphalaria glabrata*[PG066].

Plant germination inhibition. Water extracts of dried bark, dried leaves and dried stem, at a concentration of 500.0 gm/liter, produced weak activity on *Cuscuta reflexa* seeds after 6 days of exposure to the extract[PG052].

Plant growth inhibition. Water extracts of dried leaves, dried bark and dried stem, at a concentration of 500.0 gm/liter, produced weak activity on *Cuscuta reflexa*. Seedling length, weight and dry weight were measured after 6 days of exposure to the extract[PG052].

Semen coagulation. Ethanol/water (1:1) extract of the aerial parts, at a concentration of 2.0%, was inactive on rat semen[PG092].

Smooth muscle relaxant activity. Methanol extract of dried leaves, at variable concentration, was active on guinea pig ileum[PG042]. Water extract of dried fruits was active on rat ileum[PG058].

Spasmogenic activity. Water extract of dried leaves, administered by gastric intubation to rats at a concentration of 20.0 ml/kg, was active on the small intestine. Extract of paste made from fresh leaves was used[PG020].

Spasmolytic activity. Butanol extract of dried leaves, at a concentration of 0.2 mg/ml, was active on guinea pig ileum. There was 100.0% reduction in contraction vs ACh-induced contractions, and 95.72% reduction vs KCl-induced contractions. The isopentyl alcohol extract, at a concentration of 0.2 mg/ml, was active on guinea pig ileum. There was an 83.60% reduction in contraction vs ACh-induced contractions, and 77.80% reduction vs KCl-induced contractions. Butanol extract of dried stem bark, at a concentration of 0.2 mg/ml, was active on guinea pig ileum. An 82.50% reduction in contraction was observed vs ACh-induced contractions and 52.70% reduction vs KCl-induced contractions. The isopentyl alcohol extract produced a 48.10% reduction in contraction on guinea pig ileum vs KCl-induced contractions and 67.40% reduction on pigeon ileum vs ACh-induced contractions[PG050]. Hexane extract of dried leaves, at a concentration of 0.5 mg/ml, and methanol and water extracts, at concentrations of 1.0 mg/ml, were active on guinea pig ileum vs electrically induced contractions[PG048].

Spermicidal effect. Ethanol/water (1:1) extract of the aerial parts was inactive in rats[PG092].

Spontaneous activity reduction. Methanol extract of dried leaves, administered by gastric intubation to mice at a dose of 3.3 mg/kg, was active; when administered intraperitoneally to mice the ED_{90} was 4.1 mg/kg[PG040].

Toxicity assessment (quantitative). Ethanol/water (1:1) extract of the aerial parts, administered to intraperitoneally to mice, produced LD_{50} 0.188 gm/kg[PG092].

Xanthine oxidase inhibition. Ethanol (70%) extract of dried leaves was active, IC_{50} 16.0 mcg/ml[PG041].

REFERENCES

PG001 Davis, P. L., K. A. Munroe and A. G. Selnine. Laboratory bioassay of volatile naturally occurring compounds against the Caribbean fruit fly. **Proc Fla State Hort Soc** 1976; 89: 174.

PG002 Haddock, R. L. Some medicinal plants of Guam including English and Guamanian common names. Report Regional Tech Mtg Med Plants, Papeete, Tahiti, Nov, 1973, South Pacific Commissioner, Noumea, New Caledonia 1974; 79pp.

PG003 Varshney, I. P., G. Badhwar, A. A. Khan and A. Shrivastava. Saponins and sapogenins of *Sesbania grandiflora* seeds, *Albizzia lebbek* pods and *Psidium guajava* fruits. **Indian J Appl Chem** 1971; 34: 214.

PG004 Steenis-Kruseman, M. J. Van. Select Indonesian medicinal plants. **Organiz Sci Res Indonesia Bull** 1953; 18: 1.

PG005 Chang, C. L. and M. T. Peng. In vitro inactivation of gonadotropins by Psidium root extract. **Taiwan I Hsueh Hui Tsa Chih** 1973; 72: 379.

PG006 Fester, G. A., J. A. Retamar, A. I. A. Ricciardi and L. R. Fonseca. Essential oils from Argentina plants. XI. **Rev Fac Ing Quim** 1959; 28: 9.

PG007 Griffiths, L. A. On the distribution of gentisic acid in green plants. **J Exp Biol** 1959; 10: 437.

PG008 Burkhill, I. H. Dictionary of the Economic Products of the Malay Peninsula.

Ministry of Agriculture and Cooperatives, Kuala Lumpur, Malaysia. Volume II, 1966.

PG009 Misra, K. and T. R. Seshadri. Chemical components of the fruits of *Psidium guajava*. **Phytochemistry** 1968; 7: 641–645.

PG010 Seshadri, T. R. and K. Vasishta. Polyphenols of the leaves of *Psidium guajava* quercetin, guaijaverin, leucocyanidin and amritoside. **Phytochemistry** 1965; 4: 989–992.

PG011 Seshadri, T. R. and K. Vasishta. Polyphenols of the stem bark of *Psidium guajava* - The constitution of a new ellagic acid glycoside (amritoside). **Phytochemistry** 1965; 4: 317–326.

PG012 Lowry, J. B. The distribution and potential taxonomic value of alkylated ellagic acids. **Phytochemistry** 1968; 7(10): 1803–1813.

PG013 Pangsrinongsa, S. and C. Sambhandharaksa. Vitamin C content in some local fruits. **J Pharm Ass Siam** 1949; 2(5): 213–219.

PG014 Kakiuchi, N., M. Hattori, T. Namba, M. Nishizawa and T. Yamagishi. Inhibitory effect of tannins on reverse transcriptase from RNA tumor virus. **J Nat Prod** 1985; 48(4): 614–621.

PG015 Okuda, T., T. Yoshida, T. Hatano, K. Yazaki, Y. Ikegami and T. Shingu. Guavins A, C and D, complex tannins from *Psidium guajava*. **Chem Pharm Bull** 1987; 35(1): 443–446.

PG016 Tanaka, T., N. Ishida, M. Ishimatsu, G. I. Nonaka and I. Nishioka. Tannins and related compounds. CXVI. Six new complex tannins, guajavins, psidinins and psiguavin from the bark of *Psidium guajava* L. **Chem Pharm Bull** 1992; 40(8): 2092–2098.

PG017 Ortiz de Montellano, B. Empirical Aztec medicine. **Science** 1975; 188: 215–220.

PG018 Hsu, F. L. and J T. Cheng. Investigation in rats of the antihyperglycaemic effect of plant extracts used in Taiwan for the treatment of diabetes mellitus. **Phytother Res** 1992; 6(2): 108–111.

PG019 Holdsworth, D. K. Traditional medicinal plants of Rarotonga, Cook Islands. Part II. **Int J Pharmacog** 1991; 29(1): 71–79.

PG020 Lutterodt, G. D. Inhibition of microlax-induced experimental diarrhoea with narcotic-like extracts of *Psidium guajava* leaf in rats. **J Ethnopharmacol** 1992; 37(2): 151–157.

PG021 Grove, I. S. and S. Bala. Studies on antimutagenic effects of guava (*Psidium guajava*) in *Salmonella typhimurium*. **Mutat Res** 1993; 300(1): 1–3.

PG022 Villarreal, M. L., D. Alonso and G. Melesio. Cytotoxic activity of some Mexican plants used in traditional medicine. **Fitoterapia** 1992; 63(6): 518–522.

PG023 Obasi, B. N. B., C. A. Igboechi, D. C. Anuforo and K. N. Aimufua. Effects of extracts of *Newbouldia laevis*, *Psidium guajava* and *Phyllanthus amarus* on gastrointestinal tract. **Fitoterapia** 1993; 64(3): 235–238.

PG024 Gessler, M. C., M. H. H. Nkunyak, L. B. Mwasumbi, M. Heinrich and M. Tanner. Screening of Tanzanian medicinal plants for antimalarial activity. **Acta Tropica** 1994; 56(1): 65–77.

PG025 Caceres, A., M. Torres, S. Ortiz, F. Cano and E. Jauregui. Plants used in Guatemala for the treatment of gastrointestinal disorders. IV. Vibriocidal activity of five American plants used to treat infections. **J Ethnopharmacol** 1993; 39(1): 73–75.

PG026 Zamora-Martinez, M. C. and C. N. P. Pola. Medicinal plants used in some rural populations of Oaxaca, Puebla and Veracruz, Mexico. **J Ethnopharmacol** 1992; 35(3) 229–257.

PG027 Matsuo, T., N. Hanamure, K. Shimoi, Y. Nakamura and I. Tomita. Identification of (+)-gallocatechin as a bio-antimutagenic compound in *Psidium guajava* leaves. **Phytochemistry** 1994; 36(4): 1027–1029.

PG028 Singh, J., A. K. Dubey and N. N. Tripathi. Antifungal activity of *Mentha spicata*. **Int J Pharmacog** 1994; 32(4): 314–319.

PG029 Bassols, F. and E. P. Demole. The occurrence of pentane-2-thiol in guava fruit. **J Essent Oil Res** 1994; 5(5): 481–483.

PG030 Caceres, A., L. Figueroa, A. M. Taracena and B. Samayoa. Plants used in Guatemala for the treatment of respiratory diseases. 2. Evaluation of activity of 16 plants against gram-positive bacteria. **J Ethnopharmacol** 1993; 39(1): 77–82.

PG031   Lozoya, X., M. Meckes, M. Abou-Aaid, J. Tortoriello, C. Nozzolillo and J. T. Arnason. Quercetin glycosides in *Psidium guajava* L. leaves and determination of a spasmolytic principle. **Arch Med Res** 1994; 25(1): 11–15.

PG032   Hussam, T. S., S. H. Nasralla and A. K. N. Chaudhuri. Studies on the antiinflammatory and related pharmacological activities of *Psidium guajava*. A preliminary report. **Phytother Res** 1995; 9(2): 118–122.

PG033   Lutete, T., K. Kambu, D. Ntondele, K. Cimanga and N. Luki. Antimicrobial activity of tannins. **Fitoterapia** 1994; 65(3): 276–278.

PG034   Awasthi, A. K. Ethnobotanical studies on the Negrito Islanders of Andaman Islands, India - The Great Andamanese. **Econ Bot** 1991; 45(2): 274–280.

PG035   Kapadia, G. J., E. B. Chung, B. Ghosh, Y. N. Shukla, S. P. Basak, J. F. Morton and S. N. Pradhan. Carcinogenicity of some folk medicinal herbs in rats. **J Nat Cancer Inst** 1978; 60: 683–686.

PG036   Trivedi, K. K. and K. Misra. Chemical investigation of *Psidium guajava* roots. **Curr Sci** 1984; 53(14): 746–747.

PG037   Cuellar Cuellar, A., R. Arteaga Lara and J. Perez Zayas. *Psidium guajava* L. phytochemical screening and study of the essential oil. **Rev Cubana Farm** 1984; 18(1): 92–99.

PG038   Idstein, H., C. Bauer and P. Schreier. Volatile acids from tropical fruits: Cherimoya (*Annona cherimolia*, Mill.), guava (*Psidium guajava*, L.), mango (*Manigfera indica*, L., var. Alphonso), papaya (*Carica papaya*, L.). **Z Lebensmunters Forsch** 1985; 180(5): 394–397.

PG039   Jain, A. K., K. Shimoi, Y. Nakamura, I. Tomita and T. Kada. Preliminary study on the desmutagenic and antimutagenic effect of some natural products. **Curr Sci** 1987; 56(24): 1266–1269.

PG040   Lutterodt, G. D. and A. Maleque. Effects on mice locomotor activity of a narcotic-like principle from *Psidium guajava* leaves. **J Ethnopharmacol** 1988; 24(2/3): 219–231.

PG041   Theoduloz, C., L. Franco, E. Ferro and G. Schmeda Hirschmann. Xanthine oxidase inhibitory activity on Paraguayan Myrtaceae. **J Ethnopharmacol** 1988; 24(2/3): 179–183.

PG042   Lutterodt, G. D. Inhibition of gastrointestinal release of acetylcholine by quercetin as a possible mode of action of *Psidium guajava* leaf extracts in the treatment of acute diarrhoeal disease. **J Ethnopharmacol** 1989; 25(3): 235–247.

PG043   Le Grand, A. Anti-infectious phytotherapy of the tree-savannah, Senegal (Western Africa) III: A review of the phytochemical substances and antimicrobial activity of 43 species. **J Ethnopharmacol** 1989; 25(3): 315–338.

PG044   Mair, A. G. R., M. Pandiyan and H. Venkasubramanian. Polyphenolic compounds from flowers of *Psidium guajava*. **Fitoterapia** 1987; 58(3): 204–205.

PG045   Quansah, N. Ethnomedicine in the Maroantsetra region of Madagascar. **Econ Bot** 1988; 42(3): 370–375.

PG046   Reddy, M. B., K. R. Reddy and M. N. Reddy. A survey of medicinal plants of Chenchu Tribes of Andhra Pradesh, India. **Int J Crude Drugs Res** 1988; 26(4): 189–196.

PG047   Weenen, H., M. H. H. Nkunya, D. H. Bray, et al. Antimalarial compounds containing an α,β-unsaturated carbonyl moiety from Tanzanian medicinal plants. **Planta Med** 1990; 56(4): 368–370.

PG048   Lozoya, X., G. Becerril and M. Martinez. Intraluminal perfusion model of in vitro guinea pig's ileum as a model of study of the antidiarrheic properties of the guava (*Psidium guajava*) **Arch Invest Med** (Mex) 1990; 21: 155–162.

PG049   Caceres, A., B. R. Lopez, M. A. Giron and H. Logemann. Plants used in Guatemala for the treatment of dermatophytic infections. I. Screening for anti-mycotic activity of 44 plant extracts. **J Ethnopharmacol** 1991; 31(3): 263–276.

PG050   Kambu, K., L. Tona, S. Kaba, K. Cimanga and N. Mukala. Antispasmodic activity of extracts proceeding of plant antidiarrheic traditional preparations used in Kinshasa, Zaire. **Ann Pharm Fr** 1990; 48(4): 200–208.

PG051 Ji, X. D., Q. L. Pu, H. M. Garraffo and L. K. Pannell. The essential oil of the leaves of *Psidium guajava* L. **J Essent Oil Res** 1991; 3(3): 187–189.

PG052 Chauhan, J. S., N. K. Singh and S. V. Singh. Screening of higher plants for specific herbicidal principle active against dodder, *Cuscuta reflexa* Roxb. **Indian J Exp Biol** 1989; 27(10): 877–884.

PG053 Caceres, A., E. Jauregu, D. Herrera and H. Logemann. Plants used in Guatemala for the treatment of dermatomucosal infections. 1. Screening of 38 plant extracts for anticandidal activity. **J Ethnopharmacol** 1991; 33(3): 277–283.

PG054 Wilson III, C. W. and P. E. Shaw. Terpene hydrocarbons from *Psidium guajava*. **Phytochemistry** 1978; 17: 1435–1436.

PG055 Mishra, C. S. and K. Misra. Chemical constituents of *Psidium guajava* heartwood. **J Indian Chem Soc** 1981; 58: 201–202.

PG056 Oliveros-Belardo, L., R. M. Smith and J. M. Robinson. Chemical study of the essential oil from the fruit peelings of *Psidium guajava* L., Philippine variety. **Abstr 23rd Annual Meeting American Society of Pharmacognosy** August 1–5 1982 Pittsburgh PA 1982; 23: Abstr-43.

PG057 Nagar, P. K. and T. R. Rao. Studies on endogenous cytokinins in guava (*Psidium guajava* L.). **Ann Bot (London)** 1981; 48: 845–852.

PG058 Apisariyakul, A. and V. Anantasarn. A pharmacological study of the Thai medicinal plants used as cathartics and antispasmodics. **Abstr 10th Conference of Science and Technology Thailand Chiengmai Univ**, Thailand 1984; 452,453.

PG059 Osman, A. M., Y. M. El-Garby and A. E. Sheta. Chemical examination of local plants. Part VII. *Psidium guajava* leaf extracts. **Egypt J Chem** 1975; 18: 347.

PG060 Gupta, M. P., T. D. Arias, M. Correa and S. S. Lamba. Ethnopharmacognostic observations on Panamanian medicinal plants. Part 1. **Q J Crude Drug Res** 1979; 17(3/4): 115–130.

PG061 Adu-Tutu, M., Y. Afful, K. Asante-Appiah, D. Lieberman, J. B. Hall and M. Elvin-Lewis. Chewing stick usage in Southern Ghana. **Econ Bot** 1979; 33: 320–328.

PG062 Medina, F. R. and R. Woodbury. Terrestrial plants molluscicidal to Lymnaeid hosts of *Fasciliasis hepatica* in Puerto Rico. **J Agr Univ Puerto Rico** 1979; 63: 366–376.

PG063 Okuda, T., T. Yoshida, T. Hatano, K. Yazaki and M. Ashida. Tannins and related compounds in Myrtaceae. Ellagitannins of the Casuarinaceae, Stachyuraceae and Myrtaceae. **Phytochemistry** 1982; 21: 2871–2874.

PG064 Cheng, J. T. and R. S. Yang. Hypoglycemic effect of guava juice in mice and human subjects. **Amer J Chin Med** 1983; 11(1/4): 74–76.

PG065 Rao, R. R. and N. S. Jamir. Ethnobotanical studies in Nagaland. I. Medicinal plants. **Econ Bot** 1982; 36: 176–181.

PG066 Rouquayrol, M. Z., M. C. Fonteles, J. E. Alencar, F. Jose de Abreu and A. A. Craveiro. Molluscicidal activity of essential oils from Northeastern Brazilian plants. **Rev Brasil Pesq Med Biol** 1980; 13: 135–143.

PG067 Okuda, T., T. Hatano and K. Yazaki. Guavin B, an ellagitannin of novel type. **Chem Pharm Bull** 1984; 32(9): 3787–3788.

PG068 Balick, M. J. Ethnobotany of Palms in the Neotropics. Advances on Economic Botany in the Neotropics G. T. Prance and J. A. Kallunki (Eds) New York Botanical Garden, Bronx, N. Y. 1984; 1: 9–23pp.

PG069 Lopez Abraham, A. N., N. M. Rojas Hernandez and C. A. Jimenez Misas. Potential antineoplastic activity of Cuban plants. IV. **Rev Cubana Farm** 1981; 15(1): 71–77.

PG070 Arnold, H. J. and M. Gulumian. Pharmacopoeia of traditional medicine in Venda. **J Ethnopharmacol** 1984; 12(1): 35–74.

PG071 Kargbo, T. K. Traditional practices affecting the health of women and children in Africa. **Unpublished Manuscript** 1984.

PG072 Goh, S. H., E. Soepadmo, P. Chang, U. Barnerjee et al. Studies on Malaysian medicinal plants. Preliminary results.

Proc 5th **Asian Symposium on Medicinal Plants and Spices**, South Korea 1984; August 20–24. 5: 473–483.

PG073 Ishii, R., K. Yoshikawa, H. Minakata, H. Komura and T. Kada. Specificities of bio-antimutagens in plant kingdom. **Agr Biol Chem** 1984; 48(10): 2587–2591.

PG074 Holdsworth, D. Phytomedicine of the Madang Province, Papua, New Guinea. Part I. Karkar Island. **Int J Crude Drug Res** 1984; 22(3): 111–119.

PG075 Whistler, W. A. Traditional and herbal medicine in the Cook Islands. **J Ethnopharmacol** 1985; 13(3): 239–280.

PG076 Trivedi, K. K. and K. Misra. Chemical investigation of *Psidium guajava* roots. **Curr Sci** 1984; 53(14): 746–747.

PG077 Velazco, E. A. Herbal and traditional practices related to maternal and child health care. **Rural Reconstruction Review** 1980; 35–39.

PG078 Tiwari, K. C., R. Majumder and S. Bhattacharjee. Folklore medicines from Assam and Arunachal Pradesh (District Tirap). **Int J Crude Res** 1979; 17(2): 61–67.

PG079 Khan, M. R., G. Ndaalio, M. H. H. Nkunya, H. Wevers. Studies on the rationale of African traditional medicine. Part II. Preliminary screening of medicinal plants for anti-gonoccoci activity. **Pak J Sci Ind Res** 1978; 27(5/6): 189–192.

PG080 Singh, Y. N. Traditional medicine in Fiji. Some herbal folk cures used by Fiji Indians. **J Ethnopharmacol**. 1986; 15(1): 57–88.

PG081 Maruyama, Y., H. Matsuda, R. Matsuda, M. Kubo, T. Hatano and T. Okuda. Study on *Psidium guajava* L. (1). Antidiabetic effect and effective components of the leaf of *Psidium guajava* L. (Part 1). **Shoyakugaku Zasshi** 1985; 39(4): 261–269.

PG082 Weniger, B., M. Rouzier, R. Daguilh, D. Henrys, J. H. Henrys and R. Anthon. Popular medicine of the Central Plateau of Haiti. 2. Ethnopharmacological inventory. **J Ethnopharmacol** 1986; 17(1): 13–30.

PG083 Kloss, H., F. W. Thiongo, J. H. Ouma and A. E. Butterworth. Preliminary evaluation of some wild and cultivated plants from snail control in Machakos District, Kenya. **J Trop Med Hyg** 1987; 90(4): 197–204.

PG084 Chiang, H. C., S. H. Lee and S. I. Guo. Active principles of hypoglycemic effect from *Psidium guajava*. Part II. **Asian J Pharm Suppl** 1986; 6(8): 58–.

PG085 Verpoorte, R. and P. P. Dihal. Medicinal plants of Surinam. IV. Antimicrobial activity of some medicinal plants. **J Ethnopharmacol** 1987; 21(3): 315–318.

PG086 Yang, L. L., K. Y. Yen, Y. Kiso and H. Kikino. Antihepatotoxic actions of Formosan plant drugs. **J Ethnopharmacol** 1987; 19(1): 103–110.

PG087 Ramirez, V. R., L. J. Mostacero, A. E. Garcia, C. F. Mejia, P. F. Pelaez, C. D. Medina and C. H. Miranda. Vegetales empleados en medicina tradicional Norperuana. **Banco Agrario Del Peru & NACL Univ Trujillo**, Peru, June 1988; 54pp.

PG088 Maikere-Faniyo, R., L. Van Puyvelde, A. Mutwewingabo and F. X. Habiyaremye. Study on Rwandese medicinal plants used in the treatment of diarrhea 1. **J Ethnopharmacol** 1989; 26(2): 101–109.

PG089 Darias, V., L. Brando, R. Rabanal, C. Sanchez Mateo, R. M. Gonzalez Luis and A. M. Hernandez Perez. New contribution to the ethnopharmacological study of the Canary Islands. **J Ethnopharmacol** 1989; 25(1): 77–92.

PG090 Misas, C. A. J., N. M. R. Hernandez and A. N. L. Abraham. Contribution to the biological evaluation of Cuban plants. II. **Rev Cub Med Trop** 1979; 31: 13–19.

PG091 Macleod, A. J. and N. G. de Troconis. Volatile flavour components of guava. **Phytochemistry** 1982; 21(6): 1339–1342.

PG092 Dhawan, B. N., G. K. Patnaik, R. P. Rastogi, K. K. Singh and J. S. Tandon. Screening of Indian plants for biological activity. VI. **Indian J Exp Biol** 1977; 15: 208–219.

PG093 Osman, A. M., M. E. G. Younes and A. E. Sheta. Triterpenoids of the leaves of *Psidium guajava*. **Phytochemistry** 1974; 13: 2015.

PG094 Collier, W. A. and L. Van de Piji. The antibiotic action of plants, especially the higher plants, with results with

Indonesian plants. **Chron Nat** 1949; 105: 8.

PG095   Logan, M. H. Digestive disorders and plant medicine in Highland Guatemala. **Anthropos** 1973; 68: 537–543.

PG096   Sasaki, S., H. C. Chiang, K. Habaguchi, T. Yamada, K. Nakanishi, S. Matsueda, H. Y. Hsu and W. N. Wu. The constituents of medicinal plants in Taiwan. **Yakugaku Zasshi** 1966; 86: 869–870.

PG097   Mueller-Oerlinghausen, B., W. Ngamwathana and P. Kanchanapee. Investigation into Thai medicinal plants said to cure diabetes. **J Med Assoc Thailand** 1971; 54: 105–111.

PG098   Malcolm, S. A. and E. A. Sofowora. Antimicrobial activity of selected Nigerian folk remedies and their constituent plants. **Lloydia** 1969; 32: 512–517.

PG099   Peng, M. T., H. C. Lee and H. S. Lin. Effect of Psidium root on the reproductive organs of rats and mice. **Tohoku J Exp Med** 1955; 62: 287–297.

PG100   Re, L., S. Barocci, C. Capitani, C. Vivani, M. Ricci, L. Rinaldi, G. Paolucci, A. Scarpantonio, O. S. Leon-Fernandez nad M. A. Morales. Effects of some natural extracts on the acetylcholine release at the mouse neuromuscular junction. **Pharmacol Res** 1999; 39(3): 239–245.

PG101   Jaiarj, P., P. Khoohaswan, Y. Wongkrajang, P. Peungvicha, P. Suriyawong, M. L. Saraya nad O. Ruangsomboon. Anticough and antimicrobial activities of *Psidium guajava* Linn. leaf extract. **J Ethnopharmacol** 1999; 67(2): 203–212.

PG102   Gnan, S. O. and M. T. Demello. Inhibition of *Staphylococcus aureus* by aqueous Goiaba extracts. **J Ethnopharmacol** 1999; 68(1-3): 103–108.

PG103   Shaheen, H. M., B. H. Ali, A. A. Alqarawi and A. K. Bashir. Effect of *Psidium guajava* leaves on some aspects of central nervous system in mice. **Phytother Res** 2000; 14(2): 107–111.

PG104   Tijet, N., U. Waspi, D. J. Gaskin, P. Hunziker, B. L. Muller, E. N. Vulfson, A. Slusarenko, A. R. Brash and I. M. Whitehead. Purification, molecular cloning, and expression of the gene encoding fatty acid 13-hydroperodie lyase from guava fruit (*Psidium guajava*). **Lipids** 2000; 35(7): 709–720.

PG105   Viera, R. H., Dd, Rodrigues, F. A. Goncalves, F. G. Menezes, J. S. Aragao and O. V. Sousa. Microbial effect of medicinal plant extracts (*Psidium guajava* Linn and *Carica papaya* Linn.) upon bacterial isolated from fish muscle and known to induce diarrhea in children. **Rev Inst Med Trop Sao Paulo** 2001; 43(3): 145–148.

PG106   Jimenez-Escrig, A., M. Rincon, R. Pulido and F. Saura-Calixto. Guava fruit (*Psidium guajava* L.) as a new source of antioxidant dietary fiber. **J Agri Food Chem** 2001; 49(11): 5489–5493.

25 | Punica granatum

L.

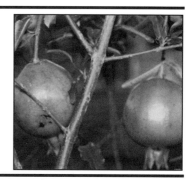

Common Names

Anar	Fiji	Pomegranate	Guyana
Anar	Nepal	Pomegranate	India
Dadima	India	Pomegranate	Madeira
Darim	India	Pomegranate	Mexico
Darim	Nepal	Pomegranate	Nepal
Darinko bokra	Nepal	Pomegranate	Turkey
Delum	Japan	Pomegranate	USA
Delun	Sri Lanka	Pomegranate	West Indies
Granada	Cuba	Posnar	India
Granada	Guatemala	Qsur roman	Morocco
Granada	Peru	Ranato	Italy
Granado	Canary Islands	Roma	Madeira
Granado	Mexico	Roman	Egypt
Granatum	India	Roman	Ethiopia
Grenade	Rodrigues Islands	Romeira	Madeira
Grenadier	Tunisia	Romman amruj	Morocco
Grenadillo	Belize	Romman	Jordan
Gul armini	Pakistan	Romman	Tunisia
Mathalanarakom	India	Ruman	Oman
Melograno	Italy	Seog-ryu	Oman
Mkoma manga	East Africa	Sham-al-rumman	Arabic countries
Nar	Turkey	Shih liu pi	China
Pomegranate	Egypt	Thab thim	Thailand
Pomegranate	England	Thapthim	Thailand
Pomegranate	Greece	Zakuro	Thailand

BOTANICAL DESCRIPTION

The plant is an erect shrub of the PUNICACEAE family, up to 3 meters high, much branched from the base, having branchlets slender, often ending in a spine. Leaves are simple, oblong-lanceolate, 1–9 by 0.5–2.5 cm; consisting of obtuse or marginate apex, base acute, shiny, glabrous. Flowers are showy, orange red, about 3 cm in diameter; 1–5 borne at branch tips, the others solitary in the highest leaf-axils, sessile or subsessile. Consisting of calyx 2–3 cm long,

From: *Medicinal Plants of the World, vol. 1: Chemical Constituents, Traditional and Modern Medicinal Uses, 2nd ed.*
By: Ivan A. Ross © Humana Press Inc., Totowa, NJ

tubular, lobes erect to recurved, 5–9, thick, coriaceous; petals the same number as the calyx lobes, rounded or very obtuse; from edge hypanthium; filament-free; inferior ovary, ovules numerous; style 1, stigma capitate. Fruit is a globose berry, crowded by persistent calyx-lobes, having leathery pericarp filled with numerous seeds, which are surrounded by pink and red, transparent, juicy, acidic, pleasant-tasting pulp. They are propagated by seeds or layering, in ordinary garden soil, with regular watering.

ORIGIN AND DISTRIBUTION

Pomegranate is one of the oldest drugs known. It is mentioned in the Ebers papyrus of Egypt written in about 1550 BC, and is included in many Ayurvedic texts. Pomegranate is native of Iran and is extensively cultivated as a fruit-tree or ornamental, or for medicinal purposes in Mediterranean region such as Spain, Morocco, Egypt, Afghanistan, and Iran. It is commonly found in the tropics and subtropics.

TRADITIONAL MEDICINAL USES

Arabic countries. Dried fruit peel is used as a contraceptive in the form of a pessary in Unani medicine[PG066].

Argentina. Decoction of dried pericarp is taken orally for diarrhea, and to treat respiratory and urinary tract infections[PG033].

Belize. Hot water extract of dried leaves is used externally for "women's problems". Leaves are boiled and the liquid is used for washing[PG063].

Canary Islands. Hot water extract of fresh root bark is taken orally as an anthelmintic[PG092].

China. Dried entire plant is used externally for burns and to promote eschar formation in burn treatment[PG086].

Europe. Hot water extract of root bark is taken orally as an emmenagogue[PG006].

East Africa. Hot water extract of pounded or soaked root is taken orally for tapeworm infestations[PG022].

Ethiopia. Extract of dried fruit is used for skin lesions[PG036]. Leaves, crushed in water, are taken orally to expel tapeworms[PG062]. Hot water extract of root bark is taken orally as an emmenagogue[PG006].

Fiji. Fresh juice of *Punica granatum* and *Cynodon dactylon* leaf juice is taken orally for cold and running nose. Fresh fruit juice is taken orally for jaundice and for diarrhea[PG078]. Water extract of dried fruit peel is taken orally for diabetes. Rind is ground with water and taken first thing in the morning. Decoction of dried seed is taken orally for syphilis[PG078].

Greece. Water extract of fruit peel is used a vaginal suppository with or without oak gall to be applied for some hours and removed immediately after coitus[PG003]. Decoction of dried fruit peel is taken orally to treat tracheobronchitis. The dried peel is boiled in water[PG034].

Guatemala. Hot water extract of dried fruit is used externally for wounds, ulcers, bruises and sores, mouth lesions, stomatitis, leucorrhea, and vaginitis. For conjunctivitis, the extract is applied ophthalmically[PG089].

India. Dried root is used as an abortifacient. Three parts *Allium cepa* seeds, 3 parts of *Punica granatum* root, 2 parts of *Cajanus cajan* and red lead oxide are taken with honey orally[PG080]. Fresh entire plant, made into a paste, is used for snakebite. The paste is applied to the bite; juice is dropped into the nostrils, ears and navel[PG073]. Fresh plant juice is used for snakebite. Plant is made into a paste and applied to bite; juice is dropped into the nostrils, ears and navel[PG073]. Hot water extract of dried bark and fruit is taken orally for leprosy, leucorrhea and menorrhagia[PG090]. Hot water extract of root bark is taken orally as an anthelmintic[PG097]. Olive oil extract of dried fruit is used externally to prevent premature graying of hair. The mixture contains *Terminalia arjuna*, *Aglaia roxburghiana*, *Jasminum officianales*, *Indigofera tinctoria*, *Tinospora cordifolia*,

Pterocarpus marsupium, Eclipta alba, Pandanus tectorius, Oroxylum indicum, Valeriana hardwickii, Terminalia chebula, Terminalia bellerica, Emblica officinales, Punica granatum, Nelumbium speciosum and *Sesamum indicum*[PG093]. Powdered immature fruit is taken orally for peptic ulcers. A half-teaspoon of powder is added to soft porridge and taken every morning[PG049]. Dried unripe fruit is taken orally for dysentery. Tender fruits or rinds of mature fruits are boiled in milk and made into a paste that is given internally[PG067]. Fruit juice is taken orally for high fever with loss of senses[PG040]. Water extract of dried fruit peel is taken orally for diarrhea[PG026]. Poultice of fruit peel and *Tamarix gallicia* bark is applied twice in 24 hours to the breasts to abate flaccidity. Hot water extract of dried fruit peel, mixed with aromatics, is taken orally for treating diarrhea and dysentery[PG076].

Indonesia. Hot water extracts of dried fruit peel[PG076] and root bark[PG006] are taken orally as abortifacients[PG076].

Italy. Hot water extract of dried fruit peel is used for inflammations[PG046].

Malaysia. Extract of dried fruit is taken orally by pregnant women for childbirth disorders[PG071]. Hot water extract of leaves is taken orally for irregular menses[PG008].

Mexico. Hot water extract of fruit peel is taken orally to stop excessive bleeding during menses[PG041].

Peru. Hot water extract of dried bark is taken orally by pregnant women to prevent abortion, for bloody dysentery and as an antidiarrheal. Hot water extract of dried root is taken orally for abortion, as an antidiarrheal and for bloody dysentery[PG088].

Sri Lanka. Hot water extract of fresh fruit is taken orally as a cooling agent and for dysentery[PG074].

Thailand. Hot water extract of dried root is taken orally as an anthelmintic. Hot water extract of dried fruit peel is taken orally for diarrhea and dysentery[PG102].

Tunisia. Extract of the dried bark is taken orally to treat ulcers[PG068].

USA. Hot water extract of dried root bark is used as a vaginal douche. For diarrhea, steep a teaspoon of bark in a cup of boiling water, cool and drink one cup a day. The extract is also taken orally as a remedy for tapeworm[PG103].

West Indies. Fruit peel, mixed and dry, ground with fowl gizzard and white flour, is eaten as porridge for tapeworm[PG061].

CHEMICAL CONSTITUENTS
(ppm unless otherwise indicated)

3-O-methyl-3,4-methylenedioxyellagic acid: Heartwood[PG112]
2-(2-Propenyl)-delta-piperideine: Bk[PG027]
1,2,4,6-Tetra-O-galloyl-beta-D-glucose: Lf[PG012]
1,2,3,4,6-Penta-O-galloyl-beta-D-glucose: Lf[PG102]
Apigenin-4'-O-beta-D-glucoside: Lf[PG018]
Betulinic acid: Bk, Lf[PG096]
Brevifolin carboxylic acid: Lf[PG017]
Callistephin: Sd Coat, Fr Pe[PG020]
Casuariin: Bk 940[PG014]
Casuarinin: Bk 0.32%[PG014], PC 3.8[PG030]
Chrysanthemin: Fr Pe[PG020], Sd Ct[PG020]
Coniine: Pl[PG011]
Corilagin: Lf 473.7[PG012,PG017], PC 4[PG030]
Coumestrol: Sd[PG045]
Cyanidin: Fl, Lf[PG044]
Cyanidin-3,5-diglucoside: Sd Ct[PG043]
Cyanin: Fr Pe[PG020], Sd Ct[PG020,PG043]
Daidzein: Sd[PG045]
Delphin: Sd Ct[PG020,PG043]
Delphinidin; Fl, Lf[PG044]
Delphinidin-3-0-beta-D-glucoside: Sd Ct[PG020]
Delphinidin-3-glucoside: Sd Ct[PG043]
Ellagic acid: Bk[PG009], Lf[PG017], PC[PG030], Fr Pe[PG065]
Ellagic acid,3'-0-methyl-3-4-methyl: Bk[PG009]
Ellagic acid,3-3'-4-tri-0-methyl: Bk[PG009]
Ellagic acid,3-3'-di-0-methyl: Bk[PG009]
Enedioxy: Bk[PG009]
Estrone: Sd 4.0 mcg/kg-17.0 mg/kg[PG064,PG045]
Fluoride: Cortex 5.8[PG091]
Friedelin: Bk[PG059]

Gallagyldilactone: PC[PG030]

Gallic acid: PC 0.09–4.00%[PG030]

Genistein: Sd[PG045]

Genistin: Sd[PG045]

Granatin A: Fr Pe[PG083], Lf 1.3%[PG012], PC[PG013,PG030]

Granatin B: Fr Pe[PG057,PG083], Lf 1.72%[PG012,PG017], PC[PG030]

Heneicosanoic acid: Sd oil 5.0%[PG085]

Hygrine: Bk 2.0%[PG027]

Isopelletierine: Bk[PG011]

Lauric acid, 4-methyl: Sd oil 0.5%[PG085]

Luteolin-3'-0-beta-D-glucoside: Lf[PG018]

Luteolin-3'-0-beta-D-xylopyranoside: Lf[PG018]

Luteolin-4'-0-beta-D-glucoside: Lf[PG018]

Mannitol: Lf 0.547%[PG012]

Methyl pelletierine: Rt Bk[PG011]

Methyl isopelletierine: Bk[PG011]

N-methyl pelletierine: Bk, Br[PG027]

Nonadecanoic acid: Sd oil 5.9%[PG085]

Nor-hygrine: Bk 0.7%[PG027]

Nor-pseudopelletierine: Bk, Br[PG027]

Palmitic acid: Sd oil 10.4%[PG085]

Pectin: Fr Pe[PG055]

Pedunculagin: Bk 82.4[PG015], PC 4[PG030]

Pelargonin: Fr Pe, Sd Ct[PG020]

Pelletierine: Bk 21.6%[PG027,PG011], St 48.7%[PG027], Br 49.6%[PG027]

Polyphenols: Fr Pe[PG070]

Pseudopelletierine: Bk 44.3%[PG027]

Punicacortein A: Bk 28[PG014]

Punicacortein B: Bk 27[PG014]

Punicacortein C: Bk 1100[PG014]

Punicacortein D: Bk 62[PG014]

Punicafolin: Lf 137[PG012,PG017]

Punicalagin: Bk 0.14%[PG015], Fr Pe[PG042], PC[PG013,PG030]

Punicalin: Bk 880[PG015], Fr Pe[PG042], PC[PG013]

Punicic acid: Sd oil 33.3%[PG086]

Punigluconin: Bk 140[PG014]

Pyridine,N-(2'-5'-dihydroxy-phenyl): Lf[PG018]

Sedridine: Bk 0.3%[PG027]

Stearic acid: Sd oil 5.9%[PG085]

Stearic acid,13-methyl: Sd oil 1.5%[PG085]

Strictinin: Lf 63[PG0112]

Tannin: Bk[PG016,PG056]

Tellimagrandin 1: PC 26[PG030]

Tricosanoic acid: Sd oil 4.9%[PG085]

Unicalin: PC[PG030]

Xanthoxylin: Lf[PG017]

PHARMACOLOGICAL ACTIVITIES AND CLINICAL TRIALS

Abortifacient effect. Ethanol (95%) extract of fruit, administered orally to rats at a dose of 200.0 mg/kg, was inactive[PG099].

Allergenic activity. Fruit, taken orally by human adults, was active. A case was reported of tongue angioedema following ingestion of the fruit. An IgE-mediated mechanism could not be demonstrated[PG051].

Analgesic activity. Ethanol/water (1:1) extract of the aerial parts, administered intraperitoneally to mice at a dose of 0.125 mg/kg, was inactive vs tail pressure method[PG094].

Anthelmintic activity. Chloroform extract of dried root and stem, administered to mice by gastric intubation at a dose of 250.0 mg/kg for 3 days, was active on *Hymenolepsis nana* and inactive on *Nippostrongylus brasiliense* and *Syphacia obvelata*[PG084]. Methanol extract of fruit peel, administered orally to mice at a dose of 120.0 mg/kg, was active on *Hymenolepis diminuta*. Eighty seven percent clearance of worms was observed in 2 days[PG095]. Water extract of dried fruitpeel, at a concentration of 10.0 ml/plate, was active on *Ascaris galli*, *Pheritima posthuma*, and *Taenia solium*[PG028].

Antiamoebic activity. Alkaloid fraction of dried root, at a concentration of 1.0 mg/ml in broth culture, was inactive on *Entamoeba histolytica* and *Entamoeba invadens*. The water extract, at a concentration of 2.0 ml and tannin fraction, at a concentration of 10.0 mcg/ml, were active on *Entamoeba histolytica* and *Entamoeba invadens*. One hundred percent growth was inhibited[PG024].

Antiancylostomiasis activity. Hot water extract of root bark, ingested by human adults, was inactive. Two ounces of bark is boiled in 2 pints water until half of it is evaporated. Four ounces are given at hourly doses of 1 ounce, with the last dose followed by magnesium sulfate. Thirteen patients were treated[PG097].

Antiascariasis activity. Ethanol (95%) extract of the epicarp was active on earthworm. Paralysis occurred in 18 hours with a death rate of 50%[PG021].

Antibacterial activity. Acidic-ethanol extract, dichloromethane extract, methanol extract washed in petroleum ether, and the acidic extract made alkaline then washed with dichloromethane of the dried fruit, at a doses of 0.20 ml/disc on agar plate, were inactive on *Pseudomonas aeruginosa*, *Salmonella gallinarum* and *Staphylococcus albus*. Strong activity was produced on *Escherichia coli*, *Klebsiella pneumoniae* and *Proteus vulgaris*. Water extract of dried fruit, at a dose of 0.20 ml/disc on agar plate, was inactive on *Escherichia coli*, *Salmonella gallinarum* and *Pseudomonas aeruginosa*, and produced strong activity on *Klebsiella pneumoniae*, *Proteus vulgaris* and *Staphylococcus albus*[PG036]. Decoction of dried pericarp, on agar plate, was active on *Pseudomonas aeruginosa*[PG033]. Ethanol (80%) extract of dried aerial parts, at a concentration of 100.0 mcg/ml on agar plate, was active on *Bacillus anthracis*, *Proteus vulgaris* and *Salmonella paratyphi* A; inactive on *Escherichia coli*, *Klebsiella pneumoniae*, *Pseudomonas aeruginosa*, *Shigella sonnei*, *Staphylococcus aureus* and *Vibrio cholera*[PG075]. Ethanol (95%) extract of dried fruit peel, at a concentration of 10.0 mg/ml on agar plate, was inactive on *Corynebacterium diphtheriae* and *Diplococcus pneumonia*, and produced weak activity on *Staphylococcus aureus*, *Streptococcus pyogenes* and *Streptococcus viridans*. The water extract was inactive on *Corynebacterium diptheriae* and *Diplococcus pneumonia*; produced weak activity on *Staphylococcus aureus*, *Streptococcus pyogenes*, and *Streptococcus viridans*[PG054]. Ethanol (95%) extract of dried fruit peel, at a concentration of 100.0 mg/disc on agar plate, was active on *Bacillus subtilis*, *Salmonella typhosa* and *Shigella dysenteriae*; inactive on *Escherichia coli* and produced strong activity on *Staphylococcus aureus*. The water extract, at a concentration

of 20.0 mg/disc on agar plate, was inactive on *Bacillus subtilis*, *Escherichia coli*, *Salmonella typhosa*, *Shigella dysenteriae*, and *Staphylococcus aureus*. Dose expressed as dry weight of plant material[PG058]. Ethanol/water (1:1) extract of the aerial parts, at a concentration greater than 25.0 mcg/ml on agar plate, was inactive on *Bacillus subtilis*, *Escherichia coli*, *Salmonella typhosa*, *Staphylococcus aureus*, and *Agrobacterium tumefaciens*[PG094]. Hot water extract of dried entire plant, at a concentration of 62.5 mg/ml on agar plate, was active on *Escherichia coli* and *Staphylococcus aureus*[PG031]. Saline extract of leaves, at a concentration of 1:40 on agar plate, was active on *Staphylococcus aureus* and inactive on *Pasteurella pestis*[PG098]. Acetone extract of dried leaves, on agar plate, was active on *Escherichia coli*, *Pseudomonas aeruginosa*, *Salmonella newport*, *Salmonella typhosa*, *Sarcina lutea*, *Serratia marcescens*, *Shigella flexneri*, *Shigella flexneri* 3A, *Staphylococcus albus*, and *Staphylococcus aureus*. Ethanol (95%) extract, on agar plate, was active on *Escherichia coli*, *Pseudomonas aeruginosa*, *Salmonella* B, *Salmonella newport*, *Salmonella typhosa*, *Sarcina lutea*, *Serratia marcescens*, *Shigella flexneri*, *Shigella flexneri* 3A, *Staphylococcus albus*, and *Staphylococcus aureus*. Water extract, on agar plate, was active on *Escherichia coli*, *Pseudomonas aeruginosa*, *Salmonella* B, *Salmonella newport*, *Salmonella typhosa*, *Serratia marcescens*, *Shigella flexneri*, and *Staphylococcus albus*; inactive on *Sarcina lutea*, *Shigella flexneri* 3A, and *Staphylococcus aureus*[PG025]. Seed oil, on agar plate, was active on *Klebsiella pneumonia*, *Salmonella paratyphi*, and *Shigella flexneri*[PG007]. Acetone extract of dried stem, on agar plate, was active on *Escherichia coli*, *Pseudomonas aeruginosa*, *Salmonella* B, *Salmonella newport*, *Salmonella typhosa*, *Sarcina lutea*, *Serratia marcescens*, *Shigella flexneri*, *Shigella flexneri* 3A, *Staphylococcus albus*, and *Staphylococcus aureus*. The water extract was active on *Escherichia coli*, *Pseudomonas aeruginosa*, *Salmonella* B, *Sal-*

monella newport, Salmonella typhosa, Serratia marcescens, Shigella flexneri, and Staphylococcus albus, and inactive on Sarcina lutea, Shigella flexneri 3A, and Staphylococcus aureus[PG025]. Tincture of dried fruit, at a concentration of 30.0 microliters/disc (extract of 10 gram plant material in 100 ml ethanol) on agar plate, was inactive on Escherichia coli, Pseudomonas aeruginosa and Staphylococcus aureus[PG089]. Successive petroleum ether, chloroform, methanol, and water extracts of the fruit were tested in vitro for their antibacterial activities. The methanolic extract was found to be the most effective against all the microorganisms tested[PG110].

Anticonvulsant activity. Ethanol/water (1:1) extract of aerial parts, administered intraperitoneally to mice at a dose of 0.125 mg/kg, was inactive vs electroshock-induced convulsions[PG094].

Antidiabetic effect. Ethanol (50%) extract of the male abortive flowers, administered orally to normal, glucose-fed hyperglycemic, and alloxan-induced diabetic rats, produced significant blood glucose lowering effect[PG108].

Antidiarrheal activity. Decoction of dried fruit peel, administered intragastrically to rats at a dose of 500.0 mg/kg, was active vs castor oil-induced diarrhea. Ethanol (95%) extract, administered intragastrically to rats at a dose of 50.0 mg/kg, was active. The extract reduced fecal output. At a dose of 500.0 mg/kg, weak activity was produced vs castor oil-induced diarrhea[PG026]. Decoction of fruit peel, administered orally to children, was active. The infantile diarrhea was treated with Kexieding capsule, composed of 5 herbs, including roasted ginger, clove and fruit peel of Punica granatum. Of the 234 infants and 71 children treated, 281 (92%) were cured in 1–3 days and 9 (3%) were significantly improved. The total effective rate was 95%. Bacteria caused only 9 of 79 severe cases; one who manifested symptoms of bacterial dysentery and bloody-mucoid stools was ultimately cured with Baitouweng mixture[PG052].

Methanol extract of the seed, administered orally to rats, produced significant inhibitory activity against castor oil induced diarrhea and PGE2 induced enteropooling in rats. The extract also indicated a significant reduction in gastro-intestinal motility in charcoal meal tests in rats[PG107].

Antifertility effect. Fruit peel, in the ration of guinea pigs of both sexes at a dose of 18.0 gm/kg and in the ration of female rats, was active[PG002].

Antifungal activity. Ethanol/water (1:1) extract of aerial parts, at a concentration greater than 25.0 mcg/ml on agar plate, was inactive on Microsporum canis, Trichophyton mentagrophytes, and Aspergillus niger[PG094]. Hot water extract of dried entire plant, at a concentration of 62.5 mg/ml on agar plate, was active on Aspergillus niger[PG031].

Anti-inflammatory activity. Ethanol (80%) extract of dried fruit peel, administered by gastric intubation to male rats at a dose of 100.0 mg/kg, produced weak activity vs carrageenin-induced pedal edema. Twenty-three percent inhibition of edema was observed[PG046]. Ethanol/water (1:1) extract of aerial parts, administered orally to rats at a dose of 0.125 mg/kg, was inactive vs carrageenin-induced pedal edema. Animals were dosed 1 hour before carrageenin injections[PG094].

Antimalarial activity. Methanol extract of dried leaves was inactive on Plasmodium falciparum, MIC > 25.0 mcg/ml[PG029].

Antimutagenic activity. Methanol extract of dried fruit, at a concentration of 50.0 microliters/disc on agar plate, was inactive on Bacillus subtilis NIG-1125, His Met, and Escherichia coli B/R-WP2-TRP[PG072].

Antimycobacterial activity. Ethanol (95%) extract of dried aerial parts, at a concentration of 1:50 on agar plate, produced weak activity on Mycobacterium tuberculosis[PG010].

Antinematodal activity. Water extract of a commercial sample of pericarp, at a concentration of 10.0 mg/ml, was inactive on

Toxacara canis. The methanol extract produced weak activity[PG053].

Antioxidant effect. Methanol extract of fruit, at a concentration of 50.0 microliters, was active[PG088]. Fermented juice and seed oil produced strong antioxidant activity close to that of butylated hydroanisole and *Thea sinensis*, and significantly great than that of red wine (*Vitis vitifera*) Flavonoids extracted from cold pressed seed oil produced 31–44% inhibition of sheep cyclo-oxygenase and 69–81% inhibition of soybean lipoxygenases. Flavonoids extracted from the fruit peel produced 21–30% inhibition of soybean lipooxygenase though no significant inhibition of sheep cyclo-oxygenase[PG106].

Antispasmodic activity. Ethanol/water (1:1) extract of aerial parts was inactive on the guinea pig ileum vs ACh- and histamine-induced spasms[PG094].

Antiuremic activity. Decoction of dried bark in the drinking water of rats at a dose of 150.0 mg/kg was active vs casein/adenine-induced renal failure. Urea, creatinine, methylguanidine, and guanidinosuccinic acid were assayed[PG035].

Antiviral activity. Hot water extract of dried root bark, at a concentration of 0.1 mg/ml in cell culture, was active on Herpes simplex 1 virus and measles virus; a concentration of 0.5 mg/ml was active on poliovirus 1; when administered intragastrically to mice at a dose of 5.0 mg/animal, was active on Herpes simplex 1 virus[PG032]. Water extract of fruit, in cell culture, was active on Coxsackie B5 virus, Herpes simplex virus, influenza virus (Lee), poliovirus 1, and REO virus Type 1[PG023].

Antiyeast activity. Acid-ethanol extract, and dichloromethane extract, methanol extract and washing in petroleum ether, and acidic extract made alkaline, then washed with dichloromethane of dried fruit, at a concentration of 0.20 ml/disc on agar plate, were inactive on *Candida albicans*. Strong activity was produced with dichloromethane extract and petroleum ether extract washed with methanol, and acidic extract made alkaline, then extracted with dichloromethane[PG036]. Ethanol (95%) extract of dried fruit peel, at a concentration of 100.0 mg/disc on agar plate, produced strong activity on *Candida albicans*. The water extract, at a concentration of 20.0 mg/disc, was inactive. Dose expressed as dry weight of plant material[PG098]. Ethanol/water (1:1) extract of aerial parts, at a concentration greater than 25.0 mcg/ml on agar plate, was inactive on *Candida albicans* and *Cryptococcus neoformans*[PG094]. Tincture of dried fruit, at a concentration of 30.0 microliters/disc (extract of 10 grams plant material in 100 ml ethanol) on agar plate, was inactive on *Candida albicans*[PG089].

Barbiturate potentiation. Ethanol/water (1:1) extract of aerial parts, administered intraperitoneally to mice at a dose of 0.125 mg/kg, was inactive[PG094].

Cytotoxic activity. Acetone extract of dried bark, at a concentration of 5.0%, was equivocal by cylinder plate method on CA-Ehrlich ascites, 21 mm inhibition. Ether extract, at a concentration of 5.0%, was inactive by cylinder plate method on CA-Ehrlich ascites, 15 mm zone of inhibition was produced. Water extract, at a concentration of 5.0%, was inactive by cylinder plate method on CA-Ehrlich ascites, 0 mm inhibition[PG101]. Hot water extract of fruit peel, at a dose of 120.0 mcg/ml in cell culture, was active on CA-JTC-26. The inhibition rate was 59%[PG050]. Methanol/water (1:1) extract of bark, in cell culture, was active on CA-9KB, $ED_{50} < 20.0$ mcg/ml[PG104]. Water extract of dried pericarp, at a concentration of 120.0 mcg/ml in cell culture, was active on CA-Mammary-Microalveolar and Cells-Human-Embryonic HE-1[PG047].

Diuretic activity. Ethanol/water (1:1) extract of serial parts, administered intraperitoneally to saline-loaded male rats, was active. Urine was collected for 4 hours after the treatment[PG094].

Embryotoxic effect. Acetone, hot water, and methanol extracts of dried root, administered by gastric intubation to pregnant rats at doses of 150.0 mg/kg, were inactive. Rats were dosed on days 1–7[PG079]. Ethanol (95%) extract of fruit, administered orally to female rats at a dose of 200.0 mg/kg, was inactive[PG099]. Methanol and acetone extracts of dried entire plant, administered by gastric intubation to pregnant rats at doses of 200.0 mg/kg, were inactive. Dosing was done on days 1–7[PG081].

Estrogenic effect. Dried seed extract, administered subcutaneously at variable dosage levels to ovariectomized mice, was active. Activity was equivalent to 4.0–17.0 mcg estrone/kg[PG064]. Seed oil, administered intraperitoneally to mice at a dose of 0.4 ml/animal, produced strong activity. A dose of 0.5 ml/animal, administered intraperitoneally to rabbits and subcutaneously to ovariectomized rats was active. The unsaponifiable fraction administered intraperitoneally to female rabbits at a dose of 250.0 mg/animal was active[PG005].

Feeding deterrent (insect). Seed oil, at a concentration of 1.0% in the ration, was inactive on *Anthonomus grandis*[PG087].

Gastroprotective effect. Aqueous extract of the fruit peel was investigated in the rat against ethanol-induced damage. The extract produced 100% precipitation of ovine hemoglobin in vitro. Oral administration induced a significant decrease in gastric lesions. The observed protection was more pronounced when the test solution was given at the same time with ethanol. The acid content of the stomach was significantly increased by extracts prepared in ethanol[PG105].

Glutamate-pyruvate stimulation. Tannin fraction (hydrolyzable) of pericarp, administered intraperitoneally to mice at a dose of 20.0 ml/kg, was active. Solutions equal to 0.5% gallotannin were injected; daily dosing for 2 days followed by sacrifice and examination on days 3, 5, and 9[PG060].

Hepatotoxic activity. Tannin fraction (hydrolyzable) of pericarp, administered intra-peritoneally to mice at a dose of 20.0 ml/kg, was active. Solutions equal to 0.5% gallotannin were injected; daily dosing for 2 days followed by sacrifice and examination on days 3, 5, and 9, showed severely damaged liver parenchyma[PG060].

Hypoglycemic activity. Ethanol/water (1:1) extract of aerial parts, administered orally to rats at a dose of 250.0 mg/kg, was inactive. Less than 30% drop in blood sugar level was observed[PG094]. Flower, administered orally to male rats at a dose of 4.0 gm/animal, was active[PG019].

Hypothermic activity. Ethanol/water (1:1) extract of aerial parts, administered intraperitoneally to mice at a dose of 0.125 mg/kg, was active[PG094].

Intestinal antisecretory activity. Decoction of dried fruit peel, administered intragastrically to rats, was active vs $MgSO_4$-induced enteropooling. The ethanol (95%) extract, at a dose of 500.0 mg/kg, was active vs $MgSO_4$-induced enteropooling[PG026].

Immunomodulatory activity. Aqueous suspension of the fruit rind powder, administered orally to rabbits at a dose of 100 mg/kg, stimulated the cell-mediated and humoral components of the immune system. There was an increase in antibody titer to typhoid-H antigen. It also enhanced the inhibition of leukocyte migration in Leucocyte Migration Inhibition test and induration of skin in delayed hypersensitivity test with Purified Protein Derivative[PG111].

Molluscicidal activity. Ethanol (95%) and water extracts of dried root, at concentrations of 1000 ppm, produced weak activity on *Biomphalaria glabrata* and *Biomphalaria straminea*[PG100]. The bark produced both time and dose dependent effect on the snail *Lymnaea acuminata*. The 24 hour LC_{50} of the column purified bark was 4.39 mg/l. The ethanol extract at 24 hours was LC_{50} 22.42 mg/l[PG109].

Plant growth inhibitor. Hot water extract of bark, at a concentration of 2.0 gm/liter, was active. The number of fronds of *Lemna paucicostata* that were greater than 1 mm in length was 57% of control[PG048].

Plant root growth stimulant. Hot water extract of bark, at a concentration of 2.0 gm/liter, was active. Root length in *Brassica rapa* was 121% of control, and the number of roots in *Cucumis sativus* more than 5 mm in length, was 554% of control[PG048].

Plaque formation suppressant. Water extract of a commercial sample of pericarp was inactive on *Streptococcus mutans*, $IC_{50} >$ 1000 mcg/ml. Methanol extract was active, IC_{50} 60.0 mcg/ml. Methanol/water (1:1) extract was active, IC_{50} 370.0 mcg/ml[PG082]. Water, methanol and methanol/water (1:1) extracts of dried bark, at concentrations of 1.0, 0.5 and 1.0 mg/ml, respectively, were active on *Streptococcus mutans*[PG077].

Prostaglandin synthetase inhibition. Hot water extract of a commercial sample of pericarp, at a concentration of 750.0 mcg/ml, showed weak activity on rabbit microsomes[PG059].

Protease (HIV) inhibition. Water extract of dried pericarp, at a concentration of 200.0 mcg/ml, was equivocal. The methanol extract was inactive[PG037].

Semen coagulation. Ethanol/water (1:1) extract of aerial parts, at a concentration of 2.0%, was inactive on rat sperm[PG094].

Spermicidal effect. Ethanol/water (1:1) extract of aerial parts was inactive on rat sperm[PG094].

Toxicity assessment (quantitative). Ethanol/water (1:1) extract of aerial parts, administered intraperitoneally to mice, produced LD_{50} 0.25 gm/kg[PG094].

Tyrosinase inhibition. Methanol/water (1:1) extract of dried pericarp, at a concentration of 330.0 mcg/ml, produced weak activity, 35.3% inhibition[PG039]. Methanol/water (1:1) extract of dried root bark, at a concentration of 330.0 mcg/ml, produced weak activity, 29.7% inhibition[PG039].

Uterine relaxation effect. Seed oil, administered intraperitoneally to mice at a dose of 0.2 ml/animal, was active[PG004].

Uterine stimulant effect. Water extract of fruit peel was active on the uterus of non-pregnant rats[PG001].

REFERENCES

PG001   Dhawan, B. N. and P. N. Saxena. Evaluation of some indigenous drugs for stimulant effect on the rat uterus. A preliminary report. **Indian J Med Res** 1958; 46(6): 808–811.

PG002   Gujraj, M. L., D. R. Varma and K. N. Sareen. Oral contraceptives. Part 1. Preliminary observations on the antifertility effect of some indigenous drugs. **Indian J Med Res** 1960; 48: 46–51.

PG003   Jochle, W. Biology and pathology of reproduction in Greek mythology. **Contraception** 1971; 4: 1–13.

PG004   Sharaf, A. Food plants as a possible factor in fertility control. **Qual Plant Mater Veg** 1969; 17: 153.

PG005   Sharaf, A. and S. A. R. Nigm. The oestrogenic activity of pomegranate seed oil. **J Endocrinol** 1964; 29: 91.

PG006   Watt, J. M. and M. G. Breyer-Brandwijk. The Medicinal and Poisonous Plants of Southern and Eastern Africa. 2nd Ed, E. S. Livingstone, Ltd., London, 1962.

PG007   Chopra, C. L., M. C. Bhatia and I. C. Chopra. In vitro antibacterial activity of oils from Indian medicinal plants. **J Amer Pharm Assoc Sci Ed** 1960; 49: 780.

PG008   Burkhill, I. H. Dictionary of the Economic Products of the Malay Peninsula. Ministry of Agriculture and Cooperatives, Kuala Lumpur, Malaysia. Volume II, 1966.

PG009   Lowry, J. B. The distribution and potential taxonomic value of alkylated ellagic acids. **Phytochemistry** 1968; 7(10): 1803–1813.

PG010   Wang, V. F. L. In vitro antibacterial activity of some common Chinese herbs on *Mycobacterium tuberculosis*. **Chin Med J** 1950; 68: 169–172.

PG011   Willaman, J. J. and B. G. Schubert. Alkaloid bearing plants and their contained alkaloids.. ARS, USDA, Tech

Bull 1234, Supt Documents, Govt Print Off, Washingont DC, 1961.

PG012 Tanaka, T., G. I. Nonaka and I. Nishioka. Punicafolin, an ellagitannin from the leaves of Punica granatum. **Phytochemistry** 1985; 24(9): 2075–2078.

PG013 Kakiuchi, N., M. Hattori, T. Namba, M. Nishizawa and T. Yamagishi. Inhibitory effect of tannins on reverse transcriptase from RNA tumor virus. **J Nat Prod** 1985; 48(4): 614–621.

PG014 Tanaka, T., G. I. Nonaka and I. Nishioka. Tannins and related compounds. XLI. Isolation and characterization of novel ellagitannins, punicacorteins A, B, C and D, and punigluconin from the bark of Punica granatum L. **Chem Pharm Bull** 1986; 34(2): 656–663.

PG015 Tanaka, T., G. I. Nonoka and I. Nishioka. Tannins and related compounds. XL. Revision of the structures of punicalin and punicalagin, and isolation and characterization of 2-O-galloylpunicalin from the bark of Punica granatum L. **Chem Pharm Bull** 1986; 34(2): 650–655.

PG016 Anon. Tannins. **Patent-Japan Kokai Tokkyo Koho**-58 1983; 154,571: 10pp.

PG017 Nawwar, M. A. M., S. A. M. Hussein and I. Merfort. NMR spectral analysis of polyphenols from Punica granatum. **Phytochemistry** 1994; 36(3): 793–798.

PG018 Nawwar, M. A. M., S. A. M. Hussein and I. Merfort. Leaf phenolics of Punica granatum. **Phytochemistry** 1994; 37(4): 1175–1177.

PG019 Kazmi, H., M. Aslan, Z. U. Khan and M. I. Bureny. A report on the trial of a Unani prescription for diabetes. **Rawal Med** 1974; 3(2): 67.

PG020 Du, C. T., P. L. Wang and F. J. Francis. Anthocyanins of pomegranate, Punica granatum. **J Food Sci** 1975; 40: 417.

PG021 Kaleysa Raj, R. Screening of indigenous plants for anthelmintic action against human Ascaris lumbricoides: Part II. **Indian J Physiol Pharmacol** 1975; 19: 47–49.

PG022 Kokwaro, J. O. Medicinal Plants of East Africa. East Afr Literature Bureau, Niarobi, 1976.

PG023 Konowalchuk, J. and J. I. Speirs. Antiviral activity of fruit extracts. **J Food Sci** 1976; 41: 1013.

PG024 Segura, J. J., L. H. Morales-Ramos and J. Verde-Star. Growth inhibition of Entamoeba histolytica and E. invadens produced by the root of Granade (Punica granatum L.) **Arch Invest Med (Mex)** 1990; 21(3): 235–239.

PG025 Misas, C. A. J., N. M. R. Hernandez and A. M. L. Abraham. Contribution to the biological evaluation of Cuban plants. IV. **Rev Cub Med Trop** 1979; 31(1): 29–35.

PG026 Pillai, N. R. Anti-diarrheal activity of Punica granatum in experimental animals. **Int J Pharmacog** 1992; 30(3): 201–204.

PG027 Neuhofer, H., L. Witte, M. Gorunovic and F. Czygan. Alkaloids in the bark of Punica granatum L. (pomegranate) from Yugoslavia. **Pharmazie** 1993; 48(5): 389–391.

PG028 Hukkeri, V. I., G. A. Kalyani, B. C. Hatpaki and F. V. Manvi. In vitro anthelmintic activity of aqueous extract of fruit rind of Punica granatum. **Fitoterapia** 1993; 64(1): 69,70.

PG029 Ayudhaya, T. D., W. Nutakul, U. Khunanek et al., Study on the in vitro antimalarial activity of some medicinal plants against Plasmodium falciparum. **Bull Dept Med Sci** 1987; 29: 22–38.

PG030 Satomi, H., K. Umemura, A. Ueno, T. Hatano, T. Okuda and T. Noro. Carbonic anhydrase inhibitors from the pericarps of Punica granatum L. **Biol Pharm Bull** 1993; 16(8): 787–790.

PG031 Anesini, C. and C. Perez. Screening of plants used in Argentine folk medicine for antimicrobial activity. **J Ethnopharmacol** 1993; 39(2): 119–128.

PG032 Kurokawa, M., H. Ochiai, K. Nagasaka, M. Neki, H. X. Xu, S. Kadota, S. Sutardio, T. Matsumoto, T. Namba and K. Shiraki. Antiviral traditional medicines against Herpes Simplex Virus (HSV-1), Poliovirus, and Measles virus in vitro and their therapeutic efficacies for HSV-1 infection in mice. **Antiviral Res** 1993; 22(2/3): 175–188.

PG033 Perez, C. and C. Anesini. Inhibition of Pseudomonas aerguinosa by Argentinean medicinal plants. **Fitoterapia** 1994; 65(2): 169–172.

PG034 Malamas, M. and M. Marselos. The tradition of medicinal plants in Zagori,

Epirus (Northwestern Greece). **J Ethnopharmacol** 1992; 37(3): 197–203.

PG035 Yokozawa, T., K. Jujioka, H. Oura, T. Tanaka, G. Nonaka and I. Nishioka. Confirmation that tannin-containing crude drugs have a uremic toxin-decreasing action. **Phytother Res** 1995; 9(1): 1–5.

PG036 Desta, B. Ethiopian traditional herbal drugs. Part ll: Antimicrobial activity of 63 medicinal plants. **J Ethnopharmacol** 1993; 39(2): 129–139.

PG037 Kusumoto, I. T., T. Nakabayashi, H. Kida, H. Miyashiro, M. Hattori, T. Namba and K. Shimotohno. Screening of various plant extracts used in Ayurvedic medicine for inhibitory effect on human immunodeficiency virus type 1 (HIV-1) protease. **Phytother Res** 1995; 9(3): 180–184.

PG038 Kim, S. Y., J. H. Kim, S. K. Kim, M. J. Oh and M. Y. Jung. Antioxidant activities of selected Oriental herb extracts. **J Amer Oil Chem Soc** 1994; 71(6): 633–640.

PG039 Iida, K., K. Hase, K. Shimomura, S. Sudo, S. Kadota and T. Namba. Potent inhibitors of tyrosinase activity and melanin biosynthesis from *Rheum officinale*. **Planta Med** 1995; 61(5): 425–428.

PG040 Singh, V. K. and Z. A. Ali. Folk medicines in primary health care: Common plants used for the treatment of fevers in India. **Fitoterapia** 1994; 65(1): 68–74.

PG041 Latorre, D. L. and F. A. Latorre. Plants used by the Mexican Kickapoo Indians. **Econ Bot** 1977; 31: 340–357.

PG042 Mayer, W., A. Gorner and K. Andra. Pinicalagin and punicalin, two tannins from pomegranate peel. **Justus Liebigs Ann Chem** 1977; 1976–.

PG043 Santagati, N. A., R. Duro and F. Duro. Study on pigments present in pomegranate seeds. **Riv Merceol** 1984; 23(2): 247–254.

PG044 Kirillova, V. V. and Z. T. Kondzhariya. Nature of the tannins of some subtropical plants. **Chem Nat Comp** 1988; 23(4): 507–508.

PG045 Moneam, N. M. A., A. S. El Sharaky and M. M. Badreldin. Oestrogen content of pomegranate seeds. **J Chromatogr** 1988; 438(2): 438–442.

PG046 Mascolo, N., G. Autore, F. Capasso, A. Menghini and M. P. Fasulo. Biological screening of Italian medicinal plants for anti-inflammatory activity. **Phytother Res** 1987; 1(1): 28–31.

PG047 Sato, A. Studies on anti-tumor activity of crude drugs. I. The effects of aqueous extracts of some crude drugs in short-term screening test. **Yakugaku Zasshi** 1989; 109(6): 407–423.

PG048 Shimomura, H., Y. Sashida and H. Nakata. Plant growth regulating activities of crude drugs and medicinal plants. **Shoyakugaku Zasshi** 1981; 35(3): 173–179.

PG049 Nagaraju, N. and K. N. Rao. A survey of plant crude drugs of Rayalaseema, Andhra Pradesh, India. **J Ethnopharmacol** 1990; 29(2): 137–158.

PG050 Sato, A. Cancer chemotherapy with Oriental medicine. I. Antitumor activity of crude drugs with human tissue cultures in In vitro screening. **Int J Orient Med** 1990: 15(4): 171–183.

PG051 Igea, J, M., J. Cuesta, M. Cuevas, L. M. Elias, C. Marcos, M. Lazaro and J. A. Comparied. Adverse reaction to pomegranate ingestion. **Allergy** 1991; 46(6): 472–474.

PG052 Zheng, Y. Z. and N. Zhang. Treatment of 305 cases of infantile diarrhea with kexieding capsule. **Fujian J Traditional Chinese Med** 1988; 19(3): 13–14.

PG053 Kiuchi, F., N. Nakamura, N. Miyashita, S. Nishizawa, Y. Tsuda and K. Kondo. Nematocidal activity of some anthel-mintics, traditional medicines, and spices by a new assay method using larvae of *Toxacara canis*. **Shoyakugaku Zasshi** 1989; 43(4): 279–287.

PG054 Naovi, S. A. H., M. S. Y. Khan and S. B. Vohora. Anti-bacterial, anti-fungal and anthelmintic investigations on Indian medicinal plants. **Fitoterapia** 1991; 62(3): 221–228.

PG055 Yuldasheva, N. P., D. A. Rakhimov and Z. F. Ismailov. The pectin of the rind of the fruit of *Punica granatum*. **Chem Nat Comp** 1978; 14(3): 328.

PG056 Okuda, T., K. Mori and R. Murakami. Constituents of *Geranium thunbergii* VI. Differences of tannin activity caused by structural differences. 2. Colorimetry with methylene blue. **Yakugaku Zasshi** 1977; 97: 1273–1278.

PG057 Okuda, T., T. Hatano, H. Nitta and R. Fujii. Hydrolysable tannins having enantiomeric dehydrohexanhydroxydiphenoyloup: Revised structure of terchebin and structure of granatin B. **Tetrahedron Lett** 1980; 21: 4361–4364.

PG058 Avirutnant, W. and A. Pongpan. The antimicrobial activity of some Thai flowers and plants. **Mahidol Univ J Pharm Sci** 1983; 10(3): 81–86.

PG059 Chandler, R. F. and S. N. Hooper. Friedelin and associated triterpenoids. **Phytochemistry** 1979; 18: 711–724.

PG060 Anon. Studies on the toxic effects of certain burn escharotic herbs. **Chung-Hua I Hsueh Tsa Chih** (New series) 1978; 4: 388.

PG061 Ayensu, E. S. Medicinal plants of the West Indies. **Unpublished Manuscript** 1978; 110pp.

PG062 Wilson, R. T. and W. G. Mariam. Medicine and magic in Central Tigre: A contribution to the ethnobotany of the Ethiopian plateau. **Econ Bot** 1979; 33: 29–34.

PG063 Arnason, T., F. Uck, J. Lambert and R. Hebda. Maya medicinal plants of San Jose Succotz, Belize. **J Ethnopharmacol** 1980; 2(4): 345–364.

PG064 Hoelscher, M. Exposure to phytoestrogens may surpass DES residues. **Feedstuffs** 1979; 51: 54–68.

PG065 Nair, A. G. R., R. Gunasegaran and B. S. Joshi. Chemical investigation of certain South Indian plants. **Indian J Chem Ser B** 1982; 21: 979–980.

PG066 Razzack, H. M. A. The concept of birth control in Unani medical literature. **Unpublished Manuscript** 1980; 64pp.

PG067 John, D. One hundred useful raw drugs of the Kani Tribes of Trivandrum Forest Division, Kerala, India. **Int J Crude Drug Res** 1984; 22(1): 17–39.

PG068 Boukef, K., H. R. Souissi and G. Balansard. Contribution to the study on plants used in traditional medicine in Tunisia. **Plant Med Phytother** 1982; 16(4): 260–279.

PG069 Kiuchi, F., M. Shibuya, T. Kinoshita and U. Sankawa. Inhibition of prostaglandin biosynthesis by the constituents

of medicinal plants. **Chem Pharm Bull** 1983; 31(10): 3391–3396.

PG070 Botrus, D., T. F. Zykina, L. I. Kostinskaya and G. A. Golovchenko. Polyphenol compounds in pomegranate. **Izv Vyssh Uchebn Zaved Pishch Tekhnol** 1984; 3: 117–119.

PG071 Goh, S. H., E. Soepadmo, P. Chang, U. Barnerjee et al. Studies on Malaysian medicinal plants. Preliminary results. **Proc 5ᵗʰ Asian Symposium on Medicinal Plants and Spices**, South Korea 1984; August 20–24. 5: 473–483.

PG072 Ishii, R., K. Yoshikawa, H. Minakata, H. Komura and T. Kada. Specificities of bio-antimutagens in plant kingdom. **Agr Biol Chem** 1984; 48(10): 2587–2591.

PG073 Jain, S. P. and H. S. Puri. Ethnomedical plants of Jaunsar-Bawar Hills, Uttar Pradesh, India. **J Ethnopharmacol** 1984; 12(2): 213–222.

PG074 Arseculeratne, S. N., A. A. L. Gunatilaka and R. G. Panabokke. Studies on medicinal plants of Sri Lanka. Part 14. Toxicity of some traditional medicinal herbs. **J Ethnopharmacol** 1985; 13(3): 323–335.

PG075 Aynehchi, Y., M. H. Salehi Sormaghi, M. Shirudi and E. Souri. Screening of Iranian plants for antimicrobial activity. **Acta Pharm Suecica** 1982; 19(4): 303–308.

PG076 Said, M. Potential of herbal medicines in modern medical therapy. **Ancient Sci Life** 1984; 4(1): 36–47.

PG077 Namba, T., M. Tsunezaku, Y. Takehana, S. Nunome et al., Studies on dental caries prevention by traditional Chinese medicines. IV. Screening of crude drugs for anti-plaque action and effects on *Artemisia capillaris* spikes on adherence of *Streptococcus mutans* to smooth surfaces and synthesis of glucan. **Shoyakugaku Zasshi** 1984; 38(3): 253–263.

PG078 Singh, Y. N. Traditional medicine in Fiji. Some herbal folk cures used by Fiji Indians. **J Ethnopharmacol** 1986; 15(1): 57–88.

PG079 Prakash, A. O. Potentialities of some indigenous plants for antifertility activity. **Int J Crude Drug Res** 1986; 24(1): 19–24.

PG080   Venkataraghavan, S. and T. P. Sundaresan. A short note on contraceptive in Ayurveda. **J Sci Res Pl Med** 1981; 2(1/2): 39.

PG081   Prakesh, A. O., S. Shukla, S. Mathur, V. Saxena and R. Mathur. Evaluation of some indigenous plants for anti-implantation activity in rats. **Probe** 1986; 25(2): 151–155.

PG082   Namba, T., M. Tsunezuka, N. Kakiuchi, D. M. R. B. Dissanayake, U. Pilapitiya, K. Saito and M. Hattori. Studies on dental caries prevention by traditional medicines (Part VII). Screening of Ayurvedic medicines for anti-plaque action. **Shoyakugaku Zasshi** 1985; 39(2): 146–153.

PG083   Kakiuchi, N., M. Hattori, M. Nishizawa, T, Yamagishi, T. Okuda and T. Namba. Studies on dental caries prevention by traditional medicines. VIII. Inhibitory effect of various tannins on glucan synthesis by glucosyltransferase from *Streptococcus mutans*. **Chem Pharm Bull** 1986; 34(2): 720–725.

PG084   Singhal, K. C. Anthelmintic activity of *Punica granatum* and *Artemisia siversiana* against experimental infections in mice. **Indian J Pharmacol** 1984; 15(2): 119–122.

PG085   Batra, A., B. K. Mehta and M. M. Bokadia. Fatty acid composition of *Punica granatum* seed oil. **Acta Pharm Jugosl** 1986; 36(1): 63–66.

PG086   Siang, S. T. Use of combined traditional Chinese and Western medicine in the management of burns. **Panminerva Med** 1983; 25(3): 197–202.

PG087   Jacobson, M., M. M. Crystal, and R. Kleiman. Effectiveness of several poly-unsaturated seed oils as boll weevil feeding deterrents. **J Amer Oil Chem Soc** 1981; 58(11): 982–983.

PG088   Ramirez, V. R., L. J. Mostacero, A. E. Garacia, C. F. Mejia, P. F. Pelaez, C. D. Medina and C. H. Miranda. Vegetales empleados in medicina tradicional Norperauna. **Banco Agrario del Peru & Nacl Univ Trujillo**, Peru, June, 1988 1988: 54pp.

PG089   Caceres, A., L. M. Giron, S. R. Alvarado, and M. F. Torres. Screening of antimicrobial activity of plants popularly used in Guatemala for the treatment of dermatomucosal diseases. **J Ethnopharmacol** 1987; 20(3): 223–237.

PG090   Singh, V. P., S. K. Sharma, and V. S. Khare. Medicinal plants from Ujjain District Madhya Pradesh. Part II. **Indian Drugs Pharm Ind** 1980; 5: 7–12.

PG091   Sakai, T., K. Kobashi, M. Tsunezuka, M. Hattori and T. Namba. Studies on dental caries prevention by traditional Chinese medicines (Part VI). On the fluoride contents in crude drugs. **Shoyakugaku Zasshi** 1985; 39(2): 165–169.

PG092   Darias, V., L. Brando, R. Rabanal, C. Sanchez Mateo, R. M. Gonzalez Luis and A. M. Hernandez Perez. New contribution to the ethnopharmacological study of the Canary Islands. **J Ethnopharmacol** 1989; 25(1): 77–92.

PG093   Kumar, D. S. and Y. S. Prabhakar. On the ethnomedical significance of the Arjun tree, *Terminalia arjuna* (Roxb.) Wight & Arnot. **Indian J Homoeopath Med** 1984; 19(3): 114–120.

PG094   Dhawan, B. N., G. K. Patnaik, R. P. Rastogi, K. K. Singh and J. S. Tandon. Screening of Indian plants for biological activity. VI. **Indian J Exp Biol** 1977; 15: 208–219.

PG095   Kim, N. D. Anthelmintics in crude drugs on the drugs for tapeworms. **Yakhak Hoe Chi** 1974; 19: 87.

PG096   Pavanasasivam, G. and M. U. S. Sultanbawa. Betulinic acid in the Dilleniaceae and a review of its natural distribution. **Phytochemistry** 1974; 13: 2002B.

PG097   Caius, J. F. and K. S. Mhaskar. The correlation between the chemical composition of anthelmintics and their therapeutic value in connection with the hookworm inquiry in the Madras presidency. XIX. Drugs allied to thyme. **Indian J Med Res** 1923; 11: 353.

PG098   Collier, W. A. and L. Van de Piji. The antibiotic action of plants, especially the higher plants, with results with Indonesian plants. **Chron Nat** 1949; 105: 8.

PG099   Prakash, A. O. and R. Mathur. Screening of Indian plants for antifertility activity. **Indian J Exp Biol** 1976; 14: 623–626.

PG100   Pinheiro de Sousa, M. and M. Z. Rouquayrol. Molluscicidal activity of plants from Northeast Brazil. **Rev Bras Fpesq Med Biol** 1974; 7(4): 389–394.

PG101 Ueki, H., M. Kaibara, M. Sakagawa and S. Hayashi. Antitumor activity of plant constituents. I. **Yakugaku Zasshi** 1961; 81: 1641–1644.

PG102 Wasuwat, S. A list of Thai medicinal plants, ASRCT, Bangkok, Report No. 1 on Res. Project. 17. A.S.R.C.T. Bangkok Thailand 1967; 17: 22pp.

PG103 Anon. The Herbalist. Hammond Book Company, Hammond, Indiana, 1931; 400pp.

PG104 Anon. Unpublished data, National Cancer Institute. National Cancer Inst. Central Files 1976.

PG105 Gharzouli, K., S. Khennouf, S. Amira and A. Gharzouli. Effects of aqueous extracts from *Quercus ilex* L. root bark, *Punica granatum* L. Fruit peel and *Artemisia herba-alba* Asso leaves on ethanol-induced gastric damage in rats. **Phytother Res** 1999; 1391): 42–45.

PG106 Schubert, S. Y., E. P. Lanksy and I. Neeman. Antioxidant and eicosanoid enzyme inhibition properties of pomegranate seed oil and fermented juice flavonoids. **J Ethnopharmacol** 1999; 66(1): 11–17.

PG107 Das, A. K., S. C. Mandal, S. K. Banerjee, S. Sinha, J. Das, B. P. Saha and M. Pal. Studies on antimalarial activity of *Punica granatum* seed extract in rats. **J Eth-nopharmacol** 1999; 68 (1–3): 205–208.

PG108 Jafri, M. A., K. Aslam, K. Javed and S. Singh. Effect of *Punica granatum* Linn. (flowers) on blood glucose level in normal and alloxan-induced diabetic rats. **J Ethnopharmacol** 2000; 70(3): 309–314.

PG109 Tripathi, S. M. and D. K. Singh. Molluscicidal activity of *Punica granatum* bark and *Canna indica* root. **Braz J Med Biol Res** 2000; 33(11): 1351–1355.

PG110 Prashant, D., M. K. Asha and A. Amit. Antibacterial activity of *Punica granatum*. **Fitoterapia** 2001; 72(2): 171–173.

PG111 Gracious Ross, R., S. Selvasubramanian and S. Jayasundar. Immunomodulatory activity of *Punica granatum* in rabbits-A preliminary study. **J Ethnopharmacol** 2001; 78(1): 85–87.

PG112 el-Toumy, S. A., M. S. Marouk and H. W. Rauwald. Ellagi- and gallotannins from *Punica granatum* heartwood. **Pharmazie** 2001; 56(10): 823–824.

26 | Syzygium cumini
(Linn.) Skeels

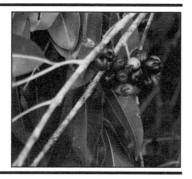

Common Names

Alla naeredu	India	Jamun	India
Azeitona	Brazil	Jamun	Nepal
Jam	India	Java plum	Brazil
Jaman	India	Java plum	India
Jaman	Pakistan	Java plum	Nepal
Jamblon	Rodrigues Islands	Java plum	West Indies
Jambol	West Indies	Luk-wa	Thailand
Jambolan	Brazil	Madan	Japan
Jambolan	India	Malabar plum	Brazil
Jambolana	Nepal	Malak rose-apple	Brazil
Jambolao	Brazil	Naeredu	India
Jambu	India	Naval	India
Jambul	India	Negresse	India
Jambul	USA	Rotra	Madagascar
Jamdlan	India	Tete	West Indies
Jamoon	Guyana	Wa	Thailand
Jamoon	India	Waa	Thailand

BOTANICAL DESCRIPTION

A smooth tree of the MYRTACEAE family, 4–15 meters in height. Leaves leathery oblong-ovate to elliptic or obovate and 6–12 cm long, the tip being broad and shortly pointed. The panicles are borne mostly from the branchlets below the leaves, often being axillary or terminal, and are 4–6 cm long. The flowers are numerous, scented, pink or nearly white, without stalks, and borne in crowded fascicles on the ends of the branchlets. The calyx is funnel-shaped, about 4 mm long, and 4-toothed. The petals cohere and fall together as a small disk. The stamens are very numerous and as long as the calyx. Fruit is oval to elliptic; 1.5–3.5 cm long, dark purple or nearly black, luscious, fleshy and edible; it contains a single large seed.

ORIGIN AND DISTRIBUTION

The original home of *Syzygium cumini* is India or the East Indies. It is found in Thailand, the Philippines, Madagascar and some other countries. The plant has been successfully introduced into many

From: *Medicinal Plants of the World, vol. 1: Chemical Constituents, Traditional and Modern Medicinal Uses, 2nd ed.*
By: Ivan A. Ross © Humana Press Inc., Totowa, NJ

other tropical countries such as the West Indies, East and West Africa and some subtropical regions including Florida, California, Algeria and Israel.

TRADITIONAL MEDICINAL USES

Brazil. Decoction of dried leaves is taken orally to treat diabetes[SC018].

India. Bark paste and curd is taken orally 3 times a day for 2 days to cure dysentery[SC023]. Decoction[SC011] and fluidextract[SC011] of dried bark is taken orally for diabetes. Ten grams of dried leaves of *Zanthoxylum armatum* are boiled in 8 liters of water along with 125 gm of a mixture of equal parts of the bark of *Acacia nilotica*, *Mangifera indica* and *Syzygium cumini* until the quantity of water is reduced to 2 liters. Fifty milliliters of the decoction is taken twice a day after meals[SC033]. Hot water extract of dried bark is taken orally for dysentery, indigestion and as a blood purifier[SC048]. Decoction of dried bark is taken orally for venereal ulcers. *Terminalia arjuna*, *Pongamia pinnata*, *Vateria indica*, *Syzygium cumini*, *Ficus benghalensis*, *F. religiosa*, *F. racemosa*, *F. talbotii* and *Azadirachta indica* are used[SC057]. Fruits are taken orally to cure gastrointestinal complaints[SC024]. Hot water extract of dried fruits is used externally as an astringent and orally for stomach ulcers and to reduce acidity[SC048]. Hot water extract of dried fruits and seeds is taken orally for diabetes[SC009]. Leaves are taken orally for leucorrhea; 2 young leaves are chewed with cold water for 3–4 days[SC024]. Decoction of dried seeds is taken orally for diabetes[SC011] and the fluidextract is taken orally as an antiinflammatory[SC011]. The hot water extract is taken orally as an antipyretic[SC028]. For diabetes, 100–250 mg seed powder is taken orally 3 times a day with water[SC030]. Decoction of dried seeds is taken orally for diarrhea; the seeds are taken together with *Cassia auriculata*[SC031]. Hot water extract of dried seeds, taken orally, is prescribed in Ayurvedic medicine for diabetes[SC045]. It is also used as an astringent in

dysentery and diarrhea, and to reduce urinary sugars in diabetes[SC051]. Leaf juice is taken orally to treat diabetes. The juice is taken mixed with milk every morning[SC025]. Fresh leaf juice is taken orally for stomach pain[SC049]. Seeds are taken orally for diabetes[SC019]. Stembark juice, mixed with buttermilk, is taken orally every day for constipation and to stop bloody discharge in the feces[SC025].

Pakistan. Hot water extract of dried aerial parts is used for diabetes[SC050]. Seeds are taken orally for diarrhea, diabetes, dysentery and blood pressure[SC017].

Thailand. Dried stembark is taken orally as a cardiotonic, CNS stimulant and for fainting[SC043]. Hot water extract of dried bark is taken orally as an antipyretic[SC062]. Hot water extract of dried seeds is taken orally for diabetes[SC060]. Leaf ash is used externally to relieve itching caused by centipede bite. Decoction of the root is taken orally as an antiemetic and to increase lactation in new mothers[SC053].

USA. Fluidextract of seeds is reputed to be valuable for diabetes[SC003].

West Indies. Seeds are used for diabetes[SC044].

CHEMICAL CONSTITUENTS
(ppm unless otherwise indicated)

1-Galloyl glucose: Sd[SC017]
3-6-Hexahydroxy-diphenoyl glucose: Sd[SC017]
3-Galloyl glucose: Sd[SC017]
4-6-Hexahydroxy-diphenoyl glucose: Sd[SC017]
6-Galloyl glucose: Sd[SC017]
Acetophenone, 2-6-dihydroxy-4-methoxy: Fl[SC027]
Alanine: Lf[SC001]
Alpha copanene: St EO 2.15%[SC041]
Alpha humulene: Lf EO 2.80%, St EO 6.51%, Fr EO 2.30%[SC041]
Alpha pinene: Lf EO 30.10%, St EO 18.56%, Fr EO 30.89%[SC041]
Alpha terpinene: Lf EO[SC038]
Alpha terpineol: Lf EO[SC038]
Astragalin: St Bk[SC016]
Beta caryophyllene: Lf EO 2.50%, Fr EO 0.40%[SC041]

Beta phellandrene: Lf EO[SC038]

Beta pinene: Lf EO 20.50%, St EO 12.61%, Fr EO 10.81%[SC041]

Beta sitosterol: Lf [SC001], St Bk 600[SC006,SC016]

Betulinic acid: Lf [SC001], St Bk 0.11%[SC006,SC016]

Borneol acetate: Lf EO 2.20%, St EO 1.46%, Fr EO 0.32%[SC041]

Borneol: Lf EO[SC038]

Bornylene: Lf EO[SC038]

Camphene: St EO 1.31%, Fr EO 1.0%[SC041]

Cinnamic acid methyl ester: Lf EO[SC038]

Cis ocimene: Lf EO 9.0%, St EO 14.83%, Fr EO 18.50%[SC041]

Citric acid: Fr[SC040], Lf[SC001]

Clycolic acid: Lf[SC001]

Corilagin: Sd[SC017]

Cuminaldehyde: Lf EO[SC038]

Cyanin: Fr[SC040]

Daucosterol: St Bk[SC016]

Delphinidin-3-0-beta-D-gentiobioside: Fr[SC015]

Delta cadinene: St EO 1.46%[SC041]

Dotriacontan-1-ol: Lf[SC001]

Ellagic acid: Sd[SC011,SC017,SC006], St Bk[SC016]

Ellagic acid,3-3-4-tri-o-methyl: Sd, Bk[SC017]

Ellagic acid,3-3-di-o-methyl: Sd, Bk[SC017]

Epi friedelanol: St Bk 600[SC006]

Eugenin: St Bk 20[SC006]

Eugenol: Lf EO[SC038]

Friedelanol: St Bk[SC016]

Friedelin: St Bk 800[SC006,SC016]

Fructose: Fr[SC040], Lf[SC001]

Gallic acid: Bk[SC011], Sd[SC011,SC014,SC017], St Bk[SC016]

Gamma cadinene: St EO 0.64%[SC041]

Gamma terpinene: St EO 0.65%[SC041]

Glucose: Fr[SC040], Lf[SC001]

Glycine: Lf[SC001]

Hentriacontan-1-ol: Lf[SC001]

Heptacosan-1-ol: Lf[SC001]

Hexahydroxy diphenic acid: Sd[SC017]

Iso rhamnetin 3-0-rutinoside: Rt[SC036]

Jambolin: Sd[SC011]

Kaempferol: St Bk[SC016]

Leucine: Lf[SC001]

Limonene: Lf EO 8.50%, St EO 6.48%, Fr EO 4.50%[SC041]

Malic acid: Fr[SC040]

Malvidin-3-0-beta-D-laminaribioside: Fr[SC015]

Mannose: Fr[SC040]

Maslinic acid: Lf[SC001]

Methyl xanthoxylin: Fl[SC027]

Montanyl alcohol: Lf[SC001]

Myrcene: Fr EO 3.82%, St EO 4.28%[SC041]

Myricetin-3-0-beta-D-glucoside: Rt[SC013]

Myricetin-3-0-robinoside: Rt[SC013]

N-Dotriacontane: Lf[SC001]

N-Hentriacontane: Lf[SC001]

N-Heptacosane: Lf[SC001]

N-Hexacosane: Lf[SC001]

N-Nonacosane: Lf[SC001]

N-Octacosane: Lf[SC001]

N-Tetratriacontane: Lf[SC001]

N-Triacontane: Lf[SC001]

N-Tritriacontane: Lf[SC001]

Octacosan-1-ol: Lf[SC001]

Oleanolic acid: Fl 0.5%[SC056], Sd[SC006]

Oxalic acid: Lf[SC001]

Petunidin-3-0-beta-D-gentibioside: Fr[SC015]

Quercetin: Sd[SC017], St Bk[SC016]

Rutin: Lf 1.5%[SC046]

Sucrose: St Bk[SC016]

Taxifolin: Sd[SC017]

Terpinolene: Lf EO[SC038], St EO 0.96%[SC041]

Tetratriacontan-1-ol: Lf[SC001]

Trans ocimene: Lf EO 9.50%, St EO 12.24%, Fr EO 12.10%[SC041]

Triacontan-1-ol: Lf[SC001]

Tritriancontan-1-ol: Lf[SC001]

Tyrosine: Lf[SC001]

PHARMACOLOGICAL ACTIVITIES AND CLINICAL TRIALS

Abortifacient effect. Ethanol/water (1:1) extract of the aerial parts, administered orally to rats at a dose of 200.0 mg/kg, was inactive[SC058].

Analgesic activity. Ethanol/water (1:1) extract of the aerial parts, administered intraperitoneally to mice at a dose of 0.375 mg/kg, was inactive vs tail pressure method[SC058]. Methanol extract of dried seeds, administered intraperitoneally to mice at a dose of 25.0 mg/kg, was active vs acetic acid-induced writhing, results significant at $P < 0.001$ level[SC051].

Antiaggression effect. Methanol extract of dried seeds, administered intraperitoneally to mice at a dose of 150.0 mg/kg, was active vs foot shock-induced aggression, results significant at $P < 0.01$ level[SC051].

Antibacterial activity. Ethanol (95%) and water extracts of dried fruit, at concentrations of 100.0 and 20 mg/disc, respectively, (expressed as dry weight of the fruit) on agar plate, were inactive on *Bacillus subtilis*, *Escherichia coli*, *Salmonella typhosa*, *Shigella dysenteriae* and *Staphylococcus aureus*[SC042]. Ethanol/water (1:1) extract of the aerial parts, at a concentration > 25.0 mcg/ml on agar plate, was inactive on *Bacillus subtilis*, *Escherichia coli*, *Salmonella typhosa*, *Staphylococcus aureus* and the plant pathogen *Agro-bacterium tumefaciens*[SC058]. Saline extract of leaves, at a concentration of 1:80 on agar plate, was active on *Staphylococcus aureus*[SC059].

Antibradykinin activity. Methanol extract of dried seeds, administered intraperitoneally to mice, was active vs bradykinin-induced pedal edema[SC028].

Anticlastogenic activity. Fruit juice, administered intraperitoneally to mice at a dose of 50.0 ml/kg, was active on mice marrow cells vs mitomycin C-, tetracycline- and dimethylnitrosamine-induced micronuclei[SC021].

Anticonvulsant activity. Ethanol/water (1:1) extract of the aerial parts, administered intraperitoneally to mice at a dose of 0.375 mg/ml, was inactive vs electroshock-induced convulsions[SC058]. Methanol extract of dried seeds, administered intraperitoneally to mice at a dose of 150.0 mg/kg, was inactive vs strychnine-induced convulsions[SC051].

Antifungal activity. Ethanol/water (1:1) extract of the aerial parts, at a concentration > 25.0 mcg/ml on agar plate, was inactive on *Microsporum canis*, *Trichophyton mentagrophytes* and *Aspergillus niger*[SC058].

Antihistamine activity. Ethanol/water (1:1) extract of dried bark, at a concentration of 0.01 gm/ml, was active on guinea pig ileum[SC062]. Methanol extract of dried seeds, administered intraperitoneally to rats, was active vs histamine-induced pedal edema[SC028].

Antihyperglycemic activity. Decoction of the aerial parts, taken orally by adults at a dose 500.0 mg/person, was active. It also produced oliguria, and patients complained of pain in the loins. The symptoms disappeared after 1 week of treatment[SC012]. Powdered commercial sample of seeds, administered by gastric intubation to rats at a dose of 53.2 mg/kg, was active. Effect was seen in streptozotocin-induced diabetic animals challenged with glucose after having received daily dose of extract for 1 week. This dose was inactive vs glucose-induced hyperglycemia[SC035]. Ethanol (95%) and hot water extracts of dried seeds, administered orally and intravenously to human adults at variable dosage levels, were active[SC007]. When administered intragastrically to rats at a dose of 50.0 mg/kg, the extract was active vs alloxan-induced hyperglycemia[SC010]. Ethanol (95%) extract of dried seeds, administered intraperitoneally to rats at a dose of 75.0 mg/animal, was inactive vs treptozotocin-induced hyperglycemia[SC054]. The hot water extract, administered intragastrically to rabbits at a dose of 10.0 gm/kg (dry weight of seeds), was active vs alloxan-induced hyperglycemia[SC060]. Seeds, administered by gastric intubation to rabbits at a dose of 1.0 gm/kg, were active[SC045]. Seeds, administered orally to human adults at a dose of 4–24 gm/person, were active when administered to 28 diabetic patients, results significant at $P < 0.05$ level[SC026]. Hot water extracts of dried fruit pulp, administered by gastric intubation to dogs at a dose of 150.0 gm/kg (expressed as dry weight of the fruit), and to rabbits at a dose of 50.0 gm/kg, were inactive vs alloxan-induced hyperglycemia[SC008]. Teas prepared from the leaves, administered to orally to 30 non-diabetic young volunteers submitted to a glucose tolerance test, did not produce any antihyperglycemic activity. In animal experiments, the effect of increasing doses of the

extract administered for 2 weeks, on the post-prandial blood glucose level of normal rats and rats with streptozotocin-induced diabetes mellitus did not produce any activity[SC063].

Anti-implantation effect. Ethanol/water (1:1) extract of the aerial parts, administered orally to rats at a dose of 100.0 mg/kg, was inactive[SC058].

Anti-inflammatory activity. Chloroform extract of dried seeds, administered intrapaw to rats at a dose of 2.5 mg/paw, was active vs carrageenin-induced pedal edema. The extract, administered intraperitoneally to rats at a dose of 100.0 mg/kg, was active vs turpentine-induced joint edema, carrageenin-, PGE-1-, histamine-, serotonin-, bradykinin- and hyaluronidase-induced pedal edema. A dose of 25.0 mg/kg was active vs formalin-, carrageenin- and kaolin-induced pedal edema, and adjuvant- and formaldehyde-induced arthritis[SC028]. Ethanol/water (1:1) extract of the aerial parts, administered orally to rats at a dose of 0.375 mg/kg, was inactive vs carrageenin-induced pedal edema. Animals were dosed 1 hour before carrageenin injections[SC058]. Ethanol extract of the bark, administered orally to rats at a dose of 10.125 gm/kg, produced significant activity in carrageenin, kaolin-carrageenin, and formaldehyde-induce paw edema and cotton pellet granuloma tests[SC064].

Antipyretic activity. Chloroform[SC032] and methanol[SC028] extracts of dried seeds, administered intraperitoneally to rats at doses of 50.0 mg/kg, were active vs yeast-induced pyrexia.

Antispasmodic activity. Ethanol/water (1:1) extract of the aerial parts was inactive on guinea pig ileum vs ACh- and histamine-induced spasms[SC058]. Ethanol/water (1:1) extract of dried bark, at a concentration of 0.01 gm/ml, was active on guinea pig ileum[SC062].

Antitoxic activity. Methanol extract of dried seeds, administered intraperitoneally to mice at a dose of 50.0 mg/kg, was active. The extract antagonized amphetamine toxicity[SC051].

Antiviral activity. Ethanol/water (1:1) extract of dried entire plant, at a concentration of 0.1 mg/ml in cell culture, was inactive on Ranikhet virus and vaccinia virus. For Ranikhet virus, infected chorioallantoic membrane viral titre decreased 10% and for vaccinia virus, 0%[SC020]. The extract, when injected into chick embryo at a dose of 1.0 mg/animal, was inactive on Ranikhet and vaccinia viruses. Infected chick embryo viral titre decreased 10% and 0%, respectively[SC020]. Ethanol/water (1:1) extract of the aerial parts, at a concentration of 50.0 mcg/ml in cell culture, was inactive on Ranikhet and vaccinia viruses[SC058]. Water extract of the bark was active on potato X virus[SC002].

Antiyeast activity. Ethanol (95%) and water extracts of dried fruit, at concentrations of 100.0 and 20.0 mg/disc respectively (expressed as dry weight of the fruit) on agar plate, were inactive on *Candida albicans*[SC042]. Ethanol/water (1:1) extract of the aerial parts, at a concentration greater than 25.0 mcg/ml on agar plate, was inactive on *Candida albicans* and *Cryptococcus neoformans*[SC058].

Barbiturate potentiation. Methanol extract of dried seeds, administered intraperitoneally to mice at a dose of 25.0 mg/kg, was active, results significant at $P < 0.001$ level[SC051].

Capillary permeability decrease. Chloroform extract of dried seeds, administered intraperitoneally to rats at a dose of 50.0 mg/kg, was active[SC032].

Cathepsin B induction. Seeds, administered by gastric intubation to Rhesus monkeys at a dose of 240.0 mg/animal daily for 15 days, were active. When administered to rats at a dose of 170.0 mg/animal, produced weak activity, and were active at a dose of 510.0 mg/animal[SC039].

CNS depressant activity. Methanol extract of dried seeds, administered intraperitoneally to mice at a dose of 25.0 mg/kg, was active[SC051].

Conditioning avoidance response decrease. Methanol extract of dried seeds, administered intraperitoneally to mice at a dose of 150.0 mg/kg, was active, results significant at $P < 0.001$ level[SC051].

Death. Methanol extract, administered intraperitoneally to mice at a dose of 400.0 mg/kg, was inactive[SC051].

Diuretic activity. Ethanol/water (1:1) extract of the aerial parts, administered intraperitoneally to rats at a dose of 0.187 mg/kg, was inactive. Urine was collected for 4 hours postdrug from saline-loaded animals[SC058]. Water extract of dried leaves, administered by gastric intubation to rats at a concentration of 2.5%, was active. Animals were given water or 2.5% solution of *Syzygium cumini*. Quantity of solution equaled 5% of body weight. Urinary excretion was 59% for controls, and 68% for 2.5% group. No changes in sodium or potassium excretion were observed[SC029].

Estrogenic effect. Methanol extract of leaves, administered subcutaneously to mice, was active[SC004].

Fish poison. Water extract of fresh bark was active, LD_{50} 0.18%[SC055].

Hypoglycemic activity. Ethanol (95%) and water extracts of dried seeds, administered intragastrically to rabbits at variable dosage levels, were active. Hot water extract, administered intragastrically to dogs at a dose of 20.0 gm/kg (dry weight of seed), was inactive. A dose of 10.0 gm/kg, administered intragastrically to rabbits, was active[SC008]. Seeds, administered by gastric intubation to rats at doses of 170.0, 240.0 and 510.0 mg/animal daily for 15 days were active[SC039]. Ethanol/water (1:1) extract of the aerial parts, administered orally to rats at a dose of 250.0 mg/kg, was inactive. Less than 30% drop in blood sugar level was observed[SC058]. Hot water extract of dried fruit pulp, administered by gastric intuba-

tion to dogs at a dose of 200.0 gm/kg (expressed as dry weight of fruit pulp), was inactive, and to rabbits, at a dose of 50.0 gm/kg, was active[SC008]. Water extract of dried fruit and seeds, administered orally to rabbits at a dose of 10.0 mg/kg, was active. Drop in blood sugar of 15 mg relative to inert-treated controls indicated positive results[SC009].

Hypotensive activity. Ethanol/water (1:1) extract of dried bark, administered intravenously to dogs at variable dosage levels, was inactive[SC062].

Hypothermic activity. Ethanol/water (1:1) extract of the aerial parts, administered intraperitoneally to mice at a dose of 0.375 mg/kg, was inactive[SC058]. Methanol extract of dried seeds, administered intraperitoneally to mice at a dose of 50.0 mg/kg, was active, results significant at $P < 0.001$ level[SC051].

Leukocyte migration inhibition. Chloroform extract of dried seeds, administered intraperitoneally to rats at a dose of 50.0 mg/kg, was active vs carrageenin-induced pleurisy[SC032].

Molluscicidal activity. Ethanol (95%) and water extracts, at concentrations of 10,000 ppm, were inactive on *Biomphalaria glabrata* and *Biomphalaria straminea*[SC061]. Water, saturated with essential oil of fresh leaves, at a concentration of 1:10, was inactive on *Biomphalaria glabrata*[SC047].

Natriuretic activity. Water extract of dried leaves, administered by gastric intubation to rats at a concentration of 2.5%, was inactive. Animals were given water or 2.5% solution of *Syzygium cumini*. The quantity of solution equaled 5% of body weight. Urinary excretion was 59% for controls and 68% for the 2.5% group. No changes in sodium or potassium excretion were found[SC029].

Nematocidal activity. Decoction of a commercial sample of bark, at a concentration of 10.0 mg/ml, was inactive on *Toxacara canis*[SC034]. Water and methanol extracts of dried seeds, at concentrations of 5.0 and 1.0

mg/ml, respectively, were inactive on *Toxacara canis*[SC037].

Plaque formation suppressant. Water, methanol and methanol/water (1:1) extracts of a commercial sample of bark were active on *Streptococcus mutans*, IC_{50} 260.0, 120.0 and 380.0 mcg/ml, respectively[SC052].

Polygalacturonase inhibition. Hot water extract of bark produced weak activity. Hot water extract of leaves was active[SC005].

Prostaglandin inhibition. Methanol extract of dried seeds, administered intraperitoneally to rats, was active vs PGE-1-induced pedal edema[SC028].

Protease (HIV) inhibition. Water extract of dried bark, at a dose of 200.0 mcg/ml, produced weak activity; the methanol extract was active[SC022].

Protopectinase inhibition. Hot water extract of bark was inactive, and of leaves was active[SC005].

Semen coagulation. Ethanol/water (1:1) extract of aerial parts, at a concentration of 2.0%, was inactive on rat semen[SC058].

Skeletal muscle relaxant effect. Methanol extract of dried seeds, administered intraperitoneally to mice at a dose of 100.0 mg/kg, was active vs Rotarod test, results significant at $P < 0.02$ level[SC051].

Spermicidal effect. Ethanol/water (1:1) extract of the aerial parts was inactive on rat sperm[SC058].

Spontaneous activity reduction. Methanol extract of dried seeds, administered intraperitoneally to mice at a dose of 25.0 mg/kg, was active, results significant at $P < 0.001$ level[SC051].

Toxic effect. Ethanol/water (1:1) extract of dried stembark, administered by gastric intubation and subcutaneously to mice at a dose of 10.0 gm/kg (dry weight of stembark), was inactive[SC043].

Toxicity assessment. Ethanol (95%) extract of dried seeds, administered intravenously to mice, produced LD_{50} 0.4 gm/kg, and 4.0 gm/kg with intragastric administration[SC007]. Ethanol/water (1:1) extract of the aerial parts, administered intraperitoneally to mice, produced LD_{50} 0.75 gm/kg[SC058].

Weight increase. Powdered commercial sample of seeds, administered by gastric intubation to rats at a dose of 53.2 mg/kg, was active. Animals were dosed daily for 1 week[SC035].

REFERENCES

SC001   Gupta, G. S. and D. P. Sharma. Triterpenoids and other constituents of *Eugenia jambolana* leaves. **Phytochemistry** 1974; 13: 2013.

SC002   Singh, R. Inactivation of potato virus X by plant extracts. **Phytopathol Mediterr** 1971; 10: 211.

SC003   Anon. Lilly's Handbook of Pharmacy and Therapeutics. 5th Rev, Eli Lilly and Co., Indianapolis, 1898.

SC004   Ray, B. N. and A. K. Pal. Estrogenic activity of tree leaves as animal feed. **Indian J Physiol Allied Sci** 1967; 20: 6.

SC005   Prasad, V. and S. C. Gupta. Inhibitory effect of bark and leaf decoction on the activity of pectic enzymes of *Alternaria tennis*. **Indian J Exp Biol** 1967; 5: 192.

SC006   Sengupta, P. and P. B. Das. Terpenoids and related compounds. Part IV. Triterpenoids from the stem-bark of *Eugenia jambolana*. **J Indian Chem Soc** 1965; 42: 255.

SC007   Anon. Hypoglycemic medicament based on *Syzygium jambolanum* (Java Plum). **Patent-Fr M**-6114 1968; 4pp.

SC008   Shorti, D. S., M. Kelkar, V. K. Deshmukh and R. Aiman. Investigation of the hyperglycemic properties of *Vinca rosea*, *Cassia auriculata* and *Eugenia jambolana*. **Indian J Med Res** 1963; 51(3): 464–467.

SC009   Jain, S. R. and S. N. Sharma. Hypoglycaemic drugs of Indian indigenous origin. **Planta Med** 1967; 15(4): 439–442.

SC010   Sigogneau-Jagodzinski, M., P. Bibal-Prot, M. Chanez, P. Boiteau and A. R. Ratsimamanga. Contribution to a study of the hypoglycemic and antidiabetic extract of Madagascar Rotra (*Eugenia jambolana* Lamarck). **CR Acad Sci Ser D** 1967; 264(8): 1119–1123.

SC011   Steinmetz, E. F. A botanical drug from the tropics used in the treatment of diabetes mellitus. **Acta Phytother** 1961; 7: 23–25.

SC012   Khan, A. H. and A. Burney. A preliminary study of the hypoglycaemic properties of indigenous plants. **Pak J Med Res** 1962; 2: 100–116.

SC013   Vaishnava, M. M., A. K. Tripathy and K. R. Gupta. Flavonoids from *Syzygium cumini* roots. **Fitoterapia** 1992; 63(3): 259–260.

SC014   Desai, H. K., D. H. Gawad, T. R. Govindachari, et al. Chemical investigation of some Indian plants: Part VIII. **Indian J Chem** 1975; 13: 97–98.

SC015   Jain, M. C. and T. R. Seshadri. Anthocyanins of *Eugenia jambolana* fruits. **Indian J Chem** 1975; 13: 20.

SC016   Bhargava, K. K., T. R. Seshadri and R. Dayal. Chemical components of *Eugenia jambolana* stem bark. **Curr Sci** 1974; 43: 645.

SC017   Bhatia, I. S. and K. L. Bajaj. Chemical constituents of the seeds and bark of *Syzygium cumini*. **Planta Med** 1975; 28: 346.

SC018   Teixeira, C. C., F. D. Fuchs, R. M. Blotta, A. P. Da Costa, D. G. Mussnich and G. G. Ranquetat. Plants employed in the treatment of diabetes mellitus. Results of an ethnopharmacological survey in Porto Alegre, Brazil. **Fitoterapia** 1992; 63(4): 320–322.

SC019   Reddy, M. B., K. R. Reddy and M. N. Reddy. A survey of plant crude drugs of Anantapur District, Andhra Pradesh, India. **Int J Crude Drug Res** 1989; 27(3): 145–155.

SC020   Rana, N. S. and M. N. Ioshi. Investigation on the antiviral activity of ethanolic extracts of Syzygium species. **Fitoterapia** 1992; 63(3): 542–544.

SC021   Lim-Sylianco, C. Y., J. A. Concha, A. P. Jocano and C. M. Lim. Antimutagenic effects of expressions from twelve medicinal plants. **Philippine J Sci** 1986; 115(1): 23–30.

SC022   Kusumoto, I. T., T. Nakabayashi, H. Kida, H. Miyashiro, M. Hattori, T. Namba and K. Shimotohno. Screening of various plant extracts used in Ayurvedic medicine for inhibitory effect on human immunodeficiency virus type 1 (HIV-1) protease. **Phytother Res** 1995; 9(3): 180–184.

SC023   Singh, K. K. and J. K. Maheshwari. Traditional phytotherapy of some medicinal plants used by the Tharus of the Nainital District, Uttar Pradesh, India. **Int J Pharmacog** 1994; 32(1): 51–58.

SC024   Anis, M. and M. Iqbal. Medicinal plantlore of Aligarh, India. **Int J Pharmacog** 1994; 32(1): 59–64.

SC025   Bhandary, M. J., K. R. Chandrashekar and K. M. Kaveriappa. Medical ethnobotany of the Siddis of Uttar Kannada District, Karnataka, India. **J Ethnopharmacol** 1995; 47(3): 149–158.

SC026   Bhatt, H. V., O. P. Gupta and P. S. Gupta. Hypoglycaemia induced by *Syzygium cumini* Linn. seeds in diabetes mellitus. **Asian Med J** 1983; 26(7): 489–491.

SC027   Linde, H. About two phenols in cloves. **Arch Pharm (Weinheim)** 1983; 26(7): 489–491.

SC028   Mahapatra, P. K., D. Chakraborty and A. K. N. Chaudhuri. Antiinflammatory and antipyretic activities of *Syzygium cumini*. **Planta Med** 1986; 6: 540–A.

SC029   Silva-Netto, C. R., R. A. Lopes and G. L. Pozetti. Changes in urinary volume and sodium and potassium excretion in rats submitted to Jambolao (*Syzygium jambolanum*) solution load. **Rev Fac Odont Ribeirao Preto** 1989; 23(2): 213–215.

SC030   Shah, G. L. and G. V. Gopal. Ethnomedical notes from the tribal inhabitants of the North Gujarat (India). **J Econ Taxon Botany** 1985; 6(1): 193–201.

SC031   Reddy, M. B., K. R. Reddy and M. N. Reddy. A survey of medicinal plants of Chenchu Tribes of Andhra Pradesh, India. **Int J Crude Drugs Res** 1988; 26(4): 189–196.

SC032   Chaudhuri, A. K. N., S. Pal, A. Gomes and S. Bhattacharya. Anti-inflammatory and related actions of *Syzygium cumini* seed extract. **Phytother Res** 1990; 4(1): 5–10.

SC033   Alam, M. M., M. B. Siddiqui and W. Husain. Treatment of diabetes through herbal drugs in rural India. **Fitoterapia** 1990; 61(3): 240–242.

SC034   Kiuchi, F., M. Hioki, N. Nakamura, N. Miyashita, Y. Tsuda and K. Kondo. Screening of crude drugs used in Sri Lanka for nematocidal activity on the larva of *Toxacara canis*. **Shoyakugaku Zasshi** 1989; 43(4): 288–293.

SC035   Al-Zaid, M. M., M. A. M. Hassan, N. Badir and K. A. Gumaa. Evaluation of blood glucose lowering activity of three plant diet additives. **Int J Pharmacog** 1991; 29(2): 81–88.

SC036   Vaishnava, M. M. and K. R. Gupta. Isorhamnetin 3-o-rutinoside from *Syzygium cumini* Linn. **J Indian Chem Soc** 1990; 67(9): 785–786.

SC037   Ali, M. A., M. Mikage, F. Kiuchi, Y. Tsuda and K. Kondo. Screening of crude drugs used in Bangladesh for nematocidal activity on the larva of *Toxacara canis*. **Shoyakugaku Zasshi** 1991; 45(3): 206–214.

SC038   Khanna, R. K. Chemical examination of the essential oil from the leaves of *Syzygium cumini* Skeel. **Indian Perfum** 1991; 35(2): 112–115.

SC039   Bansal, R., N. Ahmad and J. R. Kidwai. Effect of oral administration of *Eugenia jambolana* seeds & chloropropamide on blood glucose level & pancreatic cathepsin B in rats. **Indian J Biochem Biophys** 1981; 18: 377.

SC040   Bobbio-Adilma, F. O. and R. P. Scamparini. Carbohydrates, organic acids and anthocyanin of *Eugenia jambolana* Lamarck. **Ind Aliment (Pinerolo, Italy)** 1982; 21: 296–298.

SC041   Craveiro, A. A., C. H. S. Andrade, F. J. A. Matos, J. W. Alencar and M. I. L. Machado. Essential oil of *Eugenia jambolana* Lamk. **J Nat Prod** 1983; 46(4): 591–592.

SC042   Avirutnant, W. and A. Pongpan. The antimicrobial activity of some Thai flowers and plants. **Mahidol Univ J Pharm Sci** 1983; 10(3): 81–86.

SC043   Mokkhasmit, M., K. Swatdimongkol and P. Satrawaha. Study on toxicity of Thai medicinal plants. **Bull Dept Med Sci** 1971; 12(2/4): 36–65.

SC044   Ayensu, E. S. Medicinal plants of the West Indies. **Unpublished Manuscript** 1978; 110pp.

SC045   Kedar, P. and C. H. Chakrabarti. Effects of Jambolan seed treatment on blood sugar, lipid and urea in streptozotocin induced diabetes in rabbits. **Indian J Physiol Pharmacol** 1983; 27(2): 135–140.

SC046   Shaft, N. and M. Ikram. Quantitative survey of rutin-containing plants. Part 1. **Int J Crude Drug Res** 1982; 20(4): 183–186.

SC047   Rouquayrol, M. Z., M. C. Fonteles, J. E. Alencar, F. Jose de Abreu and A. A. Craveiro. Molluscicidal activity of essential oils from Northeastern Brazilian plants. **Rev Brasil Pesq Med Biol** 1980; 13: 135–143.

SC048   Deka, L., R. Majumdar and A. M. Dutta. Some Ayurvedic important plants from District Kamrup (Assam). **Ancient Sci Life** 1983; 3(2): 108–115.

SC049   Sebastian, M. K. and M. M. Bhandari. Medico-ethno botany of Mount Abu, Rajasthan, India. **J Ethnopharmacol** 1984; 12(2): 223–230.

SC050   Said, M. Potential of herbal medicines in modern medical therapy. **Ancient Sci Life** 1984; 4(1): 36–47.

SC051   Chakraborty, D., P. K. Mahapatra and A. K. Nag Chaudhuri. A neurospsychopharmacological study of *Syzygium cumini*. **Planta Med** 1986; 2: 139–143.

SC052   Namba, T., M. Tsunezuka, N. Kakiuchi, D. M. R. B. Dissanayake, U. Pilapitiya, K. Saito and M. Hattori. Studies on dental caries prevention by traditional medicines (Part V11). Screening of Ayurvedic medicines for anti-plaque action. **Shoyakugaku Zasshi** 1985; 39(2): 146–153.

SC053   Anderson, E. F. Ethnobotany of Hill tribes of Northern Thailand. II. Lahu medicinal plants. **Econ Bot** 1986; 40(4): 442–450.

SC054   Chakraborty, T. and G. Poddar. Herbal drugs in diabetes–Part I: Hypoglycaemic activity of indigenous plants in streptozotocin (STZ) induced diabetic rats. **J Inst Chem (India)** 1984; 56(1): 20–22.

SC055   Kulakkattolickal, A. Piscicidal plants of Nepal. Preliminary toxicity screening using grass carp (*Ctenopharyngodon idella*) fingerlings. **J Ethnopharmacol** 1987; 21(1): 1–9.

SC056   Rajasekaran, M., J. S. Bapna, S. Lakshmanan, A. G. Ramachandran Nair, A. J. Veliath and M. Panchanadam. Antifertility effect in male rats of oleanolic acid, a triterpene from *Eugenia jambolana* flowers. **J Ethnopharmacol** 1988; 24(1): 115–121.

SC057   Kumar, D. S. and Y. S. Prabhakar. On the ethnomedical significance of the Arjun tree, *Terminalia arjuna* (Roxb.) Wight & Arnot. **Indian J Homoeopath Med** 1984; 19(3): 114–120.

SC058   Dhawan, B. N., G. K. Patnaik, R. P. Rastogi, K. K. Singh and J. S. Tandon. Screening of Indian plants for biological activity. VI. **Indian J Exp Biol** 1977; 15: 208–219.

SC059   Collier, W. A. and L. Van de Piji. The antibiotic action of plants, especially the higher plants, with results with Indonesian plants. **Chron Nat** 1949; 105: 8.

SC060   Mueller-Oerlinghausen, B., W. Ngamwathana and P. Kanchanapee. Investigation into Thai medicinal plants said to cure diabetes. **J Med Assoc Thailand** 1971; 54: 105–111.

SC061   Pinheiro de Sousa, M. and M. Z. Rouquayrol. Molluscicidal activity of plants from Northeast Brazil. **Rev Bras Fpesq Med Biol** 1974; 7(4): 389–394.

SC062   Mokkhasmit, M., K. Swasdimongkol, W. Ngarmwathana and U. Permphiphat. Pharmacological evaluation of Thai medicinal plants. (Continued). **J Med Assoc Thailand** 1971; 54(7): 490–504.

SC063   Teixeira, C. C., C. A. Rava, P. Mallman da Silva, R. Melchior, R. ARgenta, F. Anselmi, C. R. Almeida and F. D. Fuchs. Absence of antihyperglycemic effect of jambolan in experimental and clinical models. **J Ethnopharmacol** 2000; 71(1–2): 343–347.

SC064   Muruganandan, S., K. Srinivasan, S. Chandra, S. K. Tandan, J. Lai and V. Raviprakash. Anti-inflammatory activity of *Syzgium cumini* bark. **Fitoterapia** 2001; 72(4): 369–375.

27 | Tamarindus indica
L.

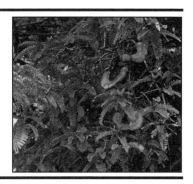

Common Names

Ajagbon	Nigeria	Tamarind	Guyana
Ambliki	India	Tamarind	India
Amli	Fiji	Tamarind	Indonesia
Ambali	India	Tamarind	Japan
Asam jawa	Indonesia	Tamarind	West Indies
Asam jawa	Malaysia	Tame tamarind	West Indies
Asem	Indonesia	Tamarinde	Guinea
Cheench	India	Tamarindo	Brazil
Cinca	India	Tamarindo	Canary Islands
Dakhar	Senegal	Tamarindo	Cuba
Hamer	Saudi Arabia	Tamarindo	Guatemala
Icheku oyibo	Nigeria	Tamarindo	Indonesia
Imli	Fiji	Tamarindo	Madagascar
Imli	India	Tamarindo	Nicaragua
Kaju asam	Indonesia	Tamarindo	Peru
Makham	Thailand	Tamarindo	Puerto Rico
Manhan	China	Tamarini	Guinea
Mkwaju	Tanzania	Tamparanu	Nicaragua
Ntemi	Guinea	Tamrand	Nicaragua
Ntomi	Guinea	Tateli	India
Pokok asam jawa	Malaysia	Tetul	India
Slim	Nicaragua	Timer hendi	Morocco
Tamarin	Rodrigues Islands	Tombi	Guinea
Tamarin des indes	West Indies	Tombinyi	Guinea
Tamarind	Bangladesh	Tsaniya	Nigeria

BOTANICAL DESCRIPTION

A large tree of the LEGUMINOSAE family, up to 30 meters high, having spreading branches; bark, brownish-gray and flaked. Leaves are even-pinnate, consisting of 10–18 pairs of small leaflets, rather closed together; petioles and rachis 5–12 cm long; leaflets oblong, 8–30 by 3–9 mm, opposite, pink or reddish when young, membranous and glabrous with obtuse or rounded apex and the base unequal. Inflorescence is in terminal raceme, yellowish-orange or pale

From: *Medicinal Plants of the World, vol. 1: Chemical Constituents, Traditional and Modern Medicinal Uses, 2nd ed.*
By: Ivan A. Ross © Humana Press Inc., Totowa, NJ

green; consisting of calyx-tube narrow turbinate, with 4 imbricate segments, 1 cm long; petals 3, unequal, upper cordate, about 1 cm long, 2 lateral ones, narrowed towards the base; fertile stamens 3, base connate; ovary linear, about 7 mm long, pubescent, on a stalk adnate to the calyx-tube. Pods are oblong, slightly curved, 5–15 by 1–2.5 cm, reddish brown. Seeds are glossy, dark brown, embedded in a thick, sticky, acid brown pulp.

ORIGIN AND DISTRIBUTION

Native of tropical Africa, now pantropic. It is cultivated for the edible fruits and as an ornamental and shade tree.

TRADITIONAL MEDICINAL USES

Brazil. Decoction of dried fruit is taken orally for fevers[TI016].

Canary Islands. Dried fruit is eaten as a choleretic[TI058].

China. Fresh fruit is used as a food[TI049].

Colombia. Hot water extract of dried fruit is taken orally as an abortive[TI056].

Dominican Republic. Water extract of dried leaves is taken orally to treat liver complaints[TI024].

Fiji. Dried fruit pulp is taken orally for sore throat and diarrhea. Dried leaves, in a poultice with mustard oil are applied on the affected area for sprains. For eye troubles, leaves soaked in water are applied as a poultice. Infusion of dried bark, fruit and leaves is taken orally for piles. Infusion of dried fruit is taken orally to induce vomiting[TI051].

Guatemala. Hot water extract of dried fruit is taken orally as a sudorific and febrifuge, for urinary tract infections and infections of the skin and mucosa; externally, it is used for skin eruptions and erysipelas[TI057]. Hot water extract of dried fruit pulp is used for ringworm and skin fungal diseases[TI034].

Guinea. Water extract of bark is taken orally by women after childbirth, and together with the bark of *Afzelia africana*, as a remedy for troubles during pregnancy[TI001].

India. Externally, bark is used as an astringent. Orally, it is used as a tonic and febrifuge, and the ash obtained by heating the bark with salt in an earthen pot, is mixed with water and taken orally for colic and indigestion, as a gargle for sore throat and a mouthwash for apthous sores[TI025]. Hot water extract of dried bark is taken orally for paralysis and as a tonic[TI048]. Fruit juice, mixed with *Calotropis gigantea* latex, is taken orally to relieve menstrual pains[TI035]. Hot water extract of dried leaves is taken orally for inflammatory swellings and urinary discharges[TI048]. Leaf juice is taken orally to treat encephalitis. Four drops of leaf juice and three drops of latex from *Calotropis gigantea* are taken daily for 8 days. For rheumatic arthritis, leaf juice, latex of *Calotropis gigantea*, goat milk and sesame oil is applied externally[TI018].

Indonesia. Water extract of fruit is taken orally as an abortifacient[TI002].

Ivory Coast. Hot water extract of leaf and root is taken orally to treat sleeping sickness. The decoction, and decoction of leaves and roots of *Afzelia africana* and *Ficus* species is taken orally and also used as a vapor bath[TI063].

Madagascar. Hot water extract of the trunk bark is taken orally for amenorrhea[TI065].

Malaysia. Hot water extract of root, mixed with several other plants, is taken orally for amenorrhea[TI006].

Nigeria. Fresh leaves, ground with the leaves of *Prosopis africana* in equal proportions, are taken orally with water to treat malaria fever. Cold water and 1.5 teaspoonfuls of crushed potash are added to 1–2 handfuls of leaves and left until an extract is obtained. The extract is used as a laxative[TI017]. Hot water extracts of the dried bark and husk of the pods, and the leaves and bark of *Diospyros mespiliformis* are taken orally for leprosy[TI039].

Peru. Hot water extract of dried fruit peel is taken orally as a laxative[TI055].

Saudi Arabia. Dried fruit is taken orally in the traditional medicine[TI068].

Senegal. Hot water extract of dried stem bark is taken orally medicinally[TI050]. Externally, it is used as a cicatrizant[TI052].

Sudan. Dried fruit pulp is taken orally as a purgative, for malaria and bacterial infections[TI011].

Tanzania. Decoction of dried leaves is taken orally to treat malaria[TI020]. Decoction of hot water extract of dried bark and root is taken orally with *Stereospermum kunthianum* bark and root for the treatment of leprosy[TI039]. Decoction of root is taken orally for distended painful abdomen and dysentery. Juice from fresh leaves is taken orally for bloody diarrhea[TI059].

Thailand. Hot water extract of dried fruit pulp is taken orally as an expectorant. Hot water extract of dried leaves is taken orally as a cathartic. Hot water extract of dried seed is taken orally as an anthelmintic[TI067].

West Indies. Fruit pulp is taken orally as a laxative[TI038].

CHEMICAL CONSTITUENTS

(ppm unless otherwise indicated)

3-4-Dihydroxy phenyl acetate: Sd[TI023]
Alpha humulene: Fr Pu 2.0%[TI022]
Alpha murolene: Fr Pu[TI022]
Alpha pinene: Fr Pu[TI022]
Alpha copaene: Fr Pu 0.6%[TI022]
Alpha oxo-glutaric acid: Fr, Lf, Fl[TI013]
Arabinose: Fr[TI070]
Arachidic acid: Sd oil[TI007,TI026]
Aromadendrene: Fr Pu 90%[TI022]
Ascorbic acid: Fr 24–585, Lf 600[TI069]
Ash: Fl 3.5%, Lf 2.6–7.3%[TI069], Fr 2.7–3.94%[TI071], Sd 2.5–3.2%[TI070]
Behenic acid: Sd oil[TI007,TI026]
Benzoic acid,3-4-dihydroxy methyl ester: Sd[TI023]
Beta caryophyllene: Fr Pu 0.5%[TI022]
Beta pinene: Fr Pu[TI022]
Beta carotene: Fl 10, Fr 0–1, Lf 2–110[TI069]
Beta elemene: Fr Pu 0.3%[TI022]
Calcium pectate: Fr[TI070]
Calcium tartrate: Fr[TI070]

Carbohydrate: Fl 75%, Lf 70.6–75.0%[TI069], Fr 62.5–92.5%[TI069,TI071], Sd 65.1–74.0%[TI070]
Carvacrol: Fr Pu 0.5%[TI022]
Cellulose: Fr 1.8–3.2%[TI072]
Chlorine: Lf 940[TI070]
Citric acid: Fr[TI070]
Copper: Lf 21[TI070]
D-Arabinose: Sd[TI070]
D-Galactose: Sd[TI070]
D-Glucose: Sd[TI070]
D-Xylose: Sd[TI070]
Epi-catechin: Sd[TI023]
Fat: Fl 9%, Fr 0.3–0.9%, Lf 3.6–4.4%[TI069], Sd 6.0–7.4%[TI070]
Fiber: Fl 6%, Lf 5.7–18.6%[TI069], Fr 3.1–7.4%[TI071], Sd 0.7–4.3%[TI070]
Fructose: Fr 9–12%[TI070]
Furfural: Fr Pu 3.0%[TI022]
Galactose: Fr[TI070]
Galacturonic acid: Fr[TI070]
Gamma cadinene: Fr Pu 0.4%[TI022]
Glucose: Fr 21–28%[TI070]
Glyoxylic acid: Fr, Lf, Fl[TI013]
HCN: Pl[TI073]
Hordenine: Bk[TI070]
Invert sugars: Fr 30–40%[TI070]
Iron: Fl 70[TI069], Fr 13–109[TI070,TI071], Lf 52–88[TI069,TI070]
Isoorientin: Lf 10[TI009]
Isovitexin: Lf 5[TI009]
Lactic acid: Fr[TI070]
Lauric acid: Sd oil[TI007,TI026]
Lignoceric acid: Sd oil[TI007,TI026]
Linalool: Fr Pu 0.10%[TI022]
Linoleic acid: Fr 590–860[TI071], Sd oil 2.7–3.4%[TI070]
Linolenic acid: Sd oil[TI012,TI026]
Lysine: Fr 1390–2026[TI071]
Magnesium: Fr 920–1341[TI071], Lf 710[TI070]
Malic acid: Fr 1%, Lf 1.5%[TI070]
Methionine: Fr 140–204[TI071]
Methoxyl: Fr[TI070]
Methyl glutamic acid: Sprout[TI070]
Methyleneglutamic acid: Sprout[TI070]
Methyleneglutamine: Sprout[TI070]
Mucilage: Sd[TI027]
MUFA: Fr 1810–2640[TI071]
Myrcene: Fr Pu[TI022]
Myristic acid: Sd oil[TI007,TI026]
N-Octadecane: Fr Pu 0.15%[TI022]
Niacin: Fr 16–33[TI071], Fl 60, Lf 66[TI069]

Oleic acid: Sd oil[TI007,TI012,TI026]
Orientin: Lf 12.5[TI009]
Oxalic acid: Fr, Lf 1960[TI070]
Oxaloacetic acid: Fr, Lf, Fl[TI013]
Oxalosuccinic acid: Fr, Lf, Fl[TI013]
P-Cresol: Fr[TI069]
Palmitic acid: Sd oil[TI007,TI026]
Pantothenic acid: Fr 1–2[TI071]
Pectin: Sd[TI027]
Pentosan: Fr 4.2–4.8%[TI070,TI072]
Phenol: Fr[TI069]
Phlobotannin: Sd[TI070]
Phosphorus: Fl 2200, Lf 1000–2281 [TI069],
　　Fr 1130–1647[TI071], Sd 2370[TI070]
Pipecolinic acid: Fr[TI070]
Potassium: Fr 0.6–1.5%[TI069,TI071], Fl 1.27%,
　　Lf 1.197%[TI069]
Potassium oxide: Fr 1032–7654[TI072]
Proline: Fr[TI070]
Protein: Fl 12.5%, Lf 14.1–22.4%[TI069],
　　Fr 2.8–11.7%[TI069,TI071], Sd 17.1–20.1%[TI070]
PUFA: Fr 590–860[TI071]
Pyridoxine: Fr 1–2[TI069,TI071]
Quinic acid: Fr[TI070]
Riboflavin: Fl 6[TI069], Fr 1–3[TI071],
　　Lf 1–5[TI069,TI070]
SFA: Fr 2720–3965[TI071]
Sodium: Fl 250, Lf 351[TI069],
　　Fr 49–743[TI069,TI071]
Stearic acid: Sd oil[TI007]
Succinic acid: Fr[TI070]
Sulfur: Lf 630[TI070]
Tamarind xyloglucan: Fr[TI019]
Tamarindienal: Fr Pu[TI011]
Tamarindus galactoxyloglucan: Sd[TI010]
Tannin: Sd[TI070]
Tartaric acid: Fr[TI032]
Thiamin: Fl 4, Lf 4[TI069], Fr 2–9[TI071]
Tryptophan: Fr 180–262[TI071]
Uronic acid: Fr[TI070]
Uzarigenen-3-O-beta-D-xylopyranosyl(1(2)-
　　alpha-L-rhamnopyranoside: Sd[TI075]
Vitexin: Lf 28.5[TI009]
Water: Fr 31.4%[TI071]

PHARMACOLOGICAL ACTIVITIES AND CLINICAL TRIALS

Allergenic activity. Powdered commercial sample of fruit produced weak activity. Reactions to patch tests occurred most commonly in patients who were regularly exposed to the substance, or who already had dermatitis on the fingertips. Previously unexposed patients had few reactions, i.e., no irritant reactions[TI028].

Antibacterial activity. Acetone extract of commercial sample of fruit, on agar plate, was active on *Salmonella typhimurium*. The ethanol (70%) extract was active on *Bacillus cereus, Bacillus megaterium, Escherichia coli, Pseudomonas aeruginosa, Salmonella typhimurium, Staphylococcus albus* and *Staphylococcus aureus*[TI045]. Tincture of dried fruit, at a concentration of 30.0 microliters/disc on agar plate, was active on *Escherichia coli*. Extract of 10 gm dried fruit in 100 ml ethanol was used[TI057]. Ethanol (95%) and hot water extracts of dried root bark, on agar plate, were inactive on *Escherichia coli* and *Staphylococcus aureus*[TI066]. Ethanol (95%) extract of fruit, on agar plate, was active on *Bacillus subtilis, Escherichia coli, Salmonella typhosa, Staphylococcus aureus* and *Vibrio cholera*[TI062]. Ethanol (95%) extract of dried fruit, on agar plate, was active on *Escherichia coli* and inactive on *Staphylococcus aureus*. The hot water extract was active on *Escherichia coli* and equivocal on *Staphylococcus aureus*. Ethanol (95%) extract of dried leaves, on agar plate, was active on *Staphylococcus aureus* and inactive on *Escherichia coli*. The hot water extract was active on *Staphylococcus aureus* and *Escherichia coli*[TI066]. Methanol extract of dried stem bark, at a concentration of 10.0 mg/ml, was active on several Gram-negative organisms and inactive on Gram-positive organisms. A concentration of 15.0 mg/ml was active on *Sarcina lutea*[TI050].

Antifungal activity. Acetone and ethanol (95%) extracts of dried leaves, at a concentration of 50% on agar plate, were inactive on *Neurospora crassa*. The water extract was active. Acetone and water extracts of dried bark, at a concentration of 50% on agar plate, were inactive. The ethanol (95%) extract was active. Acetone and water extracts of dried stem, at a concentration of 50%, were inactive and the ethanol (95%) extract, at a concentration of 50% on agar plate, was active on *Neurospora crassa*[TI046]. Ethanol (70%) extract of commercial sample of fruit, on agar plate, was active on several fungi[TI045]. Ethanol (95%) extract of fruit, on agar plate, was active on *Trichophyton mentagrophytes* and *Trichophyton rubrum*[TI062]. Ethanol/water (1:1) extract of dried fruit, at a concentration of 333.0 mg/ml (expressed as dry weight of plant) on agar plate, was active on *Aspergillus fumigatus*, *Aspergillus niger*, *Penicillium digitatum*, *Rhizopus nigricans* and *Trichophyton mentagrophytes*. At concentrations of 333.0 and 500.0 mg/ml, the extract was inactive on *Aspergillus niger* and *Botrytis cinerea*[TI060]. At 500 mg/ml, the extract was active on *Aspergillus fumigatus*, *Fusarium oxysporum*, *Penicillium digitatum*, *Rhizopus nigricans* and *Trichophyton mentagrophytes*, and inactive on *Botrytis cinerea*[TI053]. Hot water extract of dried fruit pulp, at a concentration of 1.0 ml in broth culture, was active on *Microsporum canis*, *Epidermophyton floccosum* and *Trichophyton mentagrophytes* var. granulare, and inactive on *Microsporum gypseum* and *Trichophyton mentagrophytes* var. algodonosa[TI034]. Water extract of fresh leaves, on agar plate, produced strong activity on *Ustilago nuda*[TI047].

Antihepatotoxic effect. Hot water extract of dried leaves, at a concentration of 1.0 mg/plate in cell culture, was active on hepatocytes when measured by leakage of LDH and ASAT[TI024].

Antiinflammatory activity. Aqueous, ethanol, and chloroform extracts of the leaves, administered to mice with ear edema induced by arachidonic acid and to rats with subplantar edema induced by carrageenan topically and intraperitoneally, respectively, produced weak activity[TI074].

Antilithic activity. Dried fruit pulp, ingested by human adults at a dose of 3.0 gm/day, was inactive. Tamarind intake did not affect crystallization rates of calcium or oxalate in urine samples from normal or stone-forming subjects[TI029].

Antimalarial activity. Ethyl acetate and petroleum ether extracts of dried leaves were active on *Plasmodium falciparum*, ED_{50} 70.0 and 90.0 mcg/ml, respectively. The ethanol (95%) and water extracts were inactive, ED_{50} > 500 mcg/ml[TI0203]. Methanol extract of dried fruit was inactive on *Plasmodium falciparum* vs hypoxanthine uptake by Plasmodia, IC_{50} > 499 mcg/ml[TI031].

Antinematodal activity. Water extract of commercial sample of pulp, at a concentration of 10.0 mg/ml, was inactive and the methanol extract produced weak activity on *Toxacara canis*[TI037].

Antioxidant activity. Methanol extract of fresh seeds, at a concentration of 0.2 mg/well, produced strong activity by thiocyanate assay[TI021].

Antischistosomal activity. Water extract, at a concentration of 100.0 ppm, was active on *Schistosoma mansoni*[TI033].

Antiviral activity. Ethanol (80%) extract of freeze dried fruit, at variable concentration in cell culture, was equivocal on Herpes virus Type 1; inactive on adenovirus, coxsackie B2 virus, measles virus, polio virus I and Semlicki-forest virus vs plaque inhibition[TI044]. Ethanol/water (1:1) extract of flowers, at a concentration of 50.0 mcg/ml in cell culture, produced weak activity on Ranikhet virus[TI003]. Water extract of bark was active on potato X virus[TI005].

Antiyeast activity. Ethanol/water (1:1) extract of dried fruit, at a concentration of 333.0 mg/ml (expressed as dry weight of plant) on agar plate, was inactive on *Saccharomyces pastorianus* and *Candida albicans*[TI053]. Tincture of dried fruit, at a concentration of 30.0 microliters/disc on agar plate, was inactive on *Candida albicans*. Extract of 10 gm dried fruit in 100 ml ethanol was used[TI057].

Cytotoxic activity. Ethanol/water (1:1) extract of flowers, in cell culture, was inactive on CA-9KB, $ED_{50} > 20.0$ mcg/ml[TI003].

Diuretic activity. Decoction of dried fruit, administered nasogastrically to rats at a dose of 1.0 gm/kg, produced strong activity[TI054].

Embryotoxic effect. Ethanol/water (1:1) extract of dried fruit, administered to rats by gastric intubation at a dose 100.0 mg/kg, was inactive[TI043].

Hepatic mixed function oxidase inhibition. Dried fruit, in the ration of rats at a dose of 2.5 mg%, was active[TI030].

Hypotensive activity. Hot water extract of dried root, administered intravenously to rats at a dose of 1.0 ml/animal, was inactive[TI036].

Juvenile hormone activity. Acetone extract of stem was active[TI014].

Lipid peroxide formation inhibition. Hot water extract of dried leaves, at a concentration 1.0 mg/plate in cell culture, was active on hepatocytes when monitored by reduction of malonaldehyde[TI024].

Molluscicidal activity. Aqueous slurry (homogenate) of fresh entire plant (fruits, leaves and roots) was inactive on *Lymnaea columella* and *Lymnaea cubensis*, $LD_{100} > 1M$ ppm[TI042]. Methanol extract of dried seeds, at a concentration of 100.0 ppm, was equivocal on *Bulinus globosus*. Ten percent mortality was observed[TI041]. Water and methanol extracts of dried fruit pulp were active (assayed after 24 hours exposure) on *Bulinus truncatus*, LC_{50} 400.0 ppm and 300.0 ppm, respectively[TI015].

Mutagenic activity. Dried fruit, at a concentration of 0.1 mg/plate on agar plate, was active on *Salmonella typhimurium* TA1535 and inactive on *S. typhimurium* TA1537, TA1538 and TA98[TI061].

Plant germination inhibition. Chloroform extract of dried leaves produced weak activity vs *Amaranthus spinosus* (20% inhibition). Ethanol (95%) extract, at a concentration of 8000 ppm, was active vs Allium roots[TI064]. Chloroform extract of dried seeds was active vs *Amaranthus spinosus* (36% inhibition) [TI040].

Polygalacturonase inhibition. Hot water extract of bark and leaves was active[TI008].

Protopectinase inhibition. Hot water extract of bark and leaves was active[TI008].

Radical scavenging effect. Hot water extract of dried leaves, at a concentration of 250.0 mg/liter, was active. When measured by decoloration of diphenylpicryl hydroxyl radical solution, 57% decoloration was observed[TI024].

Spasmolytic activity. Ethanol (95%) extract of fresh leaves and stem, at a concentration of 3.3 ml/liter, was active on guinea pig ileum. Water extract, administered intraperitoneally to guinea pig at a concentration of 33.0 ml/liter, was active on the ileum[TI004].

Toxicity assessment (quantitative). Ethanol/water (1:1) extract of flowers, administered orally to mice, produced a maximum tolerated dose of 1.0 gm/kg[TI003].

Vasodilator activity. Ethanol (95%) extract of fresh leaves and stem, at a concentration of 0.33 ml/liter, was active on the isolated rat hindquarter [TI004].

REFERENCES

TI001 Vasileva, B. Plantes Medicinales de Guinee. Conarky, Republique de Guinee, 1969.

TI002 Garcia-Barriga, H. Flora Medicinal de Colombia. Volume 1. Universidad Nacional, Bogota, 1974.

TI003 Dhar, M. L., M. M. Dhar, B. N. Mehrotra and C. Ray. Screening of Indian plants for biological activity. Part 1. **Indian J Exp Biol** 1968; 6: 232–247.

TI004 Feng, P. C., L. J. Haynes, K. E. Magnus, J. R. Plimmer and H. S. A. Sherrat. Pharmacological screening of some West Indian medicinal plants. **J Pharm Pharmacol** 1962; 14: 556–561.

TI005 Singh, R. Inactivation of potato virus X by plant extracts. **Phytopathol Mediterr** 1971; 10: 211.

TI006 Gimlette, J. D. A Dictionary of Malayan Medicine, Oxford Univ. Press., New York, USA, 1939.

TI007 Badami, R. C. and C. D. Daulatabad. Component acids of *Tamarindus indica*, *Peltophorum ferrugineum*, and *Albizzia julibrassin.* **J Karnatak Univ** 1969; 14: 2.

TI008 Prasad, V. and S. C. Gupta. Inhibitory effect of bark and leaf decoction on the activity of pectic enzymes of *Alternaria tennis.* **Indian J Exp Biol** 1967; 5: 192.

TI009 Bhatia, V. K., S. R. Gupta and T. R. Seshadri. C-glycosides of tamarind leaves. **Phytochemistry** 1966; 5: 177–181.

TI010 Gidley, M. J., P. J. Lillford, D. W. Rowlands, P. Lang, M. Dentini, V. Grescenzi, et al. Structure and solution properties of tamarind-seed polysaccharide. **Carbohydr Res** 1991; 214(2): 299–314.

TI011 Imbabi, E. S., K. E. Ibrahim, B. M Ahmed, I. M. Abulefuthu and P. Hulbert. Chemical characterization of tamarind bitter principle, tamarindineal. **Fitoterapia** 1992; 63(6): 537–538.

TI012 Haq, Q. N., M. N. Nabi and M. Kiamuddin. Oil from tamarind seed (*Tamarindus indica*). **Bangladesh J Sci Ind Res** 1973; 8: 42.

TI013 Mukherjee, D. and M. M. Laloraya. Keto acids in leaves, developing flowers and fruits of *Tamarindus indica*. **Plant Biochem J** 1974; 1: 53.

TI014 Prabhu, V. K. K. and M. John. Juvenomimetic activity in some plants. **Experientia** 1975; 31: 913.

TI015 Imbabi, E. S. and I. M. Abu-Al-Futuh. Investigation of the molluscicidal activity of *Tamarindus indica*. **Indian J Pharmacy** 1992; 30(2): 157–160.

TI016 Brandao, M., M. Botelho and E. Krettli. Antimalarial experimental chemotherapy using natural products. **Cienc Cult** 1985; 37(7): 1152–1163.

TI017 Bhat, R. B., E. O. Eterjere and V. T. Oladipo. Ethnobotanical studies from Central Nigeria. **Econ Bot** 1990; 44(3): 382–390.

TI018 Reddy, M. B., K. R. Reddy and M. N. Reddy. A survey of plant crude drugs of Anantapur District, Andhra Pradesh, India. **Int J Crude Drug Res** 1989; 27(3): 145–155.

TI019 York, W. S., L. K. Harvey, R. Guillen, P. Albersheim and A. G. Darvill. Structural analysis of tamarind seed xyloglucan oligosaccharides using beta-galactosidase digestion and spectroscopic methods. **Carbohydr Res** 1993; 248(1): 285–301.

TI020 Gessler, M. C., M. H. H. Nkunyak, L. B. Mwasumbi, M. Heinrich and M. Tanner. Screening Tanzanian medicinal plants for antimalarial activity. **Acta Tropica** 1994; 56(1): 65–77.

TI021 · Tsuda, T., Y. Makino, H. Kato, T. Osawa and S. Kawakishi. Screening for antioxidative activity of edible pulses. **Biosci Biotech Biochem** 1993; 57(9): 1606–1608.

TI022 Sagrero-Nieves, L., J. P. Bartley and A. Provis-Schwede. Supercritical fluid extraction of the volatile constituents from tamarind (*Tamarindus indica* L.). **J Essent Oil Res** 1994; 6(5): 547–548.

TI023 Tsuda, T., M. Watanabe, K. Ohshima, A. Yamamoto, S. Kawakishi and T. Osawa. Antioxidative components isolated from the seed of tamarind (*Tamarindus indica* L.). **J Agr Food Chem** 1994; 42(12): 2671–2674.

TI024 Joyeux, M., F. Mortier and J. Fleurentin. Screening of antiradical, antilipoper-oxidant and hepatoprotective effects of nine plant extracts used in Caribbean folk medicine. **Phytother Res** 1995; 9(3): 228–230.

TI025 Khan, M. A., T. Khan and Z. Ahmad. Barks used as source of medicine in Madhya Pradesh, India. **Fitoterapia** 1994; 65(5): 444–446.

TI026 Pitke, P. M., P. P. Singh and H. C. Srivastava. Fatty acid composition of tamarind kernel oil. **J Amer Oil Chem Soc** 1977; 54: 592.

TI027 Karawya, M. S., G. M. Wassel, H. H. Baghdadi and N. M. Ammar. Mucilages and pectins of Opuntia, Tamarindus and Cydonia. **Planta Med** 1980; 38: 68–75.

TI028 Seetharam, K. A. and J. S. Pasricha. Condiments and contact dermatitis of the finger tips. **Indian J Dermatol Venereol Leprol** 1987; 53(6): 325–328.

TI029 Singh, P. P., P. Hada, I. Narula and S. K. Gupta. In vivo effect of tamarind (*Tamarindus indica* L.) on urolith inhibitory activity in urine. **Indian J Exp Biol** 1988; 25(12): 863–865.

TI030 Sambaiah, K. and K. Srinivasan. Influence of spices and spice principles on hepatic mixed function oxygenase system in rats. **Indian J Biochem Biophys** 1989; 26(4): 254–258.

TI031   Weenen, H., M. H. H. Nkunya, D. H. Bray, et al. Antimalarial compounds containing an α,β-unsaturated carbonyl moiety from Tanzanian medicinal plants. **Planta Med** 1990; 56(4): 368–370.

TI032   Anasuya, A. and M. Sasikala. Tamarind ingestion and lithogenic properties of urine: Study in men. **Nutr Res** 1990; 10(10): 1109–1117.

TI033   Elsheikh, S. H., A. K. Bashir, S. M. Suliman and M. E. Wassila. Toxicity of certain Sudanese plant extracts on Cercariae and Miracidia of Schistosoma mansoni. **Int J Crude Drug Res** 1990; 28(4): 241–245.

TI034   Caceres, A., B. R. Lopez, M. A. Giron and H. Logemann. Plants used in Guatemala for the treatment of dermatophytic infections. I. Screeening for anti-mycotic activity of 44 plant extracts. **J Ethnopharmacol** 1991; 31(3): 263–276.

TI035   Nagaraju, N. and K. N. Rao. A survey of plant crude drugs of Rayalaseema, Andhra Pradesh, India. **J Ethnopharmacol** 1990; 29(2): 137–158.

TI036   Carbajal, D., A. Casaco, L. Arruzazabala, R. Gonzalez and V. Fuentes. Pharmacological screening of plant decoctions commonly used in Cuban folk medicine. **J Ethnopharmacol** 1991; 33(1/2): 21–24.

TI037   Kiuchi, F., N. Nakamura, N. Miyashita, S. Nishizawa, Y. Tsuda and K. Kondo. Nematocidal activity of some anthelmintics, traditional medicines, and spices by a new assay method using larvae of Toxacara canis. **Shoyakugaku Zasshi** 1989; 43(4): 279–287.

TI038   Ayensu, E. S. Medicinal plants of the West Indies. **Unpublished Manuscript** 1978; 110pp.

TI039   Nwude, N. and O. O. Ebong. Some plants used in the treatment of leprosy in Africa. **Leprosy Rev** 1980; 51: 11–18.

TI040   Rizvi, S. J. H., D. Mukerji and S. N. Mathur. A new report of a possible source of natural herbicide. **Indian J Exp Biol** 1980; 18: 777–781.

TI041   Sofowora, E. A. and C. O. Adewunmi. Preliminary screening of some plant extracts for molluscicidal activity. **Planta Med** 1980; 39: 57–65.

TI042   Medina, F. R. and R. Woodbury. Terrestrial plants molluscicidal to Lymnaeid hosts of Fasciliasis hepatica in Puerto Rico. **J Agr Univ Puerto Rico** 1979; 63: 366–376.

TI043   Prakash, A. O., R. B. Gupta and R. Mathur. Effect of oral administration of forty-two indigenous plant extracts on early and late pregnancy in albino rats. **Probe** 1978; 17(4): 315–323.

TI044   Van den Berghe, D. A., M. Ieven, F. Mertens, A. J. Vlietinck and E. Lammens. Screening of higher plants for biological activities. II. Antiviral activity. **J Nat Prod** 1978; 41: 463–467.

TI045   Ross, S. A., S. E. Megalla, D. W. Bishay and A. H. Awad. Studies for determining antibiotic substances in some Egyptian plants. Part 1. Screening for antimicrobial activity. **Fitoterapia** 1980; 51: 303–308.

TI046   Lopez Abraham, A. N., N. M. Rojas Hernandez and C. A. Jimenez Misas. Potential antineoplastic activity of Cuban plants. IV. **Rev Cubana Farm** 1981; 15(1): 71–77.

TI047   Singh, K. V. and R. K. Pathak. Effect of leaves extracts of some higher plants on spore germination of Ustilago maydes and U. nuda. **Fitoterapia** 1984; 55(5): 318–320.

TI048   Deka, L., R. Majumdar and A. M. Dutta. Some Ayurvedic important plants from District Kamrup (Assam). **Ancient Sci Life** 1983; 3(2): 108–115.

TI049   Pei, S. J. Preliminary study of ethnobotany in Xishuang Banna, People's Republic of China. **J Ethnopharmacol** 1985; 13(2): 121–137.

TI050   Laurens, A., S. Mboup, M. Tignokpa, O. Sylla and J. Masquelier. Antimicrobial activity of some medicinal species of Dakar markets. **Pharmazie** 1985; 40(7): 482–485.

TI051   Singh, Y. N. Traditional medicine in Fiji. Some herbal folk cures used by Fiji Indians. **J Ethnopharmacol** 1986; 15(1): 57–88.

TI052   Tignokpa, M., A. Laurens, S. Mboup and O. Sylla. Popular medicinal plants of the markets of Dakar (Senegal). **Int J Crude Drug Res** 1986; 24(2): 75–80.

TI053   Guerin, J. C. and H. P. Reveillere. Antifungal activity of plant extracts used in therapy. l. Study of 41 plant extracts against 9 fungi species. **Ann Pharm Fr** 1984; 42(6): 553–559.

TI054   Caceres, A., L. M. Giron and A. M. Martinez. Diuretic activity of plants used for treatment of urinary aliments in Guatemala. **J Ethnopharmacol** 1987; 19(3): 233–245.

TI055   Ramirez, V. R., L. J. Mostacero, A. E. Garcia, C. F. Mejia, P. F. Pelaez, C. D. Medina and C. H. Miranda. Vegetales empleados en medicina tradicional Norperuana. **Banco Agrario Del Peru & NACL Univ Trujillo**, Peru, June 1988; 54pp.

TI056   Gonzalez, F and M. Silva. A survey of plants with antifertility properties described in the South American folk medicine. **Abstr Princess Congress I**, Bangkok, Thailand, Dec. 1987; 20pp.

TI057   Caceres, A., L. M. Giron, S. R. Alvarado, and M. F. Torres. Screening of antimicrobial activity of plants popularly used in Guatemala for the treatment of dermatomucosal diseases. **J Ethnopharmacol** 1987; 20(3): 223–237.

TI058   Darias, V., L. Brando, R. Rabanal, C. Sanchez Mateo, R. M. Gonzalez Luis and A. M. Hernandez Perez. New contribution to the ethnopharmacological study of the Canary Islands. **J Ethnopharmacol** 1989; 25(1): 77–92.

TI059   Chabra, S. C., R. L. A. Mahunnah and E. N. Mshiu. Plants used in traditional medicine in Eastern Tanzania. I. Pteridophytes and angiosperms (Acanthaceae to Canellaceae). **J Ethnopharmacol** 1987; 21(3): 253–277.

TI060   Guerin, J. C. and H. P. Reveillere. Antifungal activity of plant extracts used in therapy. I. Study of 41 plant extracts against 9 fungi species. **Ann Pharm Fr** 1984; 42(6): 553–559.

TI061   Sivaswamy, S. N., B. Balchandran, S. Balanehru and V. M. Sivaramakrishnan. Mutagenic activity of South Indian food items. **Indian J Exp Biol** 1991; 29(8): 730–737.

TI062   Ray, P. G. and S. K. Majumdar. Antimicrobial activity of some Indian plants. **Econ Bot** 1976; 30: 317–320.

TI063   Kerharo, J. Historic and ethnopharmacognostic review on the belief and traditional practices in the treatment of sleeping sickness in West Africa. **Bull Soc Med Afr Noire Lang Fr** 1974; 19: 400.

TI064   Rathore, J. S. and S. K. Mishra. Inhibition of root elongation by some plant extracts. **Indian J Biochem Biophys** 1971; 9: 523–524.

TI065   Roig y Mesa, J. T. Plantas Medicinales, Aromaticas o Venenosas de Cuba. Ministerio de Agricultura, Republica de Cuba, Havana, 1945; 872pp.

TI066   George, M. and K. M. Pandalai. Investigations on plant antibiotics. Part IV. Further search for antibiotic substances in Indian medicinal plants. **Indian J Med Res** 1949; 37: 169–181.

TI067   Wasuwat, S. A list of Thai medicinal plants, ASRCT, Bangkok, Report No. 1 on Res. Project. 17. ASRCT Bangkok Thailand 1967; 17: 22pp.

TI068   Miles, S. B. The Countries and Tribes of the Persian Gulf. Frank Cass & Co. Ltd., London, 1966; 390–399pp.

TI069   Duke, James A. Handbook of Phytochemical Constituents of GRAS Herbs, CRC Press, LLC, 1992: 585–587pp.

TI070   The Wealth of India. 11 Volumes. Council of Scientific and Industrial Research, New Delhi, 1948–1976.

TI071   USDA Agricultural Handbook, No. 8. USDA, Washington, DC, Volumes 8–1 through 8–16, 1963–1986.

TI072   List, P. H. and Horhammer, L. Hager's Handbuch der Pharmazeutischen Praxis, Volumes 2–6, Springer-Verlag, Berlin, 1969–1979.

TI073   Watt, J. M. and Breyer-Brandwijk, M. G., The Medicinal and Poisonous Plants of Southern and Eastern Africa. 2nd Ed., E. & S. Livingstone, Ltd. Edinburgh, 1962, 1457pp.

TI074   Rimbau, V., C. Cerdan, R. Vila and J. Iglesias. Antiinflammatory activity of some extracts from plants used in the traditional medicine of north-African countries (II). **Phytother Res** 1999; 13(2): 128–132.

TI075   Yadava, R. N. and S. Yadav. A new cardenolide uzarigenen-3-O-beta-D-xylopyranosyl(1→2)-alpha-L-rhamnopyranoside. **J Asian Nat Prod Res** 1999; 1(4): 245–249.

Glossary

Abortifacient. Anything used to cause abortion.

Acaulescent. More or less stemless, the stem often subterranean.

Accessory. Fruit formed from the expanded dome-like receptacle of a single flower, covered with numerous achenes, known only in the strawberry.

Achene Seed. and pericarp attached only at the funiculus, the seed usually tightly enclosed by the fruit wall.

Acicular. Needle-shaped.

Acuminate. An acute apex in which the sides are concave and taper to an extended point.

Acute. Apex formed by two straight margins, meeting at less than 90 degrees.

Aggregate. Fruit formed from the many separate dry or fleshy fruits of a single flower, as in the raspberry.

Alkaloid. A basic organic nitrogenous compound of plant origin that is pharmacologically active and bitter tasting; certain alkaloids, such quinine, atropine, codeine, and scopolamine, are used in medicine.

Allergenic. A substance capable of inducing an allergic response.

Alternate. One leaf at a node.

Alveolate. Resembles the surface of a honeycomb.

Amblyopia. Impaired vision.

Amenorrhea. An abnormal suppression or nonoccurrence of menstruation.

Amoebicidal. A substance that destroys amoebas.

Analgesic. Pain reliever that does not induce loss of consciousness.

Angina Disease. of the heart signaled by acute constricting pains in the chest.

Angiosperm. Flower-bearing plants; ovules are enclosed in an ovary that forms the fruit after fertilization.

Ankylostomiasis. A hookworm disease, common in tropical countries.

Anodyne. A soothing pain-easing agent.

Anthelmintic. Causes removal or death of worms in the body.

Anthers. The pollen-bearing part of a stamen.

Anthrax. A carbuncle.

Anti-inflammatory. Reduces inflammation

Antidiabetic. A medicine counteracting or checking diabetes.

Antidote. Remedy counteracting the effects of a poison.

Antifebrile. A substance that reduces fever.

Antileukemic. Acts against a disorder and generally fatal condition of the blood and blood making tissues, characterized by a persistent excess of leukocytes.

Antinephritic. Counteracts kidney disease.

Antipyretic. Agent that relieves or reduces fever.

From: *Medicinal Plants of the World, vol. 1: Chemical Constituents, Traditional and Modern Medicinal Uses, 2nd ed.* By: Ivan A. Ross © Humana Press Inc., Totowa, NJ

Antiscorbutic. A remedy for scurvy.

Antiseptic. Prevents infection or putrefaction; a disinfecting agent.

Antispasmodic. Prevents or cures spasms, as in epilepsy.

Antitumor. Refers to tumor growth-inhibiting properties, usually referred to in connection with cancer.

Aperient. A mild laxative.

Apetalous. Without petals.

Aphrodisiac. Agents that stimulate sexual desire.

Aphtha. (plural, aphthae) An ulcer of the mucous membrane, usually oral.

Apiculate. Terminates in a short sharp flexible point.

Arachnoid. Slender white loosely tangled hairs; cobwebby.

Arboreous. Trees with well-developed trunk.

Arcuate. An uncommon pattern in which the major veins curve gently upward.

Aristate. An abrupt hard bristle-like point.

Astringent. A substance that checks the discharge of mucus, serum etc., by causing contraction of the tissue.

Athlete's Foot. A fungal infection of the foot, causing itching, blisters, and cracking of the skin.

Attenuate. The apex drawn out into a long gradual taper.

Auriculate. Has a pair of rounded lobes that somewhat resemble the human ear.

Axils. The cavity or angle formed by the junction of the upper side of a leaf stalk or branch with a stem or branch.

Bactericide. Anything that destroys bacteria.

Barbellate. Hairs with barbs down the sides.

Berry. Entire soft pericarp, as in the tomato or grape.

Biliousness. Popular term used to describe conditions marked by general malaise, giddiness, vomiting, headache, indigestion, constipation, and so forth.

Blade. Lamina, the flattened expanded portion; a few leaves are bladeless.

Bract. A leaf much reduced in size, particularly if it is associated with a flower or inflorescence.

Bronchiectasias. A chronic inflammation or degenerative condition of one or more bronchioles.

Bronchitis. An inflammation of the tubes in the lungs.

Bulb. An upright series of overlapping leaf bases attached to a small basal stem, as in the onion.

Caespitose. Growing in tufts, mats, or clumps.

Calceolate. Slipper-shaped.

Calculus. Stone concretion in some part of the body

Calyx. The outermost series of leaf-like parts of a flower, individually called sepals.

Canescent. With a dense mat of gray-white hairs.

Carbuncle. An extensive dangerous form of boil having a flat surface that discharges pus from multiple points and occupies several inches of skin surface.

Carcinogen. A substance which causes cancer.

Cardiac. Products that have an effect upon the heart.

Carminative. A substance that prevents formation of or promotes expulsion of gas from the alimentary tract; relieves flatulence.

Catarrh. Excessive secretion from an inflamed mucous membrane, especially of the air passages of the throat and head.

Cathartic. Producing evacuation of the bowels.

Caudate. The apex tail-like.

Caulescent. Aerial stem or stems evident.

Cercaricidal. Affected by a larval parasitic trematode worm.

Cholalogue. A drug that stimulates the flow of bile by the liver.

Chronic. Diseases that are of long duration, either mild or acute.

Ciliate. Hairs along the margins only.

Ciliate. With fine hairs on the margin.

Clambering. Spreads over undergrowth or objects, usually without the aid of twinning stems or tendrils.

Clasping. The bases partly to completely surrounding the stem.

Claw. A long narrow stalk-like base of a petal or sepal.

Cleft. Indented about halfway to the midrib or base of the blade.

Climbing. Ascends upon other plants or objects by means of special structures.

Colic. Pain resulting from excessive or sudden abdominal spasmodic contractions of muscles in the intestine walls, bile ducts, ureter, or any obstruction, twisting, or distention of any of the hollow organs or tubes following the stretching of the walls by gas or solid substances.

Coma. Stupor; abnormally deep sleep.

Comose. With a tuft of hairs at the apex of a seed or at the base of a floret in a grass spikelet.

Complete. A flower that has all four series.

Conjunctivitis. Inflammation of the mucous membrane lining of the eyelids and covering of the anterior part of the eyeball.

Constipation. A morbid inactivity of the bowels.

Consumption. A general term used to describe the wasting of tissues, including but not limited to, tuberculosis.

Contact dermatitis. Local allergic reaction provoked by skin contact with chemical substances that act as antigens or haptens.

Contraceptive. Prevents conception by chemical or physical means.

Cordate. Of the shape of the stylized heart with the petiole attached between the basal lobes.

Corm. An upright, hard, or fleshy stem surrounded by dry scaly leaves, as in the gladiolus bulb.

Corniculate. Bears a small horn-like protuberance, as in the milkweed flower.

Corona. Any outgrowth situated between the corolla and the androecium, as in milkweeds.

Crenate. Scalloped, with blunt teeth.

Cruciform. Cross-shaped, as in the sepals and petals of the mustard family.

Cuneate. Wedge-shaped.

Cupule. A series of fused bracts that form a cup beneath the true fruit, as in the acorn.

Cuspidate. A sharp-pointed tip formed by abruptly and sharply concave sides.

Cyanogenic. Capable of producing hydrocyanic acid (HCN).

Cystitis. Inflammation of the urinary bladder.

Decoction. A liquid preparation obtained by boiling medicinal plant substances in water and extracting drugs by straining the preparation.

Decumbent. Stems lying upon the ground with their ends turned up.

Decussate. Opposite leaves that alternate at right angles to one another at successive nodes, thereby forming four rows of leaves.

Dehiscent. A fruit that opens by sutures, pores, or caps.

Deltoid. Of the shape of an equilateral triangle.

Demulcent. Substances used for their soothing and protective action; allays irritation of surfaces, especially mucous membranes.

Dengue. Infective eruptive fever causing acute pains in joints.

Dentate. Has coarse angular teeth directed outward at right angles to the margin.

Denticulate. Finely dentate.

Depilatory. Removes hair.

Diabetes. Metabolic disorder affecting insulin production and resulting in faulty carbohydrate metabolism.

Diaphoretic. Drugs that promote perspiration as a result of stimulation of the sweat glands.

Diarrhea. Abnormal frequency and fluidity of stool discharges.

Dicotyledon. An angiosperm having two cotyledons (seed leaves); usually the leaves are net-veined, and floral parts are in fours or fives.

Didymous. A strongly lobed fruit, thus appearing as a pair.

Dioecious. A species in which any particular plant bears either staminate or pistillate flowers, but not both; the species is composed of separate staminate and pistillate plants.

Diuretic. Agent that increases urine flow by acting on the kidneys.

Divaricate. Extremely divergent, more or less at a right angle.

Divergent. Broadly spreading.

Divided. Indented to the midrib or base of the blade.

Doubly serrate. The serrations themselves serrate.

Dropsy. A leakage of the watery part of the blood into any of the tissues or cavities of the body.

Drupe. Exocarp and mesocarp fleshy, endocarp bony; the seed and endocarp constitute a **pyrene**; mango.

Dull. Not shining; lacking luster.

Dysentery. Inflammation of the bowel with evacuation of mucous and blood in the stool.

Dysmenorrhea. Abnormal pains during the menstruation period. The pain may be either spasmodic or continuous.

Dyspepsia. Difficult or painful digestion, generally chronic.

Dysuria. Difficult, painful, or incomplete urination.

Ecbolic. Causing contraction of the uterus and thus inducing abortion or promoting parturition.

Echinate. With straight, often comparatively large, prickle-like hairs.

Eczema. Noncontagious itching; inflammatory skin eruption characterized by papules, vesicles, and pustules that may also be associated with edema, scaling, or exudation.

Elephantiasis. A chronic enlargement of the cutaneous and subcutaneous tissues. It is most common in the tropics and results from obstruction of the lymphatics.

Elliptic. Oval, the ends rounded and is widest at the middle.

Emarginate. With a shallow notch at the apex.

Emetic. A drug or an agent having the power to empty the stomach by vomiting.

Emmenagogue. Applied to drugs which have the power of stimulating the menstrual discharge.

Emollient. A substance applied externally to soften the skin, or internally, to soothe an irritated or inflamed surface.

Empacho. An infant disease resulting in diarrhea, pale stools, and sour vomit, attributed to diet of mother during pregnancy.

Emphysema. Enlargement of air vesicles in the lungs; swelling of connective tissues of the body caused by to the presence of air.

Endocarp. The innermost layer of the fruit wall; it may be soft, papery, or bony.

Endosperm. The albumin of a seed.

Enema. A liquid preparation injected into the rectum, resulting in complete emptying of the large bowel in minutes.

Enteritis. Acute or chronic intestinal inflammation.

Entire. Not in any way indented, the margin featureless.

Epidermis. True skin of a plant below the cuticle.

Epilepsy. A chronic nervous affliction characterized by loss of consciousness and/or muscular convulsions, sometimes accompanied by paroxysmic seizures.

Epiphyte. A plant growing nonparasitically upon another.

Erose. Gnawed, as if chewed upon.

Erysipelas. An acute inflammation disease of the skin caused by infection by various strains of *Streptococcus* and accompanied by fever.

Erythrasma. A chronic contagious dermatitis caused by an actinomycete and affecting warm moist areas.

Erythrocytes. Red blood cells formed in red bone marrow.

Essential. Applied to volatile oils of plants, marked by characteristic odor; also applied to fatty acids believed by nutritionists to be necessary for health.

Estrogenic effect. The effect of female steroidal hormones in promoting ovulation and secondary sexual characteristics.

Evacuant. A medicine or purgative that empties an organ, especially the bowel.

Exanthema. A disease accompanied by eruptions of the skin, such as measles or scarlet fever.

Exocarp. The outermost layer of the fruit wall; it may be the "skin" of the fruit, a leathery or hard rind.

Expectorant. A medicine promoting secretion of bronchial mucus and facilitating the ejection of phlegm from the lungs by coughing.

Extract. A pharmaceutical preparation obtained by dissolving the active constituents of a drug with a suitable solvent, evaporating the solvent, and adjusting to proscribe standards.

Falcate. Sickle-shaped.

Fascicled. Clustered.

Febrifuge. A drug tending to reduce fever.

Fibrosis. Morbid increase of fibrous tissue in the body; fibroid degeneration of blood capillaries.

Fibrositis. Inflammation of fibrous tissue.

Filariasis. A disease caused by parasitic worms.

Filiform. Thread-like.

Fimbriate. As in ciliate, but coarser and longer.

Fimbriate. Fringed, the hairs coarser than in ciliate.

Flatulence. The presence of an excessive amount of gas in stomach and intestine.

Flavonoid. A group of organic compounds responsible for a great number of colors in fruits and flowers. In the past, they were often used in conjunction with mordants for the dyeing of fabrics.

Floccose. With tufts of soft hairs that rub off easily.

Fruticose. Shrubby, with more than one major stem.

Fumigate. Applying smoke or vapor to affected part.

Funiculus. The seed stalk.

Galactogogue. An agent that induces or increases the secretion of milk.

Gastritis. Inflammation of the stomach.

Gastrointestinal. Pertaining to the stomach and intestines.

Genito-urinary. Relating to the genital and the urinary organs or functions.

Germicidal. A substance that kills germs and microorganisms in general.

Gingivitis. Inflammation of the gums.

Glabrate. Hairy at first, but then glabrous.

Glabrous. Without hairs.

Glandular. Hairs with swollen tips; gland-bearing.

Glaucoma. Group of diseases characterized by increasing intraocular pressures causing defects in vision.

Glaucous. Covered with a whitish waxy bloom.

Glochidiate. Hairs barbed at the tip only, as in the hairs of certain cacti.

Glossitis. Inflammation of the tongue.

Glycoside. Naturally occurring substance consisting of sugars combined with nonsugars such as a flavonoid, coumarine, steroid, terpene, and so forth (aglycones).

Gonorrhea. A venereal disease that causes inflammation of the mucous membranes of the urethra and adjacent cavities.

Gout. A condition or uric acid metabolism. It occurs in paroxysms and is characterized by painful inflammation of parts of the joints and an excessive amount of uric acid in the blood.

Hastate. More or less arrowhead-shaped, but with the basal lobes divergent.

Haustoria. Roots or suckers found in parasitic plants.

Head. Capitulum, a dense spherical or rounded inflorescence of sessile flowers, as in the Compositae family.

Helicoid cyme. A one-sided coiled inflorescence resembling a fiddlehead, as in most members of the *Boraginaceae* family.

Hemolytic. An agent capable of destroying blood cells.

Hemorrhoids. An enlarged and often dilated blood vessel or vein of the anal canal or the lower portion of the alimentary tract.

Hemostatic. An agent that arrests hemorrhage.

Hepatitis. Inflammation of the liver.

Hernia. Protrusion of an organ through its containing wall. It may occur in any part of the body, but is especially associated with the abdominal cavity.

Herpes. Skin disease with patches of distinct vesicles.

Hesperidium. Ovary superior; septations conspicuous, these lined with fleshy hairs, restricted to the citrus fruits.

Hip. A vase-like leathery hypanthium containing several achenes; restricted to the rose.

Hirsute. With rough or coarse, more or less erect hairs.

Hirtellous. Minutely hirsute.

Hispid. With long rigid bristly hairs.

Hives. Any of various skin diseases, especially urticaria.

Hydrocele. An accumulation of fluid in bag-like cavities in the body.

Hydrolysis. The addition of water of a molecule of water to a chemical compound accompanied by a splitting of that compound into usually two fragments; hydrolysis is normally facilitated by the presence of small amounts of acids; for example, the degradation of starch into simple sugars achieved by prolonged heating of an acidified starch slurry in water.

Hypertension. Abnormally high constrictive tension in blood vessels, usually revealed as high blood pressure.

Hypoglycemia. Deficiency of normal glucose levels in the body; low blood sugar.

Imbricate. Overlapping.

Incised. Deeply and sharply cut.

Inflorescence. Axes along which all the buds are flower buds.

Infusion. The extract obtained from steeping of plant material in water, for example, tea.

Integument (Bot.) The skin of a seed.

Involucre. A set of separate or fused bracts associated with a fruit, as in the walnut.

Jaundice. Yellowness of the skin, mucus membranes and secretions, as a result of bile pigments in the blood.

Keel. A structure resembling the bottom of a boat, as in the two fused lower petals of many legume flowers.

Laciniate. Slashed into narrow pointed segments.

Lacrimation. The excessive secretion of tears.

Lactagogue. An agent that induces the secretion and flow of milk.

Lactation. The formation and secretion of milk.

Lanate. Woolly or cottony.

Lanceolate. Lance-shaped, several times longer than wide; the sides curved, with the blade broadest below the middle.

Laryngitis. Inflammation of the larynx.

Laxative. A gentle bowel stimulant.

Lectin. Protein that effects agglutination, precipitation, or other phenomena resembling the action of a specific antibody.

Leprosy. A chronic disease of the skin and nerves characterized by whitish pigmentation.

Leukopenia. An abnormally low number of leukocytes (white blood cells) in the blood.

Leukorrhea. A white or yellowish mucopurulent vaginal discharge.

Liana. A twining or climbing plant with rope-like woody stems.

Lianas. Woody plants with elongate flexible, nonsupporting stems.

Linear. Several times longer than wide, the sides more or less parallel.

Liniment. An agent or substance applied to the skin by gentle friction or by brisk rubbing, meant to relieve superficial pain.

Lobed. Indented about one-fourth to almost half way to the midrib or base of the blade.

Loch. A syrupy medication having a local action in the mucus membrane of the throat.

Lodicule. The highly reduced perianth of the grasses.

Lumbago. Muscular rheumatism; a general term for backache in the lumbar region.

Lustrous. Shining.

Lyrate. With a series of pinnate lobes and a larger terminal lobe.

Malaria. An acute, usually chronic, disease caused by protozoa belonging to the genus *Plasmodium* and transmitted by *Anopheles* mosquito. It is characterized by intermittent fever, anemia, and debility, and in its acute form, by chills, high fever, and profuse sweating at regular intervals.

Mange. A contagious skin disease characterized by itching and hair loss, caused by parasitic mites.

Marasmus. A wasting away of the body, associated with inadequate food.

Masticatory. A substance chewed to increase salivation.

Mealy. Swollen hairs which collectively form a covering resembling cooking meal.

Meningitis. A disease of the membranes enveloping the brain and spinal cord.

Menorrhagia. Excessive menstrual flow.

Mesocarp. The middle layer of the fruit wall, often the fleshy edible portion.

Metrorrhagia. Bleeding between periods.

Migraine. A recurring and intensely painful headache, often accompanied by vomiting, giddiness, and disturbance of the vision.

Molluscicidal. An agent that destroys a variety of skin diseases.

Monocotyledon. Angiosperms having one cotyledon (seed leaf); the leaves are usually parallel-veined, and floral parts are in threes.

Monoecious. A species in which any plant bears both ataminate and pistillate flowers.

Mucronate. Possessing a hard short abrupt point.

Multiple. Fruit derived from the fusion of an entire inflorescence, as in the pineapple.

Net. A complex venation pattern of major and minor veins that form a network or reticulum.

Neuralgia. An acute paroxysmal pain along the course of and over the local distribution of a nerve.

Obcordate. As in the cordate leaf, but the petiole attached at the point of the heart.

Oblanceolate. As in the lanceolate leaf, but the petiole attached at the narrow end.

Oblique. Asymmetrical; unequal-sided.

Oblong. About two or three times longer than broad; rectangular with rounded corners.

Obovate. As in ovate, but the petiole attached at the narrow end.

Obtuse. Apex formed by two lines that meet at more than a right angle.

Oliguria. A deficiency in the excretion of urine.

Ophthalmia. Inflammation of the eyeball or the conjunctiva of the eye.

Opposite. Two leaves at a node.

Orbicular. Circular or nearly so.

Oval. Broadly elliptic, the length less than twice the width.

Ovate. The shape of the longitudinal section through a chicken's egg, with the petiole attached at the broad end.

Oxytocic. Stimulating movements of the uterus.

Palmate. The major veins radiating from a common point at the base of the blade, as in the maples.

Palpitation. A rapid pulsation or throbbing of the heart.

Panicle. A loose compound flower cluster produced by irregular branching.

Papillate. Pimple-like hairs or pimple-like protuberance.

Parallel. Several to many veins of about the same size (the midrib sometimes more conspicuous) and parallel to one another, as in many monocots.

Parasiticide. Any agent that destroys parasites.

Parted. Indented nearly all the way to the midrib or the base of the blade.

Parturient. Applied to substances used during childbirth.

Parturition. The act of childbirth

Pediculicide. An agent for treatment of the feet.

Pediculosis. The condition of being infected with lice.

Peduncle. The stalk supporting a single flower in an inflorescence.

Pepo. A berry with a leathery rind, derived from an inferior ovary; use is often restricted to the squash family.

Perfect. A flower with both stamens and carpels, without regard to the state of the perianth.

Perfoliate. The condition of a sessile leaf when the base completely encircles the stem.

Pericarp. The fruit wall, made up of the endocarp, mesocarp, and exocarp; the wall of the ripened ovary of a flower.

Peristalsis. Wavelike muscular contractions of the intestines.

Petioles. The stalk that supports the lamina; if missing, the leaf is sessile.

Phagocytosis. The destruction and absorption of bacteria or microorganisms by phagocytes.

Pharynx. The throat; the joint opening of the gullet and windpipe.

Phthisis. A wasting disease of the lungs; difficulty in breathing.

Phyllode. A leaflike petiole of a bladeless leaf, as in some *Acacia*.

Phyllode. A petiole that develops into a flattened expansion taking the place of a leaf.

Phytoalexin. An antimicrobial compound produced in a plant in response to fungal infection.

Piles. A synonym for hemorrhoids.

Pilose. With sparse slender soft hairs.

Pinnae. A single leaflet of a pinnate leaf.

Pinnate. Having the shape or arrangement of a feather. Prominent midvein with a series of major veins arising at about 30–45 degrees angles along its length.

Pistillate. A unisexual (female) flower in which only carpels are present, the stamens being rudimentary or suppressed.

Pitted. Covered with small cavities.

Pityriasis. A skin disease in which the epidermis sheds thin scales as dandruff.

Pleurisy. Inflammation of the pleura membrane enveloping the lung.

Pneumonia. Refers to a large number conditions that include the inflammation or passive congestion of the lungs, resulting in portions of the lung becoming solid.

Pome. Ovary inferior, surrounded by fleshy tissue, usually interpreted as a hypanthium, as in the apple or pear.

Postpartum. After childbirth.

Poultice. A mass of material applied to sore or inflamed part of the body for the purpose of supplying heat and moisture or acting as a local stimulant.

Prickly Heat. Heat rash; irritation of the skin caused by heat.

Prolapse. The descent of an organ or viscus of the body from its natural position.

Prophylactic. Operating to ward off or protect against a disease.

Prostrate. Lying flat upon the ground; typically without adventitious roots.

Proteolytic. Cause splitting of proteins into smaller products during digestion.

Prothallus. The first or false thallus formed in the germination of the sexually produced spores in ferns; a delicate cellular structure bearing the sexual organs.

Pruritus. Localized or generalized itching due to the irritation of sensory nerve endings.

Psoriasis. A noncontagious inflammatory skin disease characterized by reddish patches and white scales.

Pterygium. A triangular fleshy mass of thickened conjunctiva occurring at the inner side of the eyeball causing a disturbance to vision.

Puberulent. Minutely canescent.

Pubescent. Downy; the hairs short soft and erect.

Pulmonary. Pertaining to or affecting the lungs.

Punctate. Dotted with pinpoint impressions or translucent dots.

Purgative. Drugs which evacuate the bowels; more drastic than a laxative.

Pyorrhea. A purulent discharge that contains or consists of pus.

Quinones. Organic compounds based on benzene where two hydrogen atoms have been replaced in the same ring by two oxygen atoms. Quinones are usually highly colored and are often responsible for the yellow and red colors of some seeds, bark and woods etc.

Rank. A vertical row of leaves.

Reniform. Kidney-shaped or bean-shaped.

Repent. Trailing, stems prostrate, creeping or sprawling, and often rooting at the node.

Resolvent. Medicine that reduces swelling or inflammation.

Restorative. A remedy that is efficient in restoring health and strength.

Resupinate. Inverted because of a 180 degrees twist in a petiole or pedicel.

Reticulate. Netted with regular slightly elevated lines.

Revolute. The margin rolled toward the lower side of the blade.

Rheumatism. A general term for painful inflammation of muscle, tendon, joint, bone, or nerve, resulting in discomfort.

Rhizome. Horizontal underground stem distinguished from a root by scale-like leaves and axillary buds. Horizontal stem with reduced scaly leaves, as in many grasses.

Ringworm. A common contagious disease produced by fungi that affects the skin, hair, or nails.

Rosette. A radiating leaf cluster at or near the base of the plant.

Rostulate. In rosettes.

Rounded. The apex gently curved.

Rubefacient. Applied to counter irritants to the skin; substances that produce blisters or inflammation.

Rugose. Wrinkled.

Runcinate. Coarsely-toothed, the teeth pointing toward the base of the leaf, as in the dandelion.

Sagittate. Arrowhead-shaped.

Saponin. A substance characterized by the ability to form emulsions and soapy lathers.

Scabies. A contagious skin disease caused by a mite that burrows in the horny layer of the skin.

Scabrous. Rough to the touch because of coarse stiff ascending hairs.

Scapose. Bearing a flower or inflorescence on a leafless flowering stem.

Scrofula. A tuberculous condition of the lymphatic glands characterized by enlarged suppurating abscess and cheese-like degeneration.

Scurfy. Covered with minute scales.

Scurvy. A nutritional disorder caused by deficiency of vitamin C; characterized by extreme weakness, spongy gums, and a tendency to develop hemorrhages under the skin, from the mucus membranes, and under the periosteum.

Sedative. An agent that quiets nervous excitement.

Septum. An internal partition within the fruit.

Sericeous. Silky; the hairs long, fine, and appressed.

Serrate. With coarse saw-like teeth that point forward.

Serrulate. Finely serrate.

Setaceous. Bristly.

Sheath. The basal portion of a leaf that surrounds the stem.

Shingles. A virus that lives in the nerves and affects one specific part of the body.

Shrubs. Woody perennials with more than one principal stem arising from the ground.

Sinate. Wavy in and out, in the plane of the blade.

Soporific. Inducing sleep.

Sori. Clusters of spore cases in ferns.

Spadix. A spike or head of flowers with a fleshy axis, usually enclosed within a bract.

Spasmodic. Periodic sharp attacks marked by spasms.

Spatulate. Spoon-shaped.

Spine. A leaf or portion of a leaf that is sharp-pointed, the most common examples being paired stipular spines; not to be confused with **thorns**, which are modified stems or **prickles**, which are mere outgrowths of the epidermis, as in the cultivated rose.

Spinose. With a spine at the tip.

Sporangium. A spore case in which asexual spores are produced.

Spreading. Oriented outward and more or less diverging from the point of origin.

Staminate. A unisexual (male) flower in which stamens are present, the carpels being rudimentary or suppressed.

Steam-distillation. The process of isolating the volatile principles from a material by passing steam through it (or boiling it with water) and condensing the steam to recover the usually insoluble volatile substance.

Stimulant. Anything that quickens or promotes the activity of some physiological process.

Stipe. A stalk or support.

Stipules. A pair of appendages located at the base of the petiole where it joins the stem; often short-lived and seen only as stipule scars; if not formed, the leaf is exstipulate.

Stolon. A trailing runner or rootstock by which grasses may propagate.

Stomachic. Applied to drugs given for disorders of the stomach.

Striated. Marked with longitudinal lines.

Stricture. Abnormal narrowing of a tubular organ; sometimes a result of inflammation.

Strigose. Hairs sharp, appressed, rigid, and often swollen at the base.

Style. The stalk between the ovary and the stigma.

Styptic. Substances that clot the blood and thus stop bleeding.

Subulate. Slender and tapering to a point, as in the awl, a tool used to make holes in leather.

Sudorific. Producing copious perspiration.

Suffruticose. Plants woody at the base but herbaceous above.

Sulcate. Furrowed with longitudinal lines.

Suppository. A small solid medication that is inserted into a bodily orifice other than the mouth.

Syconium. A hollow vase-like inflorescence with the flowers lining the inside; restricted to the fig.

Syphilis. A venereal disease, characterized by a variety of lesions, caused by *Treponema pallidum*.

Tachycardia. Abnormally rapid heart action as a disease.

Tannin. Astringent principle of many plants.

Tapeworm. A parasitic worm of the class Cestoidea; a segmented an ribbon-like flatworm. It develops in the alimentary canals or vertebrates.

Tendril. A twining leaf or portion of a leaf, as in the leaflets of the sweet pea; tendrils may also be of stem origin.

Tetanus. An acute infectious disease caused by a bacillus and characterized by rigid spasmodic contractions of various voluntary muscles especially of the jaw.

Thrush. A mycotic disease of the upper digestive tract (mouth, lips, and throat) resulting from infection by the fungus *Candida albicans*. It occurs especially in children and is characterized by small whitish spots on the tip and sides of the tongue.

Tisane. A medical decoction or tea of herbs drunk as a beverage or for its mildly medicinal effect.

Tomentose. Densely and softly matted.

Tonic. A drug or an agent given to improve the normal tone of an organ or of the patient generally.

Trachoma. A contagious virus disease of the eye characterized by granular conjunctivitis.

Trees. Woody perennials with a single main stem or trunk.

Truncate. The apex appearing chopped off.

Tuber. An enlarged fleshy tip of an underground stem, as in the Irish potato.

Tuberculate. Warty.

Tuberculosis. An infectious disease caused by the tubercle bacillus. It may affect any tissue of the body, but especially occurs in the lungs.

Tumor. Generally any abnormal swelling of the body other than those caused by direct injury is considered a tumor.

Turion. A swollen scaly offshoot of a rhizome.

Twining. Coiling around plants or objects as a means of support.

Typhus. An infectious disease caused by the *Rickettsia* microorganism, characterized by high fever and delirium.

Ulcer. An interruption of continuity of a surface with an inflamed base. Any open sore other than a wound.

Umbel. An indeterminate inflorescence in which a number of nearly equal peduncles radiate from a small area at the top of a very short axis, giving an umbrella-like appearance.

Uncinate. Hooked hairs.

Undulate. Wavy perpendicular to the plane of the blade.

Uremia. Condition of the blood caused by retention of urinary matter normally eliminated by the kidneys.

Varicose. Abnormally dilated or knotted blood vessels.

Velutinous. Velvety; the hairs dense, firm, and straight.

Venereal. Pertaining to, or produced by, sexual intercourse.

Vermicide. Substance that kills worms.

Vermifuge. Substance that kills or expels intestinal worms.

Verticel. An axillary whorl of flowers radiating in many directions, as in several members of the mint family (*Labiatae*).

Vertigo. Any of a group of disorders in which dizziness is experienced.

Vesicant. A blistering agent; any agent or drug that produces blisters on the skin.

Vesicatory. Any substance capable of causing blisters.

Villous. Shaggy; the hairs long, slender, soft, but not matted.

Vine. Herbaceous plants with elongate, flexible, nonself-supporting stems.

Viscera. Internal organs of the body, especially in the abdomen and thorax.

Viscid. Sticky.

Vitiligo. A skin disease characterized by whitish nonpigmented areas surrounded by hyperpigmented borders.

Vulnerary. A remedy used for treating wounds.

Wart. A common skin tumor caused by a virus infection. It is contagious from case to case or from skin area to skin area in the same individual.

Whitlow. An old general term for any suppurative inflammation on a finger or toe.

Whorled. Three or more leaves at a node.

Yaws. An infectious, nonvenereal tropical disease caused by *Treponema pertenus*. It is characterized by an initial lesion (the mother-yaw), followed by further multiple lesions of the skin. It is also known as *Framboesia*.

Yellow Fever. A tropical epidemic disease caused by mosquito-borne viral infection.

Index

A

Abrus precatorius, 15–25
  botanical description, 16
  chemical constituents, 17–19
  common names, 15
  origin and distribution, 16
  pharmacological activities and clinical
    trials, 19–25
  traditional medicinal uses, 16–17
African cucumber, 337–354
Aging
  Allium sativum, 39
AIDS therapeutic effect
  Allium sativum, 38
Allergenic activity
  Allium sativum, 39
  Carica papaya, 151
  Curcuma longa, 231
  Mangifera indica, 319
  Persea americana, 386
  Punica granatum, 434
  Tamarindus indica, 458
Allium sativum, 33–77
  botanical description, 34
  chemical constituents, 36–38
  common names, 33
  origin and distribution, 34
  pharmacological activities and clinical
    trials, 38–77
  traditional medicinal uses, 34–36
Aloe vera, 103–122
  botanical description, 104
  chemical constituents, 106–108
  common names, 103
  origin and distribution, 104
  pharmacological activities and clinical
    trials, 108–122
  traditional medicinal uses, 104–106
Alternate
  defined, 2
Ampalaya, 337–354

Analgesic activity
  Abrus precatorius, 19
  Allium sativum, 39
  Aloe vera, 108
  Annona muricata, 136
  Carica papaya, 151
  Cassia alata, 168
  Cymbopogon citratus, 199
  Cyperus rotundus, 213
  Hibiscus rosa-sinensis, 258
  Jatropha curcas, 280
  Lantana camara, 292
  Momordica charantia, 343
  Moringa pterygosperma, 371
  Mucuna pruriens, 308
  Persea americana, 386
  Phyllanthus niruri, 396
  Portulaca oleracea, 407
  Psidium guajava, 419
  Punica granatum, 434
  Syzygium cumini, 447
Androgenic effect
  Carica papaya, 151
  Hibiscus rosa-sinensis, 258
Anesthetic activity
  Aloe vera, 108–109
Annona muricata, 133–138
  botanical description, 133
  chemical constituents, 134–136
  common names, 133
  origin and distribution, 133
  pharmacological activities and clinical
    trials, 136–138
  traditional medicinal uses, 134
Antiaging activity
  Allium sativum, 39
Antiallergenic activity
  Allium sativum, 39
Antiasthmatic activity
  Aloe vera, 109
  Curcuma longa, 231–232

Antiatherosclerotic activity
  Allium sativum, 40
Antibacterial activity
  Abrus precatorius, 19
  Allium sativum, 40–41
  Aloe vera, 109
  Annona muricata, 136
  Carica papaya, 151–152
  Cassia alata, 168–169
  Catharanthus roseus, 180
  Curcuma longa, 232
  Cymbopogon citratus, 199–200
  Cyperus rotundus, 214
  Hibiscus sabdariffa, 269
  Jatropha curcas, 280–281
  Lantana camara, 292–293
  Mangifera indica, 319–320
  Manihot esculenta, 330
  Momordica charantia, 343–344
  Moringa pterygosperma, 371–372
  Persea americana, 386
  Phyllanthus niruri, 396
  Portulaca oleracea, 407–408
  Psidium guajava, 419–420
  Punica granatum, 434–436
  Syzygium cumini, 448
  Tamarindus indica, 458
Anticancer activity
  Aloe vera, 109
Anticarcinogenic effect
  Allium sativum, 41–42
  Momordica charantia, 344
Anticonvulsant activity
  Abrus precatorius, 19
  Allium sativum, 42
  Annona muricata, 136–137
  Carica papaya, 152
  Cassia alata, 169
  Curcuma longa, 232
  Cymbopogon citratus, 200
  Cyperus rotundus, 214
  Hibiscus rosa-sinensis, 258
  Jatropha curcas, 281
  Lantana camara, 293
  Momordica charantia, 344
  Moringa pterygosperma, 372
  Portulaca oleracea, 408

Psidium guajava, 420
Punica granatum, 436
Syzygium cumini, 448
Antidepressant activity
  Annona muricata, 137
Antidiabetic effect
  Aloe vera, 110
  Mangifera indica, 320
  Mucuna pruriens, 308
  Punica granatum, 436
Antidiarrheal activity
  Abrus precatorius, 19
  Allium sativum, 42
  Cyperus rotundus, 214
  Jatropha curcas, 281
  Phyllanthus niruri, 396
  Psidium guajava, 420–421
  Punica granatum, 436
Antidiuretic activity
  Catharanthus roseus, 180–181
Antiedema activity
  Allium sativum, 42
  Carica papaya, 152
  Curcuma longa, 232
  Hibiscus sabdariffa, 269
  Persea americana, 386
  Psidium guajava, 421
Antiestrogenic effect
  Allium sativum, 42
  Carica papaya, 152
  Hibiscus rosa-sinensis, 258–259
Antifertility effect
  Abrus precatorius, 19–20
  Aloe vera, 110
  Carica papaya, 152–153
  Catharanthus roseus, 181
  Hibiscus rosa-sinensis, 259
  Jatropha curcas, 281
  Manihot esculenta, 330
  Momordica charantia, 344
  Moringa pterygosperma, 372
  Portulaca oleracea, 408
  Punica granatum, 436
Antifungal activity
  Abrus precatorius, 20
  Allium sativum, 42–44
  Aloe vera, 110

Annona muricata, 137
Cassia alata, 169–170
Catharanthus roseus, 181
Curcuma longa, 232–233
Cymbopogon citratus, 200
Cyperus rotundus, 215
Hibiscus rosa-sinensis, 259
Hibiscus sabdariffa, 269–270
Jatropha curcas, 281
Lantana camara, 293
Mangifera indica, 320
Manihot esculenta, 330–331
Momordica charantia, 344–345
Moringa pterygosperma, 372
Persea americana, 386
Phyllanthus niruri, 396
Portulaca oleracea, 408
Psidium guajava, 421
Punica granatum, 436
Syzygium cumini, 448
Tamarindus indica, 458–459
Antihemorrhagic activity
Lantana camara, 293
Antihepatotoxic activity
Annona muricata, 137
Carica papaya, 153
Curcuma longa, 233
Cyperus rotundus, 215
Antihistamine activity
Cassia alata, 170
Cyperus rotundus, 215
Momordica charantia, 345
Moringa pterygosperma, 372
Syzygium cumini, 448
Antihypercholesterolemic activity
Allium sativum, 44–46
Aloe vera, 110
Catharanthus roseus, 181
Curcuma longa, 233
Momordica charantia, 345
Antihyperglycemic activity
Allium sativum, 44, 46
Aloe vera, 110
Cassia alata, 170
Catharanthus roseus, 181
Curcuma longa, 233
Mangifera indica, 320

Momordica charantia, 345–347
Phyllanthus niruri, 396
Psidium guajava, 421
Syzygium cumini, 448–449
Antihyperlipemic activity
Allium sativum, 46–47
Manihot esculenta, 331
Antihypertensive activity
Allium sativum, 47
Catharanthus roseus, 181
Cyperus rotundus, 215
Hibiscus sabdariffa, 270
Mucuna pruriens, 308
Persea americana, 387
Portulaca oleracea, 408
Antihypertriglyceridemic effect
Allium sativum, 47
Hibiscus sabdariffa, 270
Anti-inflammatory activity
Abrus precatorius, 20
Allium sativum, 48
Aloe vera, 111
Cassia alata, 170
Catharanthus roseus, 181
Curcuma longa, 233–234
Cymbopogon citratus, 200
Cyperus rotundus, 215
Hibiscus rosa-sinensis, 259
Hibiscus sabdariffa, 270
Jatropha curcas, 281
Mangifera indica, 320–321
Moringa pterygosperma, 372
Mucuna pruriens, 308
Portulaca oleracea, 408
Psidium guajava, 421
Punica granatum, 436
Syzygium cumini, 449
Tamarindus indica, 459
Anti-ischemic effect
Curcuma longa, 234
Antimalarial activity
Annona muricata, 137
Carica papaya, 153
Catharanthus roseus, 181
Cyperus rotundus, 215
Mangifera indica, 321
Momordica charantia, 348

Moringa pterygosperma, 372–373
Persea americana, 387
Phyllanthus niruri, 397
Psidium guajava, 421–422
Punica granatum, 436
Tamarindus indica, 459
Antimicrobial activity
    Allium sativum, 48
Antimycobacterial activity
    Allium sativum, 49
    Aloe vera, 112
    Carica papaya, 153
    Curcuma longa, 235
    Cymbopogon citratus, 201
    Mangifera indica, 321
    Momordica charantia, 348
    Moringa pterygosperma, 373
    Portulaca oleracea, 408
    Psidium guajava, 422
    Punica granatum, 436
Antineoplastic effect
    Allium sativum, 49
Antinephrotic activity
    Allium sativum, 49
Antiovulatory effect
    Hibiscus rosa-sinensis, 259
Antioxidant activity
    Allium sativum, 49–50
    Carica papaya, 153–154
    Cyperus rotundus, 215
    Tamarindus indica, 459
Antiparasitic activity
    Annona muricata, 137
    Jatropha curcas, 281–282
Antiparkinson activity
    Mucuna pruriens, 308–309
Anti-PMS activity
    Psidium guajava, 419
Antiprotozoan activity
    Allium sativum, 50–51
Antispasmodic activity
    Abrus precatorius, 20–21
    Carica papaya, 153
    Cassia alata, 170
    Catharanthus roseus, 182
    Curcuma longa, 235
    Cymbopogon citratus, 201

Cyperus rotundus, 216
Hibiscus rosa-sinensis, 260
Jatropha curcas, 282
Moringa pterygosperma, 373
Mucuna pruriens, 309
Phyllanthus niruri, 397
Psidium guajava, 422
Punica granatum, 437
Syzygium cumini, 449
Antispermatogenic effect
    Abrus precatorius, 21
    Allium sativum, 51
    Carica papaya, 153
    Catharanthus roseus, 182
    Curcuma longa, 235
    Cymbopogon citratus, 201
    Momordica charantia, 348–349
    Portulaca oleracea, 408
Antistress activity
    Cymbopogon citratus, 201
Antithrombotic effect
    Allium sativum, 51
Antitoxic activity
    Allium sativum, 51–52
Antitumor activity
    Abrus precatorius, 21
    Allium sativum, 52–53
    Aloe vera, 112
    Annona muricata, 137
    Carica papaya, 153
    Cassia alata, 170
    Catharanthus roseus, 182
    Curcuma longa, 235
    Cyperus rotundus, 216
    Jatropha curcas, 282
    Mangifera indica, 321
    Manihot esculenta, 331
    Momordica charantia, 349
    Moringa pterygosperma, 373
    Phyllanthus niruri, 397
    Portulaca oleracea, 408
Antiulcer activity
    Allium sativum, 53
    Aloe vera, 112
    Carica papaya, 153–154
    Curcuma longa, 235
    Momordica charantia, 349

Moringa pterygosperma, 373
Portulaca oleracea, 408
Antiviral activity
    Abrus precatorius, 21
    Allium sativum, 53
    Aloe vera, 113
    Annona muricata, 137
    Carica papaya, 154
    Catharanthus roseus, 182
    Curcuma longa, 235
    Cyperus rotundus, 216
    Hibiscus rosa-sinensis, 260
    Hibiscus sabdariffa, 270
    Jatropha curcas, 282
    Mangifera indica, 321
    Manihot esculenta, 331
    Momordica charantia, 349
    Moringa pterygosperma, 373
    Phyllanthus niruri, 397–398
    Portulaca oleracea, 408
    Psidium guajava, 422
    Punica granatum, 437
    Syzygium cumini, 449
    Tamarindus indica, 459
Antiyeast activity
    Allium sativum, 53–54
    Aloe vera, 113
    Carica papaya, 154
    Cassia alata, 170
    Curcuma longa, 235–236
    Cymbopogon citratus, 201
    Cyperus rotundus, 216
    Hibiscus sabdariffa, 270
    Jatropha curcas, 282
    Mangifera indica, 321
    Manihot esculenta, 331
    Momordica charantia, 349
    Moringa pterygosperma, 373
    Persea americana, 387
    Portulaca oleracea, 408
    Psidium guajava, 422
    Punica granatum, 437
    Syzygium cumini, 449
    Tamarindus indica, 459
Aphrodisiac activity
    Mucuna pruriens, 309
Aphthous stomatitis effect
    Aloe vera, 113–114

Asthmatic activity
    Aloe vera, 109
    Curcuma longa, 231–232
Atherosclerotic activity
    Allium sativum, 40, 54–55

B

Bacteria. *See* Antibacterial activity
Bacterial stimulant activity
    Allium sativum, 55
Balsam pear, 337–354
Barbados aloe, 103–122
Barbiturate potentiation
    Allium sativum, 55
    Cassia alata, 170
    Cymbopogon citratus, 202
    Cyperus rotundus, 216–217
    Hibiscus rosa-sinensis, 260
    Jatropha curcas, 282
    Persea americana, 387
    Punica granatum, 437
    Syzygium cumini, 449
Barbiturate sleeping time decrease
    Moringa pterygosperma, 374
Bitter gourd, 337–354
Bitter melon, 337–354
Black reed, 197–204
Blade
    defined, 2
Bowen mango, 315–324
Burn wound effect
    Aloe vera, 114

C

Cancer activity
    Aloe vera, 109
Carcinogenesis inhibition
    Allium sativum, 55–56
    Curcuma longa, 236
    Moringa pterygosperma, 374
Carcinogenic activity
    Allium sativum, 41–42
    Momordica charantia, 344
    Psidium guajava, 422
Cardiac depressant activity
    Aloe vera, 114
    Annona muricata, 137

Cardiac effect
  Jatropha curcas, 282
Cardiotonic activity
  Catharanthus roseus, 182
  Curcuma longa, 236
Cardiotoxic activity
  Allium sativum, 56
Cardiovascular effects
  Allium sativum, 56
Carica papaya, 143–156
  botanical description., 144–145
  chemical constituents, 148–150
  common names, 143
  origin and distribution, 145
  pharmacological activities and clinical
    trials, 150–156
  traditional medicinal use, 145–148
Carilla, 337–354
Cassia alata, 165–172
  botanical description, 165–166
  chemical constituents, 167
  common names, 165
  origin and distribution, 166
  pharmacological activities and clinical
    trials, 167–172
  traditional medicinal uses, 166–167
Catharanthus roseus, 175–185
  botanical description, 175
  chemical constituents, 177–179
  common names, 175
  origin and distribution, 176
  pharmacological activities and clinical
    trials, 179–185
  traditional medicinal uses, 176–177
Chemical constituents
  abbreviations, 14
Chemopreventive effect
  Allium sativum, 57
  Hibiscus sabdariffa, 270
Cholesterol inhibition
  Allium sativum, 57
Chronotropic effect
  Allium sativum, 58
Citronella, 197–204
Coagulant activity
  Allium sativum, 59
Common cold prevention
  Allium sativum, 59

Common purslane, 405–410
Compound leaves, 3
Convulsant activity. *See* Anticonvulsant
    activity
Crab's eye, 15–25
Cundeamor, 337–354
Curcuma longa, 227–242
  botanical description, 228
  chemical constituents, 230–231
  common names, 227
  origin and distribution, 228
  pharmacological activities and clinical
    trials, 231–242
  traditional medicinal uses, 228–230
Cymbopogon citratus, 197–204
  botanical description, 197
  chemical constituents, 198
  common names, 197
  origin and distribution, 198
  pharmacological activities and clinical
    trials, 199–204
Cyperus rotundus, 209–219
  botanical description, 210
  chemical constituents, 212–213
  common names, 209
  origin and distribution, 210
  pharmacological activities and clinical
    trials, 213–219
  traditional medicinal uses, 210–212
Cytotoxic activity
  Abrus precatorius, 21–22
  Allium sativum, 59–60
  Aloe vera, 115
  Annona muricata, 137–138
  Catharanthus roseus, 183
  Curcuma longa, 237
  Cyperus rotundus, 217
  Hibiscus sabdariffa, 271
  Jatropha curcas, 283
  Mangifera indica, 321–322
  Momordica charantia, 349–350
  Moringa pterygosperma, 374
  Mucuna pruriens, 309
  Phyllanthus niruri, 398
  Portulaca oleracea, 409
  Psidium guajava, 423
  Punica granatum, 437
  Tamarindus indica, 460

D

Depressant activity
  Annona muricata, 137
Dermatitis producing effect
  Allium sativum, 60
  Lantana camara, 294
  Mangifera indica, 322
Diabetic effect. *See* Antidiabetic effect
Diabetogenic activity
  Manihot esculenta, 331
Diarrhea. *See also* Antidiarrheal activity
  induction
    Aloe vera, 115
Diuretic activity
  Abrus precatorius, 22
  Allium sativum, 60
  Carica papaya, 154
  Cassia alata, 170
  Curcuma longa, 237
  Cymbopogon citratus, 202
  Cyperus rotundus, 217
  Hibiscus sabdariffa, 271
  Jatropha curcas, 283
  Momordica charantia, 350
  Moringa pterygosperma, 374
  Persea americana, 387
  Psidium guajava, 423
  Punica granatum, 437
  Syzygium cumini, 450
  Tamarindus indica, 460
Dry fruits, 12–13

E

Embryotoxic effect
  Allium sativum, 61
  Aloe vera, 116
  Cassia alata, 170
  Cymbopogon citratus, 202
  Hibiscus rosa-sinensis, 261
  Punica granatum, 438
Enzyme activity
  Lantana camara, 294–295
Estrogenic effect
  Allium sativum, 42
  Aloe vera, 116
  Carica papaya, 152
  Cyperus rotundus, 217

  Hibiscus rosa-sinensis, 258–259, 261
  Hibiscus sabdariffa, 271
  Mangifera indica, 322
  Momordica charantia, 350
  Punica granatum, 438
  Syzygium cumini, 450
Estrous cycle disruption effect
  Abrus precatorius, 22
  Cassia alata, 170
  Cymbopogon citratus, 202
  Hibiscus rosa-sinensis, 261
  Psidium guajava, 423

F

Fertility. *See also* Antifertility effect
  promotion effect
    Mucuna pruriens, 309–310
Fibrinolytic activity
  Allium sativum, 61–62
Fleshy fruits, 13–14
Food consumption reduction
  Allium sativum, 62
Fungal activity. *See* Antifungal activity

G

Garlic, 33–77
Gastric mucosal exfoliant activity
  Allium sativum, 62
Growth inhibitor activity
  Cyperus rotundus, 217
Guava, 415–424

H

Hair conditioner
  Aloe vera, 116
Hair inhibition
  Aloe vera, 116
  Lantana camara, 295
Hair stimulant
  Allium sativum, 63–64
  Cyperus rotundus, 217
Hemagglutinin activity
  Carica papaya, 154
Hematopoietic activity
  Cyperus rotundus, 217–218
Hemorrhagic activity
  Lantana camara, 293

Hepatotoxic activity
  Annona muricata, 137
  Carica papaya, 153
  Curcuma longa, 233
  Cyperus rotundus, 215
  Lantana camara, 295
Hibiscus rosa-sinensis, 253–262
  botanical description, 254
  chemical constituents, 256–257
  common names, 253
  origin and distribution, 254
  pharmacological activities and clinical
    trials, 257–262
  traditional medicinal uses, 254–256
Hibiscus sabdariffa, 267–272
  botanical description, 267–268
  chemical constituents, 268–269
  common names, 267
  origin and distribution, 268
  pharmacological activities and clinical
    trials, 269–272
  traditional medicinal uses, 268
Histamine activity. *See* Antihistamine
  activity
HIV-1 reverse transcriptase inhibition
  Momordica charantia, 351
Horseradish tree, 367–376
Hypercholesterolemic activity
  Allium sativum, 64
Hyperglycemic activity
  Catharanthus roseus, 183
  Cymbopogon citratus, 202
  Manihot esculenta, 332
  Momordica charantia, 351
  Moringa pterygosperma, 374
  Psidium guajava, 423
Hypertensive activity
  Allium sativum, 64
  Annona muricata, 138
  Cyperus rotundus, 218
  Lantana camara, 295
  Persea americana, 387
  Portulaca oleracea, 409
Hypertriglyceridemic activity
  Allium sativum, 64
Hypnotic effect

Cymbopogon citratus, 202
Hypocholesterolemic activity
  Allium sativum, 64–65
  Cymbopogon citratus, 202–203
  Moringa pterygosperma, 374–375
  Mucuna pruriens, 310
Hypoglycemic activity
  Abrus precatorius, 22
  Allium sativum, 65–66
  Aloe vera, 116–117
  Carica papaya, 154
  Cassia alata, 170–171
  Catharanthus roseus, 183
  Curcuma longa, 238
  Cyperus rotundus, 218
  Jatropha curcas, 283
  Mangifera indica, 322
  Momordica charantia, 351–352
  Moringa pterygosperma, 375
  Mucuna pruriens, 310
  Phyllanthus niruri, 398
  Portulaca oleracea, 409
  Psidium guajava, 423
  Punica granatum, 438
  Syzygium cumini, 450
Hypoglycemic effect
  Hibiscus rosa-sinensis, 261
Hypolipemic activity
  Allium sativum, 66
  Aloe vera, 117
Hypotensive activity
  Allium sativum, 66
  Aloe vera, 117
  Catharanthus roseus, 183
  Cymbopogon citratus, 203
  Momordica charantia, 352
  Syzygium cumini, 450
Hypothermic activity
  Curcuma longa, 238
  Cymbopogon citratus, 203
  Jatropha curcas, 283
  Momordica charantia, 352
  Punica granatum, 438
  Syzygium cumini, 450
Hypotriglyceridemic activity
  Allium sativum, 67

I

Immunomodulatory activity
Allium sativum, 67
Aloe vera, 117
Cymbopogon citratus, 203
Inflammation. See also Anti-inflammatory activity
induction
Carica papaya, 155
Inflorescence
types, 8–12
Insecticide activity
Abrus precatorius, 22
Allium sativum, 67
Annona muricata, 138
Carica papaya, 155
Catharanthus roseus, 184
Curcuma longa, 239
Cymbopogon citratus, 203
Lantana camara, 295–296
Mangifera indica, 322
Momordica charantia, 352–353
Insect repellent activity
Cyperus rotundus, 218
Insulin activity
Catharanthus roseus, 184
Insulin induction
Allium sativum, 67
Momordica charantia, 353
International Code of Botanical Nomenclature (ICBN), 1
Intestinal motility inhibition
Abrus precatorius, 22
Allium sativum, 68
Cymbopogon citratus, 203
Hibiscus sabdariffa, 271

J

Jambul, 445–451
Jatropha curcas, 277–284
botanical description, 278
chemical constituents, 280
common names, 277
origin and distribution, 278
pharmacological activities and clinical trials, 280–281
traditional medicinal uses, 278–280

Juvenile hormone activity
Cyperus rotundus, 218
Hibiscus rosa-sinensis, 261
Lantana camara, 296
Mangifera indica, 322
Manihot esculenta, 332
Tamarindus indica, 460

K–L

Karela, 337–354
Lantana camara, 289–298
botanical description, 290
chemical constituents, 291–292
common names, 289
origin and distribution, 290
pharmacological activities and clinical trials, 292–298
traditional medicinal uses, 290–291
Laxative effect
Cassia alata, 171
Leaf
attachment to stem, 7
bases, 7
defined, 2
margins, 4
shapes, 4
surfaces, 7–8
tips, 5–7
Lemon grass, 197–204
Leukopenic activity
Catharanthus roseus, 184
Curcuma longa, 239
Momordica charantia, 353
Lipid peroxidation effect
Allium sativum, 68–69
Lipoxygenase inhibition
Allium sativum, 69
Love bean, 15–25

M

Maiden apple, 337–354
Maiden's blush, 337–354
Malaria. See Antimalarial activity
Mangifera indica, 315–324
botanical description, 316
chemical constituents, 317–319
common names, 315

origin and distribution, 316
pharmacological activities and clinical trials, 319–324
traditional medicinal use, 316–317
Manihot esculenta, 329–334
  botanical description, 329
  chemical constituents, 330
  common names, 329
  origin and description, 329
  pharmacological activities and clinical trials, 330
  traditional medicinal uses, 329–330
Margin
  defined, 2
Mating inhibition
  Cymbopogon citratus, 203
Menstruation induction effect
  Hibiscus rosa-sinensis, 262
Metabolism
  Aloe vera, 117
Momordica charantia, 337–354
  botanical description, 338
  chemical constituents, 341–343
  common names, 337
  origin and distribution, 338
  pharmacological activities and clinical trials, 343–344
  traditional medicinal uses, 338–341
Moringa pterygosperma, 367–376
  botanical description, 368
  chemical constituents, 370–371
  common names, 367
  origin and distribution, 368
  pharmacological activities and clinical trials, 371–376
  traditional medicinal uses, 368–370
Mosquito repellent
  Cymbopogon citratus, 204
Mucuna pruriens, 305–311
  botanical description, 305
  chemical constituents, 307
  common names, 305
  origin and description, 306
  pharmacological activities and clinical trials, 307–311
  traditional medicinal uses, 306–307

Muscle activity
  Abrus precatorius, 23
  Allium sativum, 74
  Aloe vera, 119
  Annona muricata, 138
  Carica papaya, 155
  Catharanthus roseus, 184
  Cyperus rotundus, 219
  Hibiscus sabdariffa, 271
  Lantana camara, 297
  Moringa pterygosperma, 375
  Persea americana, 388
  Portulaca oleracea, 409–410
  Psidium guajava, 424
  Syzygium cumini, 451
Mutagenic activity
  Abrus precatorius, 23
  Allium sativum, 70
Mycobacterial activity. *See* Antimycobacterial activity

N–O

Neurotropic effect
  Allium sativum, 70
Opposite
  defined, 2
Ovulation inhibition effect
  Aloe vera, 118
  Curcuma longa, 240
  Cymbopogon citratus, 204
  Hibiscus rosa-sinensis, 262
  Manihot esculenta, 333

P

Papaw, 143–156
Papaya, 143–156
Parasitic activity
  Annona muricata, 137
  Jatropha curcas, 281–282
Parkinson activity
  Mucuna pruriens, 308–309
Penis erectile stimulant
  Mucuna pruriens, 311
Periwinkle, 175–185
Persea americana, 383–389
  botanical description, 384
  chemical constituents, 385–386
  common names, 383

origin and distribution, 384
pharmacological activities and clinical
 trials, 386–389
traditional medicinal uses, 384–385
Petiole
 defined, 2
Pheromone
 Lantana camara, 296
Phyllanthus niruri, 393–399
 botanical description, 393
 chemical constituents, 395
 common names, 393
 origin and description, 393–394
 pharmacological activities and clinical
  trials, 395–399
 traditional medicinal uses, 394–395
Pinnate
 defined, 2
Plant germination inhibition
 Hibiscus rosa-sinensis, 262
 Lantana camara, 296–297
 Momordica charantia, 353
 Psidium guajava, 423
 Tamarindus indica, 460
Plant growth inhibition
 Allium sativum, 71
 Cyperus rotundus, 218
 Mangifera indica, 323
 Mucuna pruriens, 311
 Psidium guajava, 424
 Punica granatum, 439
Platelet aggregation inhibition
 Allium sativum, 72–73
PMS activity
 Psidium guajava, 419
Pomegranate, 431–439
Portulaca oleracea, 405–410
 botanical description, 406
 chemical constituents, 407
 common names, 405
 origin and distribution, 406
 pharmacological activities and clinical
  trials, 407–410
 traditional medicinal uses, 406
Prayer bean, 15–25
Precatory bean, 15–25
Prostaglandin inhibition
 Allium sativum, 73

Prostate treatment
 Mucuna pruriens, 311
Prostatic effect
 Allium sativum, 73
Prothrombin time decrease
 Allium sativum, 73
Psidium guajava, 415–424
 botanical description, 416
 chemical constituents, 417–419
 common names, 415
 origin and distribution, 416
 pharmacological activities and clinical
  trials, 419–424
 traditional medicinal uses, 416–417
Punica granatum, 431–439
 botanical description, 431–432
 chemical constituents, 433–434
 common names, 431
 origin and distribution, 432
 pharmacological activities and clinical
  trials, 434–439
 traditional medicinal uses, 432–433
Purslane, 405–410

R–S
Rosary bean, 15–25
Semen coagulation
 Carica papaya, 155
 Cassia alata, 171
 Jatropha curcas, 284
 Moringa pterygosperma, 375
 Psidium guajava, 424
 Punica granatum, 439
 Syzygium cumini, 451
Senescence ameliorative effect
 Allium sativum, 73–74
Skin pigmentation effect
 Aloe vera, 119
Snake venom prophylaxis
 Allium sativum, 74
Soursop tree, 133–138
Spasmogenic activity. *See also*
  Antispasmodic activity
 Allium sativum, 74
 Catharanthus roseus, 184
 Curcuma longa, 241
 Hibiscus sabdariffa, 271
 Persea americana, 388

Portulaca oleracea, 410
Psidium guajava, 424
Spasmolytic activity. *See also*
    Antispasmodic activity
    Carica papaya, 155
    Jatropha curcas, 284
    Mangifera indica, 323
    Momordica charantia, 354
    Phyllanthus niruri, 398
    Tamarindus indica, 460
Spermatogenic activity. *See also*
    Antispermatogenic effect
    Mucuna pruriens, 311
Spermicidal effect
    Abrus precatorius, 23
    Allium sativum, 74
    Carica papaya, 155
    Cassia alata, 171
    Jatropha curcas, 284
    Momordica charantia, 355
    Moringa pterygosperma, 375
    Psidium guajava, 424
    Punica granatum, 439
    Syzygium cumini, 451
Stipules
    defined, 2
Stress activity
    Cymbopogon citratus, 201
Syzygium cumini, 445–451
    botanical description, 445
    chemical constituents, 446–447
    common names, 445
    origin and distribution, 445–446
    pharmacological activities and clinical
        trials, 447–451
    traditional medicinal uses, 446

T

Tachycardia activity
    Allium sativum, 75
Tamarindus indica, 455–460
    botanical description, 455–456
    chemical constituents, 457–458
    common names, 455
    origin and distribution, 456
    pharmacological activities and clinical
        trials, 458–460
    traditional medicinal uses, 456–457

Taste aversion
    Abrus precatorius, 23
Tauj dub, 197–204
Tauj qab, 197–204
Testosterone release stimulation
    Allium sativum, 75
Thrombin inhibition
    Allium sativum, 75
Thrombocytopenic activity
    Allium sativum, 75
Thromboplastin time increase
    Allium sativum, 75
Toxic effect
    Abrus precatorius, 23–24
    Allium sativum, 75–76
    Aloe vera, 119
    Annona muricata, 138
    Cassia alata, 171
    Catharanthus roseus, 184–185
    Curcuma longa, 241
    Cymbopogon citratus, 204
    Cyperus rotundus, 219
    Lantana camara, 297
    Mangifera indica, 323
    Manihot esculenta, 333–334
    Momordica charantia, 355
    Moringa pterygosperma, 375–376
    Mucuna pruriens, 311
    Persea americana, 388
    Portulaca oleracea, 410
    Syzygium cumini, 451
Toxicity assessment
    Carica papaya, 155
    Hibiscus rosa-sinensis, 262
    Jatropha curcas, 284
    Lantana camara, 297–298
    Phyllanthus niruri, 398
    Psidium guajava, 424
    Punica granatum, 439
    Tamarindus indica, 460
Tranquilizing effect
    Carica papaya, 155
Tumor. *See also* Antitumor activity
    promoting effect
        Allium sativum, 77
    promotion inhibition
        Carica papaya, 155–156

Mangifera indica, 323
Momordica charantia, 355
Persea americana, 388
Turmeric, 227–242

U

Ulcer activity. *See also* Antiulcer activity
Allium sativum, 77
Uterine effect
Abrus precatorius, 24–25
Allium sativum, 77
Aloe vera, 120
Annona muricata, 138
Carica papaya, 156
Catharanthus roseus, 185
Curcuma longa, 242
Mangifera indica, 323
Momordica charantia, 355
Moringa pterygosperma, 376
Persea americana, 388
Portulaca oleracea, 410
Punica granatum, 439

V

Vasodilator activity
Allium sativum, 77
Venation
defined, 2
Viral activity. *See* Antiviral activity

W–Y

Weight
Allium sativum, 77
Catharanthus roseus, 185
Curcuma longa, 242
Cymbopogon citratus, 204
Cyperus rotundus, 219
Mangifera indica, 323–324
Syzygium cumini, 451
Whorled
defined, 2
Wound healing
Allium sativum, 77
Aloe vera, 120–122
Cassia alata, 171
Moringa pterygosperma, 376
Yeast. *See* Antiyeast activity

About the Author

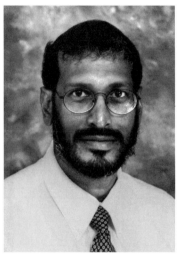

A native of Guyana, Ivan A. Ross is a biologist at the United States Food and Drug Administration. At the age of seventeen he was awarded a scholarship by the United States Agency for International Development to study agriculture at Tuskegee University. After completing his studies he returned to Guyana and was appointed to the Guyana Ministry of Agriculture. During his tour of duty, most of his time was spent in the isolated communities of the Aborigines population, incorporating modern agriculture and health care methods with the traditional system. Dr. Ross' interest in tradional medicine originated at this time. He later entered the University of Maryland, College Park, where he studied animal science and biochemisrty. In 1987 he joined the United States Department of Health and Human Services, Food and Drug Administration, as a biologist in the Division of Toxicological Research. He is an active investigator and has published several research articles, primarily dealing with food safety. Other areas of his wide-ranging experience include Lecturer of Agricultural and Rural Development at the Gambia College, Gambia, West Africa, and seminars throughtout Gambia on food safety, health awareness, and agricultural techniques. When not in the laboratory, Dr. Ross is either farming or writing.